Ethical and Regulatory Aspects
of Clinical Research

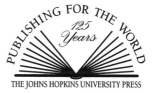

THE JOHNS HOPKINS UNIVERSITY PRESS

Ethical and Regulatory Aspects of Clinical Research

Readings and Commentary

Edited by

Ezekiel J. Emanuel, M.D., Ph.D.

Chair, Department of Clinical Bioethics, National Institutes of Health,
Bethesda, Maryland

Robert A. Crouch

Assistant Professor, Biomedical Ethics Unit,
Department of Social Studies of Medicine,
McGill University, Montreal, Quebec, Canada

John D. Arras, Ph.D.

Porterfield Professor of Biomedical Ethics and Professor of Philosophy,
University of Virginia, Charlottesville, Virginia

Jonathan D. Moreno, Ph.D.

Kornfeld Professor of Biomedical Ethics and Director,
Center for Biomedical Ethics, University of Virginia,
Charlottesville, Virginia
and

Christine Grady, R.N., Ph.D.

Head, Section on Human Subjects Research,
Department of Clinical Bioethics,
National Institutes of Health, Bethesda, Maryland

THE JOHNS HOPKINS UNIVERSITY PRESS / BALTIMORE AND LONDON

The Johns Hopkins University Press
2715 North Charles Street
Baltimore, Maryland 21218-4363
www.press.jhu.edu

Library of Congress Cataloging-in-Publication Data

Ethical and regulatory aspects of clinical research : readings and
    commentary / edited by Ezekiel J. Emanuel . . . [et al.].
        p.   ;   cm.
    Includes bibliographical references and index.
    ISBN 0-8018-7813-6 (pbk. : alk. paper)
    1. Human experimentation in medicine—Moral and ethical aspects.
2. Clinical trials—Moral and ethical aspects.   3. Medical ethics. [DNLM: 1. Ethics,
Research. 2. Research subjects. W 20.5 E832   2004]   I. Emanuel, Ezekiel J., 1957–
R853.H8E825   2004
174.28—dc21
                                                                2003012887

A catalog record for this book is available from the British Library.

For their exemplary scholarship and
commitment to the protection of
participants in research,
we dedicate this volume to
Benjamin Freedman
Jay Katz
and
Kenneth J. Ryan

Contents

Preface

Biomedical research has made spectacular strides during the past century. Thanks to the efforts of researchers in both the public and the private sectors, diseases that had struck fear and dread into the lives of our parents and grandparents—yellow fever, polio, rheumatic fever—no longer haunt our consciousness. But this power to save and ameliorate human life with new drugs, vaccines, and medical devices has inevitably raised concerns about how it is achieved and how its fruits will be distributed. The intense effort, more than a hundred years ago, to identify the cause of and treatment for yellow fever provides a telling case in point. Guiseppe Sanarelli, an Italian bacteriologist, claimed to have isolated the bacillus for yellow fever and to have infected five individuals, producing the disease in them. William Osler, the great McGill, Pennsylvania, Johns Hopkins, and Oxford University professor of medicine, condemned this research: "To deliberately inject a poison of known high degree of virulency into a human being, unless you obtain that man's sanction, is not ridiculous, it is criminal."[1] Sensitivity to the concerns raised by this controversy prompted Walter Reed to develop ethical guidelines for the research overseen by the U.S. Army's Yellow Fever Board. These guidelines included (1) self-experimentation by members of the Yellow Fever Board; (2) written agreements—the forerunner of written informed consent forms—with participants who were not members of the Yellow Fever Board; (3) payment in gold to the local workers who volunteered for the study; (4) restriction of enrollment to adults older than 24 years of age—that is, the exclusion of children as research participants; and (5) use of the phrase "with his full consent" in all journal articles about the research.

From the time of the Yellow Fever Board until the 1960s, there was relatively little public controversy over the ethics of biomedical research. Attention to the Nazi experiments in the Nuremberg doctors trial seemed more about the barbarism of an oppressive, murderous regime than about the ethics of biomedical research. Yet in the 1960s, scandals seemed to break out everywhere. Henry Knowles Beecher, professor of research in anesthesia at Harvard Medical School and Massachusetts General Hospital, a preeminent physician-researcher, wrote a landmark article that was published in 1966 in the pages of the *New England Journal of Medicine*. Entitled "Ethics and Clinical Research," his study detailed 22 cases of unethical conduct in clinical research at leading research centers, reduced simply for "reasons of space" from an original list of 50 examples. Beecher's list included many now infamous cases of unethical research: the Jewish Chronic Disease Hospital case, the Willowbrook experiment, and others.

The scandals culminated in 1972 with press reports about the U.S. Public Health Service's Tuskegee Syphilis Study. Public concern about the Tuskegee study ultimately led to the creation of the U.S. National Commission for the Protection of Human Subjects of Biomedical and Behavioral Research. The National Commission produced many reports on topics ranging from research with prisoners to the Belmont Report, a delineation of the basic ethical principles that should underlie the conduct of biomedical and behavioral research involving human subjects. It also facilitated the development of regulations that govern research with humans in the United States—the so-called Common Rule—which mandates official ethical review of research protocols by an institutional review board (IRB) and the freely given informed consent of research participants for all federally funded research.

After the creation of the National Commission and the implementation of the Common Rule it seemed that biomedical research in the United States was finally on a more secure ethical footing. The protections afforded by IRB review and informed participant consent engendered the comforting belief that scandals were a thing of the past. But by the mid-1990s controversy regarding research with humans erupted once again. Several prominent academic medical research facilities were shut down for noncompliance with U.S. regulations for the protection of research participants. Newspapers and magazines featured extended investigations of research studies gone awry; the cover of *Time* magazine pictured a human in a cage and claimed that medical testing had turned millions of people into "guinea pigs." Many features of the research landscape contributed to this renewed concern. There is a great deal more biomedical research now than there has ever been in the past. Like the economy, research has increasingly become a global affair, thus raising anew worries about possible exploitation of the poor, uneducated, and often nonwhite citizens of developing nations. Moreover, research is big business, and researchers have investments and financial entanglements of all kinds with sponsors, thus prompting worries about conflicts of interest. Genetics research—a growth industry unto itself—has raised concerns related to obtaining information about third parties and communities who never consented to the research in the first place. And empirical studies on the ethics of research have demonstrated that research participants often fail to understand the information disclosed to them, thus raising concerns about the adequacy of the protections afforded by the informed consent process.

There have been many responses to this new round of controversy, including a recognition of the need for more and better training of clinical researchers in the ethics of research. In the past there was no formal mechanism for training clinical researchers in the ethical issues endemic to their profession; they learned from their mentors, who in turn had learned from their mentors. But, like physician-patient communication, the ethical bases and requisite refinements of clinical research are no longer viewed as obvious or as things that people cannot be formally taught. Learning these things is now necessary for budding researchers.

The growing necessity of providing training in ethics for clinical researchers has outstripped the availability of quality educational materials. This book had its origins in an effort to develop a training course on the ethics of clinical research for the National Institutes of Health. When we started the course, there simply was no standard text that covered the full range of ethical issues regarding research with humans. So we had to make our own notebook. The aim was to create a comprehensive compendium of writings on the subject not only to provide the background reading assignments for the course, but also to be a reference containing the classic writings on various topics related to the ethics of clinical research. We hoped that the compendium would sit on researchers' bookshelves and be consulted as they confronted challenging issues in the design and conduct of their trials. The transition from notebook to textbook was prompted by frequent requests by those who wanted the compendium to use in their own courses.

Every book must carefully allocate the scarce resource of space. Notwithstanding our eventual inclusion of 95 selections, we could not reprint everything we wanted; the book would weigh too much—a serious health risk in itself—and cost far too much to be widely available. We have attempted to include mostly the classic writings, defined as those selections that have shaped the way a particular issue is approached and discussed and that have been the focal point for the subsequent development of other, often richer, perspectives. These are the selections that are repeatedly referenced in other articles and books. We have, however, refrained from attempting to provide an orthodox or canonical interpretation of controversial questions. On some issues a consensus has evolved, and selections encapsulating that consensus have been included. Frequently, however, the arguments advanced in the various writings clash on key points. We attempt to convey the range of reasonable perspectives on these areas of disagreement.

Each part of the book includes an introduction that provides background and a framework for the selections. Each introduction is meant to identify the key ethical issues in the specific area, summarize important insights from writings that could not be included, and highlight the key positions and arguments of those that have been included. We hope the introductions bring some order to the debates.

Making selections for a venture of this kind is, to say the least, an inexact science. Some readers of this book will conclude that some of our selections should have been left in the trash bin of history, while noting that other worthier contributions have been slighted. Furthermore, this text falls far short of being encyclopedic. We opted, for example, not to include any selections on the ethics of emergency research or on compensation for research harms. This was a consequence partly of space constraints and partly of a judgment on our part that the literature available on these topics has not yet sufficiently matured. To save space and thereby include a greater number of selections, we have edited all but a few of the writings and deleted all footnotes. It is our hope that the editing has not done violence to the arguments or the voices of the authors. In the process of selecting and pruning these topics and writings, we confronted many difficult choices, had many heated arguments, and no doubt made many errors of judgment. We take full responsibility for these, and with the assistance of our readers, we hope to rectify them in future editions.

A few comments about the in-text presentation of our editing process. When we deleted text, we indicated the deletion with bracketed ellipsis points. Periodically we inserted a bracketed note informing the reader of what we had deleted, for example, a table or a figure. We often made slight word changes or inserted parenthetical comments to clarify something in an original document and placed these clarifications in brackets, followed by "eds.," to distinguish between similar additions that the original authors or editors had made to material they quoted.

A final word about our intended audience. Our aim has been to produce a volume that is suited both to students and to scholars of research ethics, as well as to those who are actively engaged in biomedical research. We thus feel that this volume is ideally suited for an undergraduate course or a graduate seminar in research ethics. Indeed, the readings within each section have been chosen in part for their potential to engender lively classroom debates. We hope that we have provided students and teachers alike with a perspicuous overview of the substantive debates endemic to the respective areas of research addressed by the selections. In addition, however, this volume is intended to be a teaching aid and reference guide to the ethical issues confronted by physicians and researchers who conduct biomedical research. Because we believe that research ethics is a necessary part of good research practice, it is our hope that physicians and researchers will study and consult this volume ultimately in the service of improved patient care.

1. As quoted in Susan E. Lederer, *Subjected to Science* (Baltimore: Johns Hopkins University Press, 1995), 22. Osler spoke these words at a conference in 1898.

Acknowledgments and Permissions

As with any project of this scale, we have many people to thank for their assistance. Our first thanks must go to the contributors whose work makes up the bulk of this volume. Needless to say, but for their agreement to the inclusion of their writings, this volume would not exist. The publishers of the original selections have also been very generous in granting us permission to reprint excerpts from them. And they deserve a special word of thanks for often granting such permissions at discounted rates in order that we could keep the price of this volume as low as possible. We also thank our editor, Wendy Harris, of the Johns Hopkins University Press, along with three anonymous reviewers for the Press. Their comments on the original book proposal, along with Wendy's guidance throughout the production of this volume, have been extremely valuable. Close to the end of this project, we were fortunate enough to receive excellent service from Peter Strupp and his colleagues at Princeton Editorial Associates, and for this we are grateful. We also gratefully acknowledge the financial assistance provided by the Department of Clinical Bioethics, Warren G. Magnuson Clinical Center, National Institutes of Health.

We have also been very fortunate for the help we have received in preparing the volume for final submission. We thank Carrie Gumm for typing the manuscript, Jennifer Flynn for proofreading it, Chris Broom for background research early on, and both Dan Mouyard and Amy Gilbert for help during the copyediting stage. Without their help, things would have been orders of magnitude more difficult than they were.

While all of these people are responsible for helping us bring this project to fruition, we alone are responsible for any errors that remain.

We thank the following individuals for granting permission to excerpt material over which they exercise copyright control.

• George J. Annas, for permission to reprint an excerpt from his "The Changing Landscape of Human Experimentation: Nuremberg, Helsinki, and Beyond," *Health Matrix* 2 (1992): 119–40. Copyright © 1992 George J. Annas.

• Paul Lauritzen for permission to reprint an excerpt from Maura A. Ryan, "Creating Embryos for Research: On Weighing Symbolic Costs," in *Cloning and the Future of Human Embryo Research,* ed. Paul Lauritzen (New York: Oxford University Press, 2001), 50–66. Copyright © 2001 Paul Lauritzen.

• Robert J. Levine for permission to reprint an excerpt from his *Ethics and Regulation of Clinical Research,* 2nd ed. (Baltimore: Urban & Schwarzenberg, 1986). Copyright © Robert J. Levine.

We also thank the clinical investigators—who, for reasons of confidentiality, cannot be named—for permitting us to reprint their anonymized consent forms in the appendix to this volume.

We hereby thank and acknowledge the following publishers for permission to reprint or excerpt the following writings.

1. The American Association for the Advancement of Science

• Excerpted with permission from Charles Weijer and Ezekiel J. Emanuel, "Protecting Communities in Biomedical Research," *Science* 289 (2000): 1142–44. Copyright © 2000 American Association for the Advancement of Science.

• Excerpted with permission from Participants in the 2001 Conference on Ethical Aspects of Research in Developing Countries, "Fair Benefits for Research in Developing Countries," *Science* 298 (2002): 2133–34. Copyright © 2002 American Association for the Advancement of Science.

2. The American College of Physicians– American Society of Internal Medicine

• Patricia K. Woolf, "Pressure to Publish and Fraud in Science," *Annals of Internal Medicine* 104 (1986): 254–56. Copyright © 1986 American College of Physicians– American Society of Internal Medicine. Reprinted with permission.

Organizations of Medical Sciences. Reprinted with permission.

8. *Dædalus,* the Journal of the American Academy of Arts and Sciences

• Hans Jonas, "Philosophical Reflections on Experimenting with Human Subjects," *Dædalus* 98, no. 2 (Spring 1969). Reprinted by permission of *Dædalus,* the Journal of the American Academy of Arts and Sciences, from the issue entitled "Ethical Aspects of Experimentation with Human Subjects."

9. Duncker & Humblot GmbH, Berlin

• David Heyd, "Experimentation on Trial: Why Should One Take Part in Medical Research?" *Jahrbuch für Recht und Ethik* [*Annual Review of Law and Ethics*] 4 (1996): 189–204. Copyright © 1996 Duncker & Humblot GmbH, Berlin. Reprinted with permission.

10. Elsevier Science

• Nicholas A. Christakis, "Ethics Are Local: Engaging Cross-Cultural Variation in the Ethics for Clinical Research," *Social Science and Medicine* 35, no. 9 (1992): 1079–91. Reprinted with permission from Elsevier Science.

• Franklin G. Miller and Donald L. Rosenstein, "Psychiatric Symptom-Provoking Studies: An Ethical Appraisal," *Biological Psychiatry* 42, no. 5 (1997): 403–9. Copyright © 1997 by the Society of Biological Psychiatry. Reprinted by permission of Elsevier Science.

11. First Things

• The Ramsey Colloquium, "The Inhuman Use of Human Beings: A Statement on Embryo Research by the Ramsey Colloquium," *First Things* 49 (1995): 17–21. Copyright © 1995 First Things. Reprinted with permission.

12. Gale/Macmillan Reference

• Robert J. Levine, "Consent Issues in Human Research," in *Encyclopedia of Bioethics,* 2nd edition, ed. Warren T. Reich (New York: Macmillan Reference, 1995), 1241–50. Copyright © 1995 Gale/Macmillan Reference. Reprinted by permission of the Gale Group.

13. The Hastings Center

• Benjamin Freedman, "A Moral Theory of Informed Consent," *Hastings Center Report* 5, no. 4 (1975): 32–39. Copyright © 1975 The Hastings Center. Reprinted with permission.

• Allan M. Brandt, "Racism and Research: The Case of the Tuskegee Syphilis Study," *Hastings Center Report* 8, no. 6 (1978): 21–29. Copyright © 1978 The Hastings Center. Reprinted with permission.

• Harold F. Gamble, "Students, Grades, and Informed Consent," *IRB: A Review of Human Subjects Research* 4, no. 3 (1982): 7–10. Copyright © 1982 The Hastings Center. Reprinted with permission.

• Nancy R. Angoff, "Against Special Protections for Medical Students," *IRB: A Review of Human Subjects Research* 7, no. 5 (1985): 9–10. Copyright © 1985 The Hastings Center. Reprinted with permission.

• Paul S. Appelbaum, Loren H. Roth, Charles W. Lidz, Paul Benson, and William Winslade, "False Hopes and Best Data: Consent to Research and the Therapeutic Misconception," *Hastings Center Report* 17, no. 2 (1987): 20–24. Copyright © 1987 The Hastings Center. Reprinted with permission.

• Benjamin Freedman, "Cohort-Specific Consent: An Honest Approach to Phase 1 Clinical Cancer Studies," *IRB: A Review of Human Subjects Research* 12, no. 1 (1990): 5–7. Copyright © 1990 The Hastings Center. Reprinted with permission.

• Benjamin Freedman, "Placebo-Controlled Trials and the Logic of Clinical Purpose," *IRB: A Review of Human Subjects Research* 12, no. 6 (1990): 1–6. Copyright © 1990 The Hastings Center. Reprinted with permission.

• Rebecca Dresser, "Wanted: Single, White Male for Medical Research," *Hastings Center Report* 22, no. 1 (1992): 21–29. Copyright © 1992 The Hastings Center. Reprinted with permission.

• Benjamin Freedman, Abraham Fuks, and Charles Weijer, "*In loco parentis:* Minimal Risk as an Ethical Threshold for Research upon Children," *Hastings Center Report* 23, no. 2 (1993): 13–19. Copyright © 1993 The Hastings Center. Reprinted with permission.

• Sanford Leikin, "Minors' Assent, Consent, or Dissent to Medical Research," *IRB: A Review of Human Subjects Research* 15, no. 2 (1993): 1–7. Copyright © 1993 The Hastings Center. Reprinted with permission.

• Carol A. Tauer, "The NIH Trials of Growth Hormone for Short Stature," *IRB: A Review of Human Subjects Research* 16, no. 3 (1994): 1–9. Copyright © 1994 The Hastings Center. Reprinted with permission.

• Paul S. Appelbaum, "Drug-Free Research in Schizophrenia: An Overview of the Controversy," *IRB: A Review of Human Subjects Research* 18, no. 1 (1996): 1–5. Copyright © 1996 The Hastings Center. Reprinted with permission.

• Kathleen Cranley Glass, Charles Weijer, Roberta M. Palmour, Stanley H. Shapiro, Trudo M. Lemmens, and

14. The International Conference on Harmonisation Secretariat

15. The Johns Hopkins University Press

16. Lippincott, Williams & Wilkins

17. The Massachusetts Medical Society

• James L. Mills, "Data Torturing," *New England Journal of Medicine* 329 (1993): 1196–99. Copyright © 1993 Massachusetts Medical Society. All rights reserved.

• Kenneth J. Rothman and Karin B. Michels, "The Continuing Unethical Use of Placebo Controls," *New England Journal of Medicine* 331 (1994): 394–98. Copyright © 1994 Massachusetts Medical Society. All rights reserved.

• Peter Lurie and Sidney M. Wolfe, "Unethical Trials of Interventions to Reduce Perinatal Transmission of the Human Immunodeficiency Virus in Developing Countries," *New England Journal of Medicine* 337 (1997): 853–56. Copyright © 1997 Massachusetts Medical Society. All rights reserved.

• Robert D. Truog, Walter Robinson, Adrienne Randolph, and Alan Morris, "Is Informed Consent Always Necessary for Randomized, Controlled Trials?" *New England Journal of Medicine* 340 (1999): 804–7. Copyright © 1999 Massachusetts Medical Society. All rights reserved.

• Robert Michels, "Are Research Ethics Bad for Our Mental Health?" *New England Journal of Medicine* 340 (1999): 1427–30. Copyright © 1999 Massachusetts Medical Society. All rights reserved.

• Neal Dickert and Christine Grady, "What's the Price of a Research Subject? Approaches to Payment for Research Participation," *New England Journal of Medicine* 341 (1999): 198–203. Copyright © 1999 Massachusetts Medical Society. All rights reserved.

• Joseph B. Martin and Dennis L. Kasper, "In Whose Best Interest? Breaching the Academic-Industrial Wall," *New England Journal of Medicine* 343 (2000): 1646–49. Copyright © 2000 Massachusetts Medical Society. All rights reserved.

• Ezekiel J. Emanuel and Franklin G. Miller, "The Ethics of Placebo-Controlled Trials: A Middle Ground," *New England Journal of Medicine* 345 (2001): 915–19. Copyright © 2001 Massachusetts Medical Society. All rights reserved.

• Michaele C. Christian, Jacquelyn L. Goldberg, Jack Killen, Jeffrey S. Abrams, Mary S. McCabe, Joan K. Mauer, and Robert E. Wittes, "A Central Institutional Review Board for Multi-institutional Trials," *New England Journal of Medicine* 346 (2002): 1405–8. Copyright © 2002 Massachusetts Medical Society. All rights reserved.

18. The MIT Press

• Trudo Lemmens and Carl Elliott, "Justice for the Professional Guinea Pig," *American Journal of Bioethics* 1, no. 2 (2001): 51–53. Copyright © 2001 The MIT Press. Reprinted with permission.

19. The Nature Publishing Group

• Charles Weijer, Gary Goldsand, and Ezekiel J. Emanuel, "Protecting Communities in Research: Current Guidelines and Limits of Extrapolation," *Nature Genetics* 23 (1999): 275–80. Copyright © 1999 Nature Publishing Group. Reprinted with permission.

20. Oxford University Press

• Baruch A. Brody, "Conflicts of Interests and the Validity of Clinical Trials," in *Conflicts of Interest in Clinical Practice and Research,* ed. Roy G. Spece, David S. Shimm, and Allen E. Buchanan (New York: Oxford University Press, 1996), 407–17. Copyright © 1996 Oxford University Press. Reprinted with permission.

• Jonathan D. Moreno, "Convenient and Captive Populations," in *Beyond Consent: Seeking Justice in Research,* ed. Jeffrey P. Kahn, Anna C. Mastroianni, and Jeremy Sugarman (New York: Oxford University Press, 1998), 111–30. Copyright © 1998 Oxford University Press. Reprinted with permission.

21. The Russell Sage Foundation

• Jay Katz, with Alexander Morgan Capron and Eleanor Swift Glass, "The Jewish Chronic Disease Case," in their *Experimentation with Human Beings* (New York: Russell Sage Foundation, 1972), 9–10, 36–41, 63–65. Copyright © 1972 Russell Sage Foundation. Reprinted with permission.

22. The St. Louis University Law Journal

• Jay Katz, "Human Experimentation and Human Rights," *St. Louis University Law Journal* 38 (1993): 7–54. Copyright © 1993 St. Louis University Law Journal, St. Louis University School of Law. Reprinted with permission.

23. The University of Chicago Press

• American Society of Human Genetics, "Statement on Informed Consent for Genetic Research," *American Journal of Human Genetics* 59 (1996): 471–74. Copyright © 1996 by The American Society of Human Genetics. All rights reserved.

• Morris W. Foster, Deborah Bernsten, and Thomas H. Carter, "A Model Agreement for Genetic Research in Socially Identifiable Populations," *American Journal of Human Genetics* 63 (1998): 696–702. Copyright © 1998 by The American Society of Human Genetics. All rights reserved.

24. The University Publishing Group

• Charles Weijer and Robert A. Crouch, "Why Should We Include Women and Minorities in Randomized Controlled Trials?" *Journal of Clinical Ethics* 10 (1999): 100–106. Copyright © 1999 The Journal of Clinical Ethics. Reprinted with permission. <www.clinicalethics.com>

25. The World Medical Association

• The World Medical Association, The Declaration of Helsinki: Ethical Principles for Medical Research Involving Human Subjects. Adopted, most recently, by the 52nd WMA General Assembly, Edinburgh, Scotland, October 2000. Copyright © 2000 World Medical Association. Reprinted with permission.

Commonly Used Acronyms

Throughout this volume, the reader will encounter many commonly used acronyms. In each part of the book the full term is given, followed by its acronym, in parentheses in most places, but in brackets if we added them to the excerpted writings. After that, the acronym is used most of the time, except in some of the excerpted writings. Although many of these acronyms will be familiar to most readers, many may not be. Accordingly, we have produced the following table to which the reader can refer for the most commonly used acronyms, along with Web site addresses of organizations for whose names we have given the acronyms. (*Note:* For Web site addresses, "http://" is implied but not written.)

Acronym	*Full Name* *• Dates (if applicable)*	*Web Site*
ACHRE	Advisory Committee on Human Radiation Experiments (U.S.) • 1994–1995	tis.eh.doe.gov/ohre/roadmap/achre
CDC	Centers for Disease Control and Prevention (U.S.) • 1946–present	www.cdc.gov
CFR	Code of Federal Regulations (U.S.)	www.access.gpo.gov/nara/cfr/
CIOMS	Council for International Organizations of Medical Sciences • 1946–present	www.cioms.ch
DHEW	Department of Health, Education, and Welfare (U.S.) • 1953–1980	See DHHS
DHHS	Department of Health and Human Services (U.S.) • 1980–present	www.dhhs.gov

Acronym	Full Name • Dates (if applicable)	Web Site
FDA	Food and Drug Administration (U.S.) • 1968–present [in current form; originally established in 1862]	www.fda.gov
HEW	Health, Education, and Welfare	See DHEW
HHS	Health and Human Services	See DHHS
NBAC	National Bioethics Advisory Commission (U.S.) • 1995–2001	bioethics.georgetown.edu/nbac
NIH	National Institutes of Health (U.S.) • 1887–present	www.nih.gov
OHRP	Office for Human Research Protections (U.S.) • 2000–present	www.hhs.gov/ohrp
OPRR	Office for Protection from Research Risks (U.S.) • 1966–2000 (predecessor of OHRP)	See OHRP
ORI	Office of Research Integrity (U.S.) • 1992–present	ori.dhhs.gov
PHS	Public Health Service (U.S.)	www.hhs.gov/phs
USPHS	U.S. Public Health Service	See PHS
WHO	World Health Organization • 1948–present	www.who.int

Frequently Cited Research Regulations, Guidelines, and Reports

The reader may refer to the following table for frequently cited research regulations, guidelines, and reports. Many more sources could be listed, of course, but these are the documents that we believe have the most currency.[1] (*Note:* For Web site addresses, "http://" is implied but not written.)

• *Title* *Web Site*	*Date*[2] *[Date]*	*Status*	*Source Country* *or Organization*
• The Belmont Report (Report of the National Commission for the Protection of Human Subjects of Biomedical and Behavioral Research) www.hhs.gov/ohrp/humansubjects/guidance/belmont.htm	1979	R	DHEW (U.S.A.)
• The Common Rule, Title 45 (Public Welfare), Code of Federal Regulations, Part 46 (Protection of Human Subjects), Subparts A–D www.hhs.gov/ohrp/humansubjects/guidance/45cfr46.htm	2001 [1991[3]]	L	DHHS (U.S.A.)
• The Declaration of Helsinki www.wma.net/e/policy/b3.htm	2000 [1964]	G	World Medical Association (WMA)
• Ethical and Policy Issues in International Research bioethics.georgetown.edu/nbac/pubs.html	2001	R	NBAC (U.S.A.)
• Ethical and Policy Issues in Research Involving Human Participants bioethics.georgetown.edu/nbac/pubs.html	2001	R	NBAC (U.S.A.)
• Ethical Issues in Human Stem Cell Research bioethics.georgetown.edu/nbac/pubs.html	1999	R	NBAC (U.S.A.)
• The Ethics of Research Related to Healthcare in Developing Countries www.nuffieldbioethics.org/publications/pp_0000000013.asp	2002	R	Nuffield Council on Bioethics (U.K.)

• *Title* Web Site	*Date[2]* *[Date]*	*Status*	*Source Country* *or Organization*
• FDA Oversight of Clinical Investigators oig.hhs.gov/oei/reports/oei-05-99-00350.pdf	2000	R	Office of Inspector General (OIG, U.S.A.)
• Final Report: Evaluation of NIH Implementation of Section 491 of the Public Health Service Act, Mandating a Program of Protection for Research Subjects ohrp.osophs.dhhs.gov/hsp_report/hsp_final_rpt.pdf	1998	R	Bell Associates (for NIH, U.S.A.)
• The Globalization of Clinical Trials: A Growing Challenge in Protecting Human Subjects oig.hhs.gov/oei/reports/oei-01-00-00190.pdf	2001	R	OIG (U.S.A.)
• Guidelines on the Inclusion of Women and Minorities as Subjects in Clinical Research grants1.nih.gov/grants/funding/women_min/ guidelines_amended_10_2001.htm	2001 [1994]	G	NIH (U.S.A.)
• The Human Radiation Experiments: Final Report of the President's Advisory Committee tis.eh.doe.gov/ohre/roadmap/achre/report.html	1995	R	ACHRE (Department of Energy [DOE], U.S.A.)
• The ICH Harmonised Tripartite Guideline— Guideline for Good Clinical Practice (ICH-GCP Guideline) www.ich.org/pdfifpma/e6.pdf	1996	G	ICH
• Institutional Review Boards: The Emergence of Independent Boards oig.hhs.gov/oei/reports/a275.pdf	1998	R	OIG (U.S.A.)
• Institutional Review Boards: Promising Approaches oig.hhs.gov/oei/reports/a274.pdf	1998	R	OIG (U.S.A.)
• Institutional Review Boards: Their Role in Reviewing Approved Research oig.hhs.gov/oei/reports/a273.pdf	1998	R	OIG (U.S.A.)
• Institutional Review Boards: A Time for Reform oig.hhs.gov/oei/reports/a276.pdf	1998	R	OIG (U.S.A.)
• The International Ethical Guidelines for Biomedical Research Involving Human Subjects www.cioms.ch/frame_guidelines_nov_2002.htm	2002 [1993]	G	CIOMS and WHO
• The International Guidelines for Ethical Review of Epidemiological Studies www.cioms.ch/frame_1991_texts_of_guidelines.htm	1991	G	CIOMS and WHO
• The Nuremberg Code ohsr.od.nih.gov/nuremberg.php3	1947	G	Nuremberg Military Tribunal (*U.S.* v. *Karl Brandt,* et al.)

• Title Web Site	Date[2] [Date]	Status	Source Country or Organization
• Policy and Guidelines on the Inclusion of Children as Participants in Research Involving Human Subjects grants1.nih.gov/grants/guide/notice-files/not98-024.html	1998	G	NIH (U.S.A.)
• Protecting Human Research Subjects: Status of Recommendations oig.hhs.gov/oei/reports/oei-01-97-00197.pdf	2000	R	OIG (U.S.A.)
• Recruiting Human Subjects: Pressures in Industry-Sponsored Clinical Research oig.hhs.gov/oei/reports/oei-01-97-00195.pdf	2000	R	OIG (U.S.A.)
• Recruiting Human Subjects: Sample Guidelines for Practice oig.hhs.gov/oei/reports/oei-01-97-00196.pdf	2000	R	OIG (U.S.A.)
• Regulations for Institutional Review Boards (21 CFR 56) www.access.gpo.gov/nara/cfr/waisidx_00/21cfr56_00.html	2000 [1981]	L	FDA (U.S.A.)
• Regulations for the Protection of Human Subjects (21 CFR 50) www.access.gpo.gov/nara/cfr/waisidx_00/21cfr50_00.html	2000 [1980]	L	FDA (U.S.A.)
• Research Involving Human Biological Materials bioethics.georgetown.edu/nbac/pubs.html	1999	R	NBAC (U.S.A.)
• Research Involving Persons with Mental Disorders That May Affect Decisionmaking Capacity bioethics.georgetown.edu/nbac/pubs.html	1998	R	NBAC (U.S.A.)
• The Tri-Council Policy Statement: Ethical Conduct for Research Involving Humans www.pre.ethics.gc.ca/english/policystatement/policystatement.cfm	2003 [1998]	G	Canada

G = guideline (i.e., no legal force); L = legal regulation; R = report.

1. For a very thorough list of international and national research regulation documents, see Marie Hirtle, Trudo Lemmens, and Dominique Sprumont, "A Comparative Analysis of Research Ethics Review Mechanisms and the ICH Good Clinical Practice Guideline," *European Journal of Health Law* 7 (2000): 265–92.

2. The date listed *without brackets* corresponds to either (1) the date of publication of the document in question or (2) the date of the most recent change to a document that undergoes periodic revision. The date listed *within brackets* corresponds to the date that the periodically revised document first appeared or went into effect.

3. Strictly speaking, this date is correct. However, the regulations that became known as the Common Rule are the 1991 revisions of earlier research regulations promulgated in 1981 by the Department of Health and Human Services. These regulations are known as the Common Rule because they were adopted by many departments within the U.S. government; they are thus the rules common to most (but not all) of the departments within the U.S. government that engage in research with humans.

Contributors

Jeffrey S. Abrams, M.D., Senior Investigator, Clinical Investigations Branch, Clinical Therapy Evaluation Program, Division of Cancer Treatment and Diagnosis, National Cancer Institute, Bethesda, Maryland

Douglas Altman, D.Sc., Professor and Director, Centre for Statistics in Medicine, Cancer Research U.K. Medical Statistics Group, Institute of Health Sciences, Oxford, United Kingdom

Lori Andrews, J.D., Distinguished Professor of Law and Director, Institute of Science, Law, and Technology, Chicago-Kent College of Law, Illinois Institute of Technology, Chicago, Illinois

Marcia Angell, M.D., F.A.C.P., Senior Lecturer, Department of Social Medicine, Harvard Medical School, Boston, Massachusetts

Nancy R. Angoff, M.D., M.P.H., M.Ed., Assistant Professor of Internal Medicine and Associate Dean for Student Affairs, Yale University School of Medicine, New Haven, Connecticut

George J. Annas, J.D., M.P.H., Professor of Health Law, Human Rights, and Bioethics, Boston University School of Public Health, Boston, Massachusetts

Paul S. Appelbaum, M.D., A. F. Zeleznik Distinguished Professor and Chair, Department of Psychiatry, University of Massachusetts Medical School, Worcester, Massachusetts

Hadley Arkes, Ph.D., Edward N. Ney Professor of American Institutes, Department of Political Science, Amherst College, Amherst, Massachusetts

John C. Bailar III, M.D., Ph.D., Professor Emeritus, University of Chicago, Chicago, Illinois

Henry K. Beecher, M.D. (1904–1976), Henry Isaiah Dorr Professor of Anesthesia Research, Harvard Medical School, Boston, Massachusetts

Paul Benson, Ph.D., Associate Professor, Department of Sociology, University of Massachusetts Boston, Boston, Massachusetts

Matthew Berke, Ph.D., Senior Fellow, Faith and Reason Institute, Washington, D.C.

Deborah Bernsten, Ph.D., Assistant Professor of Anthropology, University of South Carolina, Beaufort, Beaufort, South Carolina

Jeffrey R. Botkin, M.D., M.P.H., Professor of Pediatrics, Adjunct Professor of Internal Medicine, Division of Medical Ethics, and Adjunct Professor of Human Genetics, University of Utah, Salt Lake City, Utah

Gerard V. Bradley, J.D., Professor, Notre Dame Law School, Notre Dame, Indiana

Allan M. Brandt, Ph.D., Amalie Moses Kass Professor of the History of Medicine, Department of Social Medicine, Harvard Medical School, Boston, Massachusetts

Baruch A. Brody, Ph.D., Leon Jaworski Professor of Biomedical Ethics and Director, Center for Medical Ethics and Health Policy, Baylor College of Medicine, Houston, Texas

Rev. James T. Burtchaell, C.S.C., Casa Santa Cruz, Phoenix, Arizona, and sometime Professor of Theology and Provost, University of Notre Dame, Notre Dame, Indiana

Rev. Francis Canavan, S.J., Ph.L., Ph.D., Professor Emeritus, Department of Political Science, Fordham University, New York, New York

Alexander Morgan Capron, LL.B., Director, Ethics, World Health Organization, Geneva, Switzerland

Thomas H. Carter, M.D., Ph.D., Associate Professor, Department of Internal Medicine, University of Iowa, Iowa City, Iowa

Sir Iain Chalmers, D.Sc., Director, U.K. Cochrane Centre, National Health Service Research and Development Programme, Oxford, United Kingdom

Nicholas A. Christakis, M.D., Ph.D., M.P.H., Professor of Medical Sociology, Department of Health Care Policy, Harvard Medical School, Boston, Massachusetts

Michaele C. Christian, M.D., Associate Director, Cancer Therapy Evaluation Program, National Cancer Institute, Bethesda, Maryland

Ellen Wright Clayton, M.D., J.D., Rosalind E. Franklin Professor and Director, Center for Genetics and Health Policy, and Professor of Pediatrics and of Law, Vanderbilt University, Nashville, Tennessee

Carl Cohen, Ph.D., L.D. (Hon.), Professor of Philosophy, University of Michigan, Ann Arbor, Michigan

Denis Cournoyer, M.D., F.R.C.P. (C), Associate Professor of Medicine and Oncology, Faculty of Medicine, McGill University, Montreal, Quebec, Canada

Rabbi David G. Dalin, Ph.D., Adjunct Scholar, Ethics and Public Policy Center, Washington, D.C., and Visiting Faculty Member, Jewish Theological Seminary, New York, New York

Midge Decter, New York, New York

Thomas S. Derr, M.Div., Ph.D., Professor of Religion and Ethics, Smith College, Northampton, Massachusetts

Neal Dickert, B.A., M.D./Ph.D. student, School of Medicine, Department of Health Policy and Management, Bloomberg School of Public Health, Johns Hopkins University, Baltimore, Maryland

Rebecca Dresser, J.D., Daniel Noyes Kirby Professor of Law and Professor of Ethics in Medicine, Washington University, St. Louis, Missouri

Harold Edgar, J.D., Julius Silver Professor of Law, Science, and Technology, Columbia University School of Law, New York, New York

Susan S. Ellenberg, Ph.D., Director, Office of Biostatistics and Epidemiology, Center for Biologics Evaluation and Research, Food and Drug Administration, Rockville, Maryland

Carl Elliott, M.D., Ph.D., Associate Professor of Philosophy and Pediatrics, Center for Bioethics, University of Minnesota, Minneapolis, Minnesota

Linda L. Emanuel, M.D., Ph.D., Buehler Professor of Geriatric Medicine and Director, Buehler Center on Aging; Principal, Education for Physicians in End-of-Life Care (EPEC) Project, Northwestern University Feinberg School of Medicine; and Professor of Health Industry Management and Director, Health Section, Ford Center on Global Citizenship, Kellogg School of Management, Northwestern University, Evanston, Illinois

Ruth R. Faden, M.P.H., Ph.D., Philip Franklin Wagley Professor of Biomedical Ethics and Executive Director, Phoebe R. Berman Bioethics Institute, Bloomberg School of Public Health, Johns Hopkins University, Baltimore, Maryland

Fr. Ernest Fortin, S.T.L., D. es L. (1923–2002), Professor, Department of Theology, Boston College, Boston, Massachusetts

Norman C. Fost, M.D., M.P.H., Professor and Director, Program in Medical Ethics, Department of History of Medicine, Department of Pediatrics, University of Wisconsin Medical School, Madison, Wisconsin

Morris W. Foster, Ph.D., Associate Professor, Department of Anthropology, University of Oklahoma Norman, Norman, Oklahoma

Benjamin Freedman, Ph.D. (1951–1997), Professor, Biomedical Ethics Unit, McGill University Faculty of Medicine, and Clinical Ethicist, Sir Mortimer B. Davis–Jewish General Hospital, Montreal, Quebec, Canada

Abraham Fuks, M.D., C.M., Dean, Faculty of Medicine, McGill University, Montreal, Quebec, Canada

Harold F. Gamble, Ph.D., Professor of Philosophy (retired), St. Louis Community College, St. Louis, Missouri

Jorge Garcia, Ph.D., Professor, Department of Philosophy, Boston College, Chestnut Hill, Massachusetts

Rabbi Marc Gellman, Ph.D., Senior Rabbi, Temple Beth Torah, Melville, New York

Robert P. George, J.D., D.Phil., McCormick Professor of Jurisprudence and Professor of Politics; and Director, James Madison Program in American Ideals and Institutions, Department of Politics, Princeton University, Princeton, New Jersey

Kathleen Cranley Glass, LL.B., B.C.L., LL.D., Associate Professor, Departments of Human Genetics and Pediatrics; Director, Biomedical Ethics Unit, McGill University Faculty of Medicine; and Clinical Ethicist, Montreal Children's Hospital, Montreal, Quebec, Canada

Mary Ann Glendon, J.D., Learned Hand Professor of Law, Harvard Law School, Cambridge, Massachusetts

Jacquelyn L. Goldberg, J.D., Administrator, Central Review Board Initiative, Cancer Therapy Evaluation Program, National Cancer Institute, Bethesda, Maryland

Gary Goldsand, M.A., Coordinator, Clinical Ethics Services, Royal Alexandra Hospital, and Adjunct Professor, John Dossetor Health Ethics Centre, Faculty of Medicine and Dentistry, University of Alberta, Edmonton, Alberta, Canada

Michael A. Grodin, M.D., F.A.A.P., Professor of Health Law, Psychiatry, Philosophy, and Medicine, Schools of Medicine, Public Health, and College of Arts and Sciences, Boston University, Boston, Massachusetts

Stanley Hauerwas, Ph.D., Gilbert T. Rowe Professor of Theological Ethics, Divinity School, Duke University, Durham, North Carolina

Deborah S. Hellman, J.D., Associate Professor, University of Maryland School of Law, Baltimore, Maryland

Samuel Hellman, M.D., A. N. Pritzker Distinguished Service Professor of Radiation and Cellular

Oncology, University of Chicago Pritzker School of Medicine, Chicago, Illinois

David Heyd, D.Phil., Chaim Perelman Professor of Philosophy, Department of Philosophy, Hebrew University, Jerusalem, Israel

John Hittinger, Ph.D., Provost and Academic Dean, Saint Mary's College of Ave Maria University, Orchard Lake, Michigan

Russell Hittinger, Ph.D., Research Professor of Law and Warren Professor of Catholic Studies, University of Tulsa College of Law, Tulsa, Oklahoma

Mark Hochhauser, Ph.D., Readability Consulting, Golden Valley, Minnesota

Franz J. Ingelfinger, M.D. (1910–1980), Professor, Section of Gastroenterology, Boston University School of Medicine, Boston, Massachusetts

Robert W. Jenson, Dr.Theol., Senior Scholar for Research, Center of Theological Inquiry, Princeton, New Jersey, and Professor Emeritus of Religion, St. Olaf College, Northfield, Minnesota

Hans Jonas, Ph.D. (1903–1993), Alvin Johnson Professor of Philosophy Emeritus, New School for Social Research, New York, New York

Eric T. Juengst, Ph.D., Associate Professor, Department of Bioethics, Case Western Reserve University School of Medicine, Cleveland, Ohio

Mary Jo Ellis Kahn, M.S.N., R.N., Representative, National Breast Cancer Coalition, Richmond, Virginia

Dennis L. Kasper, M.D., William Ellery Channing Professor of Medicine, Professor of Microbiology and Molecular Genetics, and Executive Dean for Academic Programs, Harvard Medical School; Director, Channing Laboratory; and Senior Physician, Brigham and Women's Hospital, Boston, Massachusetts

Leon R. Kass, M.D., Ph.D., Chairman, President's Council on Bioethics; Addie Clark Harding Professor, Committee on Social Thought and the College, University of Chicago; and Hertog Fellow, American Enterprise Institute, Washington, D.C.

Jay Katz, M.D., Elizabeth K. Dollard Professor Emeritus of Law, Medicine, and Psychiatry and Harvey L. Karp Professorial Lecturer in Law and Psychoanalysis, Yale Law School, New Haven, Connecticut

Muin J. Khoury, M.D., Ph.D., Director, Office of Genomics and Disease Prevention, Centers for Disease Control and Prevention, Atlanta, Georgia

Jack Killen, M.D., Assistant Director for Biodefense Research, National Institute of Allergy and Infectious Diseases, Bethesda, Maryland

Loretta M. Kopelman, Ph.D., Professor and Chair, Department of Medical Humanities, Brody School of Medicine, East Carolina University, Greenville, North Carolina

Karen Lebacqz, Ph.D., Robert Gordon Sproul Professor of Theological Ethics, Pacific School of Religion/ Graduate Theological Union, Berkeley, California

Susan E. Lederer, Ph.D., Associate Professor, Yale University School of Medicine, New Haven, Connecticut

Sanford Leikin, M.D., Emeritus Professor of Pediatrics, George Washington University School of Medicine and Health Sciences, Washington, D.C.

Trudo Lemmens, Lic.Jur., LL.M., D.C.L., Assistant Professor, Faculties of Law and Medicine, University of Toronto, Toronto, Ontario, Canada

Robert J. Levine, M.D., Professor of Medicine, Yale University School of Medicine, New Haven, Connecticut

Charles W. Lidz, Ph.D., Research Professor of Psychiatry, Center for Mental Health Services Research, University of Massachusetts Medical School, Worcester, Massachusetts

Stuart E. Lind, M.D., Professor of Medicine and Pathology, University of Oklahoma Health Sciences Center, Oklahoma City, Oklahoma

Mortimer B. Lipsett, M.D. (1921–1985), Director, National Institute of Arthritis, Diabetes, Digestive and Kidney Diseases, Bethesda, Maryland

Virginia LiVolsi, M.D., Professor of Pathology and Laboratory Medicine, University of Pennsylvania, Philadelphia, Pennsylvania

Richard R. Love, M.D., M.S., Department of Medicine, University of Wisconsin Medical School, Madison, Wisconsin

Peter Lurie, M.D., M.P.H., Deputy Director, Public Citizen's Health Research Group, Washington, D.C.

Joseph B. Martin, M.D., Ph.D., Dean, Faculty of Medicine, Harvard Medical School, Boston, Massachusetts

Joan K. Mauer, B.S., Chief, Clinical Trials Monitoring Branch, Cancer Therapy Evaluation Program, National Cancer Institute, Bethesda, Maryland

Mary S. McCabe, R.N., M.A., Director, Office of Education and Special Initiatives, National Cancer Institute, Bethesda, Maryland

Ralph McInerny, Ph.D., Michael P. Grace Professor of Medieval Studies, Department of Philosophy, University of Notre Dame, Notre Dame, Indiana

Paul McNeill, M.A., LL.B., Ph.D., Associate Professor of Ethics and Law in Medicine, School of Public Health and Community Medicine, University of New South Wales, Sydney, New South Wales, Australia

Jon F. Merz, M.B.A., J.D., Ph.D., Assistant Professor of Bioethics, Department of Medical Ethics and Center for Bioethics, University of Pennsylvania, Philadelphia, Pennsylvania

Karin B. Michels, Sc.D., M.Sc., M.P.H., Assistant Professor, Harvard Medical School, Boston, Massachusetts

Robert Michels, M.D., Walsh McDermott University Professor of Medicine and Psychiatry, Weill Medical College of Cornell University, New York, New York

Franklin G. Miller, Ph.D., Special Expert, National Institute of Mental Health, and Faculty Member, Department of Clinical Bioethics, National Institutes of Health, Bethesda, Maryland

James L. Mills, M.D., M.S., Chief, Pediatric Epidemiology Section, Division of Epidemiology, Statistics, and Prevention Research, National Institute of Child Health and Human Development, Bethesda, Maryland

David Moher, M.Sc., Director, Chalmers Research Group, Children's Hospital of Eastern Ontario Research Institute, Ottawa, Ontario, Canada

Alan Morris, M.D., Director of Research, Pulmonary Division, LDS Hospital, and Professor of Medicine and Adjunct Professor of Medical Informatics, University of Utah, Salt Lake City, Utah

Fr. Richard John Neuhaus, Editor-in-Chief, *First Things,* Institute on Religion and Public Life, New York, New York

Rabbi David Novak, Ph.D., J. Richard and Dorothy Shiff Chair of Jewish Studies, Department for the Study of Religion, University of Toronto, Toronto, Ontario, Canada

Michael Novak, M.A., George Frederick Jewett Scholar in Religion, Philosophy, and Public Policy, and Director of Social and Political Studies, American Enterprise Institute, Washington, D.C.

James Nuechterlein, Editor, *First Things,* Institute on Religion and Public Life, New York, New York

Roberta M. Palmour, Ph.D., Professor, Departments of Human Genetics and Psychiatry, McGill University, Montreal, Quebec, Canada

Adrienne Randolph, M.D., M.Sc., Assistant Professor of Pediatrics (Anaesthesia), Harvard Medical School, and Associate Director, Multidisciplinary ICU, Children's Hospital, Boston, Massachusetts

Drummond Rennie, M.D., F.R.C.P., F.A.C.P., Adjunct Professor of Medicine, Institute for Health Policy Studies, University of California San Francisco, and Deputy Editor, *JAMA,* San Francisco, California

Walter Robinson, M.D., M.P.H., Assistant Professor of Pediatrics and Social Medicine, Harvard Medical School and Children's Hospital, Boston, Massachusetts

Donald L. Rosenstein, M.D., Chief, Psychiatry Consultation-Liaison Service, and Deputy Clinical Director, National Institute of Mental Health, Bethesda, Maryland

Loren H. Roth, M.D., M.P.H., Professor of Psychiatry, University of Pittsburgh School of Medicine, Pittsburgh, Pennsylvania

David J. Rothman, Ph.D., Bernard Schoenberg Professor of Social Medicine, Columbia College of Physicians and Surgeons, and Professor of History, Columbia University, New York, New York

Kenneth J. Rothman, Dr.P.H., Professor of Epidemiology, Boston University School of Public Health, and Senior Scientist, Epidemiology and Safety Research, Ingenix, Boston, Massachusetts

Maura A. Ryan, Ph.D., Associate Professor of Christian Ethics, Department of Theology, and Associate Provost, University of Notre Dame, Notre Dame, Indiana

Pamela Sankar, Ph.D., Assistant Professor of Bioethics, Center for Bioethics, University of Pennsylvania, Philadelphia, Pennsylvania

Kenneth F. Schulz, Ph.D., M.B.A., Vice President of Quantitative Sciences, Family Health International, Research Triangle Park, North Carolina

Stanley H. Shapiro, Ph.D., Professor, Department of Epidemiology and Biostatistics, McGill University, Montreal, Quebec, Canada

David Singer, Ph.D., American Jewish Committee, New York, New York

Myriam Skrutkowska, M.Sc., Clinical Nurse Specialist, Radiation Oncology, McGill University Health Centre, Montreal, Quebec, Canada

Karen K. Steinberg, Ph.D., Chief, Molecular Biology Branch, National Center for Environmental Health, Centers for Disease Control and Prevention, Chamblee, Georgia

Eleanor Swift, LL.B., Professor, School of Law (Boalt Hall), University of California Berkeley, Berkeley, California (original work authored as Eleanor Swift Glass)

Sheila E. Taube, Ph.D., Associate Director, Cancer Diagnosis Program, Division of Cancer Treatment and Diagnosis, National Cancer Institute, Bethesda, Maryland

Carol A. Tauer, Ph.D., Professor Emerita of Philosophy, College of St. Catherine, St. Paul, Minnesota

Robert Temple, M.D., Associate Director for Medical Policy, Center for Drug Evaluation and Research, Food and Drug Administration, Rockville, Maryland

Dennis F. Thompson, Ph.D., Alfred North Whitehead Professor of Political Philosophy and Director, Center for Ethics and the Professions, Harvard University, Cambridge, Massachusetts

Elizabeth Thomson, M.S., R.N., C.G.C., F.A.A.N., Program Director, Ethical, Legal, and Social Implications of Human Genetics Research, National Human Genome Research Institute, Bethesda, Maryland

Robert D. Truog, M.D., Professor of Anesthesia, Pediatrics, and Medical Ethics, Harvard Medical School, Boston, Massachusetts

Douglas L. Weed, M.D., Ph.D., Dean, Education and Training, Division of Cancer Prevention, National Cancer Institute, Bethesda, Maryland

George Weigel, M.A., Senior Fellow and John M. Olin Chair in Religion and American Democracy, Ethics and Public Policy Center, Washington, D.C.

Charles Weijer, M.D., Ph.D., Associate Professor, Department of Bioethics, Dalhousie University School of Medicine, Halifax, Nova Scotia, Canada

Joan O. Weiss, M.S.W., Founding Director, Genetic Alliance, Washington, D.C.

Robert L. Wilken, Ph.D., William R. Kenan, Jr., Professor of the History of Christianity, Department of Religious Studies, University of Virginia, Charlottesville, Virginia

William Winslade, J.D., Ph.D., James Wade Rockwell Professor of Philosophy in Medicine, Institute for the Medical Humanities, University of Texas Medical Branch, Galveston, Texas

Robert E. Wittes, M.D., Physician-in-Chief, Memorial Hospital, Memorial Sloan-Kettering Cancer Center, New York, New York

Sidney M. Wolfe, M.D., Director, Public Citizen's Health Research Group, Washington, D.C.

Patricia K. Woolf, Ph.D., Lewis Thomas Laboratory, Princeton University, Princeton, New Jersey

Veronica Yank, M.D., Resident, Department of Medicine, Division of General Internal Medicine, University of Washington School of Medicine, Seattle, Washington

Ethical and Regulatory Aspects
of Clinical Research

Part I

Scandals and Tragedies of Research with Human Participants

Nuremberg, the Jewish Chronic Disease Hospital, Beecher, and Tuskegee

The ethical issues raised by medical experimentation with humans hinge on one question: How can the rights of individual persons be reconciled with the demands of the scientific enterprise? That the goal of all medical research is to improve human well-being only intensifies the dilemma. Medical research with humans is justifiable because it seeks knowledge that not only is of theoretical interest but also will benefit many people and society as a whole. The question is whether such a laudable collective goal can be pursued with full protection of the rights and dignity of individuals.

Medical research has increased the well-being of humans in much of the world. And it has done so in all its many guises, from early epidemiological research, such as John Snow's investigations of the cholera outbreaks in London in the mid-nineteenth century, to current studies of treatments administered in controlled settings. While interventional methods are the hallmark of sound medical research as it has been practiced at least since the 1950s, earlier examples exist. The eighteenth-century British surgeon James Lind spent six years studying scurvy in sailors aboard HMS *Salisbury*. He provided some of the sailors (but not all of them) with a diet that included fruits and vegetables. Observing the results, Lind concluded that those in the "intervention" group were more likely to remain free of scurvy than were their shipmates.[1] About 25 years later, Edward Jenner tested cowpox vaccine on his own child and on other youngsters in the neighborhood. The vaccinations protected the children from smallpox.[2] These early experiments with humans resulted in the prevention of serious disease in sailors and in future generations of children.

Yet such medical successes were not without cost. There are many examples of studies that violated the rights and dignity of the participants and, in some cases, cost them their health or even their lives. In 1897 the Italian bacteriologist Guiseppe Sanarelli announced that he had isolated the organism that caused yellow fever. To prove his claim, Sanarelli infected five persons with his isolate. Many were quick to criticize Sanarelli for his yellow fever–inducing experiments, and the harm he inflicted on his subjects was not soon forgotten.

Just three years later, the U.S. surgeon general commissioned Walter Reed to identify the cause of yellow fever, then a raging epidemic in Cuba. Largely because concerns about human experiments were running high, Reed established several safeguards. First, self-experimentation would be used, with the members of the Yellow Fever Board serving as subjects.[3] This approach was not without risk; indeed, Jesse Lazear, a member of the board, died in the experiments. Second, only adults would be enrolled. Most important, Reed designed a written contract for the local workers that clearly explained the peril of the undertaking and offered a payment of $100 to those who were willing to be exposed and another $100 to those who became ill with yellow fever. The development of this, one of the first consent forms, was prompted by the recognition that humans were being *used* in experiments, possibly at great personal risk, for the benefit of others.

The heroism of the yellow fever investigators and the development of the process for obtaining the explicit consent of the volunteers helped legitimize medical research with human beings. By the time of World War II, the need to obtain permission from would-be participants in studies was widely accepted, though apparently little thought was given to the nature of this permission in particular circumstances or to precisely what information should be disclosed to the participants. Yet just as Reed's explicit consent process was instituted in response to an earlier scandal, subsequent protective guidelines and regulations have been instituted in response to investigations that violated fundamental human rights and dignity. It is no exaggeration to say that research ethics—as a discipline that informs and responds to clinical and regulatory practice—was "born in scandal and reared in protectionism," to use Carol Levine's apt phrase.[4]

Part I of this book presents accounts and analyses of some of the most harrowing examples of the abuse of human beings in research, cases that continue to drive ethical debate and governmental policy today. Unlike the other parts of this volume, the selections presented here are not meant to engender discussion as much as to educate and inform. The question is not *whether* the examples discussed are morally justifiable, but rather *how* and *why* such events could ever have happened and, perhaps most important, how they reflect the larger social and ethical questions that have occupied clinicians, scholars, and regulators for more than 50 years.

In the aftermath of World War II, 23 Nazi doctors and bureaucrats were tried by the Allies at Nuremberg (West Germany) for using thousands of concentration camp prisoners as subjects in brutal experiments. The 1,750 victims identified in the indictment were a very small portion of those killed or injured, and the 23 defendants but a token assortment of those who conducted the experiments. In his opening statement before the Nuremberg Military Tribunal, Telford Taylor, a U.S. brigadier general and the chief counsel for the trial, outlined the studies that were performed.[5] The rationale for the experiments is impossible to understand unless one situates them within the context of Nazi Germany's overriding military aims and their efforts to achieve "racial hygiene."[6] While many of the brutalities visited on the Jews and other victims in the name of medical research are well known, they bear repeating:[7]

• *High-altitude (low-pressure) experiments:* Prisoners were put into low-pressure tanks to see how long they could survive with little oxygen. Many of those who did not die immediately were put under water until they died; autopsies followed.
• *Freezing experiments:* Prisoners were forced to remain outdoors without clothing in freezing weather for 9 to 14 hours, or were forced to remain in a bath of freezing water for three hours at a time. Rewarming of the bodies was then attempted, often without success.

• *Malaria experiments:* Prisoners were infected with malaria and then given a variety of supposedly antimalarial drugs. Many died from these drugs.
• *Mustard gas experiments:* Prisoners were deliberately wounded and the wounds then infected with mustard gas, or they were forced to inhale mustard gas. Experimentation with various treatments followed.
• *Sulfanilamide experiments:* Wounds were inflicted on prisoners, and bacterial culture, gangrene-producing culture, wood shavings, or glass shards were forced into the wounds, followed by treatment with sulfanilamide for wound infection. A control group consisted of prisoners who were subjected to the wounds and infections, but not given the sulfanilamide.
• *Typhus experiments:* Prisoners were injected with an antityphus vaccine and then infected with typhus. Prisoners in a control group were infected with typhus and received no treatment; others were infected with typhus simply to ensure that the typhus virus remained active within the prison camps.
• *Poison experiments:* Various poisons were fed to prisoners through their food. Most died immediately, and those who did not die were killed for purposes of autopsy.
• *Incendiary bomb experiments:* Prisoners were burned with phosphorus material taken from English incendiary bombs so that doctors could examine the wounds.
• *Sterilization experiments:* Because sterilization by surgical means was considered too costly and time-consuming, prisoners were subjected to chemical sterilization and x-ray sterilization experiments.

In addition to these experiments, hundreds of prisoners were killed in order to assemble a collection of skeletons for "anthropological investigation." Those killed were considered prototypes of what the Nazis called the "repulsive but characteristic subhuman."[8]

In addition to sentencing the accused the Military Tribunal judges articulated what came to be known as the Nuremberg Code (included in Part II of this volume). The Nuremberg Code, now the most widely known document on the ethics of research, included ten characteristics of acceptable research involving humans.[9]

It is at this point that our first contributors, Ruth R. Faden, Susan E. Lederer, and Jonathan D. Moreno, begin their analysis. Although now widely recognized as a landmark document, the Nuremberg Code did not provoke much of a response at the time that it was issued. Indeed, as Faden and her colleagues explain, the trial of the Nazi doctors had only modest resonance with the popular press and the medical establishment in the United States because their misdeeds were considered an anomaly attributable to a totalitarian regime of unquestionable brutality. The assumption was that researchers working in democratic countries would never do such things. Thus the Nuremberg Code was viewed as a document that was needed to restrain barbarians but was not applicable to "the rest of us."

Nonetheless, the basic tenets of the Nuremberg Code seemed to have an effect on U.S. governmental agencies. The administrators and advisors of the Atomic Energy Commission (AEC) seem to have been well aware of the trials of Nazi doctors then taking place at Nuremberg.[10] The AEC administrators were also aware of a set of secret experiments conducted during the war under the auspices of the Manhattan Project in which hospitalized patients were injected with plutonium, evidently without their knowledge.[11] The purpose of these experiments—publicly revealed only in the early 1990s—was primarily to assess and improve the safety of radiation workers and secondarily to evaluate the potential for the use of plutonium in the treatment of bone cancer. In December 1946, for example, the newly created civilian AEC suspended human studies involving the use of radioisotopes until it had the opportunity to set standards and approve the proposed research. Among the standards ultimately established by the AEC was "informed consent." This appears to have been the first time the term was used, well before its popular introduction in a 1957 malpractice case.[12]

The legitimacy of human experimentation was again questioned when research performed at the Brooklyn Jewish Chronic Disease Hospital came to light. In July 1963 a researcher at the hospital injected live cancer cells into debilitated elderly patients without their fully informed consent. The hospital was sued, and the New York state attorney general brought charges against two physicians involved in the study, Chester M. Southam and Emanuel E. Mandel. Our second selection in this part, as originally excerpted by Katz, Capron, and Glass, includes the court record of Southam's rebuttal to the charges against him, the testimony of a patient who was an unknowing subject in the study, and a news piece summarizing the findings of the trial involving Southam and Mandel.

As Southam explains, the aim of the experiment was to determine the rate of rejection of human cancer cells injected into patients. All evidence available

suggested that the cancer cells would cause an immune reaction that would lead to their expulsion from the body; the experiment thus presented no risk to the subjects. In fact, Southam argues, informing the patients of the details of the experiment would have caused them needless psychological distress, and his failure to inform them was a result of the need to minimize the risks to his subjects. Yet critics argued otherwise. Although the so-called therapeutic privilege *might* justify nondisclosure in a physician-patient relationship, the Board of Regents of the University of the State of New York argued that it could not justify nondisclosure in a researcher-participant relationship. One of the lessons that emerged from this case was that a physician-researcher may have conflicting loyalties that are of ethical importance. The Board of Regents thought so and therefore suspended the licenses of Mandel and Southam for a year. This action presaged demands for greater accountability on the part of medical researchers.

In 1966, when Henry K. Beecher, a professor of anesthesiology at Harvard Medical School, published the landmark article "Ethics and Clinical Research" in the *New England Journal of Medicine*, ethical issues in research began to take center stage. In his article, which we excerpt here, Beecher describes 22 studies that he claims violated the basic standards of ethical research with human beings. What was so shocking at the time was that these experiments were performed by respected investigators at leading medical institutions and were published in reputable medical journals. The research performed at the Jewish Chronic Disease Hospital is one case that Beecher cites. Others include a study in which investigators withheld penicillin from soldiers with strep throat infection, even though they knew there was a risk that the soldiers would develop rheumatic fever and die from valvular disease, and research on physiology that involved the insertion of a needle into the left atrium of the heart during bronchoscopy, with unknown risks and no benefits for the participants.

One of the more infamous cases Beecher discusses is the Willowbrook study, in which researchers deliberately exposed children and adolescents with disabilities to hepatitis at a New York state facility. The aim of the study was to find a preventive measure for the hepatitis that was epidemic in the institution. But critics claim that the conditions under which the children were recruited were coercive: The wards of the public facilities were closed to any new admissions due to overcrowding. Parents of the children with severe disabilities who were on the waiting list were mailed a letter indicating that their children could be admitted if they were placed in the research ward, and that they could then be transferred into the facility. Writing in his own defense, Saul Krugman, the head of the distinguished research team that conducted the study, noted that nearly every child admitted to the facility was likely to contract hepatitis anyway and that this fact mitigated the harm of deliberately exposing the children to hepatitis, as the research required.[13] Indeed, from the time that the research had been initiated at the facility the rates of hepatitis had declined substantially, making it safer than before the research started. Furthermore, Krugman argued, consent to the children's deliberate exposure in the study was obtained from their parents. In addition, the protocol had been reviewed by various university and state government entities, as well as by the Armed Forces Epidemiological Board, which funded the study. But critics argued that because the study population consisted of children with severe retardation whose parents wanted to place them in one of the few public institutions available, the consent obtained was invalid.[14] Krugman protested that the fact that the children had mental retardation was beside the point, but critics argued that it was precisely the point.

Beecher's aim was not to condemn individual researchers but rather to draw attention to serious ethical problems in the conduct of research with humans. Although the prevailing view at the time was that adherence to the Nuremberg Code was unnecessary for conscientious researchers in democracies, Beecher's examples clearly belie this belief. However, Beecher concluded that two things were indispensable for ethical research: informed consent and, more important, a virtuous investigator. His emphasis on the latter requirement suggests that Beecher himself viewed a code of research ethics as of secondary importance.

By the late 1960s medical research involving humans had undergone so many scandals and tragedies that distinguished physicians found it necessary to defend it, mainly by invoking utilitarian considerations. In *Science* Leon Eisenberg, a prominent psychiatric researcher, reminded Americans of the economic and social costs of disease and death, costs that eminently justified human experimentation in spite of the inherent limitations of the informed consent ideal.[15] In addition, citing the Reed example, Walsh McDermott wrote, "Medicine has given to society the

case for its rights in the continuation of clinical investigation." McDermott believed that "playing God" was an unavoidable responsibility, presumably one to be shouldered by clinical investigators.[16] Similarly, in 1971 Louis Lasagna posed the rhetorical question, "How many of medicine's greatest advances might have been delayed or prevented by the rigid application of some currently proposed principles to research at large?" Lasagna claimed that "for the ethical, experienced investigator no laws are needed and for the unscrupulous incompetent no laws will help."[17]

Yet only a year after Lasagna's defense of research, the wholesale violations of human rights in the Tuskegee Syphilis Study were revealed.[18] As Allan M. Brandt, our final contributor to Part I, recounts, the study was initiated in 1932 in Macon County, Alabama, in order to assess the natural course of syphilis, which had reached epidemic proportions in African American males in that area. Many researchers, Brandt points out, argued that there was no scientific rationale for the study in 1932 because the natural history of syphilis had already been elucidated by a study in Oslo at the turn of the century,[19] and treatment of latent syphilis was the standard of care. Yet over 400 men, mostly illiterate sharecroppers, were recruited for the Tuskegee study. They were not informed about the true nature of the study or about their condition, nor were their partners informed of their risk. When penicillin became publicly available in the late 1940s, the men were not given the opportunity to use it; in fact, efforts were made to ensure that the men did not receive treatment or become aware of it.

In 1972 press reports prompted the secretary of the Department of Health, Education, and Welfare to stop the study. By this time 74 of the subjects were still alive, and, as Brandt notes, "at least 28, but perhaps more than 100, had died directly from advanced syphilitic lesions." Some observers saw no particular cause for outrage over a project that had never been a secret governmental study. Others argued that the Tuskegee study exemplified a pattern of institutionalized racism in health care in a society that had been struggling with similar issues in housing, employment, and education. In the late 1970s compensation was authorized for the survivors and for the families of those who had died, but they did not receive a formal apology from the federal government until 1997. The apology, issued by President Bill Clinton, was accompanied by a $200,000 grant for the creation of the Tuskegee University National Center for Bio-ethics in Research and Health.

The Tuskegee Syphilis Study had wide repercussions. In 1974 the National Research Act became law in the United States and led to the creation of the National Commission for the Protection of Human Subjects of Biomedical and Behavioral Research, as well as the enactment of federal regulations governing research with humans. Another effect of the Tuskegee study was that it undermined the utilitarian justification of research as articulated by McDermott and Lasagna. Although there may be rare instances in which interventions can be justified on utilitarian grounds—for example, public health interventions undertaken to control an epidemic—such a justification is much harder to sustain in the case of nonemergency research with humans. Alan Donagan argued that, by the lights of the medical profession itself, the utilitarian attitudes exemplified by the Nazi experiments and the research conducted the Jewish Chronic Disease Hospital were unjustifiable. He delineated an alternative to the utilitarian justification of research in which informed consent was taken as nearly a self-evident moral obligation.[20] It is a supreme irony that in the 1960s and 1970s, a time when great advances were being made in medical research, scandals and tragedies were calling into question the ethics of such research. But as subsequent parts of the book demonstrate, this was just the beginning.

1. James Lind, *A Treatise of the Scurvy* (Edinburgh: Sands, Murray and Cochran, 1753).
2. Edward Jenner, *An Inquiry Into the Causes and Effects of Variolæ Vaccinæ* (London: Printed for the author by Sampson Low, 1798).
3. Lawrence K. Altman, *Who Goes First? The Story of Self-Experimentation in Medicine* (Berkeley: University of California Press, 1998).
4. Carol Levine, "Has AIDS Changed the Ethics of Human Subjects Research?" *Law, Medicine and Health Care* 16 (1988): 167–73.
5. Telford Taylor, "Opening Statement of the Prosecution, December 9, 1946," in *The Nazi Doctors and the Nuremberg Code,* ed. G. J. Annas and M. A. Grodin (New York: Oxford University Press, 1992), 67–93.
6. Robert N. Proctor, *Racial Hygiene* (Cambridge, Mass.: Harvard University Press, 1988); Michael Burleigh, *Ethics and Extermination* (New York: Cambridge University Press, 1997).
7. This is a summary taken from the Allies' opening statement at the Nuremberg trial; see Taylor.
8. S.S. Colonel Wolfram Sievers, as quoted in Taylor, 84.
9. A slightly abridged version of the final judgment is included in Annas and Grodin, 94–104.
10. Jonathan D. Moreno, *Undue Risk: Secret State Experiments on Humans* (New York: W. H. Freeman and Company, 2000).
11. Eileen Welsome, *The Plutonium Files* (New York: Delacorte Press, 1999).
12. *Salgo v. Leland Stanford Jr. University Board of Trustees,* 154 Cal. App.2d 560, 317 P.2d 170 (1957).
13. Saul Krugman, "The Willowbrook Hepatitis Studies Revisited: Ethical Aspects," *Reviews of Infectious Diseases* 8 (1986): 157–62.
14. David J. Rothman and Sheila M. Rothman, *The Willowbrook Wars* (New York: Harper & Row, 1984).
15. Leon Eisenberg, "The Social Imperatives of Medical Research," *Science* 198 (1977): 1105–10.
16. Walsh McDermott, "The Changing Mores of Biomedical Research: Opening Comments," *Annals of Internal Medicine* 67, Suppl. 7 (1967): 39–42.
17. Louis Lasagna, "Some Ethical Problems in Clinical Investigation," in *Human Aspects of Biomedical Innovation,* ed. Everett Mendelsohn, Judith P. Swazey, and Irene Taviss (Cambridge, Mass.: Harvard University Press, 1971), 109.
18. Susan M. Reverby, ed., *Tuskegee's Truths* (Chapel Hill: University of North Carolina Press, 2000).
19. E. Gurney Clark and Niels Danbolt, "The Oslo Study of the Natural History of Untreated Syphilis," *Journal of Chronic Diseases* 2 (1955): 311–44.
20. Alan Donagan, "Informed Consent in Therapy and Experimentation," *Journal of Medicine and Philosophy* 2 (1977): 307–29.

1   U.S. Medical Researchers, the Nuremberg Doctors Trial, and the Nuremberg Code

A Review of Findings of the Advisory Committee on Human Radiation Experiments

Ruth R. Faden, Susan E. Lederer, and Jonathan D. Moreno

The Advisory Committee on Human Radiation Experiments (ACHRE) was established by President Clinton in April 1994 in response to allegations of abuses of human subjects in government-sponsored research conducted during the cold war. The suspect research included experiments in which hospital patients were injected with plutonium and uranium, institutionalized children were administered radioactive tracers, and prisoners were exposed to testicular irradiation. In addition to investigating the facts of these and other cases, ACHRE was charged with identifying appropriate standards by which to evaluate the ethics of these experiments.

Most of the experiments we investigated had been conducted after the Nuremberg Doctors Trial and promulgation of the Nuremberg Code and involved allegations of violations of the Code's first principle requiring the voluntary and informed consent of the experimental subject. A central question before ACHRE was what role the Nuremberg Code played in the norms and practices of U.S. medical researchers. How was the Nuremberg Code viewed by U.S. medical scientists in the 1940s and 1950s, and how did they react to the Code's stringent demands? [...]

PHYSICIANS' AND RESEARCHERS' REACTIONS TO THE NEWS OF THE NUREMBERG DOCTORS TRIAL

[...] The Nuremberg Doctors Trial received limited coverage in the popular press. [David J.] Rothman has summarized the trial's *New York Times* coverage as fewer than a dozen articles from 1945 to 1947. Only the August 1947 guilty verdict appeared on page 1.

The Ethics Oral History Project [in which physicians who began their careers as medical scientists in the 1940s

and 1950s were interviewed about the norms and practices of human subjects research during that time—eds.] suggests that U.S. medical researchers, perhaps like the U.S. public generally, were not carefully following the daily developments in Nuremberg. For example, John Arnold, M.D., a researcher who during the Nuremberg Doctors Trial was involved in malaria experiments on prisoners at the Illinois State Penitentiary Stateville Branch, offered a particularly vivid (if somewhat anachronistic) recollection of the scant attention paid to the trial among U.S. medical scientists: "We were dimly aware of it. And as you ask me now, I'm astonished that we [were not] hanging on the TV at the time, watching for each twist and turn of the argument to develop. But we weren't." It might have been expected that the researchers at Stateville would have been particularly concerned with the events at Nuremberg because some of the medical defendants claimed during the trial that the wartime malaria experiments at the Illinois prison were analogous to the experiments carried out in the Nazi concentration camps.

The Nuremberg Doctors Trial was a significant event at Montefiore Hospital in New York, recalled Herbert Abrams, M.D., who was a resident at the hospital at the time of the trial: "It was surely something, at least in the environment I was in, we were aware of and that affected the thinking of everyone who was involved in clinical investigation." It seems likely, however, that the environment this young physician was in would have caused a heightened awareness of a trial dealing with Nazi medical professionals. Montefiore is a traditionally Jewish hospital that was home to many Jewish refugee physicians who had fled the terror and oppression of the Nazi regime. A trial of German physicians almost certainly would have been of particular interest in this setting.

Even among those U.S. medical researchers who might have been aware of events at Nuremberg, it seems that many did not perceive specific personal implications in the medical trial. Rothman has expressed this historical view most fully. He asserts that "the prevailing view was that [the Nuremberg medical defendants] were Nazis first, and last; by definition nothing they did, and no code drawn up in re-

Ruth R. Faden, Susan E. Lederer, and Jonathan D. Moreno, "U.S. Medical Researchers, the Nuremberg Doctors Trial, and the Nuremberg Code: A Review of Findings of the Advisory Committee on Human Radiation Experiments," *JAMA* 276 (1996): 1667–71.

sponse to them, was relevant to the United States." Katz has offered a similar summation of the immediate response of the medical community to the Nuremberg Code: "It was a good code for barbarians but an unnecessary code for ordinary physicians."

Several participants in ACHRE's Ethics Oral History Project affirmed the interpretations of Rothman and Katz, using similar language. For example, according to William Silverman, M.D., "There was a disconnect. . . . The interpretation of these Codes was that they were necessary for barbarians, but [not for] fine upstanding people." This same physician later acknowledged that U.S. researchers often did not attend to the relationship between the atrocities described at Nuremberg and their own work "for reasons of self-interest, to be perfectly frank. As I see it now I'm saddened that we didn't see the connection but that's what was done. . . . It's hard to tell you now . . . how we rationalized, but the fact is we did."

THE POPULAR PRESS

The popular press mirrored the view that human experimentation as practiced in the United States was not a morally troubling enterprise—it was as American as apple pie. Between 1948 and 1960, magazines such as the *Saturday Evening Post, Reader's Digest,* and the *American Mercury* ran "human interest" stories on "human guinea pigs." These stories generally focused on specific groups of healthy subjects—prisoners, conscientious objectors, medical students, soldiers—and described them as "volunteers." The articles explained the ordeals to which the volunteers had submitted themselves. "Among these men and women," the *New York Times* informed its Sunday readership in 1958, "you will find those who will take shots of the new vaccines, who will swallow radioactive drugs, who will fly higher than anyone else, who will watch malaria infected mosquitoes feed on their bare arms." The articles assured the public that the volunteers had plausible, often noble, reasons for volunteering for such seemingly gruesome treatment. The explanations included social redemption (especially in the case of prisoners), religious or other beliefs (particularly for conscientious objectors), the advancement of science, service to society, and thrill seeking. In sum, most articles in the popular press were uncritical about experimentation on humans and assumed that those involved had freely volunteered to participate.

However, a smaller number of press reports in the late 1940s and 1950s did suggest some tension between the words spoken at Nuremberg and the practices in the United States. As early as 1948, for example, *Science News* reported the Soviet claim that U.S. researchers were using "Nazi methods" in the conduct of prisoner experiments. Concern also began to be voiced about the dangers to volunteer "guinea pigs." In October 1954, for example, the magazine *Christian Century* called the U.S. Army to halt, at the first sign of danger, experiments at the Fitzsimmons Hospital in Denver, CO, where soldiers were called on to eat foods exposed to cobalt radiation.

It is also possible that press accounts of experiments with patients rather than healthy subjects were more inclined to be critical, even in the late 1940s. A *Saturday Evening Post* article from the January 15, 1949, issue describes how a physician with the Veterans Administration kept quiet about streptomycin trials involving veterans who were patients in the medical departments of the army, the U.S. Navy, and the Veterans Administration because of "the risk of congressional chastisement from publicity-conscious members of the House and Senate who might have screamed: 'You can't experiment on our heroes,' if it had been known that army and navy veterans of former wars were being used in medical investigation. This was a real worry of the doctors who formulated the clinical program."

EVIDENCE OF CONCERN: THE 1950s

Evidence suggests that some U.S. researchers were genuinely and deeply concerned with the issues surrounding human experimentation during the years immediately following World War II. One source of insight into the thinking of U.S. physicians engaged in clinical research during the 1950s is found in the groundbreaking work of medical sociologist Renée C. Fox, Ph.D. For two 5-month periods between September 1951 and January 1953, Fox spent long days "in continuous, direct, and intimate contact with the physicians and patients" in a metabolic research ward that she pseudonymously called "Ward F-Second." In 1959, Fox reported on the ethical dilemmas faced by the physicians conducting research on this ward. She did not suggest that the investigators under her observation were unaware of the Nuremberg Code; instead she offered a point-by-point paraphrasing of the Code, which she identified as "the basic principles governing research on human subjects which the physicians of the metabolic group [her collective term for the researchers whom she studied] were required to observe."

Rather that being unconscious or contemptuous of a set of principles intended for barbarians, Fox reported that the researchers on Ward F-Second were sometimes troubled by their inability to apply the high, but essentially unquestioned, standards enunciated at the Nuremberg Doctors Trial. She attributed the physicians' difficulty in translating their good intentions into practice as due partly to the necessarily abstract nature of all norms intended as general guides of behavior.

Sometimes private discussions among researchers about the ethical aspects of human experimentation led to public events. A good example from the early 1950s is the symposium held on October 10, 1951, at the University of California School of Medicine in San Francisco. Michael B. Shimkin, M.D., organized the symposium in response to some confidential criticism that he had received for research carried out under his direction with patients at the University of California's Laboratory of Experimental Oncology. The exact nature of this criticism is unclear from the records that remain of the episode, but Shimkin reported in a memoir that "remedial steps" were taken, including "written protocols for all new departures in clinical research, which we asked the cancer board of the medical school to review."

The organizers of the First International Congress of Neuropathology, which was held in Rome in 1952, were sufficiently concerned with ethical issues that they invited Pope Pius XII to address "The Moral Limits of Medical Methods of Research and Treatment." In a speech before 427 medical researchers from around the world (including 62 from the United States), the pope firmly endorsed the principle of obtaining consent from research subjects—whether sick or healthy. He also pointed his audience to the relatively recent lessons of the Nuremberg Doctors Trial, which he summed up as teaching that "man should not exist for the use of society; on the contrary, the community exists for the good of man." In an interview in 1961, Thomas Rivers, M.D., a prominent U.S. virus researcher, recalled that the pope's words had been influential among medical scientists working during the 1950s: "That speech had a very broad impact on medical scientists both here and abroad."

The growing significance of the Nuremberg Code can be seen by comparing 2 editions of the best-known textbook of U.S. medical jurisprudence in the mid 20th century, *Doctor and Patient and the Law*. Louis J. Regan, M.D., LL.B., offered very little in the chapter titled "Experimentation," in the 1949 edition of his book, and what he did offer made no reference to Nuremberg:

> The physician must keep abreast of medical progress, but he is responsible if he goes beyond usual and standard procedures to the point of experimentation. If such treatment is considered indicated, it should not be undertaken until consultation has been had and until the patient has signed a paper acknowledging and assuming the risk.

However, in the 1956 edition of the same text, Regan's few lines on human experimentation had been expanded to 3 pages. He presented a lengthy paraphrasing of the Nuremberg Code, and he repeated verbatim (without quotation marks) the judges' preamble to the Code, stating that "all agree" about these principles. [...]

NUREMBERG AND CLINICAL REALITY: 1959–1962

In the spring of 1959 the National Society for Medical Research (NSMR) sponsored the National Conference on the Legal Environment of Medicine, at the University of Chicago. Human experimentation was a major topic presented for discussion by the 148 conference participants, primarily medical researchers, from around the country. The published report of this conference reveals that the many researchers who gathered in Chicago understood the Nuremberg Code well enough to use it as a point of departure for discussion. As a group, the conferees acknowledged that the 10 principles of the Nuremberg Code "have become the principal guideposts to the ethics of clinical research in the western world."

Not all those in attendance, however, were entirely pleased with this state of affairs. The Committee on the Re-Evaluation of the Nuremberg Experimental Principles reported general agreement with "the spirit of these precautions" but discomfort with a number of "particulars." For example, they suggested that the absolute requirement for consent in the Code's first principle might be softened by inserting "either explicit or reasonably presumed" before the word "consent." They also added a clause that would allow for third-party permission for "those not capable of personal consent."

The discussion that took place during the 1959 NSMR conference strongly suggested that by the late 1950s many and perhaps even most U.S. medical researchers had come to recognize the Nuremberg Code as the authoritative answer to an important question: What are the rules for human experimentation? [...]

However, discomfort with the Nuremberg Code did exist and sources for this discomfort can be grouped, retrospectively, into 3 broad categories. First, some recognized the discrepancies between what they had come to know as real practices in research on patient-subjects and what they read in the lofty, idealized language of the Code. Others simply disagreed with some elements of the Code. Still others disliked the very idea of a single, concrete set of standards to guide behavior in such a complex matter as human experimentation.

Henry Beecher, M.D., the medical researcher from Harvard Medical School who was to have a profound impact on U.S. research ethics, published an article, "Experimentation in Man," in *JAMA* only a few months before the 1959 NSMR conference in Chicago. In this article, Beecher addressed a mixture of all 3 sources of discomfort with the Nuremberg Code. Beecher offered the assertion that "it is unethical and immoral to carry out potentially dangerous experiments without the subject's knowledge and consent" as the "central conclusion" of his paper. But, even with this strong statement, Beecher was not entirely satisfied with the first clause of the Code; he viewed the Nuremberg consent clause as too extreme and not squaring with the realities of clinical research.

Beecher's second form of difficulty with the Code can be found in his opinion of another Nuremberg clause, which states, in part, that a human experiment should not be "random and unnecessary in nature." Beecher cited "anesthesia, x-rays, radium, and penicillin" as important medical breakthroughs that had resulted from "random" experimentation. He further stated that he "would not know how to define experiments unnecessary in nature."

Finally, Beecher expressed skepticism in general that any Code could provide effective moral guidance for researchers working with human subjects. Near the beginning of his article, he wrote that

> [T]he problems of human experimentation
> do not lend themselves to a series of rigid
> rules. . . . In most cases, these are more likely
> to do harm than good. Rules are not going to
> curb the unscrupulous. Such abuses as have
> occurred are usually due to ignorance and in-
> experience.

Another episode involving Beecher further clarifies the medical profession's dissatisfaction with the construction of the Nuremberg Code. In the fall of 1961, Beecher and other members of the Harvard Medical School Administrative Board, the school's governing body, were presented with a set of "rigid rules" that had begun to appear in army medical research contracts. The members of the board quickly recognized the "Principles, Policies and Rules of the Surgeon General, Department of the Army, Relating to the Use of Human Volunteers in Medical Research" as little more than a restatement of the Nuremberg Code.

In view of his 1959 article, it is not surprising that Beecher was uncomfortable with the prospect of working in strict accordance with the Nuremberg Code if he were to receive funding from the army. As can be seen in the minutes of the administrative board meeting in which this matter came up for discussion, Beecher was not alone in his opposition. At the October 6, 1961, meeting of the board, when the army contract insertion was first mentioned: "[S]ome members . . . felt that with the minor changes the regulations were acceptable, while others described the regulations as vague, ambiguous and, in many instances, impossible to fulfill."

One of Beecher's fellow board members, Joseph W. Gardella, M.D., assistant dean of the medical school, produced a thorough written critique of the "Principles, Policies, and Rules of the Surgeon General" (and thus of the Nuremberg Code) following the October 1961 meeting for the consideration of the other board members. In his pa-

per, Gardella noted that the Nuremberg Code had its origin in extraordinary circumstances and was "not necessarily pertinent" to the U.S. research context. Moreover, he suggested, it was not clear that the Code was intended to refer to sick patients for whom research participation might have been beneficial. Referring specifically to the army rules, Gardella doubted the ability of the sick to understand the complex facts of their condition in a way that can make consent meaningful. The written consent requirement that the army rules added to the Nuremberg Code was seen as carrying unfortunate legal implications, undermining the trust that is the basis of the physician-patient relationship, and causing the patient-subject undue anxiety.

Gardella presented his analysis of the army rules to the other members of the Harvard Medical School Administrative Board on March 23, 1962. The minutes of that meeting document that Gardella's views were not extreme or exceptional among leading medical scientists in the early 1960s, at least at Harvard: "The members of the Board were in general agreement with the objections and criticisms expressed in [Gardella's] critique."

During this same meeting, Beecher agreed "to attempt to capture in a paragraph or so the broad philosophical and moral principles that underlie the conduct of research on human beings at the Harvard Medical School." The members of the board hoped that such a statement might satisfy the army and that it would allow Harvard, as Gardella put it, "to avert the catastrophic impact of the Surgeon General's regulation."

A few months later, Beecher had completed a document titled "Statement Outlining the Philosophy and Ethical Principles Governing the Conduct of Research on Human Beings at Harvard Medical School." At the June 8, 1962, Administrative Board meeting, Beecher's colleagues "commended" and "reaffirmed" the views expressed in Beecher's document. In this statement, as in his 1959 published paper, Beecher emphasized the significance of consent, but he also asserted that "it is folly to overlook the fact that valid, informed consent may be difficult to the point of impossible to obtain in some cases." More than consent, Beecher believed in the significance of "a special relationship of trust between subject or patient and the investigator." In the end, Beecher concluded that the only reliable foundation for this relationship was a virtuous medical researcher, with virtuous peers:

> It is this writer's point of view that the best
> approach concerns the character, wisdom, ex-
> perience, honesty, imaginativeness and sense
> of responsibility of the investigator who in all
> cases of doubt or where serious consequences
> might remotely occur, will call in his peers
> and get the benefit of their counsel. Rigid
> rules will jeopardize the Research establish-

ments of this country where experimentation in man is essential.

Available evidence suggests that, by offering Beecher's replacement for the Nuremberg Code, representatives of Harvard Medical School were able to extract a clarification during a meeting with Army Surgeon General Leonard D. Heaton, M.C., U.S.A., on July 12, 1962, that the "principles" being inserted into Harvard's research contracts with the army were "guidelines" rather than "rigid rules."

While the Harvard Medical School discussion of the army's rules took place behind closed doors and involved a policy of limited applicability, the leaders of the international medical community were simultaneously engaged in a far more visible and global attempt to bring the standards enunciated in the Nuremberg Code into line with the realities of medical research. The 1964 statement by the World Medical Association, commonly known as the Declaration of Helsinki, created 2 separate categories laying out rules for human experimentation: "Clinical Research Combined with Professional Care" and "Nontherapeutic Clinical Research." In the former category, physicians were required to obtain consent from patient-subjects only when "consistent with patient psychology." In nontherapeutic clinical research, the consent requirements were more absolute: "Clinical research on a human being cannot be undertaken without his free consent, after he has been fully informed." Another noteworthy deviation from the Nuremberg Code is the Declaration of Helsinki's allowance (in both therapeutic and nontherapeutic research) for third-party permission from a legal guardian.

As one might predict from the similarity between the changes introduced by the Declaration of Helsinki and the changes to the Nuremberg Code suggested by the U.S. participants of the NSMR conference in 1959, the World Medical Association document met with widespread approval among researchers in the United States. Organizations including the American Society for Clinical Investigation, the American Federation for Clinical Research, and the American Medical Association offered their expeditious and enthusiastic endorsements. Compared with the lofty, idealized language of the Nuremberg Code, the Declaration of Helsinki may have seemed more sensible to many researchers in the early 1960s because it offered rules that more closely resembled research practice in the clinical setting.

CONCLUSION

[. . .] At the time it was promulgated, [the Nuremberg] Code had little effect on the mainstream morality of U.S. medical researchers who used patients as their subjects and the clinic as their laboratory.

Some U.S. medical researchers who asked themselves difficult questions about their research work with patients concluded that there should be high standards of consent for subjects who are ill. That some did in fact reach this conclusion is evidence that it was not beyond the horizon of moral insight at that time. Nevertheless, they were a minority of the community of physician researchers, and the medical profession did not exhibit a willingness to reconsider its responsibilities to patients in the burgeoning world of postwar clinical research.

While a slowly increasing number of investigators reflected on the ethical treatment of human subjects during the 1950s, it was not until after the early 1960s and a series of highly publicized events connected with names like "thalidomide," "Willowbrook," and "Tuskegee" that it became apparent that a professional code, whether it originated in Nuremberg or Helsinki, did not provide sufficient protection against exploitation and abuse of human subjects of research.

---

2 The Jewish Chronic Disease Hospital Case

Jay Katz, with Alexander Morgan Capron
and Eleanor Swift Glass, eds.

In July 1963, three doctors, with approval from the director of medicine of the Jewish Chronic Disease Hospital in Brooklyn, New York, injected "live cancer cells" sub-

---

Jay Katz, with Alexander Morgan Capron and Eleanor Swift Glass, eds. *Experimentation with Human Beings* (New York: Russell Sage Foundation, 1972), 36–38, 40–41, 63–65.

cutaneously into twenty-two chronically ill and debilitated patients. The doctors did not inform the patients that live cancer cells were being used or that the experiment was designed to measure the patients' ability to reject foreign cells—a test unrelated to their normal therapeutic program.

The cancer experiment engendered a heated controversy among the hospital's doctors and led to an investigation by the hospital's grievance committee and board of directors. William A. Hyman, a member of the board who disapproved of the experiment, took the hospital to court to force disclosure of the hospital's records, claiming that the directors' approval of the experiment had not been properly obtained. As *Hyman* v. *Jewish Chronic Disease Hospital* wound its way up from the trial court through two appellate tribunals, it became clear that the legal issue involved in the suit, whether a hospital director is entitled to look at patients' medical records, only provided the backdrop for the questions really at issue which concerned the duties and obligations that the various participants in the human experimentation process should have toward one another.

Subsequently, these issues were confronted more directly when the Board of Regents of the University of the State of New York heard charges brought by the attorney general against two of the doctors involved. The board imposed sanctions, under the authority given it by New York Education Law §6514(2) to revoke, suspend, or annul the license of a practitioner of medicine upon determining "after due hearing . . . that a physician . . . is guilty of fraud or deceit in the practice of medicine [or] that a physician is or has been guilty of unprofessional conduct."

[. . .]

[What follows is the court record of Dr. Chester M. Southam's rebuttal to the charges brought against the Jewish Chronic Disease Hospital. Dr. Southam was the principal investigator of the study undertaken there.—eds.]

Rebuttal Affidavits for Respondent
Chester M. Southam, M.D.
February 4, 1964

I address myself first to the question of the measure of risk of bodily harm to the patients who were the subject of the procedures in question at the Jewish Chronic Disease Hospital. At the outset I should say that in clinical procedures neither I nor any scientist or doctor can deal in absolutes. We are always limited, at least when dealing with the human body, to speaking in terms of measurable risks. Thus, while no doctor or scientist can say as to any clinical procedure, even the simplest, that there is no possibility of untoward results, we are constantly required, both in therapeutic and in investigative procedures, to make judgments as to whether there is any unusual risk of untoward results, and if so, the degree of that risk. In terms of this standard I unhesitatingly assert that on the basis of present biological knowledge supplemented by clinical experience to date there was no practical possibility of untoward results to the patients who received injections of homotransplants in the form of tissue-cultured cells derived from other patients. The probability of any unforeseen deleterious consequences of this test is so extremely small as to be com-

parable to numerous other procedures used routinely in clinical medicine for therapeutic, diagnostic, or investigative purposes, e.g., blood transfusions, intravenous pyelograms (kidney x-rays), or tuberculin tests. The fact that these cells were tissue-cultured cancer cells did not measurably increase any risk inherent in the procedure because, being foreign to the recipient (the person injected), they bring about an immunological reaction (defense reaction, rejection reaction) that ultimately causes their destruction and elimination.

It has been known for many years that a human being will reject cells transplanted from another human being unless both are of precisely the same genetic makeup (i.e., identical twins). In fact, intensive clinical studies are now being carried on at many research centers attempting to find methods (such as treatment with certain drugs or x-ray) to overcome this rejection reaction in the hope that diseased organs, such as kidneys, might be successfully replaced. While the precise mechanisms of cell rejection are not yet known, the fact that such mechanisms exist is beyond question. The efficiency of this type of immunological reaction can be measured in terms of the time required for complete rejection of homotransplanted cells. As yet no other method of measuring this reaction has been found, and tissue-cultured cancer cells are the only kind of cells which provide sufficient reproducibility for comparison of results in different individuals at different times.

The three lines of cells derived from human cancer which were used in the studies at the Jewish Chronic Disease Hospital were derived from tumor tissues of three patients, from 4 to 12 years ago. Since that time these cells have been cultivated in sterile bottles in the laboratory in a solution of nutrients which include salts, vitamins, and blood serum. This is the process called tissue culture. After such years of growth under these artificial laboratory conditions each line of cultured cells has a high degree of uniformity and, consequently, the reaction which it will produce is highly predictable. I have had an extensive experience in homotransplantation studies in cancer patients and in healthy volunteers during the past several years.

In the early 1950s it began to appear that the defense mechanisms (i.e., the mechanism of rejection of homotransplants) of those persons who develop cancer might be in some way impaired. The most striking indication of this was the result of clinical tests on a limited number of patients with terminal cancer as reported over the signatures of myself and Drs. Rhoads and Moore in *Science*. These were all patients suffering from advanced stages of widely disseminated cancer for whom there was no known method of treatment to either inhibit their disease or prolong their lives, each of whom died as the result of his own cancer within a relatively short time. In view of the then state of knowledge the precise details of the procedure were explained and the patients freely and readily consented.

The significant result of the test was that the rate of rejection of the foreign transplants was in all cases slower than would have been expected, indicating that there was some impairment of their immunological reaction. Because these patients had far advanced cancer before the homotransplants were injected, they did not survive for long after the tests were performed. Obviously this was not the result of the test, but rather was the reason that these particular patients were selected for these earliest tests. In no case was the patient deleteriously affected by the implants. Several patients in this initial group and in subsequent groups had not rejected their transplants in the brief interval between the start of the test and their death. In fact, at autopsy a lymph node from the armpit of one of these patients contained unrejected cancer cells of the type used for the test. (These lymph nodes are in the natural route of drainage from the forearm where the test was made in this patient.)

Prior to the publication of the article in question tests were made on a number of volunteer healthy human beings in the Ohio Penitentiary. In all such cases the foreign transplants were quickly and completely rejected, as would have been expected.

After the initial tests reported in *Science,* intensive studies were undertaken, designed to increase our body of knowledge as to the immunological reaction both of normal healthy persons and those with cancer, to homotransplants of tissue-cultured lines of human cells derived from normal and tumor tissues. Between the time of the initial tests and July 16, 1963 (the date on which the injections were made in [the] Jewish Chronic Disease Hospital), approximately 600 persons had been studied by means of the techniques employed at [the] Jewish Chronic Disease Hospital, approximately 300 of whom were patients with cancer and 300 healthy, normal persons. In every healthy recipient of tissue-cultured cells, these foreign transplants were rejected with uniform promptness. Some patients with cancer rejected the cells less rapidly and after significantly varying intervals of time. Patients in the earlier stages of neoplastic disease showed normal or only slightly impaired rejection reaction. Patients in the terminal stages of cancer showed the greatest deficiency in these immunological defense mechanisms (as measured by the length of time to effect rejection) and in several such persons rejection had not been accomplished in the few weeks or months that elapsed between injection of the test cells and the patient's death from his own cancer. These patients died from the effects of their own cancer before the expected ultimate rejection of the implants. The studies also demonstrated a correlation between the rate of rejection of homotransplanted cancer cells and the patient's apparent ability to restrain his own disease, thus providing additional direct evidence that patients may have immunological (defense) mechanisms to restrain their own cancer. These results, of

course, give hope that, through further clinical research, methods of stimulating such mechanisms to greater efficacy can be developed.

The studies of healthy, normal persons at the Ohio Penitentiary, aside from demonstrating that the normal body will reject cancer cell homotransplants with the same efficiency as other types of homotransplants, further indicated the potentially highly significant fact that the body's rate of rejection increased with successive implantations of foreign cancer cells, suggesting long-run possibilities of building up the immunological mechanisms where deficiencies now occur. At present, studies are being continued to verify these scientific observations and to investigate their possible applicability to the treatment and prevention of human cancer. Such studies of human cancer can be accomplished only through the cooperation of patients and healthy volunteers.

Until the investigation conducted at the Jewish Chronic Disease Hospital, there was no direct clinical evidence that the impairment of the immunologic responses in patients with advanced cancer (as measured by the slow rate at which they rejected homotransplants) was associated with the fact that they had cancer rather than with the fact that they were in a debilitated state. This study provided direct clinical evidence that indeed the impairment was associated with the fact of cancer rather than general debilitation. The patients at [the] Jewish Chronic Disease Hospital reacted in essentially the same manner as normal, healthy human beings. I want to make perfectly clear that the question in this investigation was not whether the patients would reject the tissue-cultured cancer cell homotransplants. The only question was how fast would the body mobilize its resources of rejection. Three patients known to have cancer were also included in these tests. It was expected that rejection in the three cancer patients might be delayed, consistent with our previous experience in cancer patients, but that rejection would occur after the predicted delay unless these patients succumbed very rapidly to their own cancer.

I next turn to the question of procedures. In the early stages of this clinical research and, indeed, until the last few years a full explanation was given to the patient or healthy volunteer, including the fact that the techniques employed were not designed for his own therapy, the nature of the cultured cells involved, the general purposes of the test and the expected reaction. More recently, as our body of knowledge has increased and the course of reaction to the injections became predictable, we have simply explained that the procedure was a test which had nothing to do with treatment, that it involved the injection of foreign material, described the expected course of reaction, and that its purpose was to determine the rate at which the expected nodules would develop and then regress. In all instances in which the test was done the patients have readily given their consent, and the tests were not performed if such consent was not readily given. Unless the patient inquired, we refrained from describing the precise nature of the human cells (i.e., that they had originally been derived from tumors and then grown in tissue culture) for the reason that in my own professional judgment as well as that of my professional colleagues who had followed the course of these experiments, the precise nature of the foreign cells was irrelevant to the bodily reactions which could be expected to occur.

This course was followed, I submit, not out of any disregard for the rights or best interests of the patient nor of my responsibilities as a practitioner of medicine. It was a sincere professional judgment, based upon extensive scientific and clinical experience, that the procedures involved only the same low degree of risk inherent in many routine clinical test procedures, the patient in all such cases being informed only of the facts which are important from his standpoint. I submit that but for the highly emotion-charged term "cancer cells," this conclusion would be unquestioned by those in the medical profession who are fully cognizant of the present stage of knowledge with respect to immunological reactions.

Furthermore, in my own clinical judgment—based on fifteen years of clinical management of advanced cancer patients—to use the dreaded word "cancer" in connection with any clinical procedure on an ill person is potentially deleterious to that patient's well-being because it may suggest to him (rightly or wrongly) that his diagnosis is cancer or that his prognosis is poor. Some cancer patients do not know that their diagnosis is cancer, and even those who have been informed rarely discuss it and may even deny it. It is seldom possible for the physician to be fully cognizant of the cancer patient's extent of knowledge of and his attitude toward his disease. The doctor's choice of words in discussions with the patient has a great influence upon the patient's mental attitude. Since the initial neoplastic source of the test material employed was not germane to the reaction being studied and not, in my opinion, a cause of increased risk to the patient, I believe that such revelation is generally contraindicated in the best consideration of the patient's welfare and therefore to withhold such emotionally disturbing but medically nonpertinent details (unless requested by the patient) is in the best tradition of responsible clinical practice.

On these questions concerning procedure, I will readily submit to the judgment of my colleagues after they are fully informed.
[...]

[What follows is the court record of a patient at the Jewish Chronic Disease Hospital—eds.]

Sur-Reply Affidavit for Petitioner
Statements by Nathan Fink
[January 25, 1964]

[i] I, Mr. Nathan Fink, aged 73, make this statement, while a patient at the Brooklyn Chronic Disease Hospital.

Sometime in July or August of 1963, while a patient at the above hospital, two doctors visited me at my bedside and told me that I was to get an injection. This was supposedly a skin test, I was informed. They did not ask my approval nor consent.

A few days later, I detected a hardening under the top layer of my skin, in the area where I had previously been injected, my right thigh. This hardening enlarged about 2″ in length.

During the next six or seven weeks, I was visited by these two doctors, every second or third day, at which time, one would measure the area with a ruler, and the other one would make notations in a small book. I do not know the name of these two doctors but one of the doctors, the one who made the notations in the book, was a Filipino.

Within a period of seven weeks, the hardened area seemed to have subsided, and I was informed by the two doctors that I had a good resistance, and that the skin injection, performed upon me, had been successful.

After reading the most recent newspaper articles about the cancer injections performed on patients at this hospital, I now have reason to believe that I was one of the patients used as a guinea pig, in conjunction with this cancer experiment.

I again state that I was never given an opportunity by the doctors at this hospital to accept or refuse this injection, nor was I ever told what was the actual purpose of this experiment.

[February 1, 1964]
[ii] I recently submitted a statement regarding an injection which I was given while a patient at B.C.D. Hospital. In that statement, I advised that I believed that this injection was a cancer experiment and that I had never given any one my oral or written consent for this experiment.

I now wish to amend this statement previously submitted. About 1 month after the injection given me in July 1963, I was approached by the same 2 doctors, at which time they suggested that I sign a blank questionnaire.

I asked what this was all about and was informed that they intended to give me a new experimental pill to pep up my appetite. They further stated that my signature was necessary for them to administer this pill. Naturally, I signed this questionnaire because at this time I was actually suffering from lack of appetite.

I never was given this pill after they obtained my signature, although I asked about the pill on many occasions.

Now that I realize about the unauthorized injection given me in July 1963 and the subsequent signature taken from me, I have more reason to believe I was tricked into taking a cancer experiment with subsequent authorization.
[...]

[What follows is a news piece about this case from the journal *Science* as excerpted by Katz, Capron, and Swift. The full citation to this piece is Elinor Langer, "Human Experimentation: New York Verdict Affirms Patient's Rights," *Science* 151 (1966): 663–66.—eds.]

Human Experimentation: New York Verdict Affirms Patient's Rights
Elinor Langer
[1966—eds.]

[The] lawyers for Mandel and Southam raised two technical points of some interest. First, they claimed that, because "no clear-cut medical or professional standards were in force or were violated" by the two physicians, the attempt to find them guilty had an *ex post facto* quality. They also argued that the charges did not accurately fit the case. Testimony was introduced from well-known cancer and other professional researchers, including I. S. Ravdin, vice president for medical affairs of the University of Pennsylvania, and George E. Moore, director of Roswell Park Memorial Institute, to the effect that Southam's practices did not differ dramatically from those of other researchers. "If the whole profession is doing it," one of the lawyers remarked in an interview, "how can you call it 'unprofessional conduct'?" The lawyers also argued that the "fraud and deceit" charge was more appropriate to low-brow scoundrels, such as physicians who cheat on insurance, supply illegal narcotics, or practice medicine without a license, than to their respectable and well-intentioned clients.

To all arguments of humane motivations, extenuating circumstance, conflicting testimony, or legal ambiguities, the final answer of the Regents was very simple: It is no excuse. There was never any disagreement on the principle that patients should not be used in experiments unrelated to treatment unless they have given informed consent. But in the Regents' decision, two refinements of that principle are heavily stressed. The first is that it is the patient, and not the physician, who has the right to decide what factors are or are not relevant to his consent, regardless of the rationality of his assessment. "Any fact which might influence the giving or withholding of consent is material," the Regents said. . . .

The second principle stressed by the Regents is that the physician, when he is acting as experimenter, has no claim to the doctor-patient relationship that, in a therapeutic situation, would give him the generally acknowledged right to withhold information if he judged it in the best interest of the patient. In the absence of a doctor-patient relationship, the Regents said, "there is no basis for the exercise of their usual professional judgment applicable to patient care." Southam, in an interview, disagreed. "An experimental relation has some elements of a therapeutic relationship," he said last week. "The patients still think of you as a doctor, and I react to them as a doctor, and want to avoid frightening them unnecessarily." Mandel takes a similar position. In a letter to the editor of a medical affairs newspaper he stated: "In accordance with the age-old motto—primum non nocere—it would seem that consideration of the patient's well-being may, at times, supersede the requirement for disclosure of facts if such facts lack pertinence and may cause psychologic harm." But on this point, the Regents are clear: "No person can be said to have volunteered for an experiment unless he had first understood what he was volunteering for. Any matter which might influence him in giving or withholding his consent is material. Deliberate nondisclosure of the material fact is no different from deliberate misrepresentation of such a fact."

In closing their case, and acknowledging that the penalties imposed were severe—they might have just authorized a censure and reprimand—the Regents were pointed and succinct: "We trust that this measure of discipline will serve as a stern warning that zeal for research must not be carried to the point where it violates the basic rights and immunities of a human person."

What the impact of the case will be is by no means clear. The Regents' decision outlines clear rules for a very narrow situation and attempts to set out some broad principles as well. But it is by no means binding, and it by no means covers the variety of situations with which researchers seeking to use human subjects are faced. The question is, What will cover these situations? Codes and declarations, of which there are already several, are too general to offer specific guidance. Researchers and patients alike are too vulnerable to await a slow case-by-case accretion of specific rulings. One alternative is the development within each hospital or research institution of "ethical review committees" that could define the consent-and-disclosure requirements for each proposed experiment and see that they were adhered to. In theory, this is already taking place. During the Southam-Mandel hearings, the state attempted to prove that Southam, a recipient of a National Institutes of Health [NIH] grant, had violated regulations of the Public Health Service [PHS]. In fact, the regulations in question govern only the normal volunteer program of the NIH Clinical Center in Bethesda. The PHS response to an inquiry from New York's Attorney General made clear that the rules were not generally applicable and stated that, "in supporting extramural clinical investigations, it is the position of the Public Health Service that proper ethical and moral standards are more effectively safeguarded by the processes of review and criticism by an investigator's peers than by regulation."

That is the theory, but the trouble is it is not yet being done. And, given the tremendous growth and variety of medical research involving human beings, if it is not done by the scientific community, someone else will start to do it. The New York Regents may be only the beginning. [End of news piece—eds.]

3   Ethics and Clinical Research

HENRY K. BEECHER

Human experimentation since World War II has created some difficult problems with the increasing employment of patients as experimental subjects when it must be apparent that they would not have been available if they had been truly aware of the uses that would be made of them. Evidence is at hand that many of the patients in the examples to follow never had the risk satisfactorily explained to them, and it seems obvious that further hundreds have not known that they were the subjects of an experiment although grave consequences have been suffered as a direct result of experiments described here. There is a belief prevalent in some sophisticated circles that attention to these matters would "block progress." But, according to Pope Pius XII, ". . . science is not the highest value to which all other orders of values . . . should be subordinated."

I am aware that these are troubling charges. They have grown out of troubling practices. They can be documented, as I propose to do, by examples from leading medical schools, university hospitals, private hospitals, governmental military departments (the Army, the Navy, and the Air Force), governmental institutes (the NIH), Veterans Administration hospitals, and industry. The basis for the charges is broad.

I should like to affirm that American medicine is sound, and most progress in it soundly attained. There is, however, a reason for concern in certain areas, and I believe that the type of activities to be mentioned will do great harm to medicine unless soon corrected. It will certainly be charged that any mention of these matters does a disservice to medicine, but not one so great, I believe, as a continuation of the practices to be cited.

Experimentation in man takes place in several areas: in self-experimentation; in patient volunteers and normal subjects; in therapy; and in the different areas of *experimentation on a patient not for his benefit but for that, at least in theory, of patients in general.* The present study is limited to this last category. [. . .]

EXAMPLES OF UNETHICAL OR QUESTIONABLY ETHICAL STUDIES

These examples are not cited for the condemnation of individuals; they are recorded to call attention to a variety of

Henry K. Beecher, "Ethics and Clinical Research," *New England Journal of Medicine* 274 (1966): 1354–60.

ethical problems found in experimental medicine, for it is hoped that calling attention to them will help to correct abuses present. During ten years of study of these matters it has become apparent that thoughtlessness and carelessness, not a willful disregard of the patient's rights, account for most of the cases encountered. Nonetheless, it is evident that in many of the examples presented, the investigators have risked the health or the life of their subjects. No attempt has been made to present the "worst" possible examples; rather, the aim has been to show the variety of problems encountered. [. . .]

[Beecher discusses 22 examples, shortened from his original list of 50, all of which are included below.—eds.]

Known Effective Treatment Withheld

Example 1. It is known that rheumatic fever can usually be prevented by adequate treatment of streptococcal respiratory infections by the parenteral administration of penicillin. Nevertheless, definitive treatment was withheld, and placebos were given to a group of 109 men in service, while benzathine penicillin G was given to others.

The therapy that each patient received was determined automatically by his military serial number arranged so that more men received penicillin than received placebo. In the small group of patients studied 2 cases of acute rheumatic fever and 1 of acute nephritis developed in the control patients, whereas these complications did not occur among those who received the benzathine penicillin G.

Example 2. The sulfonamides were for many years the only antibacterial drugs effective in shortening the duration of acute streptococcal pharyngitis and in reducing its suppurative complications. The investigators in this study undertook to determine if the occurrence of the serious nonsuppurative complications, rheumatic fever and acute glomerulonephritis, would be reduced by this treatment. This study was made despite the general experience that certain antibiotics, including penicillin, will prevent the development of rheumatic fever.

The subjects were a large group of hospital patients; a control group of approximately the same size, also with exudative Group A streptococcus, was included. The latter group received only nonspecific therapy (no sulfadiazine). The total group denied the effective penicillin comprised over 500 men.

Rheumatic fever was diagnosed in 5.4 per cent of those treated with sulfadiazine. In the control group rheumatic fever developed in 4.2 per cent.

In reference to this study a medical officer stated in writing that the subjects were not informed, did not consent and were not aware that they had been involved in an experiment, and yet admittedly 25 acquired rheumatic fever. According to this same medical officer *more than 70 who had had known definitive treatment withheld* were on the wards with rheumatic fever when he was there.

Example 3. This involved a study of the relapse rate in typhoid fever treated in two ways. In an earlier study by the present investigators chloramphenicol had been recognized as an effective treatment for typhoid fever, being attended by half the mortality that was experienced when this agent was not used. Others had made the same observations, indicating that to withhold this effective remedy can be a life-or-death decision. The present study was carried out to determine the relapse rate under the two methods of treatment; of 408 charity patients 251 were treated with chloramphenicol, of whom 20, or 7.97 per cent, died. Symptomatic treatment was given, but chloramphenicol was withheld in 157, of whom 36, or 22.9 per cent, died. According to the data presented, 23 patients died in the course of this study who would not have been expected to succumb if they had received specific therapy.

Study of Therapy

Example 4. TriA (triacetyloleandomycin) was originally introduced for the treatment of infection with gram-positive organisms. Spotty evidence of hepatic dysfunction emerged, especially in children, and so the present study was undertaken on 50 patients, including mental defectives or juvenile delinquents who were inmates of a children's center. No disease other than acne was present; the drug was given for treatment of this. The ages of the subjects ranged from thirteen to thirty-nine years. "By the time half the patients had received the drug for four weeks, the high incidence of significant hepatic dysfunction . . . led to the discontinuation of administration to the remainder of the group at three weeks." [. . .] Eight patients with marked hepatic dysfunction were transferred to the hospital "for more intensive study." Liver biopsy was carried out in these 8 patients and repeated in 4 of them. Liver damage was evident. Four of these hospitalized patients, after their liver-function tests returned to normal limits, received a "challenge" dose of the drug. Within two days hepatic dysfunction was evident in 3 of the 4 patients. In 1 patient a second challenge dose was given after the first challenge and again led to evidence of abnormal liver function. Flocculation tests remained abnormal in some patients as long as five weeks after discontinuance of the drug.

Physiologic Studies

Example 5. In this controlled, double-blind study of the hematologic toxicity of chloramphenicol it was recognized that chloramphenicol is "well known as a cause of aplastic anemia" and that there is a "prolonged morbidity and high mortality of aplastic anemia" and that ". . . chloramphenicol-induced aplastic anemia can be related to dose . . . ." The aim of the study was "further definition of the toxicology of the drug. . . ."

Forty-one randomly chosen patients were given either 2 or 6 gm. of chloramphenicol per day; 12 control patients were used. "Toxic bone-marrow depression, predominantly affecting erythropoiesis, developed in 2 of 20 patients given 2.0 gm. and in 18 of 21 given 6 gm. of chloramphenicol daily." The smaller dose is recommended for routine use.

Example 6. In a study of the effect of thymectomy on the survival of skin homografts, 18 children, three and a half months to eighteen years of age, about to undergo surgery for congenital heart disease, were selected. Eleven were to have total thymectomy as part of the operation, and 7 were to serve as controls. As part of the experiment, full-thickness skin homografts from an unrelated adult donor were sutured to the chest wall in each case. (Total thymectomy is occasionally, although not usually, part of the primary cardiovascular surgery involved, and whereas it may not greatly add to the hazards of the necessary operation, its eventual effects in children are not known.) This work was proposed as part of a long-range study of "the growth and development of these children over the years." No difference in the survival of the skin homograft was observed in the 2 groups.

Example 7. This study of cyclopropane anesthesia and cardiac arrhythmias consisted of 31 patients. The average duration of the study was three hours, ranging from two to four and a half hours. "Minor surgical procedures" were carried out in all but 1 subject. Moderate to deep anesthesia, with endotracheal intubation and controlled respiration, was used. Carbon dioxide was injected into the closed respiratory system until cardiac arrhythmias appeared. Toxic levels of carbon dioxide were achieved and maintained for considerable periods. During the cyclopropane anesthesia a variety of pathologic cardiac arrhythmias occurred. When the carbon dioxide tension was elevated above normal, ventricular extrasystoles were more numerous than when the carbon dioxide tension was normal, ventricular arrhythmias being continuous in 1 subject for ninety minutes. (This can lead to fatal fibrillation.)

Example 8. Since the minimum blood-flow requirements of the cerebral circulation are not accurately known, this study was carried out to determine "cerebral hemodynamic and metabolic changes . . . before and during acute reductions in arterial pressure induced by drug administration and/or postural adjustments." Forty-four patients whose ages varied from the second to the tenth decade were involved. They included normotensive subjects, those with essential hypertension, and finally a group with malignant hypertension. Fifteen had abnormal electrocardiograms. Few details about the reasons for hospitalization are given.

Signs of cerebral circulatory insufficiency, which were easily recognized, included confusion and in some cases a nonresponsive state. By alteration in the tilt of the patient "the clinical state of the subject could be changed in a matter of seconds from one of alertness to confusion, and for the remainder of the flow, the subject was maintained in the latter state." The femoral arteries were cannulated in all subjects, and the internal jugular veins in 14.

The mean arterial pressure fell in 37 subjects from 109 to 48 mm. of mercury, with signs of cerebral ischemia. "With the onset of collapse, cardiac output and right ventricular pressures decreased sharply."

Since signs of cerebral insufficiency developed without evidence of coronary insufficiency the authors concluded that "the brain may be more sensitive to acute hypotension than is the heart."

Example 9. This is a study of the adverse circulatory responses elicited by intra-abdominal maneuvers:

> When the peritoneal cavity was entered, a deliberate series of maneuvers was carried out [in 68 patients] to ascertain the effective stimuli and the areas responsible for development of the expected circulatory changes. Accordingly, the surgeon rubbed localized areas of the parietal and visceral peritoneum with a small ball sponge as discretely as possible. Traction on the mesenteries, pressure in the area of the celiac plexus, traction on the gallbladder and stomach, and occlusion of the portal and caval veins were the other stimuli applied.

Thirty-four of the patients were sixty years of age or older; 11 were seventy or older. In 44 patients the hypotension produced by the deliberate stimulation was "moderate to marked." The maximum fall produced by manipulation was from 200 systolic, 105 diastolic, to 42 systolic, 20 diastolic; the average fall in mean pressure in 26 patients was 53 mm. of mercury.

Of the 50 patients studied, 17 showed either atrioventricular dissociation with nodal rhythm or nodal rhythm alone. A decrease in the amplitude of the T wave and elevation or depression of the ST segment were noted in 25 cases in association with manipulation and hypoten-

sion or, at other times, in the course of anesthesia and operation. In only 1 case was the change pronounced enough to suggest myocardial ischemia. No case of myocardial infarction was noted in the group studied, although routine electrocardiograms were not taken after operation to detect silent infarcts. Two cases in which electrocardiograms were taken after operation showed T-wave and ST-segment changes that had not been present before.

These authors refer to a similar study in which more alarming electrocardiographic changes were observed. Four patients in the series sustained silent myocardial infarctions; most of their patients were undergoing gallbladder surgery because of associated heart disease. It can be added further that in the 34 patients referred to above as being sixty years of age or older, some doubtless had heart disease that could have made risky the maneuvers carried out. In any event, this possibility might have been a deterrent.

Example 10. Starling's law—"that the heart output per beat is directly proportional to the diastolic filling"—was studied in 30 adult patients with atrial fibrillation and mitral stenosis sufficiently severe to require valvulotomy. "Continuous alterations of the length of a segment of left ventricular muscle were recorded simultaneously in 13 of these patients by means of a mercury-filled resistance gauge sutured to the surface of the left ventricle." Pressures in the left ventricle were determined by direct puncture simultaneously with the segment length in 13 patients and without the segment length in an additional 13 patients. Four similar unanesthetized patients were studied through catheterization of the left side of the heart transeptally. In all 30 patients arterial pressure was measured through the catheterized brachial artery.

Example 11. To study the sequence of ventricular contraction in human bundle-branch block, simultaneous catheterization of both ventricles was performed in 22 subjects; catheterization of the right side of the heart was carried out in the usual manner; the left side was catheterized transbronchially. Extrasystoles were produced by tapping on the epicardium in subjects with normal myocardium while they were undergoing thoracotomy. Simultaneous pressures were measured in both ventricles through needle puncture in this group. [. . .]

Example 12. This investigation was carried out to examine the possible effect of vagal stimulation on cardiac arrest. The authors had in recent years transected the homolateral vagus nerve immediately below the origin of the recurrent laryngeal nerve as palliation against cough and pain in bronchogenic carcinoma. Having been impressed with the number of reports of cardiac arrest that seemed to follow vagal stimulation, they tested the effects of intrathoracic vagal stimulation during 30 of their surgical procedures, concluding, from these observations in patients under satisfactory anesthesia, that cardiac irregularities and cardiac arrest due to vagovagal reflex were less common than had previously been supposed.

Example 13. This study presented a technique for determining portal circulation time and hepatic blood flow. It involved the transcutaneous injection of the spleen and catheterization of the hepatic vein. This was carried out in 43 subjects, of whom 14 were normal; 16 had cirrhosis (varying degrees), 9 acute hepatitis, and 4 hemolytic anemia.

No mention is made of what information was divulged to the subjects, some of whom were seriously ill. This study consisted in the development of a technique, not of therapy, in the 14 normal subjects.

Studies to Improve the Understanding of Disease

Example 14. In this study of the syndrome of impending hepatic coma in patients with cirrhosis of the liver certain nitrogenous substances were administered to 9 patients with chronic alcoholism and advanced cirrhosis: ammonium chloride, di-ammonium citrate, urea, or dietary protein. In all patients a reaction that included mental disturbances, a "flapping tremor," and electroencephalographic changes developed. Similar signs had occurred in only 1 of the patients before these substances were administered:

> The first sign noted was usually clouding of
> the consciousness. Three patients had a second or a third course of administration of a
> nitrogenous substance with the same results.
> It was concluded that marked resemblance
> between this reaction and impending hepatic
> coma, implied that the administration of
> these [nitrogenous] substances to patients
> with cirrhosis may be hazardous.

Example 15. The relation of the effects of ingested ammonia to liver disease was investigated in 11 with cirrhosis, and 8 miscellaneous patients. Ten of these patients had neurologic changes associated with either hepatitis or cirrhosis.

The hepatic and renal veins were cannulated. Ammonium chloride was administered by mouth. After this, a tremor that lasted for three days developed in 1 patient. When ammonium chloride was ingested by 4 cirrhotic patients with tremor and mental confusion the symptoms were exaggerated during the test. The same thing was true of a fifth patient in another group.

Example 16. This study was directed toward determining the period of infectivity of infectious hepatitis. Artificial induction of hepatitis was carried out in an institution for mentally defective children in which a mild form of hepa-

titis was endemic. The parents gave consent for the intramuscular injection or oral administration of the virus, but nothing is said regarding what was told them concerning appreciable hazards involved. [Example 16 is the Willowbrook case.—eds.]

Example 17. Live cancer cells were injected into 22 human subjects as part of a study of immunity to cancer. According to a recent review, the subjects (hospitalized patients) were "merely told they would be receiving 'some cells'"—". . . the word cancer was entirely omitted. . . ." [Example 17 is the Jewish Chronic Disease Hospital Case, a discussion of which is included in this volume.—eds.]

Example 18. Melanoma was transplanted from a daughter to her volunteering and informed mother, "in the hope of gaining a little better understanding of cancer immunity and in the hope that the production of tumor antibodies might be helpful in the treatment of the cancer patient." Since the daughter died on the day after the transplantation of the tumor into her mother, the hope expressed seems to have been more theoretical than practical, and the daughter's condition was described as "terminal" at the time the mother volunteered to be a recipient. The primary implant was widely excised on the twenty-fourth day after it had been placed in the mother. She died from metastatic melanoma on the four hundred and fifty-first day after transplantation. The evidence that this patient died of diffuse melanoma that metastasized from a small piece of transplanted tumor was considered conclusive.

Technical Study of Disease

Example 19. During bronchoscopy a special needle was inserted through a bronchus into the left atrium of the heart. This was done in an unspecified number of subjects, both with cardiac disease and with normal hearts.

The technique was a new approach whose hazards were at the beginning quite unknown. The subjects with normal hearts were used, not for their possible benefit but for that of patients in general.

Example 20. The percutaneous method of catheterization of the left side of the heart has, it is reported, led to 8 deaths (1.09 per cent death rate) and other serious accidents in 732 cases. There was, therefore, need for another method, the transbronchial approach, which was carried out in the present study in more than 500 cases, with no deaths.

Granted that a delicate problem arises regarding how much should be discussed with the patients involved in the use of a new method, nevertheless where the method is employed in a given patient for *his* benefit, the ethical problems are far less than when this potentially extremely dangerous method is used "in 15 patients with normal hearts, undergoing bronchoscopy for other reasons." Nothing was said about what was told any of the subjects, and nothing was said about the granting of permission, which was certainly indicated in the 15 normal subjects used.

Example 21. This was a study of the effect of exercise on cardiac output and pulmonary-artery pressure in 8 "normal" persons (that is, patients whose diseases were not related to the cardiovascular system), in 8 with congestive heart failure severe enough to have recently required complete bed rest, in 6 with hypertension, in 2 with aortic insufficiency, in 7 with mitral stenosis, and in 5 with pulmonary emphysema.

Intracardiac catheterization was carried out, and the catheter then inserted into the right or left main branch of the pulmonary artery. The brachial artery was usually catheterized; sometimes, the radial or femoral arteries were catheterized. The subjects exercised in a supine position by pushing their feet against weighted pedals. "The ability of these patients to carry on sustained work was severely limited by weakness and dyspnea." Several were in severe failure. This was not a therapeutic attempt but rather a physiologic study.

Bizarre Study

Example 22. There is a question whether ureteral reflux can occur in the normal bladder. With this in mind, vesi- courethrography was carried out on 26 normal babies less than forty-eight hours old. The infants were exposed to x-rays while the bladder was filling and during voiding. Multiple spot films were made to record the presence or absence of ureteral reflux. None was found in this group, and fortunately no infection followed the catheterization. What the results of the extensive x-ray exposure may be, no one can yet say. [...]

SUMMARY AND CONCLUSIONS

The ethical approach to experimentation in man has several components; two are more important than the others, the first being informed consent. [...] Secondly, there is the more reliable safeguard provided by the presence of an intelligent, informed, conscientious, compassionate, responsible investigator.

Ordinary patients will not knowingly risk their health or their life for the sake of "science." [...] When such risks are taken and a considerable number of patients are involved, it may be assumed that informed consent has not been obtained in all cases.

The gain anticipated from an experiment must be commensurate with the risk involved. An experiment is ethical or not at its inception; it does not become ethical *post hoc*—ends do not justify means. There is no ethical distinction between ends and means. [...]

---

4   Racism and Research

The Case of the Tuskegee Syphilis Study

ALLAN M. BRANDT

In 1932 the U.S. Public Health Service (USPHS) initiated an experiment in Macon County, Alabama, to determine the natural course of untreated, latent syphilis in black males. The test comprised 400 syphilitic men, as well as 200 uninfected men who served as controls. The first published report of the study appeared in 1936 with subsequent papers issued every four to six years, through the 1960s. When

Allan M. Brandt, "Racism and Research: The Case of the Tuskegee Syphilis Study," *Hastings Center Report* 8, no. 6 (1978): 21–29.

penicillin became widely available by the early 1950s as the preferred treatment for syphilis, the men did not receive therapy. In fact on several occasions, the USPHS actually sought to prevent treatment. Moreover, a committee at the federally operated Center for Disease Control decided in 1969 that the study should be continued. Only in 1972, when accounts of the study first appeared in the national press, did the Department of Health, Education and Welfare [DHEW, hereafter HEW] halt the experiment. [The DHEW is now the Department of Health and Human Services or DHHS.—eds.] At that time seventy-four of the test subjects were still alive; at least twenty-eight, but perhaps more than 100, had died directly from advanced syphilitic lesions. [...]

THE ORIGINS OF THE EXPERIMENT

In 1929, under a grant from the Julius Rosenwald Fund, the USPHS conducted studies in the rural South to determine the prevalence of syphilis among blacks and explore the possibilities for mass treatment. The USPHS found Macon County, Alabama, in which the town of Tuskegee is located, to have the highest syphilis rate of the six counties surveyed. The Rosenwald Study concluded that mass treatment could be successfully implemented among rural blacks. Although it is doubtful that the necessary funds would have been allocated even in the best economic conditions, after the economy collapsed in 1929, the findings were ignored. It is, however, ironic that the Tuskegee Study came to be based on findings of the Rosenwald Study that demonstrated the possibilities of mass treatment.

Three years later, in 1932, Dr. Taliaferro Clark, Chief of the USPHS Venereal Disease Division and author of the Rosenwald Study report, decided that conditions in Macon County merited renewed attention. Clark believed the high prevalence of syphilis offered an "unusual opportunity" for observation. From its inception, the USPHS regarded the Tuskegee Study as a classic "study in nature," rather than an experiment. As long as syphilis was so prevalent in Macon and most of the blacks went untreated throughout life, it seemed only natural to Clark that it would be valuable to observe the consequences. He described it as a "ready-made situation." Surgeon General H. S. Cumming wrote to R. R. Moton, Director of the Tuskegee Institute:

> The recent syphilis control demonstration carried out in Macon County, with the financial assistance of the Julius Rosenwald Fund, revealed the presence of an unusually high rate in this county and, what is more remarkable, the fact that 99 per cent of this group was entirely without previous treatment. This combination, together with the expected cooperation of your hospital, offers an unparalleled opportunity for carrying on this piece of scientific research which probably cannot be duplicated anywhere else in the world.

Although no formal protocol appears to have been written, several letters of Clark and Cumming suggest what the USPHS hoped to find. Clark indicated that it would be important to see how disease affected the daily lives of the men:

> The results of these studies of case records suggest the desirability of making a further study of the effect of untreated syphilis on the human economy among people now living and engaged in their daily pursuits.

It also seems that the USPHS believed the experiment might demonstrate that antisyphilitic treatment was unnecessary. As Cumming noted: "It is expected the results of this study may have a marked bearing on the treatment, or conversely the non-necessity of treatment, of cases of latent syphilis."

The immediate source of Cumming's hypothesis appears to have been the famous Oslo Study of untreated syphilis. Between 1890 and 1910, Professor C. Boeck, the chief of the Oslo Venereal Clinic, withheld treatment from almost two thousand patients infected with syphilis. He was convinced that therapies then available, primarily mercurial ointment, were of no value. When arsenic therapy became widely available by 1910, after Paul Ehrlich's historic discovery of "606," the study was abandoned. E. Bruusgaard, Boeck's successor, conducted a follow-up study of 473 of the untreated patients from 1925 to 1927. He found that 27.9 percent of these patients had undergone a "spontaneous cure," and now manifested no symptoms of the disease. Moreover, he estimated that as many as 70 percent of all syphilitics went through life without inconvenience from the disease. His study, however, clearly acknowledged the dangers of untreated syphilis for the remaining 30 percent.

Thus every major textbook of syphilis at the time of the Tuskegee Study's inception strongly advocated treating syphilis even in its latent stages, which follow the initial inflammatory reaction. In discussing the Oslo Study, Dr. J. E. Moore, one of the nation's leading venereologists wrote, "This summary of Bruusgaard's study is by no means intended to suggest that syphilis be allowed to pass untreated." If a complete cure could not be effected, at least the most devastating effects of the disease could be avoided. Although the standard therapies of the time, arsenical compounds and bismuth injection, involved certain dangers because of their toxicity, the alternatives were much worse. As the Oslo Study had shown, untreated syphilis could lead to cardiovascular disease, insanity, and premature death. [...] "Another compelling reason for treatment," noted Moore, "exists in the fact that every patient with latent syphilis may be, and perhaps is, infectious for others." In 1932, the year in which the Tuskegee Study began, the USPHS sponsored and published a paper by Moore and six other syphilis experts that strongly argued for treating latent syphilis.

The Oslo Study, therefore, could not have provided justification for the USPHS to undertake a study that did not entail treatment. Rather, the suppositions that conditions in Tuskegee existed "naturally" and that the men would not be treated anyway provided the experiment's rationale. In turn, these two assumptions rested on the prevailing medical attitudes concerning blacks, sex, and disease. For example, Clark explained the prevalence of venereal disease in Macon County by emphasizing the promiscuity among blacks:

> This state of affairs is due to the paucity of doctors, rather low intelligence of the Negro population in this section, depressed economic conditions, and the very common promiscuous sex relations of this population group which not only contribute to the spread of syphilis but also contribute to the prevailing indifference with regard to treatment.

In fact, Moore, who had written so persuasively in favor of treating latent syphilis, suggested that existing knowledge did not apply to Negroes. Although he called the Oslo Study "a never-to-be-repeated human experiment," he served as an expert consultant to the Tuskegee Study:

> I think that such a study as you have contemplated would be of immense value. It will be necessary of course in the consideration of the results to evaluate the special factor introduced by a selection of the material from negro males. Syphilis in the negro is in many respects almost a different disease from syphilis in the white.

Dr. O. C. Wenger, chief of the federally operated venereal disease clinic at Hot Springs, Arkansas, praised Moore's judgment, adding, "This study will emphasize those differences." On another occasion he advised Clark, "We must remember we are dealing with a group of people who are illiterate, have no conception of time, and whose personal history is always indefinite."

The doctors who devised and directed the Tuskegee Study accepted the mainstream assumption regarding blacks and venereal disease. The premise that blacks, promiscuous and lustful, would not seek or continue treatment, shaped the study. A test of untreated syphilis seemed "natural" because the USPHS presumed the men would never be treated; the Tuskegee Study made that a self-fulfilling prophecy. [. . .]

THE HEW FINAL REPORT

The HEW finally formed the Tuskegee Syphilis Study Ad Hoc Advisory Panel on August 28, 1972, in response to criticism that the press descriptions of the experiment had triggered. The panel, composed of nine members, five of them black, concentrated on two issues. First, was the study justified in 1932 and had the men given their informed consent? Second, should penicillin have been provided when it became available in the early 1950s? The panel was also charged with determining if the study should be terminated and assessing current policies regarding experimentation with human subjects. The group issued their report in June 1973.

By focusing on the issues of penicillin therapy and informed consent, the *Final Report* and the investigation betrayed a basic misunderstanding of the experiment's purposes and design. The HEW report implied that the failure to provide penicillin constituted the study's major ethical misjudgment; implicit was the assumption that no adequate therapy existed prior to penicillin. Nonetheless medical authorities firmly believed in the efficacy of arsenotherapy for treating syphilis at the time of the experiment's inception in 1932. The panel further failed to recognize that the entire study had been predicated on nontreatment. Provision of effective medication would have violated the rationale of the experiment—to study the natural course of the disease until death. On several occasions, in fact, the USPHS had prevented the men from receiving proper treatment. Indeed, there is no evidence that the USPHS ever considered providing penicillin.

The other focus of the *Final Report*—informed consent—also served to obscure the historical facts of the experiment. In light of the deceptions and exploitations which the experiment perpetrated, it is an understatement to declare, as the *Report* did, that the experiment was "ethically unjustified," because it failed to obtain informed consent from the subjects. The *Final Report*'s statement, "Submitting voluntarily is not informed consent," indicated that the panel believed that the men had volunteered *for the experiment*. The records in the National Archives make clear that the men did not submit voluntarily to an experiment; they were told and they believed that they were getting free treatment from expert government doctors for a serious disease. The failure of the HEW *Final Report* to expose this critical fact—that the USPHS lied to the subjects—calls into question the thoroughness and credibility of their investigation.

Failure to place the study in a historical context also made it impossible for the investigation to deal with the essentially racist nature of the experiment. The panel treated the study as an aberration, well-intentioned but misguided. Moreover, concern that the *Final Report* might be viewed as a critique of human experimentation in general seems to have severely limited the scope of the inquiry. The *Final Report* is quick to remind the reader on two occasions: "The position of the Panel must not be construed to be a general repudiation of scientific research with human subjects." The *Report* assures us that a better designed experiment could have been justified:

> It is possible that a scientific study in 1932 of untreated syphilis, properly conceived with a clear protocol and conducted with suitable

subjects who fully understood the implications of their involvement, might have been justified in the pre-penicillin era. This is especially true when one considers the uncertain nature of the results of treatment of late latent syphilis and the highly toxic nature of therapeutic agents then available.

This statement is questionable in view of the proven dangers of untreated syphilis known in 1932.

Since the publication of the HEW *Final Report,* a defense of the Tuskegee Study has emerged. These arguments, most clearly articulated by Dr. R. H. Kampmeier in the *Southern Medical Journal,* center on the limited knowledge of effective therapy for latent syphilis when the experiment began. Kampmeier argues that by 1950, penicillin would have been of no value for these men. Others have suggested that the men were fortunate to have been spared the highly toxic treatments of the earlier period. Moreover, even these contemporary defenses assume that the men never would have been treated anyway. As Dr. Charles Barnett of Stanford University wrote in 1974, "The lack of treatment was not contrived by the USPHS but was an established fact of which they proposed to take advantage." Several doctors who participated in the study continued to justify the experiment. Dr. J. R. Heller, who on one occasion had referred to the test subjects as the "Ethiopian population," told reporters in 1972:

> I don't see why they should be shocked or horrified. There was no racial side to this. It just happened to be in a black community. I feel this was a perfectly straightforward study, perfectly ethical, with controls. Part of our mission as physicians is to find out what happens to individuals with disease and without disease.

These apologies, as well as the HEW *Final Report,* ignore many of the essential ethical issues which the study poses. The Tuskegee Study reveals the persistence of beliefs within the medical profession about the nature of blacks, sex, and disease—beliefs that had tragic repercussions long after their alleged "scientific" bases were known to be incorrect. Most strikingly, the entire health of a community was jeopardized by leaving a communicable disease untreated. There can be little doubt that the Tuskegee researchers regarded their subjects as less than human. As a result, the ethical canons of experimenting on human subjects were completely disregarded.

The study also raises significant questions about professional self-regulation and scientific bureaucracy. Once the USPHS decided to extend the experiment in the summer of 1933, it was unlikely that the test would be halted short of the men's deaths. The experiment was widely reported for forty years without evoking any significant protest within the medical community. Nor did any bureaucratic mechanism exist within the government for the periodic reassessment of the Tuskegee experiment's ethics and scientific value. The USPHS sent physicians to Tuskegee every several years to check on the study's progress, but never subjected the morality or usefulness of the experiment to serious scrutiny. Only the press accounts of 1972 finally punctured the continued rationalizations of the USPHS and brought the study to an end. [. . .]

In retrospect the Tuskegee Study revealed more about the pathology of racism than it did about the pathology of syphilis; more about the nature of scientific inquiry than the nature of the disease process. The injustice committed by the experiment went well beyond the facts outlined in the press and the HEW *Final Report.* The degree of deception and damages have been seriously underestimated. As this history of the study suggests, the notion that science is a value-free discipline must be rejected. The need for greater vigilance in assessing the specific ways in which social values and attitudes affect professional behavior is clearly indicated.

Part II

Ethical and Regulatory Guidance for Research with Humans

Virtually every period of scandal in research involving humans has been followed by attempts to codify the rules that should govern such research. In Part II we include some of the most influential documents intended to guide the ethical conduct of research with humans. Although in a legal context documents are generally taken as "speaking for themselves," in fact all such writings require interpretation, especially as they are to be applied to particular cases. Many of these documents do not, in fact, have legal authority but are instead guidelines that have been adopted by various national and international bodies. Certain themes, such as participant consent and the necessity of well-designed research, have emerged since the appearance of the first of these codes, the Nuremberg Code, which was written as part of the Nuremberg doctors trial decision. However, these documents do not always speak with one voice about the way that these themes should be weighed in a moral analysis. As we shall see, some endorse the necessity of research with humans as a vital way to advance medical knowledge and ability. Others express more concern about individual participants and enumerate the many kinds of protections that should be afforded them.

What is known to posterity as the Nuremberg Code was actually the third section of the judges' decision at the Nuremberg trials following World War II. With the input of their physician advisors, Leo Alexander[1] and Andrew C. Ivy,[2] the Nuremberg judges specified ten conditions that have today become familiar, beginning with a ringing phrase, "The voluntary consent of the human subject is absolutely essential." With consent as its foundation, the code then provides an uncompromising analysis of thoroughgoing voluntariness, along with the ultimate responsibility of the experimenter. No less important are subsequent ethical requirements of the code that cannot be satisfied by consent alone. These include the importance of the scientific problem being investigated; the careful design of the study; the avoidance of death, suffering, or injury; the need to assess risk; the preparedness of the investigator to do the work; and the right of the participant to withdraw at any time.

On the whole, the Nuremberg Code remains a cogent statement of the main points of research ethics, but in practice it has exerted less influence than it might have, in spite of its routine rhetorical invocation.[3] The Nuremberg court did not provide for any interpretive or enforcement mechanism. More important, the code itself seems to prohibit many aspects of medical research that seem ethically acceptable because of its unqualified demand for voluntary consent, which prohibits almost all of pediatric, psychiatric, and emergency research. Matters were not helped by the fact that the code was drafted following a trial that stemmed from extraordinary circumstances. It was easy for critics of external interference with the medical profession to see the code as a reaction to extreme evil rather than as a guide for clinical research with humans. That is, what the Nazi doctors had done was so abhorrent that some in the medical profession were convinced that good doctors would never do such things and that therefore the code was not necessary. Nor was the code a basis for the judgment of the doctors' trial itself. The Nazi officials who were convicted in the doctors' trial were not judged based on the code, which would have been an instance of ex post facto justice. Nonetheless, it is apparent that the judges were sufficiently convinced by the Nazis' defense lawyers of the lack of ethical conventions to guide human experiments that they determined to put their ten precepts for research on record.

There has been scholarly controversy about the precise origins of and inspiration for the Nuremberg

Code, as well as its intended scope.[4] It would appear that a memorandum prepared by one of the court's expert medical consultants, Leo Alexander, was an important source of the code. An expert witness for the prosecution who represented the American Medical Association, Andrew C. Ivy, also influenced the final document. One element of Alexander's memorandum that did not find its way into the code was a paragraph that singled out mentally ill patients for receipt of additional consent from their next of kin or legal guardian. Alexander later speculated that his recommended passage was excluded because it did not apply to the cases at trial. One consequence of this omission is that, although the values expressed in the code may fairly be said to apply generally to all research participants, the only specific population to whom the code was clearly seen to apply was adult prisoners.

While the Nuremberg Code left little avenue for research involving those who could not give consent for themselves, the perceived necessity of including participants such as these, including children and those with mental illness, appears to have been one of the motivations for the World Medical Association's (WMA's) initial deliberations in 1953 on its own research ethics guidelines. This process culminated in the drafting of the WMA's 1964 Declaration of Helsinki. However, long before the declaration itself was written, in 1954, the WMA adopted a resolution that required consent by an ill participant or the person's next of kin, and "informed, free consent" in the case of healthy participants. This statement on consent was the fourth of five propositions stated in the resolution, the first three addressing the qualifications, prudence, and responsibility of the researcher, as well as respect for the individual. The last statement of the resolution confined "daring" procedures to "desperate cases."

As foreshadowed in the 1954 resolution, the 1964 Declaration of Helsinki (generally referred to as Helsinki I) allows for the sufficiency of a legal guardian's consent when a participant is unable to provide consent. The introduction of a role for a surrogate decisionmaker was a significant departure from the Nuremberg Code, which seemed to rule out, or at least did not allude to, any such indirect consent. Adding this measure was surely an effort by the WMA to establish a set of guidelines that would conform to the reality of clinical research, one that often involves the very young, those with dementia, or those in psychiatric care.

Another important difference between the Nuremberg Code and Helsinki I was the latter's distinction between therapeutic research and "nontherapeutic" or purely investigational research. By including this distinction, Helsinki I made it clear that ethical rules apply even when a research intervention is part of clinical care. The 1975 revision, Helsinki II, placed greater emphasis on informed consent than its predecessor and included independent review committees among its recommendations. Four subsequent revisions, in 1983, 1989, 1996, and 2000, addressed more specific items, such as the conformity of the review committees with the laws of the country in which the research is to be performed. The 2000 revision— which we have included in this volume—is most notable for removing the specific distinction between "therapeutic" and "nontherapeutic" research. The most recent revision enumerates further considerations that should be undertaken if a participant is also a patient, but does not define research with patients and research with nonpatients as separate sorts of research. The later Helsinki documents have been incorporated in many national and international legal statements as well as in those of professional organizations. While the 2000 revision is arguably an advance over prior versions, debate still surrounds the content of this and earlier versions.[5]

Whatever else one might say about the early research codes, they did not prevent a series of research ethics scandals in the United States that took place over about ten years, from the 1963 Brooklyn Jewish Chronic Disease Hospital case to the Tuskegee Syphilis Study, which was brought to light in 1972 (on these cases, see Part I). Although the Department of Health, Education, and Welfare (DHEW, now the Department of Health and Human Services or DHHS) first issued policies for the protection of human participants in 1966, it was not until after the discovery of the Tuskegee experiment that the National Commission for the Protection of Human Subjects of Biomedical and Behavioral Research was appointed. The National Commission operated between 1974 and 1978, and among its final products was a statement of the basic ethical principles that should guide a system of research with humans, the Belmont Report. This report claimed that three principles are "generally accepted in our cultural tradition": respect for persons, beneficence, and justice. Under each principle were described further elements that have surfaced time and again in subsequent discussions of research ethics. For example, respect for persons relates to the provision of information to research subjects, their comprehension of this information, and the voluntariness of their consent; beneficence encompasses the subtleties of risk-benefit assessment; and justice addresses how participants are selected. Though brief, the Belmont Report was a remarkably farsighted document that has provided something of a textual bedrock for the succeeding decades. It also shared with the Declaration of Helsinki the distinction between pure research and research combined with therapy, recognizing that persons with medical conditions were often the only people with whom research could be performed.

Among the National Commission's proposals were the development of general guidelines for federally funded research with humans, including the "pillars" of the system: informed participant consent and prior ethical review by an institutional review board (IRB). The National Commission also proposed specific protections for certain historically vulnerable populations: children, pregnant women, fetuses, prisoners, and persons institutionalized with mental disabilities. All but the last of these proposals became regulations in the DHHS in January 1981 (and were revised again in 1983); these were the so-called basic regulations, and they are codified as 45 Code of Federal Regulations 46 (i.e., 45 CFR 46). Further subparts of the National Commission's report were published addressing the specific protections for vulnerable populations. Except for these more specific protections, Subpart A of the DHHS rules became the basis for the 1991 Basic Policy for the Protection of Human Subjects (known as the Common Rule), which was a revision of the 1981 regulations, and to which all agencies that determined that they were bound by its provisions became signatories.

The U.S. Food and Drug Administration (FDA) is responsible for the approval and licensure of drugs and devices for sale in the United States. Although the FDA requirements are not included in this volume, they are largely in agreement with the Common Rule, particularly concerning the requirements of prior IRB review and of informed consent.

The Council for International Organizations of Medical Sciences (CIOMS), in collaboration with the World Health Organization (WHO), developed its International Ethical Guidelines for Biomedical Research Involving Human Subjects with special attention to research in developing countries, especially in response to increasingly common research on the human immunodeficiency virus/acquired immune deficiency syndrome (HIV/AIDS). Taking into account especially the Nuremberg Code and the Declaration of Helsinki, the CIOMS guidelines apply the ethical principles implicit in those documents to the particular socioeconomic and political circumstances in less developed parts of the world. The current CIOMS guidelines are the product of a 20-year effort that began in 1982 and involved consultation and review by dozens of participants from both developed and developing countries, including officials from health ministries, ethicists, philosophers, and lawyers. The first version, released in 1993, included 15 guidelines with commentary; the second version, excerpted in this volume, was issued in 2002 and includes 21 guidelines with commentary. The CIOMS guidelines open with an ethical justification of biomedical research involving human participants. It is important to consider this, since it sets the tone for the document. Research is necessary, CIOMS claims, and the guidelines are designed to protect the participants as well as the research enterprise itself.

Among the document's more interesting features is a requirement (Guideline 10) that the sponsor and the investigator "must make every effort to ensure that . . . any intervention or product developed, or knowledge generated, will be made reasonably available for the benefit of that population or community." One element of the guidelines that is sure to engender lively debate addresses the use of placebo control groups. Guideline 11 articulates three conditions in which the use of a placebo control is ethically justified: (1) when there is no established effective intervention; (2) when withholding an established effective intervention would expose subjects to, at most, temporary discomfort or delay in relief of symptoms; and (3) when use of an established effective intervention as a comparator would not yield scientifically reliable results and use of a placebo would not add any risk of serious or irreversible harm to the subjects. The commentary on Guideline 11, in which CIOMS examines the debates regarding placebo controls and defends their recommendations, is among the longest in the document, thus attesting to the complexity of the issue.

The product of an ambitious international partnership, the ICH Harmonised Tripartite Guideline—Guideline for Good Clinical Practice (ICH-GCP Guideline) was promulgated in 1996 by the International Conference on Harmonisation of Technical Requirements for Registration of Pharmaceuticals for Human Use and has been agreed upon by regulatory agencies in Europe, Japan, and the United States. The ICH-GCP Guideline delineates detailed standards for review committees, investigators, and sponsors. The guideline is intended especially for research on drugs or devices seeking regulatory approval. While it is rooted specifically in the Declaration of Helsinki along with applicable local regulations, it is far more specific than the other codes mentioned here but not necessarily wider in scope. Criticism leveled at the guideline centers on its emphasis on placebo-controlled trials as opposed to active-controlled trials—that is, studies in which new treatments or pharmaceuticals are tested against existing treatments rather than against placebo. None of the extant codes and guidelines, it seems, has failed to engender controversy on the issue of placebo controls.

Taken together, these documents provide an ethical framework that is largely consistent though still evolving in detail, especially concerning international research and research that involves vulnerable populations. An unfinished agenda that must finally accompany any code or guideline is some mechanism for its interpretation, application, and enforcement. This is surely one of the outstanding challenges for the developers of future codified systems of research ethics.

Bioethics scholars and health care lawyers have devoted significant effort to interpreting and applying these documents. For those working in the United States, the Common Rule is clearly the source of the most direct guidance, as its authority legally controls research conducted using federal funds or at an institution that has filed with the federal government an official assurance that it will abide by these rules. Nevertheless, the other documents are also often cited, especially the Nuremberg Code and the Belmont Report, although mainly for the broader philosophical context they are thought to provide. These other documents have occasionally been introduced into legal proceedings as part of an attempt to demonstrate the violation of some important ethical standard.

In some important ways the codes and guidelines are not entirely consistent. For example, the Nuremberg Code seems to rule out research with any but those able to give "voluntary consent," but research involving children and those who are demented is clearly referred to in the other sources. The 2000 revision of the Declaration of Helsinki casts doubt on whether placebo controls can be used when there is a standard therapy, but in the United States there is a strong preference for placebo controls from a scientific standpoint and a general consensus that they may ethically be employed in certain circumstances. Indeed, confu-

sion after the revision was published in 2000 prompted the WMA to publish a Note of Clarification regarding the use of placebos in October of 2001.

A failure to comply with relevant federal regulations can have serious, even dire, consequences for investigators and for their institutions. The legal status of other documents, such as "guidance documents" published by federal agencies or the other codes and statements included, is far more open to debate. But it is certain that all responsible for the well-being of human research participants, as well as all students of research ethics, should acquire familiarity with the codes and regulations included in this volume.

1. Alexander discusses the Nuremberg trials and their implication for American medicine in his "Medical Science under Dictatorship," *New England Journal of Medicine* 241 (1949): 39–47.
2. Ivy discusses the history of research with humans and offers an analysis of the use of prisoners and those with mental disabilities in research in his "The History and Ethics of the Use of Human Subjects in Medical Experiments," *Science* 108 (1948): 1–5. For Ivy's views on the Nazi war crimes, see his "Nazi War Crimes of a Medical Nature," *JAMA* 139 (1949): 131–35.
3. Leonard H. Glantz, "The Influence of the Nuremberg Code on U.S. Statutes and Regulations," in *The Nazi Doctors and the Nuremberg Code,* ed. George J. Annas and Michael A. Grodin (New York: Oxford University Press, 1992), 183–200; George J. Annas, "The Nuremberg Code in U.S. Courts: Ethics versus Expediency," ibid., 201–22; and Jonathan D. Moreno, "Reassessing the Influence of the Nuremberg Code on American Medical Ethics," *Journal of Contemporary Health Law and Policy* 13 (1997): 347–60.
4. Michael A. Grodin, "Historical Origins of the Nuremberg Code," in *The Nazi Doctors and the Nuremberg Code,* ed. Annas and Grodin, 121–44.
5. For discussions prior to the 2000 revision, see Robert J. Levine, "The Need to Revise the Declaration of Helsinki," *New England Journal of Medicine* 341 (1999): 531–34, and Troyen A. Brennan, "Proposed Revisions to the Declaration of Helsinki—Will They Weaken the Ethical Principles Underlying Human Research?" *New England Journal of Medicine* 341 (1999): 527–31. And for critical assessments of the 2000 revisions, see Heidi P. Forster, Ezekiel J. Emanuel, and Christine Grady, "The 2000 Revision of the Declaration of Helsinki: A Step Forward or More Confusion?" *The Lancet* 358 (2001): 1449–53; and Stephen M. Tollman, Hilda Bastian, Richard Doll, Laurence J. Hirsch, and Harry A. Guess, "What Are the Effects of the Fifth Revision of the Declaration of Helsinki?" *British Medical Journal* 323 (2001): 1417–23.

5   The Nuremberg Code

NUREMBERG MILITARY TRIBUNAL,
U.S. v. *KARL BRANDT*, ET AL.

1. The voluntary consent of the human subject is absolutely essential.

    This means that the person involved should have legal capacity to give consent; should be so situated as to be able to exercise free power of choice, without the intervention of any element of force, fraud, deceit, duress, overreaching, or other ulterior form of constraint or coercion; and should have sufficient knowledge and comprehension of the elements of the subject matter involved as to enable him to make an understanding and enlightened decision. This latter element requires that before the acceptance of an affirmative decision by the experimental subject there should be made known to him the nature, duration, and purpose of the experiment; the method and means by which it is to be conducted; all inconveniences and hazards reasonably to be expected; and the effects upon his health or person which may possibly come from his participation in the experiment.

    The duty and responsibility for ascertaining the quality of the consent rests upon each individual who initiates, directs, or engages in the experiment. It is a personal duty and responsibility which may not be delegated to another with impunity.

2. The experiment should be such as to yield fruitful results for the good of society, unprocurable by other methods or means of study, and not random and unnecessary in nature.

3. The experiment should be so designed and based on the results of animal experimentation and a knowledge of the natural history of the disease or other problem under study that the anticipated results will justify the performance of the experiment.

4. The experiment should be so conducted as to avoid all unnecessary physical and mental suffering and injury.

5. No experiment should be conducted where there is an *a priori* reason to believe that death or disabling injury will occur; except, perhaps, in those experiments where the experimental physicians also serve as subjects.

6. The degree of risk to be taken should never exceed that determined by the humanitarian importance of the problem to be solved by the experiment.

7. Proper preparations should be made and adequate facilities provided to protect the experimental subject against even remote possibilities of injury, disability, or death.

8. The experiment should be conducted only by scientifically qualified persons. The highest degree of skill and care should be required through all stages of the experiment of those who conduct or engage in the experiment.

9. During the course of the experiment the human subject should be at liberty to bring the experiment to an end if he has reached the physical or mental state where continuation of the experiment seems to him to be impossible.

10. During the course of the experiment the scientist in charge must be prepared to terminate the experiment at any stage, if he has probable cause to believe, in the exercise of the good faith, superior skill, and careful judgment required of him, that a continuation of the experiment is likely to result in injury, disability, or death to the experimental subject.

Nuremberg Military Tribunal, from *U.S.* v. *Karl Brandt*, et al., The Nuremberg Code, 1947.

6   The Declaration of Helsinki

*Ethical Principles for Medical Research
Involving Human Subjects*

THE WORLD MEDICAL ASSOCIATION

Adopted by the 18th WMA General Assembly, Helsinki,
June 1964 and amended by the

> 29th WMA General Assembly, Tokyo, Japan,
> October 1975

> 35th WMA General Assembly, Venice, Italy,
> October 1983

> 41st WMA General Assembly, Hong Kong,
> September 1989

> 48th WMA General Assembly, Somerset West,
> Republic of South Africa, October 1996

and the

> 52nd WMA General Assembly, Edinburgh,
> Scotland, October 2000

A. INTRODUCTION

1. The World Medical Association has developed the
   Declaration of Helsinki as a statement of ethical
   principles to provide guidance to physicians and
   other participants in medical research involving
   human subjects. Medical research involving human
   subjects includes research on identifiable human
   material or identifiable data.

2. It is the duty of the physician to promote and safeguard the health of the people. The physician's
   knowledge and conscience are dedicated to the fulfillment of this duty.

3. The Declaration of Geneva of the World Medical
   Association binds the physician with the words,
   "The health of my patient will be my first consideration," and the International Code of Medical Ethics
   declares that, "A physician shall act only in the patient's interest when providing medical care which

---

World Medical Association, Declaration of Helsinki: Ethical
Principles for Medical Research Involving Human Subjects
(Edinburgh: October 2000).

might have the effect of weakening the physical and
mental condition of the patient."

4. Medical progress is based on research which ultimately must rest in part on experimentation involving human subjects.

5. In medical research on human subjects, considerations related to the well-being of the human subject
   should take precedence over the interests of science
   and society.

6. The primary purpose of medical research involving
   human subjects is to improve prophylactic, diagnostic and therapeutic procedures and the understanding of the aetiology and pathogenesis of disease. Even
   the best proven prophylactic, diagnostic, and therapeutic methods must continuously be challenged
   through research for their effectiveness, efficiency,
   accessibility and quality.

7. In current medical practice and in medical research,
   most prophylactic, diagnostic and therapeutic procedures involve risks and burdens.

8. Medical research is subject to ethical standards that
   promote respect for all human beings and protect
   their health and rights. Some research populations
   are vulnerable and need special protection. The
   particular needs of the economically and medically
   disadvantaged must be recognized. Special attention is also required for those who cannot give
   or refuse consent for themselves, for those who
   may be subject to giving consent under duress,
   for those who will not benefit personally from the
   research and for those for whom the research is
   combined with care.

9. Research Investigators should be aware of the ethical,
   legal and regulatory requirements for research on human subjects in their own countries as well as applicable international requirements. No national ethical, legal or regulatory requirement should be
   allowed to reduce or eliminate any of the protections
   for human subjects set forth in this Declaration.

B. BASIC PRINCIPLES FOR ALL MEDICAL RESEARCH

10. It is the duty of the physician in medical research to protect the life, health, privacy, and dignity of the human subject.

11. Medical research involving human subjects must conform to generally accepted scientific principles, be based on a thorough knowledge of the scientific literature, other relevant sources of information, and on adequate laboratory and, where appropriate, animal experimentation.

12. Appropriate caution must be exercised in the conduct of research which may affect the environment, and the welfare of animals used for research must be respected.

13. The design and performance of each experimental procedure involving human subjects should be clearly formulated in an experimental protocol. This protocol should be submitted for consideration, comment, guidance, and where appropriate, approval to a specially appointed ethical review committee, which must be independent of the investigator, the sponsor or any other kind of undue influence. This independent committee should be in conformity with the laws and regulations of the country in which the research experiment is performed. The committee has the right to monitor ongoing trials. The researcher has the obligation to provide monitoring information to the committee, especially any serious adverse events. The researcher should also submit to the committee, for review, information regarding funding, sponsors, institutional affiliations, other potential conflicts of interest and incentives for subjects.

14. The research protocol should always contain a statement of the ethical considerations involved and should indicate that there is compliance with the principles enunciated in this Declaration.

15. Medical research involving human subjects should be conducted only by scientifically qualified persons and under the supervision of a clinically competent medical person. The responsibility for the human subject must always rest with a medically qualified person and never rest on the subject of the research, even though the subject has given consent.

16. Every medical research project involving human subjects should be preceded by careful assessment of predictable risks and burdens in comparison with foreseeable benefits to the subject or to others. This does not preclude the participation of healthy volunteers in medical research. The design of all studies should be publicly available.

17. Physicians should abstain from engaging in research projects involving human subjects unless they are confident that the risks involved have been adequately assessed and can be satisfactorily managed. Physicians should cease any investigation if the risks are found to outweigh the potential benefits or if there is conclusive proof of positive and beneficial results.

18. Medical research involving human subjects should only be conducted if the importance of the objective outweighs the inherent risks and burdens to the subject. This is especially important when the human subjects are healthy volunteers.

19. Medical research is only justified if there is a reasonable likelihood that the populations in which the research is carried out stand to benefit from the results of the research.

20. The subjects must be volunteers and informed participants in the research project.

21. The right of research subjects to safeguard their integrity must always be respected. Every precaution should be taken to respect the privacy of the subject, the confidentiality of the patient's information and to minimize the impact of the study on the subject's physical and mental integrity and on the personality of the subject.

22. In any research on human beings, each potential subject must be adequately informed of the aims, methods, sources of funding, any possible conflicts of interest, institutional affiliations of the researcher, the anticipated benefits and potential risks of the study and the discomfort it may entail. The subject should be informed of the right to abstain from participation in the study or to withdraw consent to participate at any time without reprisal. After ensuring that the subject has understood the information, the physician should then obtain the subject's freely-given informed consent, preferably in writing. If the consent cannot be obtained in writing, the non-written consent must be formally documented and witnessed.

23. When obtaining informed consent for the research project the physician should be particularly cautious if the subject is in a dependent relationship with the physician or may consent under duress. In that case the informed consent should be obtained by a well-

informed physician who is not engaged in the investigation and who is completely independent of this relationship.

24. For a research subject who is legally incompetent, physically or mentally incapable of giving consent or is a legally incompetent minor, the investigator must obtain informed consent from the legally authorized representative in accordance with applicable law. These groups should not be included in research unless the research is necessary to promote the health of the population represented and this research cannot instead be performed on legally competent persons.

25. When a subject deemed legally incompetent, such as a minor child, is able to give assent to decisions about participation in research, the investigator must obtain that assent in addition to the consent of the legally authorized representative.

26. Research on individuals from whom it is not possible to obtain consent, including proxy or advance consent, should be done only if the physical/mental condition that prevents obtaining informed consent is a necessary characteristic of the research population. The specific reasons for involving research subjects with a condition that renders them unable to give informed consent should be stated in the experimental protocol for consideration and approval of the review committee. The protocol should state that consent to remain in the research should be obtained as soon as possible from the individual or a legally authorized surrogate.

27. Both authors and publishers have ethical obligations. In publication of the results of research, the investigators are obliged to preserve the accuracy of the results. Negative as well as positive results should be published or otherwise publicly available. Sources of funding, institutional affiliations and any possible conflicts of interest should be declared in the publication. Reports of experimentation not in accordance with the principles laid down in this Declaration should not be accepted for publication.

C. ADDITIONAL PRINCIPLES FOR MEDICAL RESEARCH COMBINED WITH MEDICAL CARE

28. The physician may combine medical research with medical care, only to the extent that the research is justified by its potential prophylactic, diagnostic or therapeutic value. When medical research is combined with medical care, additional standards apply to protect the patients who are research subjects.

29. The benefits, risks, burdens and effectiveness of a new method should be tested against those of the best current prophylactic, diagnostic, and therapeutic methods. This does not exclude the use of placebo, or no treatment, in studies where no proven prophylactic, diagnostic or therapeutic method exists.

30. At the conclusion of the study, every patient entered into the study should be assured of access to the best proven prophylactic, diagnostic and therapeutic methods identified by the study.

31. The physician should fully inform the patient which aspects of the care are related to the research. The refusal of a patient to participate in a study must never interfere with the patient-physician relationship.

32. In the treatment of a patient, where proven prophylactic, diagnostic and therapeutic methods do not exist or have been ineffective, the physician, with informed consent from the patient, must be free to use unproven or new prophylactic, diagnostic and therapeutic measures, if in the physician's judgement it offers hope of saving life, re-establishing health or alleviating suffering. Where possible, these measures should be made the object of research, designed to evaluate their safety and efficacy. In all cases, new information should be recorded and, where appropriate, published. The other relevant guidelines of this Declaration should be followed.

Note of Clarification on Paragraph 29 of the WMA Declaration of Helsinki

The WMA is concerned that paragraph 29 of the revised Declaration of Helsinki (October 2000) has led to diverse interpretations and possible confusion. It hereby reaffirms its position that extreme care must be taken in making use of a placebo-controlled trial and that in general this methodology should only be used in the absence of existing proven therapy. However, a placebo-controlled trial may be ethically acceptable, even if proven therapy is available, under the following circumstances:

• Where for compelling and scientifically sound methodological reasons its use is necessary to determine the efficacy or safety of a prophylactic, diagnostic or therapeutic method; or

• Where a prophylactic, diagnostic or therapeutic method is being investigated for a minor condition and the patients who receive placebo will not be subject to any additional risk of serious or irreversible harm.

All other provisions of the Declaration of Helsinki must be adhered to, especially the need for appropriate ethical and scientific review.

7   The Belmont Report

*Ethical Principles and Guidelines for the Protection
of Human Subjects of Research*

THE NATIONAL COMMISSION FOR THE PROTECTION
OF HUMAN SUBJECTS OF BIOMEDICAL AND BEHAVIORAL RESEARCH

April 18, 1979
Department of Health, Education, and Welfare
["Summary," "Members of the Commission," and "Table of
Contents" omitted—eds.]

Scientific research has produced substantial social benefits.
It has also posed some troubling ethical questions. Public
attention was drawn to these questions by reported abuses
of human subjects in biomedical experiments, especially
during the Second World War. During the Nuremberg War Crime Trials, the Nuremberg code was drafted as
a set of standards for judging physicians and scientists who
had conducted biomedical experiments on concentration
camp prisoners. This code became the prototype of many
later codes intended to assure that research involving human subjects would be carried out in an ethical manner.

The codes consist of rules, some general, others specific, that guide the investigators or the reviewers of research
in their work. Such rules often are inadequate to cover complex situations; at times they come into conflict, and they
are frequently difficult to interpret or apply. Broader ethical
principles will provide a basis on which specific rules may
be formulated, criticized, and interpreted.

Three principles, or general prescriptive judgments,
that are relevant to research involving human subjects are
identified in this statement. Other principles may also be
relevant. These three are comprehensive, however, and are
stated at a level of generalization that should assist scientists, subjects, reviewers, and interested citizens to understand the ethical issues inherent in research involving human subjects. These principles cannot always be applied so
as to resolve beyond dispute particular ethical problems.
The objective is to provide an analytical framework that
will guide the resolution of ethical problems arising from
research involving human subjects.

The National Commission for the Protection of Human
Subjects of Biomedical and Behavioral Research, The
Belmont Report: Ethical Principles and Guidelines for the
Protection of Human Subjects of Research (Washington,
D.C.: Department of Health, Education, and Welfare, 1979).

This statement consists of a distinction between research and practice, a discussion of the three basic ethical
principles, and remarks about the application of these
principles.

A. BOUNDARIES BETWEEN
PRACTICE AND RESEARCH

It is important to distinguish between biomedical and behavioral research, on the one hand, and the practice of accepted therapy on the other, in order to know what activities ought to undergo review for the protection of human
subjects of research. The distinction between research and
practice is blurred partly because both often occur together
(as in research designed to evaluate a therapy) and partly
because notable departures from standard practice are often called "experimental" when the terms "experimental"
and "research" are not carefully defined.

For the most part, the term "practice" refers to interventions that are designed solely to enhance the well-being
of an individual patient or client and that have a reasonable
expectation of success. The purpose of medical or behavioral practice is to provide diagnosis, preventive treatment,
or therapy to particular individuals. By contrast, the term
"research" designates an activity designed to test an hypothesis, permit conclusions to be drawn, and thereby to
develop or contribute to generalizable knowledge (expressed, for example, in theories, principles, and statements
of relationships). Research is usually described in a formal
protocol that sets forth an objective and a set of procedures
designed to reach that objective.

When a clinician departs in a significant way from
standard or accepted practice, the innovation does not, in
and of itself, constitute research. The fact that a procedure
is "experimental," in the sense of new, untested, or different, does not automatically place it in the category of research. Radically new procedures of this description
should, however, be made the object of formal research at
an early stage in order to determine whether they are safe
and effective. Thus, it is the responsibility of medical practice committees, for example, to insist that a major innovation be incorporated into a formal research project.

Research and practice may be carried on together when research is designed to evaluate the safety and efficacy of a therapy. This need not cause any confusion regarding whether or not the activity requires review; the general rule is that if there is any element of research in an activity, that activity should undergo review for the protection of human subjects.

B. BASIC ETHICAL PRINCIPLES

The expression "basic ethical principles" refers to those general judgments that serve as a basic justification for the many particular ethical prescriptions and evaluations of human actions. Three basic principles, among those generally accepted in our cultural tradition, are particularly relevant to the ethics of research involving human subjects: the principles of respect for persons, beneficence, and justice.

1. *Respect for Persons*—Respect for persons incorporates at least two ethical convictions: first, that individuals should be treated as autonomous agents, and second, that persons with diminished autonomy are entitled to protection. The principle of respect for persons thus divides into two separate moral requirements: the requirement to acknowledge autonomy and the requirement to protect those with diminished autonomy.

An autonomous person is an individual capable of deliberation about personal goals and of acting under the direction of such deliberation. To respect autonomy is to give weight to autonomous persons' considered opinions and choices while refraining from obstructing their actions unless they are clearly detrimental to others. To show lack of respect for an autonomous agent is to repudiate that person's considered judgments, to deny an individual the freedom to act on those considered judgments, or to withhold information necessary to make a considered judgment, when there are no compelling reasons to do so.

However, not every human being is capable of self-determination. The capacity for self-determination matures during an individual's life, and some individuals lose this capacity wholly or in part because of illness, mental disability, or circumstances that severely restrict liberty. Respect for the immature and the incapacitated may require protecting them as they mature or while they are incapacitated.

Some persons are in need of extensive protection, even to the point of excluding them from activities which may harm them; other persons require little protection beyond making sure they undertake activities freely and with awareness of possible adverse consequences. The extent of protection afforded should depend upon the risk of harm and likelihood of benefit. The judgment that any individual lacks autonomy should be periodically reevaluated and will vary in different situations.

In most cases of research involving human subjects, respect for persons demands that subjects enter into the research voluntarily and with adequate information. In some situations, however, application of the principle is not obvious. The involvement of prisoners as subjects of research provides an instructive example. On the one hand, it would seem that the principle of respect for persons requires that prisoners not be deprived of the opportunity to volunteer for research. On the other hand, under prison conditions they may be subtly coerced or unduly influenced to engage in research activities for which they would not otherwise volunteer. Respect for persons would then dictate that prisoners be protected. Whether to allow prisoners to "volunteer" or to "protect" them presents a dilemma. Respecting persons, in most hard cases, is often a matter of balancing competing claims urged by the principle of respect itself.

2. *Beneficence*—Persons are treated in an ethical manner not only by respecting their decisions and protecting them from harm, but also by making efforts to secure their well-being. Such treatment falls under the principle of beneficence. The term "beneficence" is often understood to cover acts of kindness or charity that go beyond strict obligation. In this document, beneficence is understood in a stronger sense, as an obligation. Two general rules have been formulated as complementary expressions of beneficent actions in this sense: (1) do not harm and (2) maximize possible benefits and minimize possible harms.

The Hippocratic maxim "do no harm" has long been a fundamental principle of medical ethics. Claude Bernard extended it to the realm of research, saying that one should not injure one person regardless of the benefits that might come to others. However, even avoiding harm requires learning what is harmful; and, in the process of obtaining this information, persons may be exposed to risk of harm. Further, the Hippocratic Oath requires physicians to benefit their patients "according to their best judgment." Learning what will in fact benefit may require exposing persons to risk. The problem posed by the imperatives is to decide when it is justifiable to seek certain benefits despite the risks involved, and when the benefits should be foregone because of the risks.

The obligations of beneficence affect both individual investigators and society at large, because they extend both to particular research projects and to the entire enterprise of research. In the case of particular projects, investigators and members of their institutions are obliged to give forethought to the maximization of benefits and the reduction of risk that might occur from the research investigation. In the case of scientific research in general, members of the larger society are obliged to recognize the longer term benefits and risks that may result from the improvement of knowledge and from the development of novel medical, psychotherapeutic, and social procedures.

The principle of beneficence often occupies a well-defined justifying role in many areas of research involving human subjects. An example is found in research involving children. Effective ways of treating childhood diseases and fostering healthy development are benefits that serve to justify research involving children—even when individual research subjects are not direct beneficiaries. Research also makes it possible to avoid the harm that may result from the application of previously accepted routine practices that on closer investigation turn out to be dangerous. But the role of the principle of beneficence is not always so unambiguous. A difficult ethical problem remains, for example, about research that presents more than minimal risk without immediate prospect of direct benefit to the children involved. Some have argued that such research is inadmissible, while others have pointed out that this limit would rule out much research promising great benefit to children in the future. Here again, as with all hard cases, the different claims covered by the principle of beneficence may come into conflict and force difficult choices.

3. *Justice*—Who ought to receive the benefits of research and bear its burdens? This is a question of justice, in the sense of "fairness in distribution" or "what is deserved." An injustice occurs when some benefit to which a person is entitled is denied without good reason or when some burden is imposed unduly. Another way of conceiving the principle of justice is that equals ought to be treated equally. However, this statement requires explication. Who is equal and who is unequal? What considerations justify departure from equal distribution? Almost all commentators allow that distinctions based on experience, age, deprivation, competence, merit, and position do sometimes constitute criteria justifying differential treatment for certain purposes. It is necessary, then, to explain in what respects people should be treated equally. There are several widely accepted formulations of just ways to distribute burdens and benefits. Each formulation mentions some relevant property on the basis of which burdens and benefits should be distributed. These formulations are (1) to each person an equal share, (2) to each person according to individual need, (3) to each person according to individual effort, (4) to each person according to societal contribution, and (5) to each person according to merit.

Questions of justice have long been associated with social practices such as punishment, taxation, and political representation. Until recently these questions have not generally been associated with scientific research. However, they are foreshadowed even in the earliest reflections on the ethics of research involving human subjects. For example, during the 19th and 20th centuries the burdens of serving as research subjects fell largely upon poor ward patients, while the benefits of improved medical care flowed primarily to private patients. Subsequently, the exploitation of unwilling prisoners as research subjects in Nazi concentration camps was condemned as a particularly flagrant injustice. In this country, in the 1940s, the Tuskegee syphilis study used disadvantaged, rural black men to study the untreated course of a disease that is by no means confined to that population. These subjects were deprived of demonstrably effective treatment in order not to interrupt the project, long after such treatment became generally available.

Against this historical background, it can be seen how conceptions of justice are relevant to research involving human subjects. For example, the selection of research subjects needs to be scrutinized in order to determine whether some classes (e.g., welfare patients, particular racial and ethnic minorities, or persons confined to institutions) are being systematically selected simply because of their easy availability, their compromised position, or their manipulability, rather than for reasons directly related to the problem being studied. Finally, whenever research supported by public funds leads to the development of therapeutic devices and procedures, justice demands both that these not provide advantages only to those who can afford them and that such research should not unduly involve persons from groups unlikely to be among the beneficiaries of subsequent applications of the research.

C. APPLICATIONS

Applications of the general principles to the conduct of research leads to consideration of the following requirements: informed consent, risk/benefit assessment, and the selection of subjects of research.

1. *Informed Consent*—Respect for persons requires that subjects, to the degree that they are capable, be given the opportunity to choose what shall or shall not happen to them. This opportunity is provided when adequate standards for informed consent are satisfied.

While the importance of informed consent is unquestioned, controversy prevails over the nature and possibility of an informed consent. Nonetheless, there is widespread agreement that the consent process can be analyzed as containing three elements: information, comprehension and voluntariness.

Information. Most codes of research establish specific items for disclosure intended to assure that subjects are given sufficient information. These items generally include: the research procedure, their purposes, risks and anticipated benefits, alternative procedures (where therapy is involved), and a statement offering the subject the opportunity to ask questions and to withdraw at any time from the research. Additional items have been proposed, including how subjects are selected, the person responsible for the research, etc.

However, a simple listing of items does not answer the question of what the standard should be for judging how much and what sort of information should be provided. One standard frequently invoked in medical practice, namely the information commonly provided by practitioners in the field or in the locale, is inadequate since research takes place precisely when a common understanding does not exist. Another standard, currently popular in malpractice law, requires the practitioner to reveal the information that reasonable persons would wish to know in order to make a decision regarding their care. This, too, seems insufficient since the research subject, being in essence a volunteer, may wish to know considerably more about risks gratuitously undertaken than do patients who deliver themselves into the hand of a clinician for needed care. It may be that a standard of "the reasonable volunteer" should be proposed: the extent and nature of information should be such that persons, knowing that the procedure is neither necessary for their care nor perhaps fully understood, can decide whether they wish to participate in the furthering of knowledge. Even when some direct benefit to them is anticipated, the subjects should understand clearly the range of risk and the voluntary nature of participation.

A special problem of consent arises where informing subjects of some pertinent aspect of the research is likely to impair the validity of the research. In many cases, it is sufficient to indicate to subjects that they are being invited to participate in research of which some features will not be revealed until the research is concluded. In all cases of research involving incomplete disclosure, such research is justified only if it is clear that (1) incomplete disclosure is truly necessary to accomplish the goals of the research, (2) there are no undisclosed risks to subjects that are more than minimal, and (3) there is an adequate plan for debriefing subjects, when appropriate, and for dissemi-

nation of research results to them. Information about risks should never be withheld for the purpose of eliciting the cooperation of subjects, and truthful answers should always be given to direct questions about the research. Care should be taken to distinguish cases in which disclosure would destroy or invalidate the research from cases in which disclosure would simply inconvenience the investigator.

Comprehension. The manner and context in which information is conveyed is as important as the information itself. For example, presenting information in a disorganized and rapid fashion, allowing too little time for consideration, or curtailing opportunities for questioning, all may adversely affect a subject's ability to make an informed choice.

Because the subject's ability to understand is a function of intelligence, rationality, maturity, and language, it is necessary to adapt the presentation of the information to the subject's capacities. Investigators are responsible for ascertaining that the subject has comprehended the information. While there is always an obligation to ascertain that the information about risk to subjects is complete and adequately comprehended, when the risks are more serious, that obligation increases. On occasion, it may be suitable to give some oral or written tests of comprehension.

Special provision may need to be made when comprehension is severely limited—for example, by conditions of immaturity or mental disability. Each class of subjects that one might consider as incompetent (e.g., infants and young children, mentally disabled patients, the terminally ill, and the comatose) should be considered on its own terms. Even for these persons, however, respect requires giving them the opportunity to choose to the extent that they are able, whether or not to participate in research. The objections of these subjects to involvement should be honored, unless the research entails providing them a therapy unavailable elsewhere. Respect for persons also requires seeking the permission of other parties in order to protect the subjects from harm. Such persons are thus respected both by acknowledging their own wishes and by the use of third parties to protect them from harm.

The third parties chosen should be those who are most likely to understand the incompetent subject's situation and to act in that person's best interest. The person authorized to act on behalf of the subject should be given an opportunity to observe the research as it proceeds in order to be able to withdraw the subject from the research, if such action appears in the subject's best interest.

Voluntariness. An agreement to participate in research constitutes a valid consent only if voluntarily given. This element of informed consent requires conditions free of coercion and undue influence. Coercion occurs when an overt threat of harm is intentionally presented by one person to another in order to obtain compliance. Undue influence, by contrast, occurs through an offer of an excessive, unwarranted, inappropriate, or improper reward or other overture in order to obtain compliance. Also, inducements that would ordinarily be acceptable may become undue influences if the subject is especially vulnerable.

Unjustifiable pressures usually occur when persons in positions of authority or commanding influence—especially where possible sanctions are involved—urge a course of action for a subject. A continuum of such influencing factors exists, however, and it is impossible to state precisely where justifiable persuasion ends and undue influence begins. But undue influence would include actions such as manipulating a person's choice through the controlling influence of a close relative and threatening to withdraw health services to which an individual would otherwise be entitled.

2. *Assessment of Risks and Benefits*—The assessment of risks and benefits requires a careful arrayal of relevant data, including, in some cases, alternative ways of obtaining the benefits sought in the research. Thus, the assessment presents both an opportunity and a responsibility to gather systematic and comprehensive information about proposed research. For the investigator, it is a means to examine whether the proposed research is properly designed. For a review committee, it is a method for determining whether the risks that will be presented to subjects are justified. For prospective subjects, the assessment will assist the determination whether or not to participate.

The Nature and Scope of Risks and Benefits. The requirement that research be justified on the basis of a favorable risk/benefit assessment bears a close relation to the principle of beneficence, just as the moral requirement that informed consent be obtained is derived primarily from the principle of respect for persons. The term "risk" refers to a possibility that harm may occur. However, when expressions such as "small risk" or "high risk" are used, they usually refer (often ambiguously) both to the chance (probability) of experiencing a harm and the severity (magnitude) of the envisioned harm.

The term "benefit" is used in the research context to refer to something of positive value related to health or welfare. Unlike "risk," "benefit" is not a term that expresses probabilities. Risk is properly contrasted to probability of benefits, and benefits are properly contrasted with harms rather than risks of harm. Accord-

ingly, so-called risk/benefit assessments are concerned with the probabilities and magnitudes of possible harms and anticipated benefits. Many kinds of possible harms and benefits need to be taken into account. There are, for example, risks of psychological harm, physical harm, legal harm, social harm, and economic harm and the corresponding benefits. While the most likely types of harms to research subjects are those of psychological or physical pain or injury, other possible kinds should not be overlooked.

Risks and benefits of research may affect the individual subjects, the families of the individual subjects, and society at large (or special groups of subjects in society). Previous codes and Federal regulations have required that risks to subjects be outweighed by the sum of both the anticipated benefit to the subject, if any, and the anticipated benefit to society in the form of knowledge to be gained from the research. In balancing these different elements, the risks and benefits affecting the immediate research subject will normally carry special weight. On the other hand, interests other than those of the subject may on some occasions be sufficient by themselves to justify the risks involved in the research, so long as the subjects' rights have been protected. Beneficence thus requires that we protect against risk of harm to subjects and also that we be concerned about the loss of the substantial benefits that might be gained from research.

The Systematic Assessment of Risks and Benefits. It is commonly said that benefits and risks must be "balanced" and shown to be "in a favorable ratio." The metaphorical character of these terms draws attention to the difficulty of making precise judgments. Only on rare occasions will quantitative techniques be available for the scrutiny of research protocols. However, the idea of systematic, nonarbitrary analysis of risks and benefits should be emulated insofar as possible. This ideal requires those making decisions about the justifiability of research to be thorough in the accumulation and assessment of information about all aspects of the research, and to consider alternatives systematically. This procedure renders the assessment of research more rigorous and precise, while making communication between review board members and investigators less subject to misinterpretation, misinformation, and conflicting judgments. Thus, there should first be a determination of the validity of the presuppositions of the research; then the nature, probability, and magnitude of risk should be distinguished with as much clarity as possible. The method of ascertaining risks should be explicit, especially where there is no alternative to the use of such vague categories as small or slight risk. It should also be determined whether an investigator's estimates of the probability of harm or benefits are reasonable, as judged by known facts or other available studies.

Finally, assessment of the justifiability of research should reflect at least the following considerations: (i) Brutal or inhumane treatment of human subjects is never morally justified. (ii) Risks should be reduced to those necessary to achieve the research objective. It should be determined whether it is in fact necessary to use human subjects at all. Risk can perhaps never be entirely eliminated, but it can often be reduced by careful attention to alternative procedures. (iii) When research involves significant risk of serious impairment, review committees should be extraordinarily insistent on the justification of the risk (looking usually to the likelihood of benefit to the subject—or, in some rare cases, to the manifest voluntariness of the participation). (iv) When vulnerable populations are involved in research, the appropriateness of involving them should itself be demonstrated. A number of variables go into such judgments, including the nature and degree of risk, the condition of the particular population involved, and the nature and level of the anticipated benefits. (v) Relevant risks and benefits must be thoroughly arrayed in documents and procedures used in the informed consent process.

3. *Selection of Subjects*—Just as the principle of respect for persons finds expression in the requirements for consent, and the principle of beneficence in risk/benefit assessment, the principle of justice gives rise to moral requirements that there be fair procedures and outcomes in the selection of research subjects.

Justice is relevant to the selection of subjects of research at two levels: the social and the individual. Individual justice in the selection of subjects would require that researchers exhibit fairness: thus, they should not offer potentially beneficial research only to some patients who are in their favor or select only "undesirable" persons for risky research. Social justice requires that distinction be drawn between classes of subjects that ought, and ought not, to participate in any particular kind of research, based on the ability of members of that class to bear burdens and on the appropriateness of placing further burdens on already burdened persons. Thus, it can be considered a matter of social justice that there is an order of preference in the selection of classes of subjects (e.g., adults before children) and that some classes of potential subjects (e.g., the institutionalized mentally infirm or prisoners) may be involved as research subjects, if at all, only on certain conditions.

Injustice may appear in the selection of subjects, even if individual subjects are selected fairly by investigators and treated fairly in the course of research. Thus injustice arises from social, racial, sexual, and cultural biases institutionalized in society. Thus, even if individual researchers are treating their research subjects fairly, and even if institutional review boards are taking care to assure that subjects are selected fairly within a particular institution, unjust social patterns may nevertheless appear in the overall distribution of the burdens and benefits of research. Although individual institutions or investigators may not be able to resolve a problem that is pervasive in their social setting, they can consider distributive justice in selecting research subjects.

Some populations, especially institutionalized ones, are already burdened in many ways by their infirmities and environments. When research is proposed that involves risks and does not include a therapeutic component, other less burdened classes of persons should be called upon first to accept these risks of research, except where the research is directly related to the specific conditions of the class involved. Also, even though public funds for research may often flow in the same directions as public funds for health care, it seems unfair that populations dependent on public health care constitute a pool of preferred research subjects if more advantaged populations are likely to be the recipients of the benefits.

One special instance of injustice results from the involvement of vulnerable subjects. Certain groups, such as racial minorities, the economically disadvantaged, the very sick, and the institutionalized may continually be sought as research subjects, owing to their ready availability in settings where research is conducted. Given their dependent status and their frequently compromised capacity for free consent, they should be protected against the danger of being involved in research solely for administrative convenience, or because they are easy to manipulate as a result of their illness or socioeconomic condition.

8 The Common Rule, Title 45 (Public Welfare), Code of Federal Regulations, Part 46 (Protection of Human Subjects), Subparts A–D

U.S. Department of Health and Human Services,
National Institutes of Health, and
Office for Human Research Protections

SUBPART A—FEDERAL POLICY FOR THE PROTECTION OF HUMAN SUBJECTS (BASIC DHHS POLICY FOR PROTECTION OF HUMAN RESEARCH SUBJECTS)

Source: 56 FR [Federal Register] 28003, June 18, 1991.

[Detailed table of contents omitted—eds.]

§46.101 TO WHAT DOES THIS POLICY APPLY?

(a) Except as provided in paragraph (b) of this section, this policy applies to all research involving human subjects conducted, supported, or otherwise subject to regulation by any Federal Department or Agency which takes appropriate administrative action to make the policy applicable to such research. This includes research conducted by Federal civilian employees or military personnel, except that each Department or Agency head may adopt such procedural modifications as may be appropriate from an administrative standpoint. It also includes research conducted, supported, or otherwise subject to regulation by the Federal Government outside the United States.

  (1) Research that is conducted or supported by a Federal Department or Agency, whether or not it is regulated as defined in §46.102(e), must comply with all sections of this policy.

  (2) Research that is neither conducted nor supported by a Federal Department or Agency but is subject to regulation as defined in §46.102(e) must be reviewed and approved, in compliance with §46.101, §46.102, and §46.107 through §46.117 of this policy, by an Institutional Review Board (IRB) that operates in accordance with the pertinent requirements of this policy.

(b) Unless otherwise required by Department or Agency heads, research activities in which the only involvement of human subjects will be in one or more of the following categories are exempt from this policy:

  (1) Research conducted in established or commonly accepted educational settings, involving normal educational practices, such as (i) research on regular and special education instructional strategies, or (ii) research on the effectiveness of or the comparison among instructional techniques, curricula, or classroom management methods.

  (2) Research involving the use of educational tests (cognitive, diagnostic, aptitude, achievement), survey procedures, interview procedures, or observation of public behavior, unless:

   (i) information obtained is recorded in such a manner that human subjects can be identified, directly or through identifiers linked to the subjects; and (ii) any disclosure of the human subjects' responses outside the research could reasonably place the subjects at risk of criminal or civil liability or be damaging to the subjects' financial standing, employability, or reputation.

  (3) Research involving the use of educational tests (cognitive, diagnostic, aptitude, achievement), survey procedures, interview procedures, or observation of public behavior that is not exempt under paragraph (b)(2) of this section, if:

   (i) the human subjects are elected or appointed public officials or candidates for public of-

U.S. Department of Health and Human Services, National Institutes of Health, and Office for Human Research Protections, The Common Rule, Title 45 (Public Welfare), Code of Federal Regulations, Part 46 (Protection of Human Subjects) (Washington, D.C.: DHHS, revised November 13, 2001; effective December 13, 2001).

fice; or (ii) Federal statute(s) require(s) without exception that the confidentiality of the personally identifiable information will be maintained throughout the research and thereafter.

(4) Research involving the collection or study of existing data, documents, records, pathological specimens, or diagnostic specimens, if these sources are publicly available or if the information is recorded by the investigator in such a manner that subjects cannot be identified, directly or through identifiers linked to the subjects.

(5) Research and demonstration projects which are conducted by or subject to the approval of Department or Agency heads, and which are designed to study, evaluate, or otherwise examine:

   (i) Public benefit or service programs; (ii) procedures for obtaining benefits or services under those programs; (iii) possible changes in or alternatives to those programs or procedures; or (iv) possible changes in methods or levels of payment for benefits or services under those programs.

(6) Taste and food quality evaluation and consumer acceptance studies, (i) if wholesome foods without additives are consumed or (ii) if a food is consumed that contains a food ingredient at or below the level and for a use found to be safe, or agricultural chemical or environmental contaminant at or below the level found to be safe, by the Food and Drug Administration or approved by the Environmental Protection Agency or the Food Safety and Inspection Service of the U.S. Department of Agriculture.

(c) Department or Agency heads retain final judgment as to whether a particular activity is covered by this policy.

(d) Department or Agency heads may require that specific research activities or classes of research activities conducted, supported, or otherwise subject to regulation by the Department or Agency but not otherwise covered by this policy, comply with some or all of the requirements of this policy.

(e) Compliance with this policy requires compliance with pertinent Federal laws or regulations which provide additional protections for human subjects.

(f) This policy does not affect any State or local laws or regulations which may otherwise be applicable and which provide additional protections for human subjects.

(g) This policy does not affect any foreign laws or regulations which may otherwise be applicable and which provide additional protections to human subjects of research.

(h) When research covered by this policy takes place in foreign countries, procedures normally followed in the foreign countries to protect human subjects may differ from those set forth in this policy. (An example is a foreign institution which complies with guidelines consistent with the World Medical Assembly Declaration [Declaration of Helsinki amended 1989] issued either by sovereign states or by an organization whose function for the protection of human research subjects is internationally recognized.) In these circumstances, if a Department or Agency head determines that the procedures prescribed by the institution afford protections that are at least equivalent to those provided in this policy, the Department or Agency head may approve the substitution of the foreign procedures in lieu of the procedural requirements provided in this policy. Except when otherwise required by statute, Executive Order, or the Department or Agency head, notices of these actions as they occur will be published in the *Federal Register* or will be otherwise published as provided in Department or Agency procedures.

(i) Unless otherwise required by law, Department or Agency heads may waive the applicability of some or all of the provisions of this policy to specific research activities or classes of research activities otherwise covered by this policy. Except when otherwise required by statute or Executive Order, the Department or Agency head shall forward advance notices of these actions to the Office for Protection from Research Risks [OPRR, now the Office for Human Research Protections or OHRP—eds.], National Institutes of Health, Department of Health and Human Services (DHHS), and shall also publish them in the *Federal Register* or in such other manner as provided in Department or Agency procedures.[1]

§46.102 DEFINITIONS.

(a) *Department or Agency head* means the head of any Federal Department or Agency and any other officer

---

[1] Institutions with DHHS-approved assurances on file will abide by provisions of Title 45 CFR Part 46 Subparts A–D. Some of the other departments and agencies have incorpo-

or employee of any Department or Agency to whom authority has been delegated.

(b) *Institution* means any public or private entity or Agency (including Federal, State, and other agencies).

(c) *Legally authorized representative* means an individual or judicial or other body authorized under applicable law to consent on behalf of a prospective subject to the subject's participation in the procedure(s) involved in the research.

(d) *Research* means a systematic investigation, including research development, testing, and evaluation, designed to develop or contribute to generalizable knowledge. Activities which meet this definition constitute research for purposes of this policy, whether or not they are conducted or supported under a program which is considered research for other purposes. For example, some demonstration and service programs may include research activities.

(e) *Research subject to regulation,* and similar terms are intended to encompass those research activities for which a Federal Department or Agency has specific responsibility for regulating as a research activity (for example, Investigational New Drug requirements administered by the Food and Drug Administration). It does not include research activities which are incidentally regulated by a Federal Department or Agency solely as part of the Department's or Agency's broader responsibility to regulate certain types of activities whether research or non-research in nature (for example, Wage and Hour requirements administered by the Department of Labor).

(f) *Human subject* means a living individual about whom an investigator (whether professional or student) conducting research obtains

> (1) data through intervention or interaction with the individual, or
> (2) identifiable private information.

Intervention includes both physical procedures by which data are gathered (for example, venipuncture)

and manipulations of the subject or the subject's environment that are performed for research purposes. *Interaction* includes communication or interpersonal contact between investigator and subject. *Private information* includes information about behavior that occurs in a context in which an individual can reasonably expect that no observation or recording is taking place, and information which has been provided for specific purposes by an individual and which the individual can reasonably expect will not be made public (for example, a medical record). Private information must be individually identifiable (i.e., the identity of the subject is or may readily be ascertained by the investigator or associated with the information) in order for obtaining the information to constitute research involving human subjects.

(g) *IRB* means an Institutional Review Board established in accord with and for the purposes expressed in this policy.

(h) *IRB approval* means the determination of the IRB that the research has been reviewed and may be conducted at an institution within the constraints set forth by the IRB and by other institutional and Federal requirements.

(i) *Minimal risk* means that the probability and magnitude of harm or discomfort anticipated in the research are not greater in and of themselves than those ordinarily encountered in daily life or during the performance of routine physical or psychological examinations or tests.

(j) *Certification* means the official notification by the institution to the supporting Department or Agency, in accordance with the requirements of this policy, that a research project or activity involving human subjects has been reviewed and approved by an IRB in accordance with an approved assurance.

§46.103 ASSURING COMPLIANCE WITH THIS POLICY—RESEARCH CONDUCTED OR SUPPORTED BY ANY FEDERAL DEPARTMENT OR AGENCY.

(a) Each institution engaged in research which is covered by this policy and which is conducted or supported by a Federal Department or Agency shall provide written assurance satisfactory to the Department or Agency head that it will comply with the requirements set forth in this policy. In lieu of requiring submission of an assurance, individual Department or Agency heads shall accept the exis-

---

rated all provisions of Title 45 CFR Part 46 into their policies and procedures as well. However, the exemptions at 45 CFR 46.101(b) do not apply to research involving prisoners, fetuses, pregnant women, or human in vitro fertilization, Subparts B and C. The exemption at 45 CFR 46.101(b)(2), for research involving survey or interview procedures or observation of public behavior, does not apply to research with children, Subpart D, except for research involving observations of public behavior when the investigator(s) do not participate in the activities being observed.

tence of a current assurance, appropriate for the research in question, on file with the Office for Protection from Research Risks [now OHRP—eds.], National Institutes of Health, DHHS, and approved for Federalwide use by that office. When the existence of a DHHS-approved assurance is accepted in lieu of requiring submission of an assurance, reports (except certification) required by this policy to be made to Department and Agency heads shall also be made to the Office for Protection from Research Risks [now OHRP—eds.], National Institutes of Health, DHHS.

(b) Departments and agencies will conduct or support research covered by this policy only if the institution has an assurance approved as provided in this section, and only if the institution has certified to the Department or Agency head that the research has been reviewed and approved by an IRB provided for in the assurance, and will be subject to continuing review by the IRB. Assurances applicable to federally supported or conducted research shall at a minimum include:

(1) A statement of principles governing the institution in the discharge of its responsibilities for protecting the rights and welfare of human subjects of research conducted at or sponsored by the institution, regardless of whether the research is subject to Federal regulation. This may include an appropriate existing code, declaration, or statement of ethical principles, or a statement formulated by the institution itself. This requirement does not preempt provisions of this policy applicable to Department- or Agency-supported or regulated research and need not be applicable to any research exempted or waived under §46.101(b) or (i).

(2) Designation of one or more IRBs established in accordance with the requirements of this policy, and for which provisions are made for meeting space and sufficient staff to support the IRB's review and recordkeeping duties.

(3) A list of IRB members identified by name; earned degrees; representative capacity; indications of experience such as board certifications, licenses, etc., sufficient to describe each member's chief anticipated contributions to IRB deliberations; and any employment or other relationship between each member and the institution; for example: full-time employee, part-time employee, member of governing panel or board, stockholder, paid or unpaid consultant. Changes in IRB membership shall be reported to the Department or Agency head, unless in accord with §46.103(a) of this policy, the existence of a DHHS-approved assurance is accepted. In this case, change in IRB membership shall be reported to the Office for Protection from Research Risks [now OHRP—eds.], National Institutes of Health, DHHS.

(4) Written procedures which the IRB will follow (i) for conducting its initial and continuing review of research and for reporting its findings and actions to the investigator and the institution; (ii) for determining which projects require review more often than annually and which projects need verification from sources other than the investigators that no material changes have occurred since previous IRB review; and (iii) for ensuring prompt reporting to the IRB of proposed changes in a research activity, and for ensuring that such changes in approved research, during the period for which IRB approval has already been given, may not be initiated without IRB review and approval except when necessary to eliminate apparent immediate hazards to the subject.

(5) Written procedures for ensuring prompt reporting to the IRB, appropriate institutional officials, and the Department or Agency head of (i) any unanticipated problems involving risks to subjects or others or any serious or continuing noncompliance with this policy or the requirements or determinations of the IRB; and (ii) any suspension or termination of IRB approval.

(c) The assurance shall be executed by an individual authorized to act for the institution and to assume on behalf of the institution the obligations imposed by this policy and shall be filed in such form and manner as the Department or Agency head prescribes.

(d) The Department or Agency head will evaluate all assurances submitted in accordance with this policy through such officers and employees of the Department or Agency and such experts or consultants engaged for this purpose as the Department or Agency head determines to be appropriate. The Department or Agency head's evaluation will take into consideration the adequacy of the proposed IRB in light of the anticipated scope of the institution's research activities and the types of subject populations likely to be involved, the appropriateness of the proposed initial and continuing review procedures in light of the probable risks, and the size and complexity of the institution.

(e) On the basis of this evaluation, the Department or Agency head may approve or disapprove the assurance, or enter into negotiations to develop an approvable one. The Department or Agency head may limit the period during which any particular approved assurance or class of approved assurances shall remain effective or otherwise condition or restrict approval.

(f) Certification is required when the research is supported by a Federal Department or Agency and not otherwise exempted or waived under §46.101(b) or (i). An institution with an approved assurance shall certify that each application or proposal for research covered by the assurance and by §46.103 of this policy has been reviewed and approved by the IRB. Such certification must be submitted with the application or proposal or by such later date as may be prescribed by the Department or Agency to which the application or proposal is submitted. Under no condition shall research covered by §46.103 of the policy be supported prior to receipt of the certification that the research has been reviewed and approved by the IRB. Institutions without an approved assurance covering the research shall certify within 30 days after receipt of a request for such a certification from the Department or Agency, that the application or proposal has been approved by the IRB. If the certification is not submitted within these time limits, the application or proposal may be returned to the institution.

(Approved by the Office of Management and Budget under Control Number 9999-0020.)

§§46.104–46.106 [RESERVED]

§46.107 IRB MEMBERSHIP.

(a) Each IRB shall have at least five members, with varying backgrounds to promote complete and adequate review of research activities commonly conducted by the institution. The IRB shall be sufficiently qualified through the experience and expertise of its members, and the diversity of the members, including consideration of race, gender, and cultural backgrounds and sensitivity to such issues as community attitudes, to promote respect for its advice and counsel in safeguarding the rights and welfare of human subjects. In addition to possessing the professional competence necessary to review specific research activities, the IRB shall be able to ascertain the acceptability of proposed research in terms of institutional commitments and regulations, applicable law, and standards of professional conduct and practice. The IRB shall therefore include persons knowledgeable in these areas. If an IRB regularly reviews research that involves a vulnerable category of subjects, such as children, prisoners, pregnant women, or handicapped or mentally disabled persons, consideration shall be given to the inclusion of one or more individuals who are knowledgeable about and experienced in working with these subjects.

(b) Every nondiscriminatory effort will be made to ensure that no IRB consists entirely of men or entirely of women, including the institution's consideration of qualified persons of both sexes, so long as no selection is made to the IRB on the basis of gender. No IRB may consist entirely of members of one profession.

(c) Each IRB shall include at least one member whose primary concerns are in scientific areas and at least one member whose primary concerns are in nonscientific areas.

(d) Each IRB shall include at least one member who is not otherwise affiliated with the institution and who is not part of the immediate family of a person who is affiliated with the institution.

(e) No IRB may have a member participate in the IRB's initial or continuing review of any project in which the member has a conflicting interest, except to provide information requested by the IRB.

(f) An IRB may, in its discretion, invite individuals with competence in special areas to assist in the review of issues which require expertise beyond or in addition to that available on the IRB. These individuals may not vote with the IRB.

§46.108 IRB FUNCTIONS AND OPERATIONS.

In order to fulfill the requirements of this policy each IRB shall:

(a) Follow written procedures in the same detail as described in §46.103(b)(4) and to the extent required by §46.103(b)(5).

(b) Except when an expedited review procedure is used (see §46.110), review proposed research at convened meetings at which a majority of the members of the IRB are present, including at least one member whose primary concerns are in nonscientific areas. In order for the research to be approved, it shall receive the approval of a majority of those members present at the meeting.

§46.109 IRB REVIEW OF RESEARCH.

(a) An IRB shall review and have authority to approve, require modifications in (to secure approval), or disapprove all research activities covered by this policy.

(b) An IRB shall require that information given to subjects as part of informed consent is in accordance with §46.116. The IRB may require that information, in addition to that specifically mentioned in §46.116, be given to the subjects when in the IRB's judgment the information would meaningfully add to the protection of the rights and welfare of subjects.

(c) An IRB shall require documentation of informed consent or may waive documentation in accordance with §46.117.

(d) An IRB shall notify investigators and the institution in writing of its decision to approve or disapprove the proposed research activity, or of modifications required to secure IRB approval of the research activity. If the IRB decides to disapprove a research activity, it shall include in its written notification a statement of the reasons for its decision and give the investigator an opportunity to respond in person or in writing.

(e) An IRB shall conduct continuing review of research covered by this policy at intervals appropriate to the degree of risk, but not less than once per year, and shall have authority to observe or have a third party observe the consent process and the research.

(Approved by the Office of Management and Budget under Control Number 9999-0020.)

§46.110 EXPEDITED REVIEW PROCEDURES FOR CERTAIN KINDS OF RESEARCH INVOLVING NO MORE THAN MINIMAL RISK, AND FOR MINOR CHANGES IN APPROVED RESEARCH.

(a) The Secretary, HHS, has established, and published as a Notice in the *Federal Register,* a list of categories of research that may be reviewed by the IRB through an expedited review procedure. The list will be amended, as appropriate, after consultation with other departments and agencies, through periodic republication by the Secretary, HHS, in the *Federal Register.* A copy of the list is available from the Office for Protection from Research Risks [now OHRP—eds.], National Institutes of Health, DHHS, Bethesda, Maryland 20892.

(b) An IRB may use the expedited review procedure to review either or both of the following:

(1) some or all of the research appearing on the list and found by the reviewer(s) to involve no more than minimal risk,

(2) minor changes in previously approved research during the period (of one year or less) for which approval is authorized.

Under an expedited review procedure, the review may be carried out by the IRB chairperson or by one or more experienced reviewers designated by the chairperson from among members of the IRB. In reviewing the research, the reviewers may exercise all of the authorities of the IRB except that the reviewers may not disapprove the research. A research activity may be disapproved only after review in accordance with the non-expedited procedure set forth in §46.108(b).

(c) Each IRB which uses an expedited review procedure shall adopt a method for keeping all members advised of research proposals which have been approved under the procedure.

(d) The Department or Agency head may restrict, suspend, terminate, or choose not to authorize an institution's or IRB's use of the expedited review procedure.

§46.111 CRITERIA FOR IRB APPROVAL OF RESEARCH.

(a) In order to approve research covered by this policy the IRB shall determine that all of the following requirements are satisfied:

(1) Risks to subjects are minimized: (i) by using procedures which are consistent with sound research design and which do not unnecessarily expose subjects to risk, and (ii) whenever appropriate, by using procedures already being performed on the subjects for diagnostic or treatment purposes.

(2) Risks to subjects are reasonable in relation to anticipated benefits, if any, to subjects, and the importance of the knowledge that may reasonably be expected to result. In evaluating risks and benefits, the IRB should consider only those risks and benefits that may result from the research (as distinguished from risks and benefits of therapies subjects would receive even if not participating in the research). The IRB should not consider possible long-range effects of applying knowledge gained in the research (for example, the possible effects of the research on public policy) as among those research risks that fall within the purview of its responsibility.

(3) Selection of subjects is equitable. In making this assessment the IRB should take into account the purposes of the research and the setting in which the research will be conducted and should be particularly cognizant of the special problems of research involving vulnerable populations, such as children, prisoners, pregnant women, mentally disabled persons, or economically or educationally disadvantaged persons.

(4) Informed consent will be sought from each prospective subject or the subject's legally authorized representative, in accordance with, and to the extent required by §46.116.

(5) Informed consent will be appropriately documented, in accordance with, and to the extent required by §46.117.

(6) When appropriate, the research plan makes adequate provision for monitoring the data collected to ensure the safety of subjects.

(7) When appropriate, there are adequate provisions to protect the privacy of subjects and to maintain the confidentiality of data.

(b) When some or all of the subjects are likely to be vulnerable to coercion or undue influence, such as children, prisoners, pregnant women, mentally disabled persons, or economically or educationally disadvantaged persons, additional safeguards have been included in the study to protect the rights and welfare of these subjects.

§46.112 REVIEW BY INSTITUTION.

Research covered by this policy that has been approved by an IRB may be subject to further appropriate review and approval or disapproval by officials of the institution. However, those officials may not approve the research if it has not been approved by an IRB.

§46.113 SUSPENSION OR TERMINATION OF IRB APPROVAL OF RESEARCH.

An IRB shall have authority to suspend or terminate approval of research that is not being conducted in accordance with the IRB's requirements or that has been associated with unexpected serious harm to subjects. Any suspension or termination of approval shall include a statement of the reasons for the IRB's action and shall be reported promptly to the investigator, appropriate institutional officials, and the Department or Agency head.

(Approved by the Office of Management and Budget under Control Number 9999-0020.)

§46.114 COOPERATIVE RESEARCH.

Cooperative research projects are those projects covered by this policy which involve more than one institution. In the conduct of cooperative research projects, each institution is responsible for safeguarding the rights and welfare of human subjects and for complying with this policy. With the approval of the Department or Agency head, an institution participating in a cooperative project may enter into a joint review arrangement, rely upon the review of another qualified IRB, or make similar arrangements for avoiding duplication of effort.

§46.115 IRB RECORDS.

(a) An institution, or when appropriate an IRB, shall prepare and maintain adequate documentation of IRB activities, including the following:

(1) Copies of all research proposals reviewed, scientific evaluations, if any, that accompany the proposals, approved sample consent documents, progress reports submitted by investigators, and reports of injuries to subjects.

(2) Minutes of IRB meetings which shall be in sufficient detail to show attendance at the meetings; actions taken by the IRB; the vote on these actions including the number of members voting for, against, and abstaining; the basis for requiring changes in or disapproving research; and a written summary of the discussion of controverted issues and their resolution.

(3) Records of continuing review activities.

(4) Copies of all correspondence between the IRB and the investigators.

(5) A list of IRB members in the same detail as described in §46.103(b)(3).

(6) Written procedures for the IRB in the same detail as described in §46.103(b)(4) and §46.103(b)(5).

(7) Statements of significant new findings provided to subjects, as required by §46.116(b)(5).

(b) The records required by this policy shall be retained for at least 3 years, and records relating to research which is conducted shall be retained for at least 3 years after completion of the research. All records shall be accessible for inspection and copying by authorized representatives of the Department or Agency at reasonable times and in a reasonable manner.

(Approved by the Office of Management and Budget under Control Number 9999-0020.)

§46.116 GENERAL REQUIREMENTS
FOR INFORMED CONSENT.

Except as provided elsewhere in this policy, no investigator may involve a human being as a subject in research covered by this policy unless the investigator has obtained the legally effective informed consent of the subject or the subject's legally authorized representative. An investigator shall seek such consent only under circumstances that provide the prospective subject or the representative sufficient opportunity to consider whether or not to participate and that minimize the possibility of coercion or undue influence. The information that is given to the subject or the representative shall be in language understandable to the subject or the representative. No informed consent, whether oral or written, may include any exculpatory language through which the subject or the representative is made to waive or appear to waive any of the subject's legal rights, or releases or appears to release the investigator, the sponsor, the institution or its agents from liability for negligence.

(a) Basic elements of informed consent. Except as provided in paragraph (c) or (d) of this section, in seeking informed consent the following information shall be provided to each subject:

(1) a statement that the study involves research, an explanation of the purposes of the research and the expected duration of the subject's participation, a description of the procedures to be followed, and identification of any procedures which are experimental;

(2) a description of any reasonably foreseeable risks or discomforts to the subject;

(3) a description of any benefits to the subject or to others which may reasonably be expected from the research;

(4) a disclosure of appropriate alternative procedures or courses of treatment, if any, that might be advantageous to the subject;

(5) a statement describing the extent, if any, to which confidentiality of records identifying the subject will be maintained;

(6) for research involving more than minimal risk, an explanation as to whether any compensation and an explanation as to whether any medical treatments are available if injury occurs and, if so, what they consist of, or where further information may be obtained;

(7) an explanation of whom to contact for answers to pertinent questions about the research and research subjects' rights, and whom to contact in the event of a research-related injury to the subject; and

(8) a statement that participation is voluntary, refusal to participate will involve no penalty or loss of benefits to which the subject is otherwise entitled, and the subject may discontinue participation at any time without penalty or loss of benefits to which the subject is otherwise entitled.

(b) Additional elements of informed consent. When appropriate, one or more of the following elements of information shall also be provided to each subject:

(1) a statement that the particular treatment or procedure may involve risks to the subject (or to the embryo or fetus, if the subject is or may become pregnant) which are currently unforeseeable;

(2) anticipated circumstances under which the subject's participation may be terminated by the investigator without regard to the subject's consent;

(3) any additional costs to the subject that may result from participation in the research;

(4) the consequences of a subject's decision to withdraw from the research and procedures for orderly termination of participation by the subject;

(5) a statement that significant new findings developed during the course of the research which may relate to the subject's willingness to continue participation will be provided to the subject; and

(6) the approximate number of subjects involved in the study.

(c) An IRB may approve a consent procedure which does not include, or which alters, some or all of the elements of informed consent set forth above, or waive the requirement to obtain informed consent provided the IRB finds and documents that:

(1) the research or demonstration project is to be conducted by or subject to the approval of state or local government officials and is designed to study, evaluate, or otherwise examine: (i) public benefit or service programs; (ii) procedures for obtaining benefits or services under those programs; (iii) possible changes in or alternatives to those programs or procedures; or (iv) possible changes in methods or levels of payment for benefits or services under those programs; and

(2) the research could not practicably be carried out without the waiver or alteration.

(d) An IRB may approve a consent procedure which does not include, or which alters, some or all of the elements of informed consent set forth in this section, or waive the requirements to obtain informed consent provided the IRB finds and documents that:

(1) the research involves no more than minimal risk to the subjects;

(2) the waiver or alteration will not adversely affect the rights and welfare of the subjects;

(3) the research could not practically be carried out without the waiver or alteration; and

(4) whenever appropriate, the subjects will be provided with additional pertinent information after participation.

(e) The informed consent requirements in this policy are not intended to preempt any applicable Federal, State, or local laws which require additional information to be disclosed in order for informed consent to be legally effective.

(f) Nothing in this policy is intended to limit the authority of a physician to provide emergency medical care, to the extent the physician is permitted to do so under applicable Federal, State, or local law.

(Approved by the Office of Management and Budget under Control Number 9999-0020.)

§46.117 DOCUMENTATION OF INFORMED CONSENT.

(a) Except as provided in paragraph (c) of this section, informed consent shall be documented by the use of a written consent form approved by the IRB and signed by the subject or the subject's legally authorized representative. A copy shall be given to the person signing the form.

(b) Except as provided in paragraph (c) of this section, the consent form may be either of the following:

(1) A written consent document that embodies the elements of informed consent required by §46.116. This form may be read to the subject or the subject's legally authorized representative, but in any event, the investigator shall give either the subject or the representative adequate opportunity to read it before it is signed; or

(2) A short form written consent document stating that the elements of informed consent required by §46.116 have been presented orally to the subject or the subject's legally authorized representative. When this method is used, there shall be a

witness to the oral presentation. Also, the IRB shall approve a written summary of what is to be said to the subject or the representative. Only the short form itself is to be signed by the subject or the representative. However, the witness shall sign both the short form and a copy of the summary, and the person actually obtaining consent shall sign a copy of the summary. A copy of the summary shall be given to the subject or the representative, in addition to a copy of the short form.

(c) An IRB may waive the requirement for the investigator to obtain a signed consent form for some or all subjects if it finds either:

(1) That the only record linking the subject and the research would be the consent document and the principal risk would be potential harm resulting from a breach of confidentiality. Each subject will be asked whether the subject wants documentation linking the subject with the research, and the subject's wishes will govern; or

(2) That the research presents no more than minimal risk of harm to subjects and involves no procedures for which written consent is normally required outside of the research context.

In cases in which the documentation requirement is waived, the IRB may require the investigator to provide subjects with a written statement regarding the research.

(Approved by the Office of Management and Budget under Control Number 9999-0020.)

§46.118 APPLICATIONS AND PROPOSALS LACKING DEFINITE PLANS FOR INVOLVEMENT OF HUMAN SUBJECTS.

Certain types of applications for grants, cooperative agreements, or contracts are submitted to departments or agencies with the knowledge that subjects may be involved within the period of support, but definite plans would not normally be set forth in the application or proposal. These include activities such as institutional type grants when selection of specific projects is the institution's responsibility; research training grants in which the activities involving subjects remain to be selected; and projects in which human subjects' involvement will depend upon completion of instruments, prior animal studies, or purification of compounds. These applications need not be reviewed by an IRB before an award may be made. However, except for research exempted or waived under §46.101(b) or (i), no human subjects may be involved in any project supported by these awards until the project has been reviewed and approved by the IRB, as provided in this policy, and certification submitted, by the institution, to the Department or Agency.

§46.119 RESEARCH UNDERTAKEN WITHOUT THE INTENTION OF INVOLVING HUMAN SUBJECTS.

In the event research is undertaken without the intention of involving human subjects, but it is later proposed to involve human subjects in the research, the research shall first be reviewed and approved by an IRB, as provided in this policy, a certification submitted, by the institution, to the Department or Agency, and final approval given to the proposed change by the Department or Agency.

§46.120 EVALUATION AND DISPOSITION OF APPLICATIONS AND PROPOSALS FOR RESEARCH TO BE CONDUCTED OR SUPPORTED BY A FEDERAL DEPARTMENT OR AGENCY.

(a) The Department or Agency head will evaluate all applications and proposals involving human subjects submitted to the Department or Agency through such officers and employees of the Department or Agency and such experts and consultants as the Department or Agency head determines to be appropriate. This evaluation will take into consideration the risks to the subjects, the adequacy of protection against these risks, the potential benefits of the research to the subjects and others, and the importance of the knowledge gained or to be gained.

(b) On the basis of this evaluation, the Department or Agency head may approve or disapprove the application or proposal, or enter into negotiations to develop an approvable one.

§46.121 [RESERVED]

§46.122 USE OF FEDERAL FUNDS.

Federal funds administered by a Department or Agency may not be expended for research involving human subjects unless the requirements of this policy have been satisfied.

§46.123 EARLY TERMINATION OF RESEARCH SUPPORT: EVALUATION OF APPLICATIONS AND PROPOSALS.

(a) The Department or Agency head may require that Department or Agency support for any project be terminated or suspended in the manner prescribed in applicable program requirements, when the

Department or Agency head finds an institution has materially failed to comply with the terms of this policy.

(b) In making decisions about supporting or approving applications or proposals covered by this policy the Department or Agency head may take into account, in addition to all other eligibility requirements and program criteria, factors such as whether the applicant has been subject to a termination or suspension under paragraph (a) of this section and whether the applicant or the person or persons who would direct or has/have directed the scientific and technical aspects of an activity has/have, in the judgment of the Department or Agency head, materially failed to discharge responsibility for the protection of the rights and welfare of human subjects (whether or not the research was subject to Federal regulation).

§46.124 CONDITIONS.

With respect to any research project or any class of research projects the Department or Agency head may impose additional conditions prior to or at the time of approval when in the judgment of the Department or Agency head additional conditions are necessary for the protection of human subjects.

SUBPART B—ADDITIONAL PROTECTIONS FOR PREGNANT WOMEN, HUMAN FETUSES AND NEONATES INVOLVED IN RESEARCH

Source: Federal Register: November 13, 2001 (Volume 66, Number 219), Rules and Regulations, Pages 56775–56780.

§46.201 TO WHAT DO THESE REGULATIONS APPLY?

(a) Except as provided in paragraph (b) of this section, this subpart applies to all research involving pregnant women, human fetuses, neonates of uncertain viability, or nonviable neonates conducted or supported by the Department of Health and Human Services (DHHS). This includes all research conducted in DHHS facilities by any person and all research conducted in any facility by DHHS employees.

(b) The exemptions at Sec. 46.101(b)(1) through (6) are applicable to this subpart.

(c) The provisions of Sec. 46.101(c) through (i) are applicable to this subpart. Reference to State or local laws in this subpart and in Sec. 46.101(f) is intended to include the laws of federally recognized American Indian and Alaska Native Tribal Governments.

(d) The requirements of this subpart are in addition to those imposed under the other subparts of this part.

§46.202 DEFINITIONS.

The definitions in Sec. 46.102 shall be applicable to this subpart as well. In addition, as used in this subpart:

(a) "Dead fetus" means a fetus that exhibits neither heartbeat, spontaneous respiratory activity, spontaneous movement of voluntary muscles, nor pulsation of the umbilical cord.

(b) "Delivery" means complete separation of the fetus from the woman by expulsion or extraction or any other means.

(c) "Fetus" means the product of conception from implantation until delivery.

(d) "Neonate" means a newborn.

(e) "Nonviable neonate" means a neonate after delivery that, although living, is not viable.

(f) "Pregnancy" encompasses the period of time from implantation until delivery. A woman shall be assumed to be pregnant if she exhibits any of the pertinent presumptive signs of pregnancy, such as missed menses, until the results of a pregnancy test are negative or until delivery.

(g) "Secretary" means the Secretary of Health and Human Services and any other officer or employee of the Department of Health and Human Services to whom authority has been delegated.

(h) "Viable," as it pertains to the neonate, means being able, after delivery, to survive (given the benefit of available medical therapy) to the point of independently maintaining heartbeat and respiration. The Secretary may from time to time, taking into account medical advances, publish in the *Federal Register* guidelines to assist in determining whether a neonate is viable for purposes of this subpart. If a neonate is viable then it may be included in research only to the extent permitted and in accordance with the requirements of subparts A and D of this part.

§46.203 DUTIES OF IRBS IN CONNECTION WITH RESEARCH INVOLVING PREGNANT WOMEN, FETUSES, AND NEONATES.

In addition to other responsibilities assigned to IRBs under this part, each IRB shall review research covered by this subpart and approve only research which satisfies the conditions of all applicable sections of this subpart and the other subparts of this part.

§46.204 RESEARCH INVOLVING PREGNANT WOMEN OR FETUSES.

Pregnant women or fetuses may be involved in research if all of the following conditions are met:

(a) Where scientifically appropriate, preclinical studies, including studies on pregnant animals, and clinical studies, including studies on nonpregnant women, have been conducted and provide data for assessing potential risks to pregnant women and fetuses;

(b) The risk to the fetus is caused solely by interventions or procedures that hold out the prospect of direct benefit for the woman or the fetus; or, if there is no such prospect of benefit, the risk to the fetus is not greater than minimal and the purpose of the research is the development of important biomedical knowledge which cannot be obtained by any other means;

(c) Any risk is the least possible for achieving the objectives of the research;

(d) If the research holds out the prospect of direct benefit to the pregnant woman, the prospect of a direct benefit both to the pregnant woman and the fetus, or no prospect of benefit for the woman nor the fetus when risk to the fetus is not greater than minimal and the purpose of the research is the development of important biomedical knowledge that cannot be obtained by any other means, her consent is obtained in accord with the informed consent provisions of subpart A of this part;

(e) If the research holds out the prospect of direct benefit solely to the fetus then the consent of the pregnant woman and the father is obtained in accord with the informed consent provisions of subpart A of this part, except that the father's consent need not be obtained if he is unable to consent because of unavailability, incompetence, or temporary incapacity or the pregnancy resulted from rape or incest.

(f) Each individual providing consent under paragraph (d) or (e) of this section is fully informed regarding the reasonably foreseeable impact of the research on the fetus or neonate;

(g) For children as defined in Sec. 46.402(a) who are pregnant, assent and permission are obtained in accord with the provisions of subpart D of this part;

(h) No inducements, monetary or otherwise, will be offered to terminate a pregnancy;

(i) Individuals engaged in the research will have no part in any decisions as to the timing, method, or procedures used to terminate a pregnancy; and

(j) Individuals engaged in the research will have no part in determining the viability of a neonate.

§46.205 RESEARCH INVOLVING NEONATES.

(a) Neonates of uncertain viability and nonviable neonates may be involved in research if all of the following conditions are met:

(1) Where scientifically appropriate, preclinical and clinical studies have been conducted and provide data for assessing potential risks to neonates.

(2) Each individual providing consent under paragraph (b)(2) or (c)(5) of this section is fully informed regarding the reasonably foreseeable impact of the research on the neonate.

(3) Individuals engaged in the research will have no part in determining the viability of a neonate.

(4) The requirements of paragraph (b) or (c) of this section have been met as applicable.

(b) Neonates of uncertain viability. Until it has been ascertained whether or not a neonate is viable, a neonate may not be involved in research covered by this subpart unless the following additional conditions have been met:

(1) The IRB determines that:

(i) The research holds out the prospect of enhancing the probability of survival of the neonate to the point of viability, and any risk is the least possible for achieving that objective, or

(ii) The purpose of the research is the development of important biomedical knowledge which cannot be obtained by other means and there will be no added risk to the neonate resulting from the research; and

(2) The legally effective informed consent of either parent of the neonate or, if neither parent is able to consent because of unavailability, incompetence, or temporary incapacity, the legally effective informed consent of either parent's legally authorized representative is obtained in accord with subpart A of this part, except that the consent of the father or his legally authorized representative need not be obtained if the pregnancy resulted from rape or incest.

(c) Nonviable neonates. After delivery nonviable neonates may not be involved in research covered by this subpart unless all of the following additional conditions are met:

(1) Vital functions of the neonate will not be artificially maintained;

(2) The research will not terminate the heartbeat or respiration of the neonate;

(3) There will be no added risk to the neonate resulting from the research;

(4) The purpose of the research is the development of important biomedical knowledge that cannot be obtained by other means; and

(5) The legally effective informed consent of both parents of the neonate is obtained in accord with subpart A of this part, except that the waiver and alteration provisions of Sec. 46.116(c) and (d) do not apply. However, if either parent is unable to consent because of unavailability, incompetence, or temporary incapacity, the informed consent of one parent of a nonviable neonate will suffice to meet the requirements of this paragraph (c)(5), except that the consent of the father need not be obtained if the pregnancy resulted from rape or incest. The consent of a legally authorized representative of either or both of the parents of a nonviable neonate will not suffice to meet the requirements of this paragraph (c)(5).

(d) Viable neonates. A neonate, after delivery, that has been determined to be viable may be included in research only to the extent permitted by and in accord with the requirements of subparts A and D of this part.

§46.206 RESEARCH INVOLVING, AFTER DELIVERY, THE PLACENTA, THE DEAD FETUS, OR FETAL MATERIAL.

(a) Research involving, after delivery, the placenta; the dead fetus; macerated fetal material; or cells, tissue, or organs excised from a dead fetus, shall be conducted only in accord with any applicable Federal, State, or local laws and regulations regarding such activities.

(b) If information associated with material described in paragraph (a) of this section is recorded for research purposes in a manner that living individuals can be identified, directly or through identifiers linked to those individuals, those individuals are research subjects and all pertinent subparts of this part are applicable.

§46.207 RESEARCH NOT OTHERWISE APPROVABLE WHICH PRESENTS AN OPPORTUNITY TO UNDERSTAND, PREVENT, OR ALLEVIATE A SERIOUS PROBLEM AFFECTING THE HEALTH OR WELFARE OF PREGNANT WOMEN, FETUSES, OR NEONATES.

The Secretary will conduct or fund research that the IRB does not believe meets the requirements of Sec. 46.204 or Sec. 46.205 only if:

(a) The IRB finds that the research presents a reasonable opportunity to further the understanding, prevention, or alleviation of a serious problem affecting the health or welfare of pregnant women, fetuses, or neonates; and

(b) The Secretary, after consultation with a panel of experts in pertinent disciplines (for example: science, medicine, ethics, law) and following opportunity for public review and comment, including a public meeting announced in the *Federal Register,* has determined either:

  (1) That the research in fact satisfies the conditions of Sec. 46.204, as applicable; or

  (2) The following:

    (i) The research presents a reasonable opportunity to further the understanding, prevention, or alleviation of a serious problem affecting the health or welfare of pregnant women, fetuses or neonates;

    (ii) The research will be conducted in accord with sound ethical principles; and

    (iii) Informed consent will be obtained in accord with the informed consent provisions of subpart A and other applicable subparts of this part.

SUBPART C—ADDITIONAL DHHS PROTECTIONS PERTAINING TO BIOMEDICAL AND BEHAVIORAL RESEARCH INVOLVING PRISONERS AS SUBJECTS

Source: 43 FR [Federal Register] 53655, Nov. 16, 1978.

§46.301 APPLICABILITY.

(a) The regulations in this subpart are applicable to all biomedical and behavioral research conducted or supported by the Department of Health and Human Services involving prisoners as subjects.

(b) Nothing in this subpart shall be construed as indicating that compliance with the procedures set forth herein will authorize research involving prisoners as subjects, to the extent such research is limited or barred by applicable State or local law.

(c) The requirements of this subpart are in addition to those imposed under the other subparts of this part.

§46.302 PURPOSE.

Inasmuch as prisoners may be under constraints because of their incarceration which could affect their ability to make a truly voluntary and uncoerced decision whether or not to participate as subjects in research, it is the purpose of this subpart to provide additional safeguards for the protection of prisoners involved in activities to which this subpart is applicable.

§46.303 DEFINITIONS.

As used in this subpart:

(a) "Secretary" means the Secretary of Health and Human Services and any other officer or employee of the Department of Health and Human Services to whom authority has been delegated.

(b) "DHHS" means the Department of Health and Human Services.

(c) "Prisoner" means any individual involuntarily confined or detained in a penal institution. The term is intended to encompass individuals sentenced to such an institution under a criminal or civil statute, individuals detained in other facilities by virtue of statutes or commitment procedures which provide alternatives to criminal prosecution or incarceration in a penal institution, and individuals detained pending arraignment, trial, or sentencing.

(d) "Minimal risk" is the probability and magnitude of physical or psychological harm that is normally encountered in the daily lives, or in the routine medical, dental, or psychological examination of healthy persons.

§46.304 COMPOSITION OF INSTITUTIONAL REVIEW BOARDS WHERE PRISONERS ARE INVOLVED.

In addition to satisfying the requirements in §46.107 of this part, an Institutional Review Board, carrying out responsibilities under this part with respect to research covered by this subpart, shall also meet the following specific requirements:

(a) A majority of the Board (exclusive of prisoner members) shall have no association with the prison(s) involved, apart from their membership on the Board.

(b) At least one member of the Board shall be a prisoner, or a prisoner representative with appropriate background and experience to serve in that capacity, except that where a particular research project is reviewed by more than one Board only one Board need satisfy this requirement.

§46.305 ADDITIONAL DUTIES OF THE INSTITUTIONAL REVIEW BOARDS WHERE PRISONERS ARE INVOLVED.

(a) In addition to all other responsibilities prescribed for Institutional Review Boards under this part, the Board shall review research covered by this subpart and approve such research only if it finds that:

(1) the research under review represents one of the categories of research permissible under §46.306(a)(2);

(2) any possible advantages accruing to the prisoner through his or her participation in the research, when compared to the general living conditions, medical care, quality of food, amenities, and opportunity for earnings in the prison, are not of such a magnitude that his or her ability to weigh the risks of the research against the value of such advantages in the limited choice environment of the prison is impaired;

(3) the risks involved in the research are commensurate with risks that would be accepted by non-prisoner volunteers;

(4) procedures for the selection of subjects within the prison are fair to all prisoners and immune from arbitrary intervention by prison authorities or prisoners. Unless the principal investigator provides to the Board justification in writing for following some other procedures, control subjects must be selected randomly from the group of available prisoners who meet the characteristics needed for that particular research project;

(5) the information is presented in language which is understandable to the subject population;

(6) adequate assurance exists that parole boards will not take into account a prisoner's participation in the research in making decisions regarding parole, and each prisoner is clearly informed in advance that participation in the research will have no effect on his or her parole; and

(7) where the Board finds there may be a need for follow-up examination or care of participants after the end of their participation, adequate provision has been made for such examination or care, taking into account the varying lengths of individual prisoners' sentences, and for informing participants of this fact.

(b) The Board shall carry out such other duties as may be assigned by the Secretary.

(c) The institution shall certify to the Secretary, in such form and manner as the Secretary may require, that the duties of the Board under this section have been fulfilled.

§46.306 PERMITTED RESEARCH INVOLVING PRISONERS.

(a) Biomedical or behavioral research conducted or supported by DHHS may involve prisoners as subjects only if:

(1) the institution responsible for the conduct of the research has certified to the Secretary that the Institutional Review Board has approved the research under §46.305 of this subpart; and

(2) in the judgment of the Secretary the proposed research involves solely the following:

(A) study of the possible causes, effects, and processes of incarceration, and of criminal behavior, provided that the study presents no more than minimal risk and no more than inconvenience to the subjects;

(B) study of prisons as institutional structures or of prisoners as incarcerated persons, provided that the study presents no more than minimal risk and no more than inconvenience to the subjects;

(C) research on conditions particularly affecting prisoners as a class (for example, vaccine trials and other research on hepatitis which is much more prevalent in prisons than elsewhere; and research on social and psychological problems such as alcoholism, drug addiction, and sexual assaults) provided that the study may proceed only after the Secretary has consulted with appropriate experts including experts in penology, medicine, and ethics, and published notice, in the

Federal Register, of his intent to approve such research; or

(D) research on practices, both innovative and accepted, which have the intent and reasonable probability of improving the health or well-being of the subject. In cases in which those studies require the assignment of prisoners in a manner consistent with protocols approved by the IRB to control groups which may not benefit from the research, the study may proceed only after the Secretary has consulted with appropriate experts, including experts in penology, medicine, and ethics, and published notice, in the *Federal Register,* of the intent to approve such research.

(b) Except as provided in paragraph (a) of this section, biomedical or behavioral research conducted or supported by DHHS shall not involve prisoners as subjects.

SUBPART D—ADDITIONAL DHHS PROTECTIONS FOR CHILDREN INVOLVED AS SUBJECTS IN RESEARCH

Source: 48 FR [Federal Register] 9818, March 8, 1983; 56 FR [Federal Register] 28032, June 18, 1991.

§46.401 TO WHAT DO THESE REGULATIONS APPLY?

(a) This subpart applies to all research involving children as subjects, conducted or supported by the Department of Health and Human Services.

(1) This includes research conducted by Department employees, except that each head of an Operating Division of the Department may adopt such nonsubstantive, procedural modifications as may be appropriate from an administrative standpoint.

(2) It also includes research conducted or supported by the Department of Health and Human Services outside the United States, but in appropriate circumstances, the Secretary may, under paragraph (i) of §46.101 of Subpart A, waive the applicability of some or all of the requirements of these regulations for research of this type.

(b) Exemptions at §46.101(b)(1) and (b)(3) through (b)(6) are applicable to this subpart. The exemption

at §46.101(b)(2) regarding educational tests is also applicable to this subpart. However, the exemption at §46.101(b)(2) for research involving survey or interview procedures or observations of public behavior does not apply to research covered by this subpart, except for research involving observation of public behavior when the investigator(s) do not participate in the activities being observed.

(c) The exceptions, additions, and provisions for waiver as they appear in paragraphs (c) through (i) of §46.101 of Subpart A are applicable to this subpart.

§46.402 DEFINITIONS.

The definitions in §46.102 of Subpart A shall be applicable to this subpart as well. In addition, as used in this subpart:

(a) "Children" are persons who have not attained the legal age for consent to treatments or procedures involved in the research, under the applicable law of the jurisdiction in which the research will be conducted.

(b) "Assent" means a child's affirmative agreement to participate in research. Mere failure to object should not, absent affirmative agreement, be construed as assent.

(c) "Permission" means the agreement of parent(s) or guardian to the participation of their child or ward in research.

(d) "Parent" means a child's biological or adoptive parent.

(e) "Guardian" means an individual who is authorized under applicable State or local law to consent on behalf of a child to general medical care.

§46.403 IRB DUTIES.

In addition to other responsibilities assigned to IRBs under this part, each IRB shall review research covered by this subpart and approve only research which satisfies the conditions of all applicable sections of this subpart.

§46.404 RESEARCH NOT INVOLVING GREATER THAN MINIMAL RISK.

DHHS will conduct or fund research in which the IRB finds that no greater than minimal risk to children is presented, only if the IRB finds that adequate provisions are made for soliciting the assent of the children and the permission of their parents or guardians, as set forth in §46.408.

§46.405 RESEARCH INVOLVING GREATER THAN MINIMAL RISK BUT PRESENTING THE PROSPECT OF DIRECT BENEFIT TO THE INDIVIDUAL SUBJECTS.

DHHS will conduct or fund research in which the IRB finds that more than minimal risk to children is presented by an intervention or procedure that holds out the prospect of direct benefit for the individual subject, or by a monitoring procedure that is likely to contribute to the subject's well-being, only if the IRB finds that:

(a) the risk is justified by the anticipated benefit to the subjects;

(b) the relation of the anticipated benefit to the risk is at least as favorable to the subjects as that presented by available alternative approaches; and

(c) adequate provisions are made for soliciting the assent of the children and permission of their parents or guardians, as set forth in §46.408.

§46.406 RESEARCH INVOLVING GREATER THAN MINIMAL RISK AND NO PROSPECT OF DIRECT BENEFIT TO INDIVIDUAL SUBJECTS, BUT LIKELY TO YIELD GENERALIZABLE KNOWLEDGE ABOUT THE SUBJECT'S DISORDER OR CONDITION.

DHHS will conduct or fund research in which the IRB finds that more than minimal risk to children is presented by an intervention or procedure that does not hold out the prospect of direct benefit for the individual subject, or by a monitoring procedure which is not likely to contribute to the well-being of the subject, only if the IRB finds that:

(a) the risk represents a minor increase over minimal risk;

(b) the intervention or procedure presents experiences to subjects that are reasonably commensurate with those inherent in their actual or expected medical, dental, psychological, social, or educational situations;

(c) the intervention or procedure is likely to yield generalizable knowledge about the subjects' disorder or condition which is of vital importance for the understanding or amelioration of the subjects' disorder or condition; and

(d) adequate provisions are made for soliciting assent of the children and permission of their parents or guardians, as set forth in §46.408.

§46.407 RESEARCH NOT OTHERWISE APPROVABLE WHICH PRESENTS AN OPPORTUNITY TO UNDERSTAND, PREVENT, OR ALLEVIATE A SERIOUS PROBLEM AFFECTING THE HEALTH OR WELFARE OF CHILDREN.

DHHS will conduct or fund research that the IRB does not believe meets the requirements of §46.404, §46.405, or §46.406 only if:

(a) the IRB finds that the research presents a reasonable opportunity to further the understanding, prevention, or alleviation of a serious problem affecting the health or welfare of children; and

(b) the Secretary, after consultation with a panel of experts in pertinent disciplines (for example: science, medicine, education, ethics, law) and following opportunity for public review and comment, has determined either:

(1) that the research in fact satisfies the conditions of §46.404, §46.405, or §46.406, as applicable, or

(2) the following:

(i) the research presents a reasonable opportunity to further the understanding, prevention, or alleviation of a serious problem affecting the health or welfare of children;

(ii) the research will be conducted in accordance with sound ethical principles;

(iii) adequate provisions are made for soliciting the assent of children and the permission of their parents or guardians, as set forth in §46.408.

§46.408 REQUIREMENTS FOR PERMISSION BY PARENTS OR GUARDIANS AND FOR ASSENT BY CHILDREN.

(a) In addition to the determinations required under other applicable sections of this subpart, the IRB shall determine that adequate provisions are made for soliciting the assent of the children, when in the judgment of the IRB the children are capable of providing assent. In determining whether children are capable of assenting, the IRB shall take into account the ages, maturity, and psychological state of the children involved. This judgment may be made for all children to be involved in research under a particular protocol, or for each child, as the IRB deems appropriate. If the IRB determines that the capability of some or all of the children is so limited that they cannot reasonably be consulted or that the intervention or procedure involved in the research holds out a prospect of direct benefit that is important to the health or well-being of the children and is available only in the context of the research, the assent of the children is not a necessary condition for proceeding with the research. Even where the IRB determines that the subjects are capable of assenting, the IRB may still waive the assent requirement under circumstances in which consent may be waived in accord with §46.116 of Subpart A.

(b) In addition to the determinations required under other applicable sections of this subpart, the IRB shall determine, in accordance with and to the extent that consent is required by §46.116 of Subpart A, that adequate provisions are made for soliciting the permission of each child's parents or guardian. Where parental permission is to be obtained, the IRB may find that the permission of one parent is sufficient for research to be conducted under §46.404 or §46.405. Where research is covered by §46.406 and §46.407 and permission is to be obtained from parents, both parents must give their permission unless one parent is deceased, unknown, incompetent, or not reasonably available, or when only one parent has legal responsibility for the care and custody of the child.

(c) In addition to the provisions for waiver contained in §46.116 of Subpart A, if the IRB determines that a research protocol is designed for conditions or for a subject population for which parental or guardian permission is not a reasonable requirement to protect the subjects (for example, neglected or abused children), it may waive the consent requirements in Subpart A of this part and paragraph (b) of this section, provided an appropriate mechanism for protecting the children who will participate as subjects in the research is substituted, and provided further that the waiver is not inconsistent with Federal, State, or local law. The choice of an appropriate mechanism would depend upon the nature and purpose of the activities described in the protocol, the risk and anticipated benefit to the research subjects, and their age, maturity, status, and condition.

(d) Permission by parents or guardians shall be documented in accordance with and to the extent required by §46.117 of Subpart A.

(e) When the IRB determines that assent is required, it shall also determine whether and how assent must be documented.

§46.409 WARDS.

(a) Children who are wards of the State or any other agency, institution, or entity can be included in research approved under §46.406 or §46.407 only if such research is:

(1) related to their status as wards; or

(2) conducted in schools, camps, hospitals, institutions, or similar settings in which the majority of children involved as subjects are not wards.

(b) If the research is approved under paragraph (a) of this section, the IRB shall require appointment of an advocate for each child who is a ward, in addition to any other individual acting on behalf of the child as guardian or in loco parentis. One individual may serve as advocate for more than one child. The advocate shall be an individual who has the background and experience to act in, and agrees to act in, the best interests of the child for the duration of the child's participation in the research and who is not associated in any way (except in the role as advocate or member of the IRB) with the research, the investigator(s), or the guardian organization.

9 The International Ethical Guidelines for Biomedical Research Involving Human Subjects

THE COUNCIL FOR INTERNATIONAL ORGANIZATIONS
OF MEDICAL SCIENCES (CIOMS) IN COLLABORATION
WITH THE WORLD HEALTH ORGANIZATION (WHO)

GUIDELINE 1: ETHICAL JUSTIFICATION AND SCIENTIFIC VALIDITY OF BIOMEDICAL RESEARCH INVOLVING HUMAN BEINGS

The ethical justification of biomedical research involving human subjects is the prospect of discovering new ways of benefiting people's health. Such research can be ethically justifiable only if it is carried out in ways that respect and protect, and are fair to, the subjects of that research and are morally acceptable within the communities in which the research is carried out. Moreover, because scientifically invalid research is unethical in that it exposes research subjects to risks without possible benefit, investigators and sponsors must ensure that proposed studies involving human subjects conform to generally accepted scientific principles and are based on adequate knowledge of the pertinent scientific literature.

Commentary on Guideline 1

Among the essential features of ethically justified research involving human subjects, including research with identifiable human tissue or data, are that the research offers a means of developing information not otherwise obtainable, that the design of the research is scientifically sound, and that the investigators and other research personnel are competent. The methods to be used should be appropriate to the objectives of the research and the field of study. Investigators and sponsors must also ensure that all who participate in the conduct of the research are qualified by virtue of their education and experience to perform competently in their roles. These considerations should be adequately reflected in the research protocol submitted for review and clearance to scientific and ethical review committees [...] .

CIOMS in collaboration with WHO, International Ethical Guidelines for Biomedical Research Involving Human Subjects (Geneva: 2002).

GUIDELINE 2: ETHICAL REVIEW COMMITTEES

All proposals to conduct research involving human subjects must be submitted for review of their scientific merit and ethical acceptability to one or more scientific review and ethical review committees. The review committees must be independent of the research team, and any direct financial or other material benefit they may derive from the research should not be contingent on the outcome of their review. The investigator must obtain their approval or clearance before undertaking the research. The ethical review committee should conduct further reviews as necessary in the course of the research, including monitoring of the progress of the study.

Commentary on Guideline 2

Ethical review committees may function at the institutional, local, regional, or national level, and in some cases at the international level. The regulatory or other governmental authorities concerned should promote uniform standards across committees within a country, and, under all systems, sponsors of research and institutions in which the investigators are employed should allocate sufficient resources to the review process. Ethical review committees may receive money for the activity of reviewing protocols, but under no circumstances may payment be offered or accepted for a review committee's approval or clearance of a protocol.

Scientific review. According to the Declaration of Helsinki (Paragraph 11), medical research involving humans must conform to generally accepted scientific principles, and be based on a thorough knowledge of the scientific literature, other relevant sources of information, and adequate laboratory and, where indicated, animal experimentation. Scientific review must consider, inter alia, the study design, including the provisions for avoiding or minimizing risk and for monitoring safety. Committees competent to review and approve scientific aspects of research proposals must be multidisciplinary.

Ethical review. The ethical review committee is responsible for safeguarding the rights, safety, and well-being of the research subjects. Scientific review and ethical review cannot be separated: scientifically unsound research involving humans as subjects is ipso facto unethical in that it may expose them to risk or inconvenience to no purpose; even if there is no risk of injury, wasting of subjects' and researchers' time in unproductive activities represents loss of a valuable resource. Normally, therefore, an ethical review committee considers both the scientific and the ethical aspects of proposed research. It must either carry out a proper scientific review or verify that a competent expert body has determined that the research is scientifically sound. Also, it considers provisions for monitoring of data and safety.

If the ethical review committee finds a research proposal scientifically sound, or verifies that a competent expert body has found it so, it should then consider whether any known or possible risks to the subjects are justified by the expected benefits, direct or indirect, and whether the proposed research methods will minimize harm and maximize benefit. (See Guideline 8 [. . .].) If the proposal is sound and the balance of risks to anticipated benefits is reasonable, the committee should then determine whether the procedures proposed for obtaining informed consent are satisfactory and those proposed for the selection of subjects are equitable.

Ethical review of emergency compassionate use of an investigational therapy. In some countries, drug regulatory authorities require that the so-called compassionate or humanitarian use of an investigational treatment be reviewed by an ethical review committee as though it were research. Exceptionally, a physician may undertake the compassionate use of an investigational therapy before obtaining the approval or clearance of an ethical review committee, provided three criteria are met: a patient needs emergency treatment, there is some evidence of possible effectiveness of the investigational treatment, and there is no other treatment available that is known to be equally effective or superior. Informed consent should be obtained according to the legal requirements and cultural standards of the community in which the intervention is carried out. Within one week the physician must report to the ethical review committee the details of the case and the action taken, and an independent health-care professional must confirm in writing to the ethical review committee the treating physician's judgment that the use of the investigational intervention was justified according to the three specified criteria. (See also Guideline 13 [. . .].)

National (centralized) or local review. Ethical review committees may be created under the aegis of national or local health administrations, national (or centralized)

medical research councils, or other nationally representative bodies. In a highly centralized administration a national, or centralized, review committee may be constituted for both the scientific and the ethical review of research protocols. In countries where medical research is not centrally administered, ethical review is more effectively and conveniently undertaken at a local or regional level. The authority of a local ethical review committee may be confined to a single institution or may extend to all institutions in which biomedical research is carried out within a defined geographical area. The basic responsibilities of ethical review committees are:

• to determine that all proposed interventions, particularly the administration of drugs and vaccines or the use of medical devices or procedures under development, are acceptably safe to be undertaken in humans or to verify that another competent expert body has done so;

• to determine that the proposed research is scientifically sound or to verify that another competent expert body has done so;

• to ensure that all other ethical concerns arising from a protocol are satisfactorily resolved both in principle and in practice;

• to consider the qualifications of the investigators, including education in the principles of research practice, and the conditions of the research site with a view to ensuring the safe conduct of the trial; and

• to keep records of decisions and to take measures to follow up on the conduct of ongoing research projects.

Committee membership. National or local ethical review committees should be so composed as to be able to provide complete and adequate review of the research proposals submitted to them. It is generally presumed that their membership should include physicians, scientists, and other professionals such as nurses, lawyers, ethicists, and clergy, as well as lay persons qualified to represent the cultural and moral values of the community and to ensure that the rights of the research subjects will be respected. They should include both men and women. When uneducated or illiterate persons form the focus of a study they should also be considered for membership or invited to be represented and have their views expressed.

A number of members should be replaced periodically with the aim of blending the advantages of experience with those of fresh perspectives.

A national or local ethical review committee responsible for reviewing and approving proposals for externally sponsored research should have among its members or consultants persons who are thoroughly familiar with the customs and traditions of the population or community concerned and sensitive to issues of human dignity.

Committees that often review research proposals directed at specific diseases or impairments, such as HIV/AIDS or paraplegia, should invite or hear the views of individuals or bodies representing patients with such diseases or impairments. Similarly, for research involving such subjects as children, students, elderly persons, or employees, committees should invite or hear the views of their representatives or advocates.

To maintain the review committee's independence from the investigators and sponsors and to avoid conflict of interest, any member with a special or particular, direct or indirect, interest in a proposal should not take part in its assessment if that interest could subvert the member's objective judgment. Members of ethical review committees should be held to the same standard of disclosure as scientific and medical research staff with regard to financial or other interests that could be construed as conflicts of interest. A practical way of avoiding such conflict of interest is for the committee to insist on a declaration of possible conflict of interest by any of its members. A member who makes such a declaration should then withdraw, if to do so is clearly the appropriate action to take, either at the member's own discretion or at the request of the other members. Before withdrawing, the member should be permitted to offer comments on the protocol or to respond to questions of other members.

Multi-centre research. Some research projects are designed to be conducted in a number of centres in different communities or countries. Generally, to ensure that the results will be valid, the study must be conducted in an identical way at each centre. Such studies include clinical trials, research designed for the evaluation of health service programmes, and various kinds of epidemiological research. For such studies, local ethical or scientific review committees are not normally authorized to change doses of drugs, to change inclusion or exclusion criteria, or to make other similar modifications. They should be fully empowered to prevent a study that they believe to be unethical. Moreover, changes that local review committees believe are necessary to protect the research subjects should be documented and reported to the research institution or sponsor responsible for the whole research programme for consideration and due action, to ensure that all other subjects can be protected and that the research will be valid across sites.

To ensure the validity of multi-centre research, any change in the protocol should be made at every collaborating centre or institution, or, failing this, explicit inter-centre comparability procedures must be introduced; changes made at some but not all will defeat the purpose of multi-centre research. For some multi-centre studies, scientific and ethical review may be facilitated by agreement among centres to accept the conclusions of a single review committee; its members could include a representative of the ethical review committee at each of the centres at which the research is to be conducted, as well as individuals competent to conduct scientific review. In other circumstances, a centralized review may be complemented by local review relating to the local participating investigators and institutions. The central committee could review the study from a scientific and ethical standpoint, and the local committees could verify the practicability of the study in their communities, including the infrastructures, the state of training, and ethical considerations of local significance.

In a large multi-centre trial, individual investigators will not have authority to act independently, with regard to data analysis or to preparation and publication of manuscripts, for instance. Such a trial usually has a set of committees which operate under the direction of a steering committee and are responsible for such functions and decisions. The function of the ethical review committee in such cases is to review the relevant plans with the aim of avoiding abuses.

Sanctions. Ethical review committees generally have no authority to impose sanctions on researchers who violate ethical standards in the conduct of research involving humans. They may, however, withdraw ethical approval of a research project if judged necessary. They should be required to monitor the implementation of an approved protocol and its progression, and to report to institutional or governmental authorities any serious or continuing non-compliance with ethical standards as they are reflected in protocols that they have approved or in the conduct of the studies. Failure to submit a protocol to the committee should be considered a clear and serious violation of ethical standards.

Sanctions imposed by governmental, institutional, professional, or other authorities possessing disciplinary power should be employed as a last resort. Preferred methods of control include cultivation of an atmosphere of mutual trust, and education and support to promote in researchers and in sponsors the capacity for ethical conduct of research.

Should sanctions become necessary, they should be directed at the non-compliant researchers or sponsors. They may include fines or suspension of eligibility to receive research funding, to use investigational interventions, or to practise medicine. Unless there are persuasive reasons to do otherwise, editors should refuse to publish the results of research conducted unethically, and retract any articles that are subsequently found to contain falsified or fabricated data or to have been based on unethical research. Drug regulatory authorities should consider refusal to accept unethically obtained data submitted in support of an application for authorization to market a product. Such sanctions, however, may deprive of benefit not only the errant researcher or sponsor but also that segment of society intended to benefit from the research; such possible consequences merit careful consideration.

Potential conflicts of interest related to project support. Increasingly, biomedical studies receive funding from commercial firms. Such sponsors have good reasons to support research methods that are ethically and scientifically acceptable, but cases have arisen in which the conditions of funding could have introduced bias. It may happen that investigators have little or no input into trial design, limited access to the raw data, or limited participation in data interpretation, or that the results of a clinical trial may not be published if they are unfavourable to the sponsor's product. This risk of bias may also be associated with other sources of support, such as government or foundations. As the persons directly responsible for their work, investigators should not enter into agreements that interfere unduly with their access to the data or their ability to analyse the data independently, to prepare manuscripts, or to publish them. Investigators must also disclose potential or apparent conflicts of interest on their part to the ethical review committee or to other institutional committees designed to evaluate and manage such conflicts. Ethical review committees should therefore ensure that these conditions are met. See also Multi-centre research, above.

GUIDELINE 3: ETHICAL REVIEW OF EXTERNALLY SPONSORED RESEARCH

An external sponsoring organization and individual investigators should submit the research protocol for ethical and scientific review in the country of the sponsoring organization, and the ethical standards applied should be no less stringent than they would be for research carried out in that country. The health authorities of the host country, as well as a national or local ethical review committee, should ensure that the proposed research is responsive to the health needs and priorities of the host country and meets the requisite ethical standards.

Commentary on Guideline 3

Definition. The term externally sponsored research refers to research undertaken in a host country but sponsored, financed, and sometimes wholly or partly carried out by an external international or national organization or pharmaceutical company with the collaboration or agreement of the appropriate authorities, institutions, and personnel of the host country.

Ethical and scientific review. Committees in both the country of the sponsor and the host country have respon-

sibility for conducting both scientific and ethical review, as well as the authority to withhold approval of research proposals that fail to meet their scientific or ethical standards. As far as possible, there must be assurance that the review is independent and that there is no conflict of interest that might affect the judgement of members of the review committees in relation to any aspect of the research. When the external sponsor is an international organization, its review of the research protocol must be in accordance with its own independent ethical-review procedures and standards.

Committees in the external sponsoring country or international organization have a special responsibility to determine whether the scientific methods are sound and suitable to the aims of the research; whether the drugs, vaccines, devices, or procedures to be studied meet adequate standards of safety; whether there is sound justification for conducting the research in the host country rather than in the country of the external sponsor or in another country; and whether the proposed research is in compliance with the ethical standards of the external sponsoring country or international organization.

Committees in the host country have a special responsibility to determine whether the objectives of the research are responsive to the health needs and priorities of that country. The ability to judge the ethical acceptability of various aspects of a research proposal requires a thorough understanding of a community's customs and traditions. The ethical review committee in the host country, therefore, must have as either members or consultants persons with such understanding; it will then be in a favourable position to determine the acceptability of the proposed means of obtaining informed consent and otherwise respecting the rights of prospective subjects as well as of the means proposed to protect the welfare of the research subjects. Such persons should be able, for example, to indicate suitable members of the community to serve as intermediaries between investigators and subjects, and to advise on whether material benefits or inducements may be regarded as appropriate in the light of a community's gift-exchange and other customs and traditions.

When a sponsor or investigator in one country proposes to carry out research in another, the ethical review committees in the two countries may, by agreement, undertake to review different aspects of the research protocol. In short, in respect of host countries either with developed capacity for independent ethical review or in which external sponsors and investigators are contributing substantially to such capacity, ethical review in the external, sponsoring country may be limited to ensuring compliance with broadly stated ethical standards. The ethical review committee in the host country can be expected to have greater competence for reviewing the detailed plans for compliance, in view of its better understanding of the cultural and moral values of the population in which it is proposed to conduct the research; it is also likely to be in a better position to monitor compliance in the course of a study. However, in respect of research in host countries with inadequate capacity for independent ethical review, full review by the ethical review committee in the external sponsoring country or international agency is necessary.

GUIDELINE 4: INDIVIDUAL INFORMED CONSENT

For all biomedical research involving humans the investigator must obtain the voluntary informed consent of the prospective subject or, in the case of an individual who is not capable of giving informed consent, the permission of a legally authorized representative in accordance with applicable law. Waiver of informed consent is to be regarded as uncommon and exceptional, and must in all cases be approved by an ethical review committee.

Commentary on Guideline 4

General considerations. Informed consent is a decision to participate in research, taken by a competent individual who has received the necessary information; who has adequately understood the information; and who, after considering the information, has arrived at a decision without having been subjected to coercion, undue influence or inducement, or intimidation.

Informed consent is based on the principle that competent individuals are entitled to choose freely whether to participate in research. Informed consent protects the individual's freedom of choice and respects the individual's autonomy. As an additional safeguard, it must always be complemented by independent ethical review of research proposals. This safeguard of independent review is particularly important as many individuals are limited in their capacity to give adequate informed consent; they include young children, adults with severe mental or behavioural disorders, and persons who are unfamiliar with medical concepts and technology (see Guidelines 13, 14, 15).

Process. Obtaining informed consent is a process that is begun when initial contact is made with a prospective subject and continues throughout the course of the study. By informing the prospective subjects, by repetition and explanation, by answering their questions as they arise, and by ensuring that each individual understands each procedure, investigators elicit their informed consent and in so doing manifest respect for their dignity and autonomy. Each individual must be given as much time as is needed to reach a decision, including time for consultation with family members or others. Adequate time and resources should be set aside for informed-consent procedures.

Language. Informing the individual subject must not be simply a ritual recitation of the contents of a written document. Rather, the investigator must convey the information, whether orally or in writing, in language that suits the individual's level of understanding. The investigator must bear in mind that the prospective subject's ability to understand the information necessary to give informed consent depends on that individual's maturity, intelligence, education, and belief system. It depends also on the investigator's ability and willingness to communicate with patience and sensitivity.

Comprehension. The investigator must then ensure that the prospective subject has adequately understood the information. The investigator should give each one full opportunity to ask questions and should answer them honestly, promptly, and completely. In some instances the investigator may administer an oral or a written test or otherwise determine whether the information has been adequately understood.

Documentation of consent. Consent may be indicated in a number of ways. The subject may imply consent by voluntary actions, express consent orally, or sign a consent form. As a general rule, the subject should sign a consent form, or, in the case of incompetence, a legal guardian or other duly authorized representative should do so. The ethical review committee may approve waiver of the requirement of a signed consent form if the research carries no more than minimal risk—that is, risk that is no more likely and not greater than that attached to routine medical or psychological examination—and if the procedures to be used are only those for which signed consent forms are not customarily required outside the research context. Such waivers may also be approved when existence of a signed consent form would be an unjustified threat to the subject's confidentiality. In some cases, particularly when the information is complicated, it is advisable to give subjects information sheets to retain; these may resemble consent forms in all respects except that subjects are not required to sign them. Their wording should be cleared by the ethical review committee. When consent has been obtained orally, investigators are responsible for providing documentation or proof of consent.

Waiver of the consent requirement. Investigators should never initiate research involving human subjects without obtaining each subject's informed consent, unless they have received explicit approval to do so from an ethical review committee. However, when the research design involves no more than minimal risk and a requirement of individual informed consent would make the conduct of the research impracticable (for example, where the research involves only excerpting data from subjects' records), the ethical review committee may waive some or all of the elements of informed consent.

Renewing consent. When material changes occur in the conditions or the procedures of a study, and also periodically in long-term studies, the investigator should once again seek informed consent from the subjects. For example, new information may have come to light, either from the study or from other sources, about the risks or benefits of products being tested or about alternatives to them. Subjects should be given such information promptly. In many clinical trials, results are not disclosed to subjects and investigators until the study is concluded. This is ethically acceptable if an ethical review committee has approved their non-disclosure.

Cultural considerations. In some cultures an investigator may enter a community to conduct research or approach prospective subjects for their individual consent only after obtaining permission from a community leader, a council of elders, or another designated authority. Such customs must be respected. In no case, however, may the permission of a community leader or other authority substitute for individual informed consent. In some populations the use of a number of local languages may complicate the communication of information to potential subjects and the ability of an investigator to ensure that they truly understand it. Many people in all cultures are unfamiliar with, or do not readily understand, scientific concepts such as those of placebo or randomization. Sponsors and investigators should develop culturally appropriate ways to communicate information that is necessary for adherence to the standard required in the informed consent process. Also, they should describe and justify in the research protocol the procedure they plan to use in communicating information to subjects. For collaborative research in developing countries the research project should, if necessary, include the provision of resources to ensure that informed consent can indeed be obtained legitimately within different linguistic and cultural settings.

Consent to use for research purposes biological materials (including genetic material) from subjects in clinical trials. Consent forms for the research protocol should include a separate section for clinical-trial subjects who are requested to provide their consent for the use of their biological specimens for research. Separate consent may be appropriate in some cases (e.g., if investigators are requesting permission to conduct basic research which is not a necessary part of the clinical trial), but not in others (e.g., the clinical trial requires the use of subjects' biological materials).

Use of medical records and biological specimens. Medical records and biological specimens taken in the course of clinical care may be used for research without the consent of the patients/subjects only if an ethical review committee has determined that the research poses minimal risk, that the rights or interests of the patients will not be violated, that their privacy and confidentiality or anonymity are assured, and that the research is designed to answer an important question and would be impracticable if the requirement for informed consent were to be imposed. Patients have a right to know that their records or specimens may be used for research. Refusal or reluctance of individuals to agree to participate would not be evidence of impracticability sufficient to warrant waiving informed consent. Records and specimens of individuals who have specifically rejected such uses in the past may be used only in the case of public health emergencies. (See Guideline 18 Commentary, Confidentiality between physician and patient.)

Secondary use of research records or biological specimens. Investigators may want to use records or biological specimens that another investigator has used or collected for use, in another institution in the same or another country. This raises the issue of whether the records or specimens contain personal identifiers, or can be linked to such identifiers, and by whom. (See also Guideline 18 [. . .].) If informed consent or permission was required to authorize the original collection or use of such records or specimens for research purposes, secondary uses are generally constrained by the conditions specified in the original consent. Consequently, it is essential that the original consent process anticipate, to the extent that this is feasible, any foreseeable plans for future use of the records or specimens for research. Thus, in the original process of seeking informed consent a member of the research team should discuss with, and, when indicated, request the permission of, prospective subjects as to: (i) whether there will or could be any secondary use and, if so, whether such secondary use will be limited with regard to the type of study that may be performed on such materials; (ii) the conditions under which investigators will be required to contact the research subjects for additional authorization for secondary use; (iii) the investigators' plans, if any, to destroy or to strip of personal identifiers the records or specimens; and (iv) the rights of subjects to request destruction or anonymization of biological specimens or of records or parts of records that they might consider particularly sensitive, such as photographs, videotapes or audiotapes. (See also Guidelines 5 [. . .], 6 [. . .], and 7 [. . .].)

GUIDELINE 5: OBTAINING INFORMED CONSENT: ESSENTIAL INFORMATION FOR PROSPECTIVE RESEARCH SUBJECTS

Before requesting an individual's consent to participate in research, the investigator must provide the following information, in language or another form of communication that the individual can understand:

1. that the individual is invited to participate in research, the reasons for considering the individual suitable for the research, and that participation is voluntary;

2. that the individual is free to refuse to participate and will be free to withdraw from the research at any time without penalty or loss of benefits to which he or she would otherwise be entitled;

3. the purpose of the research, the procedures to be carried out by the investigator and the subject, and an explanation of how the research differs from routine medical care;

4. for controlled trials, an explanation of features of the research design (e.g., randomization, double-blinding), and that the subject will not be told of the assigned treatment until the study has been completed and the blind has been broken;

5. the expected duration of the individual's participation (including number and duration of visits to the research centre and the total time involved) and the possibility of early termination of the trial or of the individual's participation in it;

6. whether money or other forms of material goods will be provided in return for the individual's participation and, if so, the kind and amount;

7. that, after the completion of the study, subjects will be informed of the findings of the research in general, and individual subjects will be informed of any finding that relates to their particular health status;

8. that subjects have the right of access to their data on demand, even if these data lack immediate clinical utility (unless the ethical review committee has approved temporary or permanent non-disclosure of data, in which case the subject should be informed of, and given, the reasons for such non-disclosure);

9. any foreseeable risks, pain or discomfort, or inconvenience to the individual (or others) associated with participation in the research, including risks to the health or well-being of a subject's spouse or partner;

10. the direct benefits, if any, expected to result to subjects from participating in the research;

11. the expected benefits of the research to the community or to society at large, or contributions to scientific knowledge;

12. whether, when, and how any products or interventions proven by the research to be safe and effective will be made available to subjects after they have completed their participation in the research, and whether they will be expected to pay for them;

13. any currently available alternative interventions or courses of treatment;

14. the provisions that will be made to ensure respect for the privacy of subjects and for the confidentiality of records in which subjects are identified;

15. the limits, legal or other, to the investigators' ability to safeguard confidentiality, and the possible consequences of breaches of confidentiality;

16. policy with regard to the use of results of genetic tests and familial genetic information, and the precautions in place to prevent disclosure of the results of a subject's genetic tests to immediate family relatives or to others (e.g., insurance companies or employers) without the consent of the subject;

17. the sponsors of the research, the institutional affiliation of the investigators, and the nature and sources of funding for the research;

18. the possible research uses, direct or secondary, of the subject's medical records and of biological specimens taken in the course of clinical care (see also Guidelines 4 and 18 Commentaries);

19. whether it is planned that biological specimens collected in the research will be destroyed at its conclusion, and, if not, details about their storage (where, how, for how long, and final disposition) and possible future use, and that subjects have the right to decide about such future use, to refuse storage, and to have the material destroyed (see Guideline 4 Commentary);

20. whether commercial products may be developed from biological specimens, and whether the participant will receive monetary or other benefits from the development of such products;

21. whether the investigator is serving only as an investigator or as both investigator and the subject's physician;

22. the extent of the investigator's responsibility to provide medical services to the participant;

23. that treatment will be provided free of charge for specified types of research-related injury or for complications associated with the research, the nature and duration of such care, the name of the organization or individual that will provide the treatment, and whether there is any uncertainty regarding funding of such treatment;

24. in what way, and by what organization, the subject or the subject's family or dependants will be compensated for disability or death resulting from such injury (or, when indicated, that there are no plans to provide such compensation);

25. whether or not, in the country in which the prospective subject is invited to participate in research, the right to compensation is legally guaranteed;

26. that an ethical review committee has approved or cleared the research protocol.

[There is no Commentary to Guideline 5.—eds.]

GUIDELINE 6: OBTAINING INFORMED CONSENT: OBLIGATIONS OF SPONSORS AND INVESTIGATORS

Sponsors and investigators have a duty to:

• refrain from unjustified deception, undue influence, or intimidation;

• seek consent only after ascertaining that the prospective subject has adequate understanding of the relevant facts and of the consequences of participation and has had sufficient opportunity to consider whether to participate;

• as a general rule, obtain from each prospective subject a signed form as evidence of informed consent—investigators should justify any exceptions to this general rule and obtain the approval of the ethical review committee (see Guideline 4 Commentary, Documentation of consent);

• renew the informed consent of each subject if there are significant changes in the conditions or procedures of the research or if new information becomes available that could affect the willingness of subjects to continue to participate; and,

• renew the informed consent of each subject in long-term studies at pre-determined intervals, even if there are no changes in the design or objectives of the research.

Commentary on Guideline 6

The investigator is responsible for ensuring the adequacy of informed consent from each subject. The person obtaining informed consent should be knowledgeable about the research and capable of answering questions from prospective subjects. Investigators in charge of the study must make themselves available to answer questions at the request of subjects. Any restrictions on the subject's opportunity to ask questions and receive answers before or during the research undermines the validity of the informed consent.

In some types of research, potential subjects should receive counselling about risks of acquiring a disease unless they take precautions. This is especially true of HIV/AIDS vaccine research [...].

Withholding information and deception. Sometimes, to ensure the validity of research, investigators withhold certain information in the consent process. In biomedical research, this typically takes the form of withholding information about the purpose of specific procedures. For example, subjects in clinical trials are often not told the purpose of tests performed to monitor their compliance with the protocol, since if they knew their compliance was being monitored they might modify their behaviour and hence invalidate results. In most such cases, the prospective subjects are asked to consent to remain uninformed of the purpose of some procedures until the research is completed; after the conclusion of the study they are given the omitted information. In other cases, because a request for permission to withhold some information would jeopardize the validity of the research, subjects are not told that some information has been withheld until the research has been completed. Any such procedure must receive the explicit approval of the ethical review committee.

Active deception of subjects is considerably more controversial than simply withholding certain information. Lying to subjects is a tactic not commonly employed in biomedical research. Social and behavioural scientists, however, sometimes deliberately misinform subjects to study their attitudes and behaviour. For example, scientists have pretended to be patients to study the behaviour of health-care professionals and patients in their natural settings.

Some people maintain that active deception is never permissible. Others would permit it in certain circumstances. Deception is not permissible, however, in cases in which the deception itself would disguise the possibility of the subject being exposed to more than minimal risk. When deception is deemed indispensable to the methods of a study the investigators must demonstrate to an ethical review committee that no other research method would suffice; that significant advances could result from the research; and that nothing has been withheld that, if divulged, would cause a reasonable person to refuse to participate. The ethical review committee should determine the consequences for the subject of being deceived, and whether and how deceived subjects should be informed of the deception upon completion of the research. Such informing, commonly called "debriefing," ordinarily entails explaining the reasons for the deception. A subject who disapproves of having been deceived should be offered an opportunity to refuse to allow the investigator to use information thus obtained. Investigators and ethical review committees should be aware that deceiving research subjects may wrong them as well as harm them; subjects may resent not having been informed when they learn that they have participated in a study under false pretences. In some studies there may be justification for deceiving persons other than the subjects by either withholding or disguising elements of information. Such tactics are often proposed, for example, for studies of the abuse of spouses or children. An ethical review committee must review and approve all proposals to deceive persons other than the subjects. Subjects are entitled to prompt and honest answers to their questions; the ethical review committee must determine for each study whether others who are to be deceived are similarly entitled.

Intimidation and undue influence. Intimidation in any form invalidates informed consent. Prospective subjects who are patients often depend for medical care upon the physician/investigator, who consequently has a certain credibility in their eyes, and whose influence over them may be considerable, particularly if the study protocol has a therapeutic component. They may fear, for example, that refusal to participate would damage the therapeutic relationship or result in the withholding of health services. The physician/investigator must assure them that their decision on whether to participate will not affect the therapeutic relationship or other benefits to which they are entitled. In this situation the ethical review committee should consider whether a neutral third party should seek informed consent.

The prospective subject must not be exposed to undue influence. The borderline between justifiable persuasion and undue influence is imprecise, however. The researcher should give no unjustifiable assurances about the benefits, risks, or inconveniences of the research, for example, or induce a close relative or a community leader to influence a prospective subject's decision. See also Guideline 4 [...].

Risks. Investigators should be completely objective in discussing the details of the experimental intervention, the pain and discomfort that it may entail, and known risks and possible hazards. In complex research projects it may be neither feasible nor desirable to inform prospective participants fully about every possible risk. They must, however, be informed of all risks that a "reasonable person" would consider material to making a decision about whether to participate, including risks to a spouse or partner associated with trials of, for example, psychotropic or genital-tract medicaments. (See also Guideline 8 Commentary, Risks to groups of persons.)

Exception to the requirement for informed consent in studies of emergency situations in which the researcher anticipates that many subjects will be unable to consent. Research protocols are sometimes designed to address conditions occurring suddenly and rendering the patients/subjects incapable of giving informed consent. Examples are head trauma, cardiopulmonary arrest, and stroke. The investigation cannot be done with patients who can give informed consent in time and there may not be time to locate a person having the authority to give permission. In such circumstances it is often necessary to proceed with the research interventions very soon after the onset of the condition in order to evaluate an investigational treatment or develop the desired knowledge. As this class of emergency exception can be anticipated, the researcher must secure the review and approval of an ethical review committee before initiating the study. If possible, an attempt should be made to identify a population that is likely to develop the condition to be studied. This can be done readily, for example, if the condition is one that recurs periodically in individuals; examples include grand mal seizures and alcohol binges. In such cases, prospective subjects should be contacted while fully capable of informed consent, and invited to consent to their involvement as research subjects during future periods of incapacitation. If they are patients of an independent physician who is also the physician-researcher, the physician should likewise seek their consent while they are fully capable of informed consent. In all cases in which approved research has begun without prior consent of patients/subjects incapable of giving informed consent because of suddenly occurring conditions, they should be given all relevant information as soon as they are in a state to receive it, and their consent to continued participation should be obtained as soon as is reasonably possible.

Before proceeding without prior informed consent, the investigator must make reasonable efforts to locate an individual who has the authority to give permission on behalf of an incapacitated patient. If such a person can be located and refuses to give permission, the patient may not be enrolled as a subject. The risks of all interventions and procedures will be justified as required by Guideline 9 [...].

The researcher and the ethical review committee should agree to a maximum time of involvement of an individual without obtaining either the individual's informed consent or authorization according to the applicable legal system if the person is not able to give consent. If by that time the researcher has not obtained either consent or permission—owing either to a failure to contact a representative or a refusal of either the patient or the person or body authorized to give permission—the participation of the patient as a subject must be discontinued. The patient or the person or body providing authorization should be offered an opportunity to forbid the use of data derived from participation of the patient as a subject without consent or permission.

Where appropriate, plans to conduct emergency research without prior consent of the subjects should be publicized within the community in which it will be carried out. In the design and conduct of the research, the ethical review committee, the investigators, and the sponsors should be responsive to the concerns of the community. If there is cause for concern about the acceptability of the research in the community, there should be a formal consultation with representatives designated by the community. The research should not be carried out if it does not have substantial support in the community concerned. (See Guideline 8 Commentary, Risks to groups of persons.)

Exception to the requirement of informed consent for inclusion in clinical trials of persons rendered incapable of informed consent by an acute condition. Certain patients with an acute condition that renders them incapable of giving informed consent may be eligible for inclusion in a clinical trial in which the majority of prospective subjects will be capable of informed consent. Such a trial would relate to a new treatment for an acute condition such as sepsis, stroke, or myocardial infarction. The investigational treatment would hold out the prospect of direct benefit and would be justified accordingly, though the investigation might involve certain procedures or interventions that were not of direct benefit but carried no more than minimal risk; an example would be the process of randomization or the collection of additional blood for research purposes. For such cases the initial protocol submitted for approval to the ethical review committee should anticipate that some patients may be incapable of consent, and should propose for such patients a form of proxy consent, such as permission of the responsible relative. When the ethical review committee has approved or cleared such a protocol, an investigator may seek the permission of the responsible relative and enroll such a patient.

GUIDELINE 7: INDUCEMENT TO PARTICIPATE

Subjects may be reimbursed for lost earnings, travel costs, and other expenses incurred in taking part in a study; they may also receive free medical services. Subjects, particularly those who receive no direct benefit from research, may also be paid or otherwise compensated for inconvenience and time spent. The payments should not be so large, however, or the medical services so extensive as to induce prospective subjects to consent to participate in the research against their better judgment ("undue inducement"). All payments, reimbursements, and medical services provided to research subjects must have been approved by an ethical review committee.

Commentary on Guideline 7

Acceptable recompense. Research subjects may be reimbursed for their transport and other expenses, including lost earnings, associated with their participation in research. Those who receive no direct benefit from the research may also receive a small sum of money for inconvenience due to their participation in the research. All subjects may receive medical services unrelated to the research and have procedures and tests performed free of charge.

Unacceptable recompense. Payments in money or in kind to research subjects should not be so large as to persuade them to take undue risks or volunteer against their better judgment. Payments or rewards that undermine a person's capacity to exercise free choice invalidate consent. It may be difficult to distinguish between suitable recompense and undue influence to participate in research. An unemployed person or a student may view promised recompense differently from an employed person. Someone without access to medical care may or may not be unduly influenced to participate in research simply to receive such care. A prospective subject may be induced to participate in order to obtain a better diagnosis or access to a drug not otherwise available; local ethical review committees may find such inducements acceptable. Monetary and in-kind recompense must, therefore, be evaluated in the light of the traditions of the particular culture and population in which they are offered, to determine whether they constitute undue influence. The ethical review committee will ordinarily be the best judge of what constitutes reasonable material recompense in particular circumstances. When research interventions or procedures that do not hold out the prospect of direct benefit present more than minimal risk, all parties involved in the research—sponsors, investigators, and ethical review committees—in both funding and host countries should be careful to avoid undue material inducement.

Incompetent persons. Incompetent persons may be vulnerable to exploitation for financial gain by guardians. A guardian asked to give permission on behalf of an incompetent person should be offered no recompense other than a refund of travel and related expenses.

Withdrawal from a study. A subject who withdraws from research for reasons related to the study, such as unacceptable side-effects of a study drug, or who is withdrawn on health grounds, should be paid or recompensed as if full participation had taken place. A subject who withdraws for any other reason should be paid in proportion to the amount of participation. An investigator who must remove a subject from the study for wilful noncompliance is entitled to withhold part or all of the payment.

GUIDELINE 8: BENEFITS AND RISKS OF STUDY PARTICIPATION

For all biomedical research involving human subjects, the investigator must ensure that potential benefits and risks are reasonably balanced and risks are minimized.

• Interventions or procedures that hold out the prospect of direct diagnostic, therapeutic, or preventive benefit for the individual subject must be justified by the expectation that they will be at least as advantageous to the individual subject, in the light of foreseeable risks and benefits, as any available alternative. Risks of such "beneficial" interventions or procedures must be justified in relation to expected benefits to the individual subject.

• Risks of interventions that do not hold out the prospect of direct diagnostic, therapeutic, or preventive benefit for the individual must be justified in relation to the expected benefits to society (generalizable knowledge). The risks presented by such interventions must be reasonable in relation to the importance of the knowledge to be gained.

Commentary on Guideline 8

The Declaration of Helsinki in several paragraphs deals with the well-being of research subjects and the avoidance of risk. Thus, considerations related to the well-being of the human subject should take precedence over the interests of science and society (Paragraph 5); clinical testing must be preceded by adequate laboratory or animal experimentation to demonstrate a reasonable probability of success without undue risk (Paragraph 11); every project should be preceded by careful assessment of predictable risks and burdens in comparison with foreseeable benefits to the subject or to others (Paragraph 16); physician-researchers must be confident that the risks involved have been adequately assessed and can be satisfactorily managed (Paragraph 17); and the risks and burdens to the subject must be minimized, and reasonable in relation to the importance of the objective or the knowledge to be gained (Paragraph 18).

Biomedical research often employs a variety of interventions of which some hold out the prospect of direct therapeutic benefit (beneficial interventions) and others are administered solely to answer the research question (non-beneficial interventions). Beneficial interventions are justified as they are in medical practice by the expectation that they will be at least as advantageous to the individuals concerned, in the light of both risks and benefits, as any available alternative. Non-beneficial interventions are assessed differently; they may be justified only by appeal to the knowledge to be gained. In assessing the risks and benefits that a protocol presents to a population, it is appro-priate to consider the harm that could result from forgoing the research.

Paragraphs 5 and 18 of the Declaration of Helsinki do not preclude well-informed volunteers, capable of fully appreciating risks and benefits of an investigation, from participating in research for altruistic reasons or for modest remuneration.

Minimizing risk associated with participation in a randomized controlled trial. In randomized controlled trials subjects risk being allocated to receive the treatment that proves inferior. They are allocated by chance to one of two or more intervention arms and followed to a predetermined end-point. (Interventions are understood to include new or established therapies, diagnostic tests, and preventive measures.) An intervention is evaluated by comparing it with another intervention (a control), which is ordinarily the best current method, selected from the safe and effective treatments available globally, unless some other control intervention such as placebo can be justified ethically (see Guideline 11).

To minimize risk when the intervention to be tested in a randomized controlled trial is designed to prevent or postpone a lethal or disabling outcome, the investigator must not, for purposes of conducting the trial, withhold therapy that is known to be superior to the intervention being tested, unless the withholding can be justified by the standards set forth in Guideline 11. Also, the investigator must provide in the research protocol for the monitoring of research data by an independent board (Data and Safety Monitoring Board); one function of such a board is to protect the research subjects from previously unknown adverse reactions or unnecessarily prolonged exposure to an inferior therapy. Normally at the outset of a randomized controlled trial, criteria are established for its premature termination (stopping rules or guidelines).

Risks to groups of persons. Research in certain fields, such as epidemiology, genetics, or sociology, may present risks to the interests of communities, societies, or racially or ethnically defined groups. Information might be published that could stigmatize a group or expose its members to discrimination. Such information, for example, could indicate, rightly or wrongly, that the group has a higher than average prevalence of alcoholism, mental illness, or sexually transmitted disease, or is particularly susceptible to certain genetic disorders. Plans to conduct such research should be sensitive to such considerations, to the need to maintain confidentiality during and after the study, and to the need to publish the resulting data in a manner that is respectful of the interests of all concerned, or in certain circumstances not to publish them. The ethical review committee should ensure that the interests of all concerned are given due consideration; often it will be advisable to have individual consent supplemented by community consultation. [The ethical basis for the justification of risk is elaborated further in Guideline 9.]

GUIDELINE 9: SPECIAL LIMITATIONS ON RISK WHEN RESEARCH INVOLVES INDIVIDUALS WHO ARE NOT CAPABLE OF GIVING INFORMED CONSENT

When there is ethical and scientific justification to conduct research with individuals incapable of giving informed consent, the risk from research interventions that do not hold out the prospect of direct benefit for the individual subject should be no more likely and not greater than the risk attached to routine medical or psychological examination of such persons. Slight or minor increases above such risk may be permitted when there is an overriding scientific or medical rationale for such increases and when an ethical review committee has approved them.

Commentary on Guideline 9

The low-risk standard. Certain individuals or groups may have limited capacity to give informed consent either because, as in the case of prisoners, their autonomy is limited, or because they have limited cognitive capacity. For research involving persons who are unable to consent, or whose capacity to make an informed choice may not fully meet the standard of informed consent, ethical review committees must distinguish between intervention risks that do not exceed those associated with routine medical or psychological examination of such persons and risks in excess of those.

When the risks of such interventions do not exceed those associated with routine medical or psychological examination of such persons, there is no requirement for special substantive or procedural protective measures apart from those generally required for all research involving members of the particular class of persons. When the risks are in excess of those, the ethical review committee must find: (1) that the research is designed to be responsive to the disease affecting the prospective subjects or to conditions to which they are particularly susceptible; (2) that the risks of the research interventions are only slightly greater than those associated with routine medical or psychological examination of such persons for the condition or set of clinical circumstances under investigation; (3) that the objective of the research is sufficiently important to justify exposure of the subjects to the increased risk; and (4) that the interventions are reasonably commensurate with the clinical interventions that the subjects have experienced or may be expected to experience in relation to the condition under investigation.

If such research subjects, including children, become capable of giving independent informed consent during the research, their consent to continued participation should be obtained.

There is no internationally agreed, precise definition of a "slight or minor increase" above the risks associated with routine medical or psychological examination of such persons. Its meaning is inferred from what various ethical review committees have reported as having met the standard. Examples include additional lumbar punctures or bone-marrow aspirations in children with conditions for which such examinations are regularly indicated in clinical practice. The requirement that the objective of the research be relevant to the disease or condition affecting the prospective subjects rules out the use of such interventions in healthy children.

The requirement that the research interventions be reasonably commensurate with clinical interventions that subjects may have experienced or are likely to experience for the condition under investigation is intended to enable them to draw on personal experience as they decide whether to accept or reject additional procedures for research purposes. Their choices will, therefore, be more informed even though they may not fully meet the standard of informed consent. (See also Guidelines 4 [. . .], 13 [. . .], 14 [. . .], and 15 [. . .].)

GUIDELINE 10: RESEARCH IN POPULATIONS AND COMMUNITIES WITH LIMITED RESOURCES

Before undertaking research in a population or community with limited resources, the sponsor and the investigator must make every effort to ensure that:

• the research is responsive to the health needs and the priorities of the population or community in which it is to be carried out; and

• any intervention or product developed, or knowledge generated, will be made reasonably available for the benefit of that population or community.

Commentary on Guideline 10

This guideline is concerned with countries or communities in which resources are limited to the extent that they are, or may be, vulnerable to exploitation by sponsors and investigators from the relatively wealthy countries and communities.

Responsiveness of research to health needs and priorities. The ethical requirement that research be responsive to the health needs of the population or community in which it is carried out calls for decisions on what is needed to fulfil the requirement. It is not sufficient simply to determine that a disease is prevalent in the population and that new or further research is needed: the ethical requirement of "responsiveness" can be fulfilled only if successful interventions or other kinds of health benefit are made available to the population. This is applicable especially to research conducted in countries where governments lack the resources to make such products or benefits widely available. Even when a product to be tested in a particular country is much cheaper than the standard treatment in some other countries, the government or individuals in that country may still be unable to afford it. If the knowledge gained from the research in such a country is used primarily for the benefit of populations that can afford the tested product, the research may rightly be characterized as exploitative and, therefore, unethical.

When an investigational intervention has important potential for health care in the host country, the negotiation that the sponsor should undertake to determine the practical implications of "responsiveness," as well as "reasonable availability," should include representatives of stakeholders in the host country; these include the national government, the health ministry, local health authorities, and concerned scientific and ethics groups, as well as representatives of the communities from which subjects are drawn and non-governmental organizations such as health advocacy groups. The negotiation should cover the health-care infrastructure required for safe and rational use of the intervention, the likelihood of authorization for distribution, and decisions regarding payments, royalties, subsidies, technology, and intellectual property, as well as distribution costs, when this economic information is not proprietary. In some cases, satisfactory discussion of the availability and distribution of successful products will necessarily engage international organizations, donor governments and bilateral agencies, international non-governmental organizations, and the private sector. The development of a health-care infrastructure should be facilitated at the onset so that it can be of use during and beyond the conduct of the research.

Additionally, if an investigational drug has been shown to be beneficial, the sponsor should continue to provide it to the subjects after the conclusion of the study, and pending its approval by a drug regulatory authority. The sponsor is unlikely to be in a position to make a beneficial investigational intervention generally available to the community or population until some time after the conclusion of the study, as it may be in short supply and in any case cannot be made generally available before a drug regulatory authority has approved it.

For minor research studies and when the outcome is scientific knowledge rather than a commercial product, such complex planning or negotiation is rarely, if ever,

needed. There must be assurance, however, that the scientific knowledge developed will be used for the benefit of the population.

Reasonable availability. The issue of "reasonable availability" is complex and will need to be determined on a case-by-case basis. Relevant considerations include the length of time for which the intervention or product developed, or other agreed benefit, will be made available to research subjects, or to the community or population concerned; the severity of a subject's medical condition; the effect of withdrawing the study drug (e.g., death of a subject); the cost to the subject or health service; and the question of undue inducement if an intervention is provided free of charge.

In general, if there is good reason to believe that a product developed or knowledge generated by research is unlikely to be reasonably available to, or applied to the benefit of, the population of a proposed host country or community after the conclusion of the research, it is unethical to conduct the research in that country or community. This should not be construed as precluding studies designed to evaluate novel therapeutic concepts. As a rare exception, for example, research may be designed to obtain preliminary evidence that a drug or a class of drugs has a beneficial effect in the treatment of a disease that occurs only in regions with extremely limited resources, and it could not be carried out reasonably well in more developed communities. Such research may be justified ethically even if there is no plan in place to make a product available to the population of the host country or community at the conclusion of the preliminary phase of its development. If the concept is found to be valid, subsequent phases of the research could result in a product that could be made reasonably available at its conclusion. (See also Guidelines 3 [. . .], 12 [. . .], 20 [. . .], and 21 [. . .].)

GUIDELINE 11: CHOICE OF CONTROL IN CLINICAL TRIALS

As a general rule, research subjects in the control group of a trial of a diagnostic, therapeutic, or preventive intervention should receive an established effective intervention. In some circumstances it may be ethically acceptable to use an alternative comparator, such as placebo or "no treatment."

Placebo may be used:

- when there is no established effective intervention;

- when withholding an established effective intervention would expose subjects to, at most, temporary discomfort or delay in relief of symptoms;

- when use of an established effective intervention as comparator would not yield scientifically reliable results and use of placebo would not add any risk of serious or irreversible harm to the subjects.

Commentary on Guideline 11

General considerations for controlled clinical trials. The design of trials of investigational diagnostic, therapeutic, or preventive interventions raises interrelated scientific and ethical issues for sponsors, investigators, and ethical review committees. To obtain reliable results, investigators must compare the effects of an investigational intervention on subjects assigned to the investigational arm (or arms) of a trial with the effects that a control intervention produces in subjects drawn from the same population and assigned to its control arm. Randomization is the preferred method for assigning subjects to the various arms of the clinical trial unless another method, such as historical or literature controls, can be justified scientifically and ethically. Assignment to treatment arms by randomization, in addition to its usual scientific superiority, offers the advantage of tending to render equivalent to all subjects the foreseeable benefits and risks of participation in a trial.

A clinical trial cannot be justified ethically unless it is capable of producing scientifically reliable results. When the objective is to establish the effectiveness and safety of an investigational intervention, the use of a placebo control is often much more likely than that of an active control to produce a scientifically reliable result. In many cases the ability of a trial to distinguish effective from ineffective interventions (its assay sensitivity) cannot be assured unless the control is a placebo. If, however, an effect of using a placebo would be to deprive subjects in the control arm of an established effective intervention, and thereby to expose them to serious harm, particularly if it is irreversible, it would obviously be unethical to use a placebo.

Placebo control in the absence of a current effective alternative. The use of placebo in the control arm of a clinical trial is ethically acceptable when, as stated in the Declaration of Helsinki (Paragraph 29), "no proven prophylactic, diagnostic, or therapeutic method exists." Usually, in this case, a placebo is scientifically preferable to no intervention. In certain circumstances, however, an alternative design may be both scientifically and ethically acceptable, and preferable; an example would be a clinical trial of a surgical intervention, because, for many surgical interventions, either it is not possible or it is ethically unacceptable to devise a suitable placebo; for another example, in certain vaccine trials an investigator might choose to provide for those in the "control" arm a vaccine that is unrelated to the investigational vaccine.

Placebo-controlled trials that entail only minor risks. A placebo-controlled design may be ethically acceptable, and preferable on scientific grounds, when the condition for which patients/subjects are randomly assigned to placebo or active treatment is only a small deviation in physiological measurements, such as slightly raised blood pressure or a modest increase in serum cholesterol; and if delaying or omitting available treatment may cause only temporary discomfort (e.g., common headache) and no serious adverse consequences. The ethical review committee must be fully satisfied that the risks of withholding an established effective intervention are truly minor and short-lived.

Placebo control when active control would not yield reliable results. A related but distinct rationale for using a placebo control rather than an established effective intervention is that the documented experience with the established effective intervention is not sufficient to provide a scientifically reliable comparison with the intervention being investigated; it is then difficult, or even impossible, without using a placebo, to design a scientifically reliable study. This is not always, however, an ethically acceptable basis for depriving control subjects of an established effective intervention in clinical trials; only when doing so would not add any risk of serious harm, particularly irreversible harm, to the subjects would it be ethically acceptable to do so. In some cases, the condition at which the intervention is aimed (for example, cancer or HIV/AIDS) will be too serious to deprive control subjects of an established effective intervention.

This latter rationale (when active control would not yield reliable results) differs from the former (trials that entail only minor risks) in emphasis. In trials that entail only minor risks the investigative interventions are aimed at relatively trivial conditions, such as the common cold or hair loss; forgoing an established effective intervention for the duration of a trial deprives control subjects of only minor benefits. It is for this reason that it is not unethical to use a placebo-control design. Even if it were possible to design a so-called "non-inferiority," or "equivalency," trial using an active control, it would still not be unethical in these circumstances to use a placebo-control design. In any event, the researcher must satisfy the ethical review committee that the safety and human rights of the subjects will be fully protected, that prospective subjects will be fully informed about alternative treatments, and that the purpose and design of the study are scientifically sound. The ethical acceptability of such placebo-controlled studies increases as the period of placebo use is decreased, and when the study design permits change to active treatment ("escape treatment") if intolerable symptoms occur [...].

Exceptional use of a comparator other than an established effective intervention. An exception to the general rule is applicable in some studies designed to develop a therapeutic, preventive, or diagnostic intervention for use in a country or community in which an established effective intervention is not available and unlikely in the foreseeable future to become available, usually for economic or logistic reasons. The purpose of such a study is to make available to the population of the country or community an effective alternative to an established effective intervention that is locally unavailable. Accordingly, the proposed investigational intervention must be responsive to the health needs of the population from which the research subjects are recruited and there must be assurance that, if it proves to be safe and effective, it will be made reasonably available to that population. Also, the scientific and ethical review committees must be satisfied that the established effective intervention cannot be used as comparator because its use would not yield scientifically reliable results that would be relevant to the health needs of the study population. In these circumstances an ethical review committee can approve a clinical trial in which the comparator is other than an established effective intervention, such as placebo or no treatment or a local remedy.

However, some people strongly object to the exceptional use of a comparator other than an established effective intervention because it could result in exploitation of poor and disadvantaged populations. The objection rests on three arguments:

• Placebo control could expose research subjects to risk of serious or irreversible harm when the use of an established effective intervention as comparator could avoid the risk.

• Not all scientific experts agree about conditions under which an established effective intervention used as a comparator would not yield scientifically reliable results.

• An economic reason for the unavailability of an established effective intervention cannot justify a placebo-controlled study in a country of limited resources when it would be unethical to conduct a study with the same design in a population with general access to the effective intervention outside the study.

Placebo control when an established effective intervention is not available in the host country. The question addressed here is: When should an exception be allowed to the general rule that subjects in the control arm of a clinical trial should receive an established effective intervention?

The usual reason for proposing the exception is that, for economic or logistic reasons, an established effective intervention is not in general use or available in the country in which the study will be conducted, whereas the investigational intervention could be made available, given the finances and infrastructure of the country.

Another reason that may be advanced for proposing a placebo-controlled trial is that using an established effective intervention as the control would not produce scientifically reliable data relevant to the country in which the trial is to be conducted. Existing data about the effectiveness and safety of the established effective intervention may have been accumulated under circumstances unlike those of the population in which it is proposed to conduct the trial; this, it may be argued, could make their use in the trial unreliable. One reason could be that the disease or condition manifests itself differently in different populations, or other uncontrolled factors could invalidate the use of existing data for comparative purposes.

The use of placebo control in these circumstances is ethically controversial, for the following reasons:

• Sponsors of research might use poor countries or communities as testing grounds for research that would be difficult or impossible in countries where there is general access to an established effective intervention, and the investigational intervention, if proven safe and effective, is likely to be marketed in countries in which an established effective intervention is already available and it is not likely to be marketed in the host country.

• The research subjects, both active-arm and control-arm, are patients who may have a serious, possibly life-threatening, illness. They do not normally have access to an established effective intervention currently available to similar patients in many other countries. According to the requirements of a scientifically reliable trial, investigators, who may be their attending physicians, would be expected to enroll some of those patients/subjects in the placebo-control arm. This would appear to be a violation of the physician's fiduciary duty of undivided loyalty to the patient, particularly in cases in which known effective therapy could be made available to the patients.

An argument for exceptional use of placebo control may be that a health authority in a country where an established effective intervention is not generally available or affordable, and unlikely to become available or affordable in the foreseeable future, seeks to develop an affordable intervention specifically for a health problem affecting its population. There may then be less reason for concern that a placebo design is exploitative, and therefore unethical, as the health authority has responsibility for the population's health, and there are valid health grounds for testing an apparently beneficial intervention. In such circumstances an ethical review committee may determine that the proposed trial is ethically acceptable, provided that the rights and safety of subjects are safeguarded.

Ethical review committees will need to engage in careful analysis of the circumstances to determine whether the use of placebo rather than an established effective intervention is ethically acceptable. They will need to be satisfied that an established effective intervention is truly unlikely to become available and implementable in that country. This may be difficult to determine, however, as it is clear that, with sufficient persistence and ingenuity, ways may be found of accessing previously unattainable medicinal products, and thus avoiding the ethical issue raised by the use of placebo control.

When the rationale of proposing a placebo-controlled trial is that the use of an established effective intervention as the control would not yield scientifically reliable data relevant to the proposed host country, the ethical review committee in that country has the option of seeking expert opinion as to whether use of an established effective intervention in the control arm would invalidate the results of the research.

An "equivalency trial" as an alternative to a placebo-controlled trial. An alternative to a placebo-control design in these circumstances would be an "equivalency trial," which would compare an investigational intervention with an established effective intervention and produce scientifically reliable data. An equivalency trial in a country in which no established effective intervention is available is not designed to determine whether the investigational intervention is superior to an established effective intervention currently used somewhere in the world; its purpose is, rather, to determine whether the investigational intervention is, in effectiveness and safety, equivalent to, or almost equivalent to, the established effective intervention. It would be hazardous to conclude, however, that an intervention demonstrated to be equivalent, or almost equivalent, to an established effective intervention is better than nothing or superior to whatever intervention is available in the country; there may be substantial differences between the results of superficially identical clinical trials carried out in different countries. If there are such differences, it would be scientifically acceptable and ethically preferable to conduct such "equivalency" trials in countries in which an established effective intervention is already available.

If there are substantial grounds for the ethical review committee to conclude that an established effective intervention will not become available and implementable, the committee should obtain assurances from the parties concerned that plans have been agreed for making the investigational intervention reasonably available in the host country or community once its effectiveness and safety have been established. Moreover, when the study has external sponsorship, approval should usually be dependent on the sponsors and the health authorities of the host country having engaged in a process of negotiation and planning, including justifying the study in regard to local health-care needs.

Means of minimizing harm to placebo-control subjects. Even when placebo controls are justified on one of the bases set forth in the guideline, there are means of minimizing the possibly harmful effect of being in the control arm.

First, a placebo-control group need not be untreated. An add-on design may be employed when the investigational therapy and a standard treatment have different mechanisms of action. The treatment to be tested and placebo are each added to a standard treatment. Such studies have a particular place when a standard treatment is known to decrease mortality or irreversible morbidity but a trial with standard treatment as the active control cannot be carried out or would be difficult to interpret [International Conference on Harmonisation (ICH) Guideline: Choice of Control Group and Related Issues in Clinical Trials, 2000]. In testing for improved treatment of life-threatening diseases such as cancer, HIV/AIDS, or heart failure, add-on designs are a particularly useful means of finding improvements in interventions that are not fully effective or may cause intolerable side-effects. They have a place also in respect of treatment for epilepsy, rheumatism, and osteoporosis, for example, because withholding of established effective therapy could result in progressive disability, unacceptable discomfort, or both.

Second, as indicated in Guideline 8 Commentary, when the intervention to be tested in a randomized controlled trial is designed to prevent or postpone a lethal or disabling outcome, the investigator minimizes harmful effects of placebo-control studies by providing in the research protocol for the monitoring of research data by an independent Data and Safety Monitoring Board (DSMB). One function of such a board is to protect the research subjects from previously unknown adverse reactions; another is to avoid unnecessarily prolonged exposure to an inferior therapy. The board fulfils the latter function by means of interim analyses of the data pertaining to efficacy to ensure that the trial does not continue beyond the point at which an investigational therapy is demonstrated to be effective. Normally, at the outset of a randomized controlled trial, criteria are established for its premature termination (stopping rules or guidelines).

In some cases the DSMB is called upon to perform "conditional power calculations," designed to determine the probability that a particular clinical trial could ever show that the investigational therapy is effective. If that probability is very small, the DSMB is expected to recommend termination of the clinical trial, because it would be unethical to continue it beyond that point.

In most cases of research involving human subjects, it is unnecessary to appoint a DSMB. To ensure that research is carefully monitored for the early detection of adverse events, the sponsor or the principal investigator appoints an individual to be responsible for advising on the need to consider changing the system of monitoring for adverse events or the process of informed consent, or even to consider terminating the study.

GUIDELINE 12: EQUITABLE DISTRIBUTION OF BURDENS AND BENEFITS IN THE SELECTION OF GROUPS OF SUBJECTS IN RESEARCH

Groups or communities to be invited to be subjects of research should be selected in such a way that the burdens and benefits of the research will be equitably distributed. The exclusion of groups or communities that might benefit from study participation must be justified.

Commentary on Guideline 12

General considerations. Equity requires that no group or class of persons should bear more than its fair share of the burdens of participation in research. Similarly, no group should be deprived of its fair share of the benefits of research, short-term or long-term; such benefits include the direct benefits of participation as well as the benefits of the new knowledge that the research is designed to yield. When burdens or benefits of research are to be apportioned unequally among individuals or groups of persons, the criteria for unequal distribution should be morally justifiable and not arbitrary. In other words, unequal allocation must not be inequitable. Subjects should be drawn from the qualifying population in the general geographic area of the trial without regard to race, ethnicity, economic status, or gender unless there is a sound scientific reason to do otherwise.

In the past, groups of persons were excluded from participation in research for what were then considered good reasons. As a consequence of such exclusions, information about the diagnosis, prevention, and treatment of diseases in such groups of persons is limited. This has resulted in a serious class injustice. If information about the management of diseases is considered a benefit that is distributed within a society, it is unjust to deprive groups of persons of that benefit. Such documents as the Declaration of Helsinki and Guidance Points in the UNAIDS [the Joint United Nations Programme on HIV/AIDS—eds.] Guidance Document on Ethical Considerations in HIV Preventive Vaccine Research, and the policies of many national governments and professional societies, recognize the need to redress these injustices by encouraging the participation of previously excluded groups in basic and applied biomedical research.

Members of vulnerable groups also have the same entitlement to access to the benefits of investigational interventions that show promise of therapeutic benefit as persons not considered vulnerable, particularly when no superior or equivalent approaches to therapy are available.

There has been a perception, sometimes correct and sometimes incorrect, that certain groups of persons have been overused as research subjects. In some cases such overuse has been based on the administrative availability of the populations. Research hospitals are often located in places where members of the lowest socioeconomic classes reside, and this has resulted in an apparent overuse of such persons. Other groups that may have been overused because they were conveniently available to researchers include students in investigators' classes, residents of long-term care facilities and subordinate members of hierarchical institutions. Impoverished groups have been overused because of their willingness to serve as subjects in exchange for relatively small stipends. Prisoners have been considered ideal subjects for Phase I drug studies because of their highly regimented lives and, in many cases, their conditions of economic deprivation.

Overuse of certain groups, such as the poor or the administratively available, is unjust for several reasons. It is unjust to selectively recruit impoverished people to serve as research subjects simply because they can be more easily induced to participate in exchange for small payments. In most cases, these people would be called upon to bear the burdens of research so that others who are better off could enjoy the benefits. However, although the burdens of research should not fall disproportionately on socioeconomically disadvantaged groups, neither should such groups be categorically excluded from research protocols. It would not be unjust to selectively recruit poor people to serve as subjects in research designed to address problems that are prevalent in their group—malnutrition, for example. Similar considerations apply to institutionalized groups or those whose availability to the investigators is for other reasons administratively convenient.

Not only may certain groups within a society be inappropriately overused as research subjects, but also entire communities or societies may be over-used. This has been particularly likely to occur in countries or communities with insufficiently well-developed systems for the protection of the rights and welfare of human research subjects. Such over-use is especially questionable when the populations or communities concerned bear the burdens of participation in research but are extremely unlikely ever to enjoy the benefits of new knowledge and products developed as a result of the research. (See Guideline 10 [...].)

GUIDELINE 13: RESEARCH INVOLVING VULNERABLE PERSONS

Special justification is required for inviting vulnerable individuals to serve as research subjects and, if they are selected, the means of protecting their rights and welfare must be strictly applied.

Commentary on Guideline 13

Vulnerable persons are those who are relatively (or absolutely) incapable of protecting their own interests. More formally, they may have insufficient power, intelligence, education, resources, strength, or other needed attributes to protect their own interests.

General considerations. The central problem presented by plans to involve vulnerable persons as research subjects is that such plans may entail an inequitable distribution of the burdens and benefits of research participation. Classes of individuals conventionally considered vulnerable are those with limited capacity or freedom to consent or to decline to consent. They are the subject of specific guidelines in this document (Guidelines 14, 15) and include children, and persons who because of mental or behavioural disorders are incapable of giving informed consent. Ethical justification of their involvement usually requires that investigators satisfy ethical review committees that:

• the research could not be carried out equally well with less vulnerable subjects;

• the research is intended to obtain knowledge that will lead to improved diagnosis, prevention, or treatment of diseases or other health problems characteristic of, or unique to, the vulnerable class—either the actual subjects or other similarly situated members of the vulnerable class;

• research subjects and other members of the vulnerable class from which subjects are recruited will ordinarily be assured reasonable access to any diagnostic, preventive or therapeutic products that will become available as a consequence of the research;

• the risks attached to interventions or procedures that do not hold out the prospect of direct health-related benefit will not exceed those associated with routine medical or psychological examination of such persons unless an ethical review committee authorizes a slight increase over this level of risk (Guideline 9); and,

• when the prospective subjects are either incompetent or otherwise substantially unable to give informed consent, their agreement will be supplemented by the permission of their legal guardians or other appropriate representatives.

Other vulnerable groups. The quality of the consent of prospective subjects who are junior or subordinate members of a hierarchical group requires careful consideration, as their agreement to volunteer may be unduly influenced, whether justified or not, by the expectation of preferential treatment if they agree or by fear of disapproval or retaliation if they refuse. Examples of such groups are medical and nursing students, subordinate hospital and laboratory personnel, employees of pharmaceutical companies, and members of the armed forces or police. Because they work in close proximity to investigators, they tend to be called upon more often than others to serve as research subjects, and this could result in inequitable distribution of the burdens and benefits of research.

Elderly persons are commonly regarded as vulnerable. With advancing age, people are increasingly likely to acquire attributes that define them as vulnerable. They may, for example, be institutionalized or develop varying degrees of dementia. If and when they acquire such vulnerability-defining attributes, and not before, it is appropriate to consider them vulnerable and to treat them accordingly.

Other groups or classes may also be considered vulnerable. They include residents of nursing homes, people receiving welfare benefits or social assistance and other poor people and the unemployed, patients in emergency rooms, some ethnic and racial minority groups, homeless persons, nomads, refugees or displaced persons, prisoners, patients with incurable disease, individuals who are politically powerless, and members of communities unfamiliar with modern medical concepts. To the extent that these and other classes of people have attributes resembling those of classes identified as vulnerable, the need for special protection of their rights and welfare should be reviewed and applied, where relevant.

Persons who have serious, potentially disabling, or life-threatening diseases are highly vulnerable. Physicians sometimes treat such patients with drugs or other therapies not yet licensed for general availability because studies designed to establish their safety and efficacy have not been completed. This is compatible with the Declaration of Helsinki, which states in Paragraph 32: "In the treatment of a patient, where proven . . . therapeutic methods do not exist or have been ineffective, the physician, with informed consent from the patient, must be free to use unproven or new . . . therapeutic measures, if in the physician's judgement it offers hope of saving life, re-establishing health or alleviating suffering." Such treatment, commonly called "compassionate use," is not properly regarded as research, but it can contribute to ongoing research into the safety and efficacy of the interventions used.

Although, on the whole, investigators must study less vulnerable groups before involving more vulnerable groups, some exceptions are justified. In general, children are not suitable for Phase I drug trials or for Phase I or II vaccine trials, but such trials may be permissible after studies in adults have shown some therapeutic or preventive effect. For example, a Phase II vaccine trial seeking evidence of immunogenicity in infants may be justified when a vaccine has shown evidence of preventing or slowing progression of an infectious disease in adults, or Phase I research with children may be appropriate because the disease to be treated does not occur in adults or is manifested differently in children.

GUIDELINE 14: RESEARCH INVOLVING CHILDREN

Before undertaking research involving children, the investigator must ensure that:

• the research might not equally well be carried out with adults;

• the purpose of the research is to obtain knowledge relevant to the health needs of children;

• a parent or legal representative of each child has given permission;

• the agreement (assent) of each child has been obtained to the extent of the child's capabilities; and,

• a child's refusal to participate or continue in the research will be respected.

Commentary on Guideline 14

Justification of the involvement of children in biomedical research. The participation of children is indispensable for research into diseases of childhood and conditions to which children are particularly susceptible (cf. vaccine trials), as well as for clinical trials of drugs that are designed for children as well as adults. In the past, many new products were not tested for children though they were directed towards diseases also occurring in childhood; thus children either did not benefit from these new drugs or were exposed to them though little was known about their specific effects or safety in children. Now it is widely agreed that, as a general rule, the sponsor of any new therapeutic, diagnostic, or preventive product that is likely to be indicated for use in children is obliged to evaluate its safety and efficacy for children before it is released for general distribution.

Assent of the child. The willing cooperation of the child should be sought, after the child has been informed to the extent that the child's maturity and intelligence permit. The age at which a child becomes legally competent to give consent differs substantially from one jurisdiction to another; in some countries the "age of consent" established in their different provinces, states, or other political subdivisions varies considerably. Often children who have not yet reached the legally established age of consent can understand the implications of informed consent and go through the necessary procedures; they can therefore knowingly agree to serve as research subjects. Such knowing agreement, sometimes referred to as assent, is insufficient to permit participation in research unless it is supplemented by

the permission of a parent, a legal guardian, or other duly authorized representative.

Some children who are too immature to be able to give knowing agreement, or assent, may be able to register a "deliberate objection," an expression of disapproval or refusal of a proposed procedure. The deliberate objection of an older child, for example, is to be distinguished from the behaviour of an infant, who is likely to cry or withdraw in response to almost any stimulus. Older children, who are more capable of giving assent, should be selected before younger children or infants, unless there are valid scientific reasons related to age for involving younger children first.

A deliberate objection by a child to taking part in research should always be respected even if the parents have given permission, unless the child needs treatment that is not available outside the context of research, the investigational intervention shows promise of therapeutic benefit, and there is no acceptable alternative therapy. In such a case, particularly if the child is very young or immature, a parent or guardian may override the child's objections. If the child is older and more nearly capable of independent informed consent, the investigator should seek the specific approval or clearance of the scientific and ethical review committees for initiating or continuing with the investigational treatment. If child subjects become capable of independent informed consent during the research, their informed consent to continued participation should be sought and their decision respected.

A child with a likely fatal illness may object or refuse assent to continuation of a burdensome or distressing intervention. In such circumstances parents may press an investigator to persist with an investigational intervention against the child's wishes. The investigator may agree to do so if the intervention shows promise of preserving or prolonging life and there is no acceptable alternative treatment. In such cases, the investigator should seek the specific approval or clearance of the ethical review committee before agreeing to override the wishes of the child.

Permission of a parent or guardian. The investigator must obtain the permission of a parent or guardian in accordance with local laws or established procedures. It may be assumed that children over the age of 12 or 13 years are usually capable of understanding what is necessary to give adequately informed consent, but their consent (assent) should normally be complemented by the permission of a parent or guardian, even when local law does not require such permission. Even when the law requires parental permission, however, the assent of the child must be obtained.

In some jurisdictions, some individuals who are below the general age of consent are regarded as "emancipated" or "mature" minors and are authorized to consent without the agreement or even the awareness of their parents or guardians. They may be married or pregnant or be already parents or living independently. Some studies involve investigation of adolescents' beliefs and behaviour regarding sexuality or use of recreational drugs; other research addresses domestic violence or child abuse. For studies on these topics, ethical review committees may waive parental permission if, for example, parental knowledge of the subject matter may place the adolescents at some risk of questioning or even intimidation by their parents.

Because of the issues inherent in obtaining assent from children in institutions, such children should only exceptionally be subjects of research. In the case of institutionalized children without parents, or whose parents are not legally authorized to grant permission, the ethical review committee may require sponsors or investigators to provide it with the opinion of an independent, concerned, expert advocate for institutionalized children as to the propriety of undertaking the research with such children.

Observation of research by a parent or guardian. A parent or guardian who gives permission for a child to participate in research should be given the opportunity, to a reasonable extent, to observe the research as it proceeds, so as to be able to withdraw the child if the parent or guardian decides it is in the child's best interests to do so.

Psychological and medical support. Research involving children should be conducted in settings in which the child and the parent can obtain adequate medical and psychological support. As an additional protection for children, an investigator may, when possible, obtain the advice of a child's family physician, paediatrician, or other health-care provider on matters concerning the child's participation in the research. (See also Guidelines 8 [. . .], 9 [. . .], 13 [. . .].)

GUIDELINE 15: RESEARCH INVOLVING INDIVIDUALS WHO BY REASON OF MENTAL OR BEHAVIOURAL DISORDERS ARE NOT CAPABLE OF GIVING ADEQUATELY INFORMED CONSENT

Before undertaking research involving individuals who by reason of mental or behavioural disorders are not capable of giving adequately informed consent, the investigator must ensure that:

• such persons will not be subjects of research that might equally well be carried out on persons whose capacity to give adequately informed consent is not impaired;

• the purpose of the research is to obtain knowledge relevant to the particular health needs of persons with mental or behavioural disorders;

• the consent of each subject has been obtained to the extent of that person's capabilities, and a prospective subject's refusal to participate in research is always respected, unless, in exceptional circumstances, there is no reasonable medical alternative and local law permits overriding the objection; and,

• in cases where prospective subjects lack capacity to consent, permission is obtained from a responsible family member or a legally authorized representative in accordance with applicable law.

Commentary on Guideline 15

General considerations. Most individuals with mental or behavioural disorders are capable of giving informed consent; this Guideline is concerned only with those who are not capable or who because their condition deteriorates become temporarily incapable. They should never be subjects of research that might equally well be carried out on persons in full possession of their mental faculties, but they are clearly the only subjects suitable for a large part of research into the origins and treatment of certain severe mental or behavioural disorders.

Consent of the individual. The investigator must obtain the approval of an ethical review committee to include in research persons who by reason of mental or behavioural disorders are not capable of giving informed consent. The willing cooperation of such persons should be sought to the extent that their mental state permits, and any objection on their part to taking part in any study that has no components designed to benefit them directly should always be respected. The objection of such an individual to an investigational intervention intended to be of therapeutic benefit should be respected unless there is no reasonable medical alternative and local law permits overriding the objection. The agreement of an immediate family member or other person with a close personal relationship with the individual should be sought, but it should be recognized that these proxies may have their own interests that may call their permission into question. Some relatives may not be primarily concerned with protecting the rights and welfare of the patients. Moreover, a close family member or friend may wish to take advantage of a research study in the hope that it will succeed in "curing" the condition. Some jurisdictions do not permit third-party permission for subjects lacking capacity to consent. Legal authorization may be necessary to involve in research an individual who has been committed to an institution by a court order.

Serious illness in persons who because of mental or behavioural disorders are unable to give adequately informed consent. Persons who because of mental or behavioural disorders are unable to give adequately informed consent and who have, or are at risk of, serious illnesses such as HIV infection, cancer, or hepatitis should not be deprived of the possible benefits of investigational drugs, vaccines, or devices that show promise of therapeutic or preventive benefit, particularly when no superior or equivalent therapy or prevention is available. Their entitlement to access to such therapy or prevention is justified ethically on the same grounds as is such entitlement for other vulnerable groups.

Persons who are unable to give adequately informed consent by reason of mental or behavioural disorders are, in general, not suitable for participation in formal clinical trials except those trials that are designed to be responsive to their particular health needs and can be carried out only with them. (See also Guidelines 8 [...], 9 [...], and 13 [...].)

GUIDELINE 16: WOMEN AS RESEARCH PARTICIPANTS

Investigators, sponsors, or ethical review committees should not exclude women of reproductive age from biomedical research. The potential for becoming pregnant during a study should not, in itself, be used as a reason for precluding or limiting participation. However, a thorough discussion of risks to the pregnant woman and to her fetus is a prerequisite for the woman's ability to make a rational decision to enrol in a clinical study. In this discussion, if participation in the research might be hazardous to a fetus or a woman if she becomes pregnant, the sponsors/investigators should guarantee the prospective subject a pregnancy test and access to effective contraceptive methods before the research commences. Where such access is not possible, for legal or religious reasons, investigators should not recruit for such possibly hazardous research women who might become pregnant.

Commentary on Guideline 16

Women in most societies have been discriminated against with regard to their involvement in research. Women who are biologically capable of becoming pregnant have been customarily excluded from formal clinical trials of drugs, vaccines, and medical devices owing to concern about undetermined risks to the fetus. Consequently, relatively little is known about the safety and efficacy of most drugs, vaccines, or devices for such women, and this lack of knowledge can be dangerous.

A general policy of excluding from such clinical trials women biologically capable of becoming pregnant is unjust in that it deprives women as a class of persons of the benefits of the new knowledge derived from the trials. Further, it is an affront to their right of self-determination.

Nevertheless, although women of child-bearing age should be given the opportunity to participate in research, they should be helped to understand that the research could include risks to the fetus if they become pregnant during the research.

Although this general presumption favours the inclusion of women in research, it must be acknowledged that in some parts of the world women are vulnerable to neglect or harm in research because of their social conditioning to submit to authority, to ask no questions, and to tolerate pain and suffering. When women in such situations are potential subjects in research, investigators need to exercise special care in the informed consent process to ensure that they have adequate time and a proper environment in which to take decisions on the basis of clearly given information.

Individual consent of women. In research involving women of reproductive age, whether pregnant or non-pregnant, only the informed consent of the woman herself is required for her participation. In no case should the permission of a spouse or partner replace the requirement of individual informed consent. If women wish to consult with their husbands or partners or seek voluntarily to obtain their permission before deciding to enroll in research, that is not only ethically permissible but in some contexts highly desirable. A strict requirement of authorization of spouse or partner, however, violates the substantive principle of respect for persons.

A thorough discussion of risks to the pregnant woman and to her fetus is a prerequisite for the woman's ability to make a rational decision to enroll in a clinical study. For women who are not pregnant at the outset of a study but who might become pregnant while they are still subjects, the consent discussion should include information about the alternative of voluntarily withdrawing from the study and, where legally permissible, terminating the pregnancy. Also, if the pregnancy is not terminated, they should be guaranteed a medical follow-up. (See also Guideline 17 [...].)

GUIDELINE 17: PREGNANT WOMEN AS RESEARCH PARTICIPANTS

Pregnant women should be presumed to be eligible for participation in biomedical research. Investigators and ethical review committees should ensure that prospective subjects who are pregnant are adequately informed about the risks and benefits to themselves, their pregnancies, the fetus and their subsequent offspring, and to their fertility.

Research in this population should be performed only if it is relevant to the particular health needs of a pregnant woman or her fetus, or to the health needs of pregnant women in general, and, when appropriate, if it is supported by reliable evidence from animal experiments, particularly as to risks of teratogenicity and mutagenicity.

Commentary on Guideline 17

The justification of research involving pregnant women is complicated by the fact that it may present risks and potential benefits to two beings—the woman and the fetus—as well as to the person the fetus is destined to become. Though the decision about acceptability of risk should be made by the mother as part of the informed consent process, it is desirable in research directed at the health of the fetus to obtain the father's opinion also, when possible. Even when evidence concerning risks is unknown or ambiguous, the decision about acceptability of risk to the fetus should be made by the woman as part of the informed consent process.

Especially in communities or societies in which cultural beliefs accord more importance to the fetus than to the woman's life or health, women may feel constrained to participate, or not to participate, in research. Special safeguards should be established to prevent undue inducement to pregnant women to participate in research in which interventions hold out the prospect of direct benefit to the fetus. Where fetal abnormality is not recognized as an indication for abortion, pregnant women should not be recruited for research in which there is a realistic basis for concern that fetal abnormality may occur as a consequence of participation as a subject in research.

Investigators should include in protocols on research on pregnant women a plan for monitoring the outcome of the pregnancy with regard to both the health of the woman and the short-term and long-term health of the child.

GUIDELINE 18: SAFEGUARDING CONFIDENTIALITY

The investigator must establish secure safeguards of the confidentiality of subjects' research data. Subjects should be told the limits, legal or other, to the investigators' ability to safeguard confidentiality and the possible consequences of breaches of confidentiality.

Commentary on Guideline 18

Confidentiality between investigator and subject. Research relating to individuals and groups may involve the collection and storage of information that, if disclosed to third parties, could cause harm or distress. Investigators should arrange to protect the confidentiality of such information by, for example, omitting information that might lead to the identification of individual subjects, limiting access to the information, anonymizing data, or other means. During the process of obtaining informed consent the investigator should inform the prospective subjects about the precautions that will be taken to protect confidentiality.

Prospective subjects should be informed of limits to the ability of investigators to ensure strict confidentiality and of the foreseeable adverse social consequences of breaches of confidentiality. Some jurisdictions require the reporting to appropriate agencies of, for instance, certain communicable diseases or evidence of child abuse or neglect. Drug regulatory authorities have the right to inspect clinical-trial records, and a sponsor's clinical-compliance audit staff may require and obtain access to confidential data. These and similar limits to the ability to maintain confidentiality should be anticipated and disclosed to prospective subjects.

Participation in HIV/AIDS drug and vaccine trials may impose upon the research subjects significant associated risks of social discrimination or harm; such risks merit consideration equal to that given to adverse medical consequences of the drugs and vaccines. Efforts must be made to reduce their likelihood and severity. For example, subjects in vaccine trials must be enabled to demonstrate that their HIV seropositivity is due to their having been vaccinated rather than to natural infection. This may be accomplished by providing them with documents attesting to their participation in vaccine trials, or by maintaining a confidential register of trial subjects, from which information can be made available to outside agencies at a subject's request.

Confidentiality between physician and patient. Patients have the right to expect that their physicians and other health-care professionals will hold all information about them in strict confidence and disclose it only to those who need, or have a legal right to, the information, such as other attending physicians, nurses, or other health-care workers who perform tasks related to the diagnosis and treatment of patients. A treating physician should not disclose any identifying information about patients to an investigator unless each patient has given consent to such disclosure and unless an ethical review committee has approved such disclosure.

Physicians and other health-care professionals record the details of their observations and interventions in medical and other records. Epidemiological studies often make use of such records. For such studies it is usually impracticable to obtain the informed consent of each identifiable patient; an ethical review committee may waive the requirement for informed consent when this is consistent with the requirements of applicable law and provided that there are secure safeguards of confidentiality. (See also Guideline 4 Commentary: Waiver of the consent requirement.) In institutions in which records may be used for research purposes without the informed consent of patients, it is advisable to notify patients generally of such practices; notification is usually by means of a statement in patient-information brochures. For research limited to patients' medical records, access must be approved or cleared by an ethical review committee and must be supervised by a person who is fully aware of the confidentiality requirements.

Issues of confidentiality in genetic research. An investigator who proposes to perform genetic tests of known clinical or predictive value on biological samples that can be linked to an identifiable individual must obtain the informed consent of the individual or, when indicated, the permission of a legally authorized representative. Conversely, before performing a genetic test that is of known predictive value or gives reliable information about a known heritable condition, and individual consent or permission has not been obtained, investigators must see that biological samples are fully anonymized and unlinked; this ensures that no information about specific individuals can be derived from such research or passed back to them.

When biological samples are not fully anonymized and when it is anticipated that there may be valid clinical or research reasons for linking the results of genetic tests to research subjects, the investigator in seeking informed consent should assure prospective subjects that their identity will be protected by secure coding of their samples (encryption) and by restricted access to the database, and explain to them this process.

When it is clear that for medical or possibly research reasons the results of genetic tests will be reported to the subject or to the subject's physician, the subject should be informed that such disclosure will occur and that the samples to be tested will be clearly labelled.

Investigators should not disclose results of diagnostic genetic tests to relatives of subjects without the subjects' consent. In places where immediate family relatives would usually expect to be informed of such results, the research protocol, as approved or cleared by the ethical review committee, should indicate the precautions in place to prevent such disclosure of results without the subjects' consent; such plans should be clearly explained during the process of obtaining informed consent.

GUIDELINE 19: RIGHT OF INJURED SUBJECTS TO TREATMENT AND COMPENSATION

Investigators should ensure that research subjects who suffer injury as a result of their participation are entitled to free medical treatment for such injury and to such financial or other assistance as would compensate them equitably for any resultant impairment, disability, or handicap. In the case of death as a result of their participation, their depen-

dants are entitled to compensation. Subjects must not be asked to waive the right to compensation.

Commentary on Guideline 19

Guideline 19 is concerned with two distinct but closely related entitlements. The first is the uncontroversial entitlement to free medical treatment and compensation for accidental injury inflicted by procedures or interventions performed exclusively to accomplish the purposes of research (non-therapeutic procedures). The second is the entitlement of dependants to material compensation for death or disability occurring as a direct result of study participation. Implementing a compensation system for research-related injuries or death is likely to be complex, however.

Equitable compensation and free medical treatment. Compensation is owed to research subjects who are disabled as a consequence of injury from procedures performed solely to accomplish the purposes of research. Compensation and free medical treatment are generally not owed to research subjects who suffer expected or foreseen adverse reactions to investigational therapeutic, diagnostic, or preventive interventions when such reactions are not different in kind from those known to be associated with established interventions in standard medical practice. In the early stages of drug testing (Phase I and early Phase II), it is generally unreasonable to assume that an investigational drug holds out the prospect of direct benefit for the individual subject; accordingly, compensation is usually owed to individuals who become disabled as a result of serving as subjects in such studies.

The ethical review committee should determine in advance: (i) the injuries for which subjects will receive free treatment and, in case of impairment, disability, or handicap resulting from such injuries, be compensated; and (ii) the injuries for which they will not be compensated. Prospective subjects should be informed of the committee's decisions, as part of the process of informed consent. As an ethical review committee cannot make such advance determination in respect of unexpected or unforeseen adverse reactions, such reactions must be presumed compensable and should be reported to the committee for prompt review as they occur.

Subjects must not be asked to waive their rights to compensation or required to show negligence or lack of a reasonable degree of skill on the part of the investigator in order to claim free medical treatment or compensation. The informed consent process or form should contain no words that would absolve an investigator from responsibility in the case of accidental injury, or that would imply that subjects would waive their right to seek compensation for impairment, disability, or handicap. Prospective subjects should be informed that they will not need to take legal action to secure the free medical treatment or compensation for injury to which they may be entitled. They should also be told what medical service or organization or individual will provide the medical treatment and what organization will be responsible for providing compensation.

Obligation of the sponsor with regard to compensation. Before the research begins, the sponsor, whether a pharmaceutical company or other organization or institution, or a government (where government insurance is not precluded by law), should agree to provide compensation for any physical injury for which subjects are entitled to compensation, or come to an agreement with the investigator concerning the circumstances in which the investigator must rely on his or her own insurance coverage (for example, for negligence or failure of the investigator to follow the protocol, or where government insurance coverage is limited to negligence). In certain circumstances it may be advisable to follow both courses. Sponsors should seek adequate insurance against risks to cover compensation, independent of proof of fault.

GUIDELINE 20: STRENGTHENING CAPACITY FOR ETHICAL AND SCIENTIFIC REVIEW AND BIOMEDICAL RESEARCH

Many countries lack the capacity to assess or ensure the scientific quality or ethical acceptability of biomedical research proposed or carried out in their jurisdictions. In externally sponsored collaborative research, sponsors and investigators have an ethical obligation to ensure that biomedical research projects for which they are responsible in such countries contribute effectively to national or local capacity to design and conduct biomedical research, and to provide scientific and ethical review and monitoring of such research. Capacity-building may include, but is not limited to, the following activities:

• establishing and strengthening independent and competent ethical review processes/committees;

• strengthening research capacity;

• developing technologies appropriate to health-care and biomedical research;

• training of research and health-care staff; [and,]

• educating the community from which research subjects will be drawn.

Commentary on Guideline 20

External sponsors and investigators have an ethical obligation to contribute to a host country's sustainable capacity for independent scientific and ethical review and biomedical research. Before undertaking research in a host country with little or no such capacity, external sponsors and investigators should include in the research protocol a plan that specifies the contribution they will make. The amount of capacity building reasonably expected should be proportional to the magnitude of the research project. A brief epidemiological study involving only review of medical records, for example, would entail relatively little, if any, such development, whereas a considerable contribution is to be expected of an external sponsor of, for instance, a large-scale vaccine field-trial expected to last two or three years.

The specific capacity-building objectives should be determined and achieved through dialogue and negotiation between external sponsors and host-country authorities. External sponsors would be expected to employ and, if necessary, train local individuals to function as investigators, research assistants, or data managers, for example, and to provide, as necessary, reasonable amounts of financial, educational, and other assistance for capacity-building. To avoid conflict of interest and safeguard the independence of review committees, financial assistance should not be provided directly to them; rather, funds should be made available to appropriate authorities in the host-country government or to the host research institution. (See also Guideline 10 [. . .].)

GUIDELINE 21: ETHICAL OBLIGATION OF EXTERNAL SPONSORS TO PROVIDE HEALTH-CARE SERVICES

External sponsors are ethically obliged to ensure the availability of:

• health-care services that are essential to the safe conduct of the research;

• treatment for subjects who suffer injury as a consequence of research interventions; and,

• services that are a necessary part of the commitment of a sponsor to make a beneficial intervention or product developed as a result of the research reasonably available to the population or community concerned.

Commentary on Guideline 21

Obligations of external sponsors to provide health-care services will vary with the circumstances of particular studies and the needs of host countries. The sponsors' obligations in particular studies should be clarified before the research is begun. The research protocol should specify what health-care services will be made available, during and after the research, to the subjects themselves, to the community from which the subjects are drawn, or to the host country, and for how long. The details of these arrangements should be agreed by the sponsor, officials of the host country, other interested parties, and, when appropriate, the community from which subjects are to be drawn. The agreed arrangements should be specified in the consent process and document.

Although sponsors are, in general, not obliged to provide health-care services beyond that which is necessary for the conduct of the research, it is morally praiseworthy to do so. Such services typically include treatment for diseases contracted in the course of the study. It might, for example, be agreed to treat cases of an infectious disease contracted during a trial of a vaccine designed to provide immunity to that disease, or to provide treatment of incidental conditions unrelated to the study.

The obligation to ensure that subjects who suffer injury as a consequence of research interventions obtain medical treatment free of charge, and that compensation be provided for death or disability occurring as a consequence of such injury, is the subject of Guideline 19, on the scope and limits of such obligations.

When prospective or actual subjects are found to have diseases unrelated to the research, or cannot be enrolled in a study because they do not meet the health criteria, investigators should, as appropriate, advise them to obtain, or refer them for, medical care. In general, also, in the course of a study, sponsors should disclose to the proper health authorities information of public health concern arising from the research.

The obligation of the sponsor to make reasonably available for the benefit of the population or community concerned any intervention or product developed, or knowledge generated, as a result of the research is considered in Guideline 10 [. . .].

---

10   The ICH Harmonised Tripartite Guideline— Guideline for Good Clinical Practice (ICH-GCP Guideline)

THE INTERNATIONAL CONFERENCE ON HARMONISATION
OF TECHNICAL REQUIREMENTS FOR REGISTRATION
OF PHARMACEUTICALS FOR HUMAN USE

[Front matter and Section 1 omitted—eds.]

2.   THE PRINCIPLES OF ICH-GCP

2.1 Clinical trials should be conducted in accordance with the ethical principles that have their origin in the Declaration of Helsinki, and that are consistent with GCP and the applicable regulatory requirement(s).

2.2 Before a trial is initiated, foreseeable risks and inconveniences should be weighed against the anticipated benefit for the individual trial subject and society. A trial should be initiated and continued only if the anticipated benefits justify the risks.

_____

International Conference on Harmonisation of Technical Requirements for Registration of Pharmaceuticals for Human Use, ICH Harmonised Tripartite Guideline— Guideline for Good Clinical Practice (ICH-GCP Guideline) (Geneva: 1996).

2.3 The rights, safety, and well-being of the trial subjects are the most important considerations and should prevail over interests of science and society.

2.4 The available nonclinical and clinical information on an investigational product should be adequate to support the proposed clinical trial.

2.5 Clinical trials should be scientifically sound, and described in a clear, detailed protocol.

2.6 A trial should be conducted in compliance with the protocol that has received prior institutional review board (IRB)/independent ethics committee (IEC) approval/favorable opinion.

2.7 The medical care given to, and medical decisions made on behalf of, subjects should always be the responsibility of a qualified physician or, when appropriate, of a qualified dentist.

2.8 Each individual involved in conducting a trial should be qualified by education, training, and experience to perform his or her respective task(s).

2.9 Freely given informed consent should be obtained from every subject prior to clinical trial participation.

2.10 All clinical trial information should be recorded, handled, and stored in a way that allows its accurate reporting, interpretation, and verification.

2.11 The confidentiality of records that could identify subjects should be protected, respecting the privacy and confidentiality rules in accordance with the applicable regulatory requirement(s).

2.12 Investigational products should be manufactured, handled, and stored in accordance with applicable good manufacturing practice (GMP). They should be used in accordance with the approved protocol.

2.13 Systems with procedures that assure the quality of every aspect of the trial should be implemented.

3. INSTITUTIONAL REVIEW BOARD/ INDEPENDENT ETHICS COMMITTEE (IRB/IEC)

3.1 Responsibilities

3.1.1 An IRB/IEC should safeguard the rights, safety, and well-being of all trial subjects. Special attention should be paid to trials that may include vulnerable subjects.

3.1.2 The IRB/IEC should obtain the following documents: trial protocol(s)/amendment(s), written informed consent form(s) and consent form updates that the investigator proposes for use in the trial, subject recruitment procedures (e.g., advertisements), written information to be provided to subjects. Investigator's Brochure (IB), available safety information, information about payments, and compensation available to subjects, the investigator's current curriculum vitae and/or other documentation evidencing qualifications, and any other documents that the IRB/IEC may need to fulfill its responsibilities. The IRB/ IEC should review a proposed clinical trial within a reasonable time and document its views in writing, clearly identifying the trial, the documents reviewed, and the dates for the following:

  • approval/favorable opinion; modifications required prior to its approval/favorable opinion;

  • disapproval/negative opinion; and

  • termination/suspension of any prior approval/favorable opinion.

3.1.3 The IRB/IEC should consider the qualifications of the investigator for the proposed trial as documented by a current curriculum vitae and/or by any other relevant documentation the IRB/IEC requests.

3.1.4 The IRB/IEC should conduct continuing review of each ongoing trial at intervals appropriate to the degree of risk to human subjects, but at least once per year.

3.1.5 The IRB/IEC may request more information than is outlined in paragraph 4.8.10 be given to subjects when, in the judgment of the IRB/IEC, the additional information would add meaningfully to the protection of the rights, safety, and/or well-being of the subjects.

3.1.6 When a non-therapeutic trial is to be carried out with the consent of the subject's legally acceptable representative (see 4.8.12, 4.8.14), the IRB/IEC should determine that the proposed protocol and/or other document(s) adequately addresses relevant ethical concerns and meets applicable regulatory requirements for such trials.

3.1.7 Where the protocol indicates that prior consent of the trial subject or the subject's legally acceptable representative is not possible (see 4.8.15), the IRB/IEC should determine that the proposed protocol and/or other document(s) adequately addresses relevant ethical concerns and meets applicable regulatory requirements for such trials (i.e., in emergency situations).

3.1.8 The IRB/IEC should review both the amount and method of payment to subjects to assure that neither presents problems of coercion or undue influence on the trial subjects. Payments to a subject should be prorated and not wholly contingent on completion of the trial by the subject.

3.1.9 The IRB/IEC should ensure that information regarding payment to subjects, including the methods, amounts, and schedule of payment to trial subjects, is set forth in the written informed consent form and any other written information to be provided to subjects. The way payment will be prorated should be specified.

3.2 Composition, Functions, and Operations

3.2.1 The IRB/IEC should consist of a reasonable number of members, who collectively have the qualifications and experience to review and evaluate the science, medical aspects, and ethics of the proposed trial. It is recommended that the IRB/IEC should include:

(a) At least five members.

(b) At least one member whose primary area of interest is in a non-scientific area.

(c) At least one member who is independent of the institution/trial site.

Only those IRB/IEC members who are independent of the investigator and the sponsor of the trial should vote/ provide opinion on a trial-related matter. A list of IRB/IEC members and their qualifications should be maintained.

3.2.2 The IRB/IEC should perform its functions according to written operating procedures, should maintain written records of its activities and minutes of its meetings, and should comply with GCP and with the applicable regulatory requirement(s).

3.2.3 An IRB/IEC should make its decisions at announced meetings at which at least a quorum, as stipulated in its written operating procedures, is present.

3.2.4 Only members who participate in the IRB/IEC review and discussion should vote/provide their opinion and/or advise.

3.2.5 The investigator may provide information on any aspect of the trial, but should not participate in the deliberations of the IRB/IEC or in the vote/opinion of the IRB/IEC.

3.2.6 An IRB/IEC may invite nonmembers with expertise in special areas for assistance.

3.3 Procedures

The IRB/IEC should establish, document in writing, and follow its procedures, which should include:

3.3.1 Determining its composition (names and qualifications of the members) and the authority under which it is established.

3.3.2 Scheduling, notifying its members of, and conducting its meetings.

3.3.3 Conducting initial and continuing review of trials.

3.3.4 Determining the frequency of continuing review, as appropriate.

3.3.5 Providing, according to the applicable regulatory requirements, expedited review and approval/favorable opinion of minor change(s) in ongoing trials that have the approval/favorable opinion of the IRB/IEC.

3.3.6 Specifying that no subject should be admitted to a trial before the IRB/IEC issues its written approval/favorable opinion of the trial.

3.3.7 Specifying that no deviations from, or changes of, the protocol should be initiated without prior written IRB/IEC approval/favorable opinion of an appropriate amendment, except when necessary to eliminate immediate hazards to the subjects or when the change(s) involves only logistical or administrative aspects of the trial (e.g., change of monitor(s), telephone number(s)) (see 4.5.2).

3.3.8 Specifying that the investigator should promptly report to the IRB/IEC:

(a) Deviations from, or changes of, the protocol to eliminate immediate hazards to the trial subjects (see 3.3.7, 4.5.2, 4.5.4).

(b) Changes increasing the risk to subjects and/or affecting significantly the conduct of the trial (see 4.10.2).

(c) All adverse drug reactions (ADRs) that are both serious and unexpected.

(d) New information that may affect adversely the safety of the subjects or the conduct of the trial.

3.3.9 Ensuring that the IRB/IEC promptly notify in writing the investigator/institution concerning:

(a) Its trial-related decisions/opinions.

(b) The reasons for its decisions/opinions.

(c) Procedures for appeal of its decisions/opinions.

3.4 Records

The IRB/IEC should retain all relevant records (e.g., written procedures, membership lists, lists of occupations/affiliations of members, submitted documents, minutes of meetings, and correspondence) for a period of at least 3 years after completion of the trial and make them available upon request from the regulatory authority(ies). The IRB/IEC may be asked by investigators, sponsors, or regulatory authorities to provide its written procedures and membership lists.

4. INVESTIGATOR

4.1 Investigator's Qualifications and Agreements

4.1.1 The investigator(s) should be qualified by education, training, and experience to assume responsibility for the proper conduct of the trial, should meet all the qualifications specified by the applicable regulatory requirement(s), and should provide evidence of such qualifications through up-to-date curriculum vitae and/or other relevant documentation requested by the sponsor, the IRB/IEC, and/or the regulatory authority(ies).

4.1.2 The investigator should be thoroughly familiar with the appropriate use of the investigational product(s), as described in the protocol, in the current Investigator's Brochure, in the product information, and in other information sources provided by the sponsor.

4.1.3 The investigator should be aware of, and should comply with, GCP and the applicable regulatory requirements.

4.1.4 The investigator/institution should permit monitoring and auditing by the sponsor and inspection by the appropriate regulatory authority(ies).

4.1.5 The investigator should maintain a list of appropriately qualified persons to whom the investigator has delegated significant trial-related duties.

4.2 Adequate Resources

4.2.1 The investigator should be able to demonstrate (e.g., based on retrospective data) a potential for recruiting the required number of suitable subjects within the agreed recruitment period.

4.2.2 The investigator should have sufficient time to properly conduct and complete the trial within the agreed trial period.

4.2.3 The investigator should have available an adequate number of qualified staff and adequate facilities for the foreseen duration of the trial to conduct the trial properly and safely.

4.2.4 The investigator should ensure that all persons assisting with the trial are adequately informed about the protocol, the investigational product(s), and their trial-related duties and functions.

4.3 Medical Care of Trial Subjects

4.3.1 A qualified physician (or dentist, when appropriate), who is an investigator or a sub-investigator for the trial, should be responsible for all trial-related medical (or dental) decisions.

4.3.2 During and following a subject's participation in a trial, the investigator/institution should ensure that adequate medical care is provided to a subject for any adverse events, including clinically significant laboratory values, related to the trial. The investigator/institution should inform a subject when medical care is needed for intercurrent illness(es) of which the investigator becomes aware.

4.3.3 It is recommended that the investigator inform the subject's primary physician about the subject's participation in the trial if the subject has a primary physician and if the subject agrees to the primary physician being informed.

4.3.4 Although a subject is not obliged to give his/her reason(s) for withdrawing prematurely from a trial, the investigator should make a reasonable effort to ascertain the reason(s), while fully respecting the subject's rights.

4.4 Communication with IRB/IEC

4.4.1 Before initiating a trial, the investigator/institution should have written and dated approval/favorable opinion from the IRB/IEC for the trial protocol, written informed consent form, consent form updates, subject recruitment procedures (e.g., advertisements), and any other written information to be provided to subjects.

4.4.2 As part of the investigator's/institution's written application to the IRB/IEC, the investigator/institution should provide the IRB/IEC with a current copy of the Investigator's Brochure. If the Investigator's Brochure is updated during the trial, the investigator/institution should supply a copy of the updated Investigator's Brochure to the IRB/IEC.

4.4.3 During the trial the investigator/institution should provide to the IRB/IEC all documents subject to review.

4.5 Compliance with Protocol

4.5.1 The investigator/institution should conduct the trial in compliance with the protocol agreed to by the sponsor and, if required, by the regulatory authority(ies) and which was given approval/favorable opinion by the IRB/IEC. The investigator/institution and the sponsor should sign the protocol, or an alternative contract, to confirm agreement.

4.5.2 The investigator should not implement any deviation from, or changes of, the protocol without agreement by the sponsor and prior review and documented approval/favorable opinion from the IRB/IEC of an amendment, except where necessary to eliminate an immediate hazard(s) to trial subjects, or when the change(s) involves only logistical or administrative aspects of the trial (e.g., change in monitor(s), change of telephone number(s)).

4.5.3 The investigator, or person designated by the investigator, should document and explain any deviation from the approved protocol.

4.5.4 The investigator may implement a deviation from, or a change of, the protocol to eliminate an immediate hazard(s) to trial subjects without prior IRB/IEC approval/favorable opinion. As soon as possible, the implemented deviation or change, the reasons for it, and, if appropriate, the proposed protocol amendment(s) should be submitted:

(a) to the IRB/IEC for review and approval/favorable opinion,

(b) to the sponsor for agreement and, if required,

(c) to the regulatory authority(ies).

4.6 Investigational Product(s)

4.6.1 Responsibility for investigational product(s) accountability at the trial site(s) rests with the investigator/institution.

4.6.2 Where allowed/required, the investigator/institution may/should assign some or all of the investigator's/institution's duties for investigational product(s) accountability at the trial site(s) to an appropriate pharmacist or another appropriate individual who is under the supervision of the investigator/institution.

4.6.3 The investigator/institution and/or a pharmacist or other appropriate individual, who is designated by the investigator/institution, should maintain records of the product's delivery to the trial site, the inventory at the site, the use by each subject, and the return to the sponsor or alternative disposition of unused product(s). These records should include dates, quantities, batch/serial numbers, expiration dates (if applicable), and the unique code numbers assigned to the investigational product(s) and trial subjects. Investigators should maintain records that document adequately that the subjects were provided the doses specified by the protocol and reconcile all investigational product(s) received from the sponsor.

4.6.4 The investigational product(s) should be stored as specified by the sponsor (see 5.13.2 and 5.14.3) and in accordance with applicable regulatory requirement(s).

4.6.5 The investigator should ensure that the investigational product(s) are used only in accordance with the approved protocol.

4.6.6 The investigator, or a person designated by the investigator/institution, should explain the correct use of the investigational product(s) to each subject and should check, at intervals appropriate for the trial, that each subject is following the instructions properly.

4.7 Randomization Procedures and Unblinding

The investigator should follow the trial's randomization procedures, if any, and should ensure that the code is broken only in accordance with the protocol. If the trial is blinded, the investigator should promptly document and explain to the sponsor any premature unblinding (e.g., accidental unblinding, unblinding due to a serious adverse event) of the investigational product(s).

4.8 Informed Consent of Trial Subjects

4.8.1 In obtaining and documenting informed consent, the investigator should comply with the applicable regulatory requirement(s), and should adhere to GCP and to the ethical principles that have their origin in the Declaration of Helsinki. Prior to the beginning of the trial, the investigator should have the IRB/IEC's written approval/favorable opinion of the written informed consent form and any other written information to be provided to subjects.

4.8.2 The written informed consent form and any other written information to be provided to subjects should be revised whenever important new information becomes available that may be relevant to the subject's consent. Any revised written informed consent form and written information should receive the IRB/IEC's approval/favorable opinion in advance of use. The subject or the subject's legally acceptable representative should be informed in a timely manner if new information becomes available that

may be relevant to the subject's willingness to continue participation in the trial. The communication of this information should be documented.

4.8.3 Neither the investigator, nor the trial staff, should coerce or unduly influence a subject to participate or to continue to participate in a trial.

4.8.4 None of the oral and written information concerning the trial, including the written informed consent form, should contain any language that causes the subject or the subject's legally acceptable representative to waive or to appear to waive any legal rights, or that releases or appears to release the investigator, the institution, the sponsor, or their agents from liability for negligence.

4.8.5 The investigator, or a person designated by the investigator, should fully inform the subject or, if the subject is unable to provide informed consent, the subject's legally acceptable representative, of all pertinent aspects of the trial including the written information given approval/favorable opinion by the IRB/IEC.

4.8.6 The language used in the oral and written information about the trial, including the written informed consent form, should be as non-technical as practical and should be understandable to the subject or the subject's legally acceptable representative and the impartial witness, where applicable.

4.8.7 Before informed consent may be obtained, the investigator, or a person designated by the investigator, should provide the subject or the subject's legally acceptable representative ample time and opportunity to inquire about details of the trial and to decide whether or not to participate in the trial. All questions about the trial should be answered to the satisfaction of the subject or the subject's legally acceptable representative.

4.8.8 Prior to a subject's participation in the trial, the written informed consent form should be signed and personally dated by the subject or by the subject's legally acceptable representative, and by the person who conducted the informed consent discussion.

4.8.9 If a subject is unable to read or if a legally acceptable representative is unable to read, an impartial witness should be present during the entire informed consent discussion. After the written informed consent form and any other written information to be provided to subjects, is read and explained to the subject or the subject's legally acceptable representative, and after the subject or the subject's legally acceptable representative has orally consented to the subject's participation in the trial and, if capable of doing so, has signed and personally dated the informed consent form, the witness should sign and personally date the consent form. By signing the consent form, the witness attests that the information in the consent form and any other written information was accurately explained to, and apparently understood by, the subject or the subject's legally acceptable representative, and that informed consent was freely given by the subject or the subject's legally acceptable representative.

4.8.10 Both the informed consent discussion and the written informed consent form and any other written information to be provided to subjects should include explanations of the following:

(a) That the trial involves research.

(b) The purpose of the trial.

(c) The trial treatment(s) and the probability for random assignment to each treatment.

(d) The trial procedures to be followed, including all invasive procedures.

(e) The subject's responsibilities.

(f) Those aspects of the trial that are experimental.

(g) The reasonably foreseeable risks or inconveniences to the subject and, when applicable, to an embryo, fetus, or nursing infant.

(h) The reasonably expected benefits. When there is no intended clinical benefit to the subject, the subject should be made aware of this.

(i) The alternative procedure(s) or course(s) of treatment that may be available to the subject, and their important potential benefits and risks.

(j) The compensation and/or treatment available to the subject in the event of trial-related injury.

(k) The anticipated prorated payment, if any, to the subject for participating in the trial.

(l) The anticipated expenses, if any, to the subject for participating in the trial.

(m) That the subject's participation in the trial is voluntary and that the subject may refuse to participate or withdraw from the trial, at any time, without penalty or loss of benefits to which the subject is otherwise entitled.

(n) That the monitor(s), the auditor(s), the IRB/IEC, and the regulatory authority(ies) will be granted direct access to the subject's original medical records for verification of clinical trial procedures and/or data, without violating the confidentiality of the subject, to the extent permitted by the applicable laws and regulations and that, by signing a written informed consent form, the subject or the subject's legally acceptable representative is authorizing such access.

(o) That records identifying the subject will be kept confidential and, to the extent permitted by the applicable laws and/or regulations, will not be made publicly available. If the results of the trial are published, the subject's identity will remain confidential.

(p) That the subject or the subject's legally acceptable representative will be informed in a timely manner if information becomes available that may be relevant to the subject's willingness to continue participation in the trial.

(q) The person(s) to contact for further information regarding the trial and the rights of trial subjects, and whom to contact in the event of trial-related injury.

(r) The foreseeable circumstances and/or reasons under which the subject's participation in the trial may be terminated.

(s) The expected duration of the subject's participation in the trial.

(t) The approximate number of subjects involved in the trial.

4.8.11 Prior to participation in the trial, the subject or the subject's legally acceptable representative should receive a copy of the signed and dated written informed consent form and any other written information provided to the subjects. During a subject's participation in the trial, the subject or the subject's legally acceptable representative should receive a copy of the signed and dated consent form updates and a copy of any amendments to the written information provided to subjects.

4.8.12 When a clinical trial (therapeutic or non-therapeutic) includes subjects who can only be enrolled in the trial with the consent of the subject's legally acceptable representative (e.g., minors, or patients with severe dementia), the subject should be informed about the trial to the extent compatible with the subject's understanding and, if capable, the subject should sign and personally date the written informed consent.

4.8.13 Except as described in 4.8.14, a non-therapeutic trial (i.e., a trial in which there is not anticipated direct clinical benefit to the subject), should be conducted in subjects who personally give consent and who sign and date a written informed consent form.

4.8.14 Non-therapeutic trials may be conducted in subjects with consent of a legally acceptable representative provided the following conditions are fulfilled:

(a) The objectives of the trial cannot be met by means of a trial in subjects who can give informed consent personally.

(b) The foreseeable risks to the subjects are low.

(c) The negative impact on the subject's well-being is minimized and low.

(d) The trial is not prohibited by law.

(e) The approval/favorable opinion of the IRB/IEC is expressly sought on the inclusion of such subjects, and the written approval/favorable opinion covers this aspect.

Such trials, unless an exception is justified, should be conducted in patients having a disease or condition for which the investigational product is intended. Subjects in these trials should be particularly closely monitored and should be withdrawn if they appear to be unduly distressed.

4.8.15 In emergency situations, when prior consent of the subject is not possible, the consent of the subject's legally acceptable representative, if present, should be requested. When prior consent of the subject is not possible, and the subject's legally acceptable representative is not available, enrollment of the subject should require measures described in the protocol and/or elsewhere, with documented approval/favorable opinion by the IRB/IEC, to protect the rights, safety, and well-being of the subject and to ensure compliance with applicable regulatory requirements. The subject or the subject's legally acceptable representative should be informed about the trial as soon as possible and consent to continue and other consent as appropriate (see 4.8.10) should be requested.

4.9 Records and Reports

4.9.1 The investigator should ensure the accuracy, completeness, legibility, and timeliness of the data reported to the sponsor in the case report forms [CRFs] and in all required reports.

4.9.2 Data reported on the CRF, that are derived from source documents, should be consistent with the source documents or the discrepancies should be explained.

4.9.3 Any change or correction to a CRF should be dated, initialed, and explained (if necessary) and should not obscure the original entry (i.e., an audit trail should be maintained): this applies to both written and electronic changes or corrections (see 5.18.4 (n)). Sponsors should provide guidance to investigators and/or the investigators' designated representatives on making such corrections. Sponsors should have written procedures to assure that changes or corrections in CRFs made by sponsor's designated representatives are documented, are necessary, and are endorsed by the investigator. The investigator should retain records of the changes and corrections.

4.9.4 The investigator/institution should maintain the trial documents as specified in Essential Documents for the Conduct of a Clinical Trial [not included in this excerpt—

eds.] and as required by the applicable regulatory requirement(s). The investigator/institution should take measures to prevent accidental or premature destruction of these documents.

4.9.5 Essential documents should be retained until at least 2 years after the last approval of a marketing application in an ICH region and until there are no pending or contemplated marketing applications in an ICH region or at least 2 years have elapsed since the formal discontinuation of clinical development of the investigational product. These documents should be retained for a longer period however if required by the applicable regulatory requirements or by an agreement with the sponsor. It is the responsibility of the sponsor to inform the investigator/institution as to when these documents no longer need to be retained (see 5.5.12).

4.9.6 The financial aspects of the trial should be documented in an agreement between the sponsor and the investigator/institution.

4.9.7 Upon request of the monitor, auditor, IRB/IEC, or regulatory authority, the investigator/institution should make available for direct access all requested trial-related records.

4.10 Progress Reports

4.10.1 The investigator should submit written summaries of the trial status to the IRB/IEC annually, or more frequently, if requested by the IRB/IEC.

4.10.2 The investigator should promptly provide written reports to the sponsor, the IRB/IEC (see 3.3.8), and, where applicable, the institution on any changes significantly affecting the conduct of the trial, and/or increasing the risk to subjects.

4.11 Safety Reporting

4.11.1 All serious adverse events (SAEs) should be reported immediately to the sponsor except for those SAEs that the protocol or other document (e.g., Investigator's Brochure) identifies as not needing immediate reporting. The immediate reports should be followed promptly by detailed, written reports. The immediate and follow-up reports should identify subjects by unique code numbers assigned to the trial subjects rather than by the subjects' names, personal identification numbers, and/or addresses. The investigator should also comply with the applicable regulatory requirement(s) related to the reporting of unexpected serious adverse drug reactions to the regulatory authority(ies) and the IRB/IEC.

4.11.2 Adverse events and/or laboratory abnormalities identified in the protocol as critical to safety evaluations should be reported to the sponsor according to the reporting requirements and within the time periods specified by the sponsor in the protocol.

4.11.3 For reported deaths, the investigator should supply the sponsor and the IRB/IEC with any additional requested information (e.g., autopsy reports and terminal medical reports).

4.12 Premature Termination or Suspension of a Trial

If the trial is prematurely terminated or suspended for any reason the investigator/institution should promptly inform the trial subjects, should assure appropriate therapy and follow-up for the subjects, and, where required by the applicable regulatory requirement(s), should inform the regulatory authority(ies). In addition:

4.12.1 If the investigator terminates or suspends a trial without prior agreement of the sponsor, the investigator should inform the institution where applicable, and the investigator/institution should promptly inform the sponsor and the IRB/IEC, and should provide the sponsor and the IRB/IEC a detailed written explanation of the termination or suspension.

4.12.2 If the sponsor terminates or suspends a trial (see 5.21), the investigator should promptly inform the institution where applicable and the investigator/institution should promptly inform the IRB/IEC, and provide the IRB/IEC a detailed written explanation of the termination or suspension.

4.12.3 If the IRB/IEC terminates or suspends its approval/ favorable opinion of a trial (see 3.1.2 and 3.3.9), the investigator should inform the institution where applicable and the investigator/institution should promptly notify the sponsor and provide the sponsor with a detailed written explanation of the termination or suspension.

4.13 Final Report(s) by Investigator

Upon completion of the trial, the investigator, where applicable, should inform the institution; the investigator/ institution should provide the IRB/IEC with a summary of the trial's outcome, and the regulatory authority(ies) with any reports required.

5. SPONSOR

5.1 Quality Assurance and Quality Control

5.1.1 The sponsor is responsible for implementing and maintaining quality assurance and quality control systems with written standard operating procedures [SOPs] to ensure that

trials are conducted and data are generated, documented (recorded), and reported in compliance with the protocol, GCP, and the applicable regulatory requirement(s).

5.1.2 The sponsor is responsible for securing agreement from all involved parties to insure direct access (1.21) to all trial related sites, source data/documents, and reports for the purpose of monitoring and auditing by the sponsor, and inspection by domestic and foreign regulatory authorities.

5.1.3 Quality control should be applied to each state of data handling to ensure that all data are reliable and have been processed correctly.

5.1.4 Agreements, made by the sponsor with the investigator/institution and any other parties involved with the clinical trial, should be in writing, as part of the protocol or in a separate agreement.

5.2 Contract Research Organization (CRO)

5.2.1 A sponsor may transfer any or all of the sponsor's trial-related duties and functions to a CRO, but the ultimate responsibility for the quality and integrity of the trial data always resides with the sponsor. The CRO should implement quality assurance and quality control.

5.2.2 Any trial related duty and function that is transferred to and assumed by a CRO should be specified in writing.

5.2.3 Any trial-related duties and functions not specifically transferred to and assumed by a CRO are retained by the sponsor.

5.2.4 All references to a sponsor in this guideline also apply to a CRO to the extent that a CRO has assumed the trial related duties and functions of a sponsor.

5.3 Medical Expertise

The sponsor should designate appropriately qualified medical personnel who will be readily available to advise on trial related medical questions or problems. If necessary, outside consultant(s) may be appointed for this purpose.

5.4 Trial Design

5.4.1 The sponsor should utilize qualified individuals (e.g., biostatisticians, clinical pharmacologists, and physicians) as appropriate throughout all stages of the trial process, from designing the protocol and CRFs and planning the analyses to analyzing and preparing interim and final clinical trial reports.

5.4.2 For further guidance: Clinical Trial Protocol and Protocol Amendment(s) [not included in this excerpt—

eds.], the ICH Guideline for Structure and Content of Clinical Study Reports, and other appropriate ICH guidance on trial design, protocol and conduct.

5.5 Trial Management, Data Handling, and Record Keeping

5.5.1 The sponsor should utilize appropriately qualified individuals to supervise the overall conduct of the trial, to handle the data, to verify the data, to conduct the statistical analyses, and to prepare the trial reports.

5.5.2 The sponsor may consider establishing an independent data-monitoring committee (IDMC) to assess the progress of a clinical trial, including the safety data and the critical efficacy endpoints at intervals, and to recommend to the sponsor whether to continue, modify, or stop a trial. The IDMC should have written operating procedures and maintain written records of all its meetings.

5.5.3 When using electronic trial data handling and/or remote electronic trial data systems, the sponsor should:

(a) Ensure and document that the electronic data processing system(s) conforms to the sponsor's established requirements for completeness, accuracy, reliability, and consistent intended performance (i.e., validation).

(b) Maintain SOPs for using these systems.

(c) Ensure that the systems are designed to permit data changes in such a way that the data changes are documented and that there is no deletion of entered data (i.e., maintain an audit trail, data trail, edit trail).

(d) Maintain a security system that prevents unauthorized access to the data.

(e) Maintain a list of the individuals who are authorized to make data changes (see 4.1.5 and 4.9.3).

(f) Maintain adequate backup of the data.

(g) Safeguard the blinding, if any (e.g., maintain the blinding during data entry and processing).

5.5.4 If data are transformed during processing, it should always be possible to compare the original data and observations with the processed data.

5.5.5 The sponsor should use an unambiguous subject identification code [...] that allows identification of all the data reported for each subject.

5.5.6 The sponsor, or other owners of the data, should retain all of the sponsor-specific essential documents pertaining to the trial.

5.5.7 The sponsor should retain all sponsor-specific essential documents in conformance with the applicable regulatory requirement(s) of the country(ies) where the product is approved, and/or where the sponsor intends to apply for approval(s).

5.5.8 If the sponsor discontinues the clinical development of an investigational product (i.e., for any or all indications, routes of administration, or dosage forms), the sponsor should maintain all sponsor-specific essential documents for at least 2 years after formal discontinuation or in conformance with the applicable regulatory requirement(s).

5.5.9 If the sponsor discontinues the clinical development of an investigational product, the sponsor should notify all the trial investigators/institutions and all the regulatory authorities.

5.5.10 Any transfer of ownership of the data should be reported to the appropriate authority(ies), as required by the applicable regulatory requirement(s).

5.5.11 The sponsor specific essential documents should be retained until at least 2 years after the last approval of a marketing application in an ICH region and until there are no pending or contemplated marketing applications in an ICH region or at least 2 years have elapsed since the formal discontinuation of clinical development of the investigational product. These documents should be retained for a longer period however if required by the applicable regulatory requirement(s) or if needed by the sponsor.

5.5.12 The sponsor should inform the investigator(s)/institution(s) in writing of the need for record retention and should notify the investigator(s)/institution(s) in writing when the trial-related records are no longer needed.

5.6 Investigator Selection

5.6.1 The sponsor is responsible for selecting the investigator(s)/institution(s). Each investigator should be qualified by training and experience and should have adequate resources (see 4.1, 4.2) to properly conduct the trial for which the investigator is selected. If organization of a coordinating committee and/or selection of coordinating investigator(s) are to be utilized in multicentre trials, their organization and/or selection are the sponsor's responsibility.

5.6.2 Before entering an agreement with an investigator/institution to conduct a trial, the sponsor should provide the investigator(s)/institution(s) with the protocol and up-to-date Investigator's Brochure, and should provide sufficient time for the investigator/institution to review the protocol and the information provided.

5.6.3 The sponsor should obtain the investigator's/institution's agreement:

(a) to conduct the trial in compliance with GCP, with the applicable regulatory requirement(s) (see 4.1.3), and with the protocol agreed to by the sponsor and given approval/favorable opinion by the IRB/IEC (see 4.5.1);

(b) to comply with procedures for data recording/ reporting;

(c) to permit monitoring, auditing, and inspection (see 4.1.4); and

(d) to retain the trial related essential documents until the sponsor informs the investigator/institution these documents are no longer needed (see 4.9.4 and 5.5.12). The sponsor and the investigator/institution should sign the protocol, or an alternative document, to confirm this agreement.

5.7 Allocation of Duties and Functions

Prior to initiating a trial, the sponsor should define, establish, and allocate all trial-related duties and functions.

5.8 Compensation to Subjects and Investigators

5.8.1 If required by the applicable regulatory requirement(s), the sponsor should provide insurance or should indemnify (legal and financial coverage) the investigator/ the institution against claims arising from malpractice and/or negligence.

5.8.2 The sponsor's policies and procedures should address the costs of treatment of trial subjects in the event of trial-related injuries in accordance with the applicable regulatory requirement(s).

5.8.3 When trial subjects receive compensation, the method and manner of compensation should comply with applicable regulatory requirement(s).

5.9 Financing

The financial aspects of the trial should be documented in an agreement between the sponsor and the investigator/ institution.

5.10 Notification/Submission to Regulatory Authority(ies)

Before initiating the clinical trial(s), the sponsor (or the sponsor and the investigator, if required by the applicable regulatory requirement(s)) should submit any required application(s) to the appropriate authority(ies) for review, acceptance, and/or permission (as required by the applicable regulatory requirement(s)) to begin the trial(s). Any notification/submission should be dated and contain sufficient information to identify the protocol.

5.11 Confirmation of Review by IRB/IEC

5.11.1 The sponsor should obtain from the investigator/ institution:

(a) The name and address of the investigator's/institution's IRB/IEC.

(b) A statement obtained from the IRB/IEC that it is organized and operates according to GCP and the applicable laws and regulations.

(c) Documented IRB/IEC approval/favorable opinion and, if requested by the sponsor, a current copy of protocol, written informed consent form(s) and any other written information to be provided to subjects, subject recruiting procedures, and documents related to payments and compensation available to the subjects, and any other documents that the IRB/IEC may have requested.

5.11.2 If the IRB/IEC conditions its approval/favorable opinion upon change(s) in any aspect of the trial, such as modification(s) of the protocol, written informed consent form and any other written information to be provided to subjects, and/or other procedures, the sponsor should obtain from the investigator/institution a copy of the modification(s) made and the date approval/favorable opinion was given by the IRB/IEC.

5.11.3 The sponsor should obtain from the investigator/ institution documentation and dates of any IRB/IEC reapprovals/re-evaluations with favorable opinion, and of any withdrawals or suspensions of approval/favorable opinion.

5.12 Information on Investigational Product(s)

5.12.1 When planning trials, the sponsor should ensure that sufficient safety and efficacy data from nonclinical studies and/or clinical trials are available to support human exposure by the route, at the dosages, for the duration, and in the trial population to be studied.

5.12.2 The sponsor should update the Investigator's Brochure as significant new information becomes available.

5.13 Manufacturing, Packaging, Labeling, and Coding Investigational Product(s)

5.13.1 The sponsor should ensure that the investigational product(s) (including active comparator(s) and placebo, if applicable) is characterized as appropriate to the stage of development of the product(s), is manufactured in accordance with any applicable GMP, and is coded and labeled in a manner that protects the blinding, if applicable. In addition, the labeling should comply with applicable regulatory requirement(s).

5.13.2 The sponsor should determine, for the investigational product(s), acceptable storage temperatures, storage conditions (e.g., protection from light), storage times, reconstitution fluids and procedures, and devices for product infusion, if any. The sponsor should inform all involved parties (e.g., monitors, investigators, pharmacists, storage managers) of these determinations.

5.13.3 The investigational product(s) should be packaged to prevent contamination and unacceptable deterioration during transport and storage.

5.13.4 In blinded trials, the coding system for the investigational product(s) should include a mechanism that permits rapid identification of the product(s) in case of a medical emergency, but does not permit undetectable breaks of the blinding.

5.13.5 If significant formulation changes are made in the investigational or comparator product(s) during the course of clinical development, the results of any additional studies of the formulated product(s) (e.g., stability, dissolution rate, bioavailability) needed to assess whether these changes would significantly alter the pharmacokinetic profile of the product should be available prior to the use of the new formulation in clinical trials.

5.14 Supplying and Handling Investigational Product(s)

5.14.1 The sponsor is responsible for supplying the investigator(s)/institution(s) with the investigational product(s).

5.14.2 The sponsor should not supply an investigator/institution with the investigational product(s) until the sponsor obtains all required documentation (e.g., approval/favorable opinion from IRB/IEC and regulatory authority(ies)).

5.14.3 The sponsor should ensure that written procedures include instructions that the investigator/institution should follow for the handling and storage of investigational product(s) for the trial and documentation thereof. The procedures should address adequate and safe receipt, handling, storage, dispensing, retrieval of unused product from subjects, and return of unused investigational product(s) to the sponsor (or alternative disposition if authorized by the sponsor and in compliance with the applicable regulatory requirement(s)).

5.14.4 The sponsor should:

(a) Ensure timely delivery of investigational product(s) to the investigator(s).

(b) Maintain records that document shipment, receipt, disposition, return, and destruction of the investigational product(s) (see 8. Essential Documents for the Conduct of a Clinical Trial [not included in this excerpt—eds.]).

(c) Maintain a system for retrieving investigational products and documenting this retrieval (e.g., for deficient product recall, reclaim after trial completion, expired product reclaim).

(d) Maintain a system for the disposition of unused investigational product(s) and for the documentation of this disposition.

5.14.5 The sponsor should:

(a) Take steps to ensure that the investigational product(s) are stable over the period of use.

(b) Maintain sufficient quantities of the investigational product(s) used in the trials to reconfirm specifications, should this become necessary, and maintain records of batch sample analyses and characteristics. To the extent stability permits, samples should be retained either until the analyses of the trial data are complete or as required by the applicable regulatory requirement(s), whichever represents the longer retention period.

5.15 Record Access

5.15.1 The sponsor should ensure that it is specified in the protocol or other written agreement that the investigator(s)/institution(s) provide direct access to source data/documents for trial-related monitoring, audits, IRB/IEC review, and regulatory inspection.

5.15.2 The sponsor should verify that each subject has consented, in writing, to direct access to his/her original medical records for trial-related monitoring, audit, IRB/IEC review, and regulatory inspection.

5.16 Safety Information

5.16.1 The sponsor is responsible for the ongoing safety evaluation of the investigational product(s).

5.16.2 The sponsor should promptly notify all concerned investigator(s)/institution(s) and the regulatory authority(ies) of findings that could affect adversely the safety of subjects, impact the conduct of the trial, or alter the IRB/IEC's approval/favorable opinion to continue the trial.

5.17 Adverse Drug Reaction Reporting

5.17.1 The sponsor should expedite the reporting to all concerned investigator(s)/institution(s), to the IRB(s)/IEC(s), where required, and to the regulatory authority(ies) of all adverse drug reactions (ADRs) that are both serious and unexpected.

5.17.2 Such expedited reports should comply with the applicable regulatory requirement(s) and with the ICH Guideline for Clinical Safety Data Management: Definitions and Standards for Expedited Reporting.

5.17.3 The sponsor should submit to the regulatory authority(ies) all safety updates and periodic reports, as required by applicable regulatory requirement(s).

5.18 Monitoring

5.18.1 Purpose
The purposes of trial monitoring are to verify that:

(a) The rights and well-being of human subjects are protected.

(b) The reported trial data are accurate, complete, and verifiable from source documents.

(c) The conduct of the trial is in compliance with the currently approved protocol/amendment(s), with GCP, and with the applicable regulatory requirement(s).

5.18.2 Selection and Qualifications of Monitors

(a) Monitors should be appointed by the sponsor.

(b) Monitors should be appropriately trained, and should have the scientific and/or clinical knowledge needed to monitor the trial adequately. A monitor's qualifications should be documented.

(c) Monitors should be thoroughly familiar with the investigational product(s), the protocol, written informed consent form and any other written information to be provided to subjects, the sponsor's SOPs, GCP, and the applicable regulatory requirement(s).

5.18.3 Extent and Nature of Monitoring
The sponsor should ensure that the trials are adequately monitored. The sponsor should determine the appropriate extent and nature of monitoring. The determination of the extent and nature of monitoring should be based on considerations such as the objective, purpose, design, complexity, blinding, size, and endpoints of the trial. In general there is a need for on-site monitoring, before, during, and after the trial: however in exceptional circumstances the sponsor may determine that central monitoring in conjunction with procedures such as investigators' training

and meeting, and extensive written guidance can assure appropriate conduct of the trial in accordance with GCP. Statistically controlled sampling may be an acceptable method for selecting the data to be verified.

5.18.4 Monitor's Responsibilities
The monitor(s) in accordance with the sponsor's requirements should ensure that the trial is conducted and documented properly by carrying out the following activities when relevant and necessary to the trial and the trial site:

(a) Acting as the main line of communication between the sponsor and the investigator.

(b) Verifying that the investigator has adequate qualifications and resources (see 4.1, 4.2, 5.6) and remain adequate throughout the trial period, that facilities, including laboratories, equipment, and staff, are adequate to safely and properly conduct the trial and remain adequate throughout the trial period.

(c) Verifying, for the investigational product(s):

  (i) That storage times and conditions are acceptable, and that supplies are sufficient throughout the trial.
  (ii) That the investigational product(s) are supplied only to subjects who are eligible to receive it and at the protocol specified dose(s).
  (iii) That subjects are provided with necessary instruction on properly using, handling, storing, and returning the investigational product(s).
  (iv) That the receipt, use, and return of the investigational product(s) at the trial sites are controlled and documented adequately.
  (v) That the disposition of unused investigational product(s) at the trial sites complies with applicable regulatory requirement(s) and is in accordance with the sponsor.

(d) Verifying that the investigator follows the approved protocol and all approved amendment(s), if any.

(e) Verifying that written informed consent was obtained before each subject's participation in the trial.

(f) Ensuring that the investigator receives the current Investigator's Brochure, all documents, and all trial supplies needed to conduct the trial properly and to comply with the applicable regulatory requirement(s).

(g) Ensuring that the investigator and the investigator's trial staff are adequately informed about the trial.

(h) Verifying that the investigator and the investigator's trial staff are performing the specific trial functions, in accordance with the protocol and any other written agreement between the sponsor and the investigator/institution, and have not delegated these functions to unauthorized individuals.

(i) Verifying that the investigator is enrolling only eligible subjects.

(j) Reporting the subject recruitment rate.

(k) Verifying that source documents and other trial records are accurate, complete, kept up-to-date, and maintained.

(l) Verifying that the investigator provides all the required reports, notifications, applications, and submissions, and that these documents are accurate, complete, timely, legible, dated, and identify the trial.

(m) Checking the accuracy and completeness of the CRF entries, source documents and other trial-related records against each other. The monitor specifically should verify that:

   (i) The data required by the protocol are reported accurately on the CRFs and are consistent with the source documents.
   (ii) Any dose and/or therapy modifications are well documented for each of the trial subjects.
   (iii) Adverse events, concomitant medications, and intercurrent illnesses are reported in accordance with the protocol on the CRFs.
   (iv) Visits that the subjects fail to make, tests that are not conducted, and examinations that are not performed are clearly reported as such on the CRFs.
   (v) All withdrawals and dropouts of enrolled subjects from the trial are reported and explained on the CRFs.

(n) Informing the investigator of any CRF entry error, omission, or illegibility. The monitor should ensure that appropriate corrections, additions, or deletions are made, dated, explained (if necessary), and initialed by the investigator's trial staff who is authorized to initial CRF changes for the investigator. This authorization should be documented.

(o) Determining whether all are appropriately reported within the time periods required by GCP, the protocol, the IRB/IEC, the sponsor, and the applicable regulatory requirement(s).

(p) Determining whether the investigator is maintaining the essential documents.

(q) Communicating deviations from the protocol, SOPs, GCP, and the applicable regulatory requirements to the investigator and taking appropriate action designed to prevent recurrence of the detected deviations.

5.18.5 Monitoring Procedures
The monitor(s) should follow the sponsor's established written SOPs as well as those procedures that are specified by the sponsor for monitoring a specific trial.

5.18.6 Monitoring Report

(a) The monitor should submit a written report to the sponsor after each trial-site visit or trial-related communication.

(b) Reports should include the date, site, name of the monitor, and name of the investigator or other individual(s) contacted.

(c) Reports should include a summary of what the monitor reviewed and the monitor's statements concerning the significant findings/facts, deviations and deficiencies, conclusions, actions taken or to be taken, and/or actions recommended to secure compliance.

(d) The review and follow-up of the monitoring report with the sponsor should be documented by the sponsor's designated representative.

5.19 Audit

If or when sponsors perform audits, as part of implementing quality assurance, they should consider:

5.19.1 Purpose
The purpose of a sponsor's audit which is independent of and separate from routine monitoring or quality control functions, should be to evaluate trial conduct and compliance with the protocol, SOPs, GCP, and the applicable regulatory requirements.

5.19.2 Selection and Qualification of Auditors

(a) The sponsor should appoint individuals, who are independent of the clinical trials/systems, to conduct audits.

(b) The sponsor should ensure that the auditors are qualified by training and experience to conduct audits properly. An auditor's qualifications should be documented.

5.19.3 Auditing Procedures

(a) The sponsor should ensure that the auditing of clinical trials/systems is conducted in accordance with the sponsor's written procedures on what to audit, how to audit, the frequency of audits, and the form and content of the audit reports.

(b) The sponsor's audit plan and procedures for a trial audit should be guided by the importance of the trial to submissions to regulatory authorities, the number of subjects in the trial, the type and complexity of the trial, the level of risks to the trial subjects, and any identified problem(s).

(c) The observations and findings of the auditor(s) should be documented.

(d) To preserve the independence and value of the audit function, the regulatory authority(ies) should not routinely request the audit reports. Regulatory authority(ies) may seek access to an audit report on a case by case basis when evidence of serious GCP noncompliance exists, or in the course of legal proceedings.

(e) When required by applicable law or regulation, the sponsor should provide an audit certificate.

5.20 Noncompliance

5.20.1 Noncompliance with the protocol, SOPs, GCP, and/or applicable regulatory requirement(s) by an investigator/institution, or by member(s) of the sponsor's staff should lead to prompt action by the sponsor to secure compliance.

5.20.2 If the monitoring and/or auditing identifies serious and/or persistent noncompliance on the part of an investigator/institution, the sponsor should terminate the investigator's/institution's participation in the trial. When an investigator's/institution's participation is terminated because of noncompliance, the sponsor should notify promptly the regulatory authority(ies).

5.21 Premature Termination or Suspension of a Trial

If a trial is prematurely terminated or suspended, the sponsor should promptly inform the investigators/institutions, and the regulatory authority(ies) of the termination or suspension and the reason(s) for the termination or suspension. The IRB/IEC should also be informed promptly and provided the reason(s) for the termination or suspension by the sponsor or by the investigator/institution, as specified by the applicable regulatory requirement(s).

5.22 Clinical Trial/Study Reports

Whether the trial is completed or prematurely terminated, the sponsor should ensure that the clinical trial reports are prepared and provided to the regulatory agency(ies) as required by the applicable regulatory requirement(s). The sponsor should also ensure that the clinical trial reports in marketing applications meet the standards of the ICH Guideline for Structure and Content of Clinical Study Reports. (NOTE: The ICH Guideline for Structure and Content of Clinical Study Reports specifies that abbreviated study reports may be acceptable in certain cases.)

5.23 Multicentre Trials

For multicentre trials, the sponsor should ensure that:

5.23.1 All investigators conduct the trial in strict compliance with the protocol agreed to by the sponsor and, if required, by the regulatory authority(ies), and given approval/favorable opinion by the IRB/IEC.

5.23.2 The CRFs are designed to capture the required data at all multicentre trial sites. For those investigators who are collecting additional data, supplemental CRFs should also be provided that are designed to capture the additional data.

5.23.3 The responsibilities of coordinating investigator(s) and the other participating investigators are documented prior to the start of the trial.

5.23.4 All investigators are given instructions on following the protocol, on complying with a uniform set of standards for the assessment of clinical and laboratory findings, and on completing the CRFs.

5.23.5 Communication between investigators is facilitated.

[Sections 6, 7, and 8 omitted—eds.]

Part III

The Ethics of Clinical Trial Design

SECTION ONE. THE DISTINCTION BETWEEN RESEARCH AND TREATMENT

In this part of the book we investigate those elements of clinical trial design that cause ethical concerns. In passing judgment on the research protocols that come before them, the members of institutional review boards (IRBs) must, for example, carefully scrutinize the presence or absence of randomization, single or double blinding, the use of placebos as controls, and the risks and potential benefits participants can expect. Before they engage in these crucially important substantive investigations, however, they must ask whether a proposed course of medical conduct actually constitutes "research" rather than "treatment." Should a proposed course of conduct fit under the rubric of treatment, an IRB has no mandate or authority to review or comment upon its provisions, which remain a matter of private negotiation between the doctor and patient within the constraints of competent care. And even if a proposed medical intervention can legitimately be placed in the category of research, it may include distinctly therapeutic elements that should perhaps remain exempt from IRB scrutiny.

Robert J. Levine sheds much-needed light on these preliminary or threshold questions. He defines "practice" as those activities "designed solely to enhance the well-being of an individual patient or client"; by contrast, he defines "research" as a class of activities "designed to develop or contribute to generalizable knowledge." The normative standard governing practice is reasonable expectation of success. However, the presence of some, or even a great deal of, uncertainty regarding the likely results of a proposed therapeutic or diagnostic intervention does not, by itself, convert that intervention into a case of research.

Given the complexity of human diseases and the variability of individual responses to medical or surgical interventions, the practice of medicine is clouded by an ineradicable aura of uncertainty, but this should not license the oft-repeated canard that all encounters between patients and physicians constitute instances of "research" or "human experimentation." It remains true, however, that the line between practice and research can often be blurred, especially with regard to the deployment of so-called innovative or non-validated therapies. Physicians often wish to treat patients with a new drug or surgical procedure that has not yet been validated within a clinical trial. Their intention may well be exclusively therapeutic, yet they are dealing with an intervention whose safety and efficacy are difficult to predict. Are such physicians engaging in research by administering the drug or doing the procedure? Not if they are not thereby attempting to generate generalizable knowledge. Levine notes, however, that physicians contemplating the therapeutic deployment of an innovative or nonvalidated drug or diagnostic procedure *should* always conduct such practices within the context of a bona fide research program designed to test their safety and efficacy for the benefit of future patients.

Most instances of research are easy to identify, such as initial drug toxicity studies carried out on healthy volunteers or the comparison of a standard anticancer therapy with a promising new therapy. A trickier case might involve the comparison of two different antibiotics, both of which have already been approved by the U.S. Food and Drug Administration (FDA) and have already entered standard medical practice. Were a physician to administer antibiotic "A" or "B" to a patient, she would *not* have to submit her plans to an IRB; but if that physician were to decide to study the comparative benefits and side effects of these drugs by means of a controlled trial, she would be ipso facto doing research, and for that she would need the approval of an IRB.

Levine next turns to the FDA's classification of different kinds of drug studies, a proper understanding of which is crucial to an understanding of the research ethics literature. This classification scheme includes the following four categories:

• Phase I—Clinical Pharmacology: studies of the initial administration of a drug into humans, including research on toxicity, pharmacological effect, and, when appropriate, dose-response trials of safety and initial evidence of effectiveness. Most, but by no means all Phase I studies are conducted on normal human volunteers; those conducted on sick patients, such as trials of cancer drugs, can be extremely controversial. (On the ethical issues in Phase I studies, see Part III, Section Four.)

• Phase II—Clinical Investigation: initial controlled studies on efficacy and relative safety, usually conducted on a small number of patients.

• Phase III—Clinical Trials: expanded and more carefully focused studies of clinical effectiveness and safety.

• Phase IV—Postmarketing Clinical Trials: studies conducted for various reasons once a drug has already been approved for use on the market by a specified range of patients for various specified conditions.

The vast majority of literature in research focuses on Phases II and III, that is, on the design and execution of clinical trials (for safety and efficacy) prior to marketing. Phases I and IV also raise serious and important issues for conscientious researchers.[1]

Benjamin Freedman, Abraham Fuks, and Charles Weijer, probe the deeper implications for IRBs of this distinction between research and medical practice. Because the job of the IRB is to pass judgment on medical research, not standard medical treatment, these authors offer a helpful typology of research endeavors consisting of three major categories: (1) studies each of whose interventions consist of "demarcated research," such as a Phase I trial of a new compound; (2) those with a mixture of standard medical practices and specific research elements, such as a trial of two competing antinausea drugs following standard chemotherapy; and (3) those involving exclusively therapeutic practices with no demarcated research interventions, such as the trial of two already approved antibiotics mentioned earlier.

Freedman and colleagues contend that "mixed" studies, those involving elements of both treatment and research, should be disaggregated into their respective treatment and research elements. They contend that those elements of a study that are, strictly speaking, "clinical" or therapeutic, such as the use of standard chemotherapy in the comparative study of antinausea drugs described earlier, should fall outside the purview of the IRB in terms of both risk-benefit and consent analyses. So long as the nonvalidated drugs being studied cannot be judged before the trial as being better or worse than existing therapies, and so long as the risks involved with the experimental treatment are acceptable and minimized as much as possible, Freedman and colleagues conclude that such a trial is ethical. The practical import of their position is that IRBs need not and should not concern themselves with those elements of a study that fall outside the ambit of "demarcated research." So long as the chemotherapeutic regimen in our hypothetical example is accepted as reasonable medical treatment, the IRB should not trouble itself with the issue of informing prospective research participants of the risks and benefits of such standard treatments. If the chemotherapy is standard treatment, the IRB need focus only on the comparative risks and benefits of the competing antinausea drugs and the related issue of consent to their administration. The benefit of this approach for the research enterprise, according to Freedman and colleagues, is that prospective research participants need not be exposed to potentially troubling recitations of the serious risks associated with elements of some standard treatments, such as high-dose chemotherapy. To be sure, those risks need to be assessed by patients and their physicians as they consider which treatment to undergo, but they need not cloud the discussion held for the purpose of obtaining a patient's consent to a research intervention that piggybacks upon such standard treatment.

SECTION TWO. THE ETHICS OF RANDOMIZED CLINICAL TRIALS— CLINICAL EQUIPOISE

The Hippocratic tradition and recent codes of medical ethics speak clearly and emphatically concerning the physician's duty to individual patients. The tradition has emphasized the physician's covenantal duty of giving undivided loyalty to the patient, as opposed to what Paul Ramsey once called "that celebrated 'nonpatient,' the future of medical science."[2] This traditional duty of providing exclusive personal care for the individual patient is expressed in a number of applicable medical codes. For example, the American Medical Association's (AMA's) Principles of Medical Ethics state, "A physician shall, while caring for a patient, regard responsibility to the patient as paramount."[3] The AMA also recommends that when "conducting clinical investigation, the investigator should demonstrate the same concern and caution for the welfare, safety, and comfort of the person involved as is required of a physician who is furnishing medical care to a patient independent of any clinical investigation."[4] As we shall see, however, this is easier said than done.

Juxtaposed against the physician's duty of giving undivided loyalty to the individual patient is the researcher's duty—based squarely upon the larger duty to promote human welfare—to employ the most effective means for combating disease and disability, regardless of the time-honored status of standard procedures, many of which turn out to be quite useless or even harmful. This duty, implicit in the physician's Hippocratic commitment to "do no harm," is rendered explicit in the AMA's Principles of Medical Ethics, which state that "a physician shall continue to study, apply, and advance scientific knowledge. . . ."[5] The vexing ethical problem posed by this kind of rigorously scientific basis for clinical practice is that several of its defining features appear to conflict with the physician's traditional duty of providing personal care and loyalty to patients. This tension is apparent in the essential structure of the randomized clinical trial (RCT), the so-called gold standard of contemporary biomedical research.

One of the most problematic features of the RCT is the act of randomization itself, in which one of several competing treatments (including, in some cases, a placebo) is assigned by chance to each research participant. According to the advocates of RCTs, there are both scientific and ethical advantages to assigning treatments to research participants by chance. By eliminating bias in the selection and care of patient-participants, randomization helps generate scientifically valid data that will enable future patients to receive better care in the shortest possible time. Indeed, defenders of RCTs note that this disciplined procedure is *more ethical* than introducing new procedures

on the haphazard basis of clinical impressions, intuitive hunches, and historical comparisons. It is sobering to realize just how many passionately defended clinical hunches throughout the history of medicine have turned out to be literally dead wrong.

The critics of RCTs are less sanguine about the prospects of reconciling the imperatives of hard science with the physician's duty to provide personal care. Samuel Hellman and Deborah S. Hellman object to the fact that in an RCT an individual's therapy is determined not simply by an investigation into his or her physical needs and personal values, but also by the statistical requirements of the experimental design. Randomization for the sake of future patients, they claim, thus supersedes the individualized treatment of present patients. Does this not amount to a sacrifice of the individual for the sake of society at large? The Hellmans conclude that it does, and they therefore condemn RCTs for violating the central tenet of Kantian ethics: that the personhood of the individual should not be submerged in utilitarian calculations of social benefit. They urge the medical community to rely less on RCTs and to develop less morally problematic techniques for gaining valid knowledge.

One response to this dilemma is to bite the bullet and frankly admit that RCTs violate the physician's duty of giving loyalty to patients while still hoping that the ethical force of this violation can be either completely or partially neutralized. One way to do this is to claim that the participant's fully informed consent can solve the problem. Even if an RCT violates a researcher's duty to patients, those patients can let the researcher off the ethical hook by consenting to be randomized in the name of scientific progress. Another tactic is to argue that, although RCTs may expose some patient-participants to suboptimal treatment, this deviation from single-minded loyalty can be accepted by society so long as patients are not subjected to excessive risks. In other words, small losses for some patient-participants might be ethically tolerated by society if they are seen as the necessary price of medical progress that benefits everyone.

A notable problem with both of these strategies is that they explicitly acknowledge the inevitability of utilitarian tradeoffs between people as the price of scientific progress. Try as we might to minimize the harmful effects of such tradeoffs, the welfare of some people must still be sacrificed for the greater good of others. The unpleasant message conveyed by these strategies is that the ethics of clinical trial design poses a "tragic choice" between two deeply held social values, neither of which can be easily abandoned. We expect physician-researchers to place the interests of their patients above all else, yet we also demand dramatic and rapid progress in the "wars" against all manner of maladies, including cancer, acquired immune deficiency syndrome (AIDS), and spinal cord injuries.

A more morally optimistic response to this dilemma, articulated by Benjamin Freedman, attempts to reconcile the conflicting values embodied in the complex role of clinical researchers through a new theory of "clinical equipoise." Both the supporters and the detractors of RCTs agree that in order to be ethically justified, the various arms of a clinical trial must be in equipoise—that is, ex ante, before the data of the research trial are available, the researcher must have no good reasons for preferring one arm of the study to any other. According to critics like the Hellmans, such good reasons might include the individual researcher's strong hunches based upon his or her prior clinical experience, theoretical extrapolations, promising but uncontrolled early trials, or trends noticed during the early stages of a controlled trial. One problem with this account, which Freedman calls "theoretical equipoise," is that it turns equipoise into an exceedingly fragile and short-lived balance that can easily be upset and, hence, tip the ethical scales against a trial. Freedman therefore proposes an alternative understanding of the equipoise requirement: "clinical equipoise." Clinical equipoise shifts the focus from the hunches of the individual clinical researcher to the understandings of the larger community of physicians. Instead of insisting that the evidence on behalf of two treatments be *exactly balanced* and that the researchers develop no treatment preferences throughout the duration of a trial—both seemingly impossible requirements—Freedman argues for a concept of equipoise based on the existence of honest professional disagreement within the scientific community. So long as there exists a genuine dispute among clinicians as to what constitutes the "best treatment"—a dispute that *does not* require the evidence on behalf of the study interventions to be exactly balanced—an RCT is ethically permissible. Using the standard of clinical equipoise, the trial can be ethical even if a particular physician has a decided preference for one treatment over others. Indeed, Freedman adds, the original and overriding purpose of RCTs is to dispel precisely this kind of professional disagreement.

While Freedman's attempt to reconcile the demands of loyalty to patients with the rigors of RCTs is an important advance, serious problems remain. There are difficult questions concerning the nature of the community of clinical researchers upon which Freedman bases his theory. For example, some critics ask whether the relevant community includes each and every licensed physician.[6] Should one instead view the relevant community as the much smaller group of genuine experts who really have the needed clinical expertise? Moreover, critics also ask why the relevant community, defined broadly or narrowly, must reach a *unanimous* verdict in order to upset clinical equipoise.[7] Put differently, how much agreement among the members of the relevant clinical community is required for clinical equipoise to be upset? Is it ethical for clinician-researchers to recommend that their patients join a trial when the preponderance of expert opinion strongly favors, say, a new drug over standard treatment? Questions like these cast some doubt on Freedman's conclusion that the conflicting demands of ethics and science can be *fully* harmonized within the structure of an RCT. If they cannot, we might well be compelled to reconsider the unsavory possibility that perhaps the best we can do in the design of clinical trials is to *attenuate* the conflict by means of the utilitarian and informed consent-based strategies previously rejected by Freedman.

This section concludes with Robert D. Truog's essay, which might be usefully read as a response to the Hellmans' concluding appeal for the development of research design alternatives to RCTs. Focusing on the Harvard University Neonatal Extracorporeal Membrane Oxygenation (ECMO) trial as a case study in the ethics of randomization, Truog observes that the traditional RCT generates serious ethical and psychological pressures on researchers in the context of rapidly developing and potentially life-saving therapies. While Truog agrees with the utilitarian defense of RCTs in the context of non-life-threatening conditions, such as peptic ulcers and ear aches, he notes that the sacrifice of patients' well-being required by RCTs in the context of life-threatening conditions, such as potentially fatal pulmonary or cardiac failure, is simply unacceptable to most patients and physicians alike. The problem is compounded when, like ECMO, the innovative therapy in question is being perfected at a rapid rate, so that patients enrolled in a clinical trial of ECMO will not be able to benefit from subsequent and rapidly developing life-saving refinements in the technology that are occurring outside of the trial. Problems such as these lead Truog to recommend abandonment of the RCT in such circumstances in favor of large-scale multicenter prospective observational studies. The chief ethical advantage of such a study design is that it would permit clinicians to treat their patients with whatever therapy or therapeutic combination they believed to be the most efficacious. All participating researchers and institutions would then forward their data to a central registry that would analyze the data and spot trends for efficacy and safety. Although Truog concedes that this sort of innovative study design would not yield the level of rigorous statistical significance generated by RCTs, he is hopeful that sufficiently reliable conclusions can be derived from the imaginative deployment of such large databases. Noting that even the best run RCTs often fail to definitively resolve some research questions, Truog contends that the difference between his proposed method and the RCT may simply be a difference between varying degrees of confidence rather than between good science and bad.

SECTION THREE. THE ROLE OF PLACEBOS IN CLINICAL RESEARCH

Another problematic feature of many clinical trials concerns the use of placebos as controls. Whereas randomization and double blinding function to rule out possible sources of bias in the conduct of trials, placebo controls are designed to determine the genuine effectiveness of a treatment as opposed to various confounding factors, such as the psychological state of the patient. Often if patients *believe* that a certain medication will improve their condition, that fact alone can cause certain positive effects when combined with a pill, an injection, or even a surgical procedure. By designing studies with placebo controls, researchers can screen out such adventitious effects and more precisely determine the actual therapeutic benefit of a new treatment.

The use of placebo controls is usually unproblematic when researchers wish to test a new drug in the absence of a known effective treatment. Resort to placebo controls becomes ethically controversial, however, when researchers wish to introduce a new treatment as a possible successor or competitor to drugs whose use is currently standard practice. More controversial still is the use of invasive "placebo" interventions in surgical trials.[8] Supposing that re-

searchers wish to conduct a *controlled* clinical trial, they must decide what treatment, if any, the control group will receive. One option is to compare, for example, a new drug against the current standard medication; another is to compare the new drug against a placebo. The latter design can be problematic because it *seems* to conflict with Paragraph 29 of the most recent Declaration of Helsinki, which asserts that the "benefits, risks, burdens, and effectiveness of a new method should be tested against those of the best current prophylactic, diagnostic, and therapeutic methods." (The wording here is open to interpretation. The drafters of the Declaration of Helsinki inserted a Note of Clarification on Paragraph 29 of the World Medical Association [WMA] Declaration of Helsinki in which they addressed possible exceptions to the prohibition on placebos that one reading of this quotation supports. See Part II for the full text of the Declaration of Helsinki, along with the note of clarification.)

Citing the Helsinki Declaration, Kenneth J. Rothman and Karin B. Michels allege that placebos are frequently used unethically by biomedical researchers today. Citing several instances of studies that expressly withheld standard treatment from patients, Rothman and Michels argue against the supposed scientific justifications of the need to use placebos in RCTs, and conclude that the ethical burden of proof should shift to those researchers who propose to use placebo controls in place of standard therapies.

Benjamin Freedman provides additional argumentative support for the critique of the FDA's policy on placebos. Freedman begins with the interesting observation that, notwithstanding the common understanding among researchers, placebos are not without their own powerful confounding effects. Placebos have varying effects, he writes, depending on such factors as whether they are delivered via pill, capsule, or injection, and the effectiveness of various pills has been shown to be a function (believe it or not) of their color, red evoking a more powerful response than blue. Comparing any given drug against a placebo is thus not the same thing as testing it "against nothing." From this phenomenon Freedman concludes that it makes no sense for researchers to attempt to purify their studies of "confounding effects" by means of placebo controls when such effects are impossible to avoid in actual clinical practice.

In contrast to the FDA's approach, which allegedly attempts to achieve a highly purified knowledge of the actual effects of any given drug, Freedman recommends a "clinical" approach geared to producing a level of knowledge sufficient for "science in the service of healing." To be sure, Freedman concedes that there will be many situations in which resort to placebo controls will be both appropriate and necessary; but he challenges the orthodox belief that active treatment controls will usually be poor substitutes for placebo arms in clinical trials. Joining Rothman and Michels, Freedman concludes that the burden of proof should lie with those who would deprive patients of standard therapies.

The FDA's preference for placebo controls as the "gold standard" of measuring diagnostic or therapeutic efficacy is more fully articulated and defended by Robert Temple and Susan S. Ellenberg. These authors, officials at the FDA, begin with a concession: active controls are ethically preferable when no treatment or a placebo would clearly contravene patients' best interests. This is especially true, they suggest, when the standard treatment is known to prevent death or serious morbidity. But at the other end of the spectrum of harms, where treatment is not likely to affect the patient's *long-term health,* Temple and Ellenberg dismiss the notion that placebo-controlled studies would be unethical. They argue that using placebos is clearly ethical for trials on treatments for baldness or allergies or insomnia because forgoing current therapies will not result in death or serious disabilities. Consequently, they reject the invocation of the Helsinki Declaration in this context. So long as a patient will not be seriously harmed and is fully informed about the alternatives, they conclude, placebo-controlled studies can be ethical even when a standard treatment is available.

In addition to this ethical defense of some placebo studies, Temple and Ellenberg offer an important technical rationale for the FDA's preference for placebo controls. They note that a finding of "no difference" in a comparison of a new drug versus a standard treatment does not necessarily mean that the new drug is effective, even if the standard drug had been shown to be effective in previous trials. Instead, such a finding shows only either that both drugs were effective or that neither was effective. The standard drug might be effective *in general,* but it might not have been *effective in that particular trial.* They term the ability of a given study to distinguish between effective and ineffective treatments its "assay sensitivity." Temple and Ellenberg contend that studies designed with an active control and no placebo simply assume that the standard drug is going to be effective during the trial, but for a variety of common reasons it may not be. Without solid assurance of assay sensitivity (i.e., that the standard drug would have been more effective than a placebo *in similar circumstances*) Temple and Ellenberg suggest, we cannot usefully interpret the meaning of a result showing that a new drug is inferior to or indistinguishable from the standard treatment. Hence, these authors favor placebo controls of some limited size and duration even when researchers are investigating the efficacy of a new drug when a standard treatment exists. They thus conclude that the FDA's common practice of requiring placebo controls in such circumstances is justified not "merely" by efficiency concerns, such as the speed and lower cost of smaller sample sizes required by placebo controls that could be easily overridden by ethical considerations. Rather, they contend that the results of many active control "equivalency trials" of a new drug versus standard treatment cannot even be reliably interpreted in the absence of assay sensitivity and, hence, in the absence of placebo controls.

Ezekiel J. Emanuel and Franklin G. Miller conclude the debate in this section determined to tread a middle path between what they regard as the excesses of both the critics and the defenders of placebo controls. Against the claims of "placebo orthodoxy," represented here by Temple and Ellenberg, Emanuel and Miller object both to the fuzziness of these authors' criteria for justified placebo use (what counts as a "harm"?) and to their apparent willingness in some instances to permit intolerable physical and mental suffering in the name of scientific precision. Emanuel and Miller are also highly critical of the other extreme, which they term "active-control orthodoxy," represented here by Rothman and Michels, and Freedman. They contend that in many instances resort to placebo controls allows researchers to realize significant gains, more trustworthy results, effective nullification of the placebo response itself, and the exposure of fewer people to risk, without imposing significant risks on research participants. Their proposed middle way concurs with the partisans of active controls that the burden of proof rests with those who would deploy placebo controls where an established therapy already exists, but they contend that this burden can be met in the presence of compelling methodological reasons and stringent ethical-procedural safeguards.

SECTION FOUR. THE ETHICS OF PHASE I RESEARCH

No matter how promising a particular compound may look in a test tube or animal model, at some point en route to FDA approval and marketing it must first be tested in humans. These initial tests on humans are called Phase I studies. Whereas later Phase II and III studies are designed to test the efficacy and effectiveness of a given drug within expanding populations of research participants, the object of Phase I trials is to assess the toxicities and pharmacological properties of escalating doses of a drug on a very small number of participants. Most Phase I studies of medications are conducted with healthy volunteers. However, Phase I oncology and HIV/AIDS studies are too toxic to be conducted on healthy volunteers. Successive cohorts of patients are subjected to escalating doses of the drug until its effects become excessively toxic. The point just before that is labeled the "maximum tolerated dose"; at this level the drug is presumed to have the best chance of being active against the disease in question with acceptable toxicities. The maximum tolerated dose is the dose used in subsequent Phase II trials. In order to qualify for participation in such studies, patients must have a serious illness and must have failed to improve on standard therapies. In other words, those eligible for Phase I trials are often desperately sick and in the late stages of a terminal illness.

Phase I oncology trials have been questioned on various ethical grounds. Some critics argue that such standard protections as informed consent and regular IRB review are insufficient for this category of desperately ill and highly vulnerable patients, who, a priori, do not stand to gain significant, life-saving, benefit from participation. Others make the related claim that the recruitment of patient-participants into Phase I trials is tainted by the expectation of benefit when the manifest purpose of such studies, it is alleged, is merely to identify and measure a drug's toxicities. Conversely, Mortimer B. Lipsett argues that Phase I studies of cancer drugs provide clinicians with valuable information on a drug's toxic side effects and its maximum tolerated dose. Crucially, he contends that the purpose of any Phase I trial encompasses a *therapeutic intent* because the drug in question must have already been shown to cause tumor shrinkage in vitro and in animal models. Lipsett explains that patients at the National Institutes of Health (NIH) Clinical Center are told that the "chief purpose" of a clinical trial is to

find an "effective dose" of a drug. While NIH physicians must disclose to potential participants the nature of the drug's expected toxic effects, they also share their hope for favorable effects and even for a remission of the disease. Lipsett thus rejects criticisms to the effect that Phase I trials necessarily sacrifice the well-being of study participants for the benefit of future patients. He maintains that such trials offer patients benefits—such as hope, assistance to others, and reduced financial burdens—that are commensurate with risks, and that patients are fully capable of giving or withholding their informed consent. Consequently, Lipsett rebuffs the suggestion that patients in Phase I trials are exceptionally vulnerable and, hence, require an extraordinary level of IRB scrutiny.

One might respond to Lipsett by arguing that the actual intent of such studies is to discern the threshold of a drug's toxicity rather than its effectiveness. Evidence for this claim can be found in the very structure of Phase I oncology studies, which are designed to end just at that point where the drug becomes too toxic to administer.[9] Further evidence is provided by the contingent fact that the response rate of drugs in Phase I oncology trials tends to be about 5 percent.[10] Response rate includes a reduction in tumor volume, transient minimization of disease side effects, and complete remission, but these may not relate to life prolongation. Given such poor chances, and given the high toxicity of antineoplastics, one might reasonably wonder whether the possible benefits of Phase I oncology trial participation are in fact commensurate with their risks.

George J. Annas criticizes Phase I oncology studies, arguing that dying patients are especially vulnerable to exploitation and should thus be shielded by special protections. His essay can be usefully interpreted as an explicit attempt to refute Lipsett's three central claims, (1) that Phase I oncology trials are motivated by a therapeutic intent, (2) that their risk-benefit ratio is generally favorable, and (3) that standard informed consent and IRB protections suffice to shield patients from harm and abuse.

As we have seen, studies show that Phase I oncology trials rarely prove beneficial for the persons enrolled. A response rate of approximately 5 percent, plus the fact that the endpoint of Phase I trials is a showing of excessive toxicity rather than any beneficial effect, tends to bolster Annas's claim that labeling such trials "therapeutic in intent" can be dangerously misleading. Annas pointedly argues that this characterization of Phase I trails is a fantasy completely unrelated to actual probabilities. He observes that physicians often justify imposing onerous risks on dying patients because they believe that "desperate situations demand desperate remedies." This assumption leads researchers to cultivate a distorted and unrealistic notion of hope and to justify the imposition of a very unfavorable risk-benefit ratio upon patients on the ground that dying is the worst thing that could possibly happen. This ignores the fact that patients are concerned not simply with the length of their lives but also with the quality of their final days. Annas contends that the entire enterprise of Phase I trials is fueled not only by this "therapeutic misconception" shared by researchers and patients alike but also by the profit motive driving the pharmaceutical manufacturers.

Annas contends that the standard consent and IRB requirements provide insufficient protections. He therefore argues that research trials should occur only if they fulfill three conditions: (1) The research has a *reasonable probability* of benefiting the patient, (2) there is no a priori reason to believe that the trial will adversely affect the patient's quality of life, and (3) consent must be solicited, not by a researcher, but rather by a *patient rights advocate*. According to Annas, these conditions cannot be fulfilled by Phase I oncology trials, since such trials cannot benefit patients, and therefore they should be absolutely prohibited. Unfortunately, Annas never states how the information currently obtained from these trials would be obtained if they were prohibited. At what dose would efficacy trials be conducted? What toxicities should be mentioned in an informed consent form for Phase III studies?

1. John La Puma, "Physicians' Conflicts of Interest in Post-Marketing Research: What the Public Should Know, and Why Industry Should Tell Them," in *The Ethics of Research Involving Human Subjects: Facing the 21st Century*, ed. Harold Y. Vanderpool (Frederick, Md.: University Publishing Group, 1996), 203–19.

2. Paul Ramsey, *The Patient as Person* (New Haven, Conn.: Yale University Press, 1970), 11.

3. American Medical Association, Principles of Medical Ethics (adopted by the AMA House of Delegates June 17, 2001), available online at www.ama-assn.org/ama/pub/category/2512.html.

4. American Medical Association, Current Opinions of the Council on Ethical and Judicial Affairs, "E-2.07 Clinical Investigation" (issued prior to April 1977; updated June 1994 and June 1998). Available online at www.ama-assn.org/ama/pub/category/8422.html.

5. American Medical Association, Principles of Medical Ethics.

6. Fred Gifford, "Community-Equipoise and the Ethics of Randomized Clinical Trials," *Bioethics* 9 (1995):127–48.

7. Ibid.

8. Thomas B. Freeman, Dorothy E. Vawter, Paul E. Leaverton, et al., "Use of Placebo Surgery in Controlled Trials of a Cellular-Based Therapy for Parkinson's Disease," *New England Journal of Medicine* 341 (1999): 988–92; Ruth Macklin, "The Ethical Problem with Sham Surgery in Clinical Research," ibid., 992–96; Grant R. Gillett, "Unnecessary Holes in the Head," *IRB: Ethics & Human Research* 23, no. 6 (2001): 1–6; and Sam Horng and Franklin G. Miller, "Is Placebo Surgery Unethical?" *New England Journal of Medicine* 347 (2002): 137–39.

9. Benjamin Freedman, "Cohort-Specific Consent: An Honest Approach to Phase 1 Clinical Cancer Studies," *IRB: A Review of Human Subjects Research* 12, no. 1 (1990): 5–7. An excerpt from this paper is included in the appendix of this volume.

10. Christopher K. Daugherty, Donald M. Blank, Linda Janish, and Mark J. Ratain, "Quantitative Analysis of Ethical Issues in Phase I Trials," *IRB: A Review of Human Subjects Research* 22, no. 3 (2000): 6–14.

The Distinction between Research and Treatment

11   Research and Practice

ROBERT J. LEVINE

[. . .] Until recently, most regulations and ethical codes did not define such terms as "research" and "practice." Although distinguishing research from practice might not seem to present serious problems, in the legislative history of P.L. 93-348, the act that created the Commission [the U.S. National Commission for the Protection of Human Subjects of Biomedical and Behavioral Research—eds.], we find that some prominent physicians regarded this as a very important and exceedingly difficult task. Jay Katz identified ". . . drawing the line between research and accepted practice . . . (as) the most difficult and complex problem facing the Commission." Thomas Chalmers stated, "It is extremely hard to distinguish between clinical research and the practice of good medicine. Because episodes of illness and individual people are so variable, every physician is carrying out a small research project when he diagnoses and treats a patient."

Chalmers, of course, was only echoing the views of many distinguished physicians who had spoken on this issue earlier. For example, in *Experimentation with Human Subjects* Herrman Blumgart stated, "Every time a physician administers a drug to a patient, he is in a sense performing an experiment." To this Francis Moore added, ". . . every (surgical) operation of any type contains certain aspects of experimental work." Although these statements are true, they tend to obfuscate the real issue; they tend to make more difficult the task of distinguishing research from practice. The following definitions are compatible with those adopted by the Commission and incorporated subsequently in federal regulations.

The term "research" refers to a class of activities designed to develop or contribute to generalizable knowledge. Generalizable knowledge consists of theories, principles, or relationships (or the accumulation of data on

which they may be based) that can be corroborated by accepted scientific observation and inference.

The "practice" of medicine or behavioral therapy refers to a class of activities designed solely to enhance the well-being of an individual patient or client. The purpose of medical or behavioral practice is to provide diagnosis, preventive treatment, or therapy. The customary standard for routine and accepted practice is a reasonable expectation of success. The absence of validation or precision on which to base such an expectation, however, does not in and of itself define the activity in question as research. Uncertainty is inherent in therapeutic practice because of the variability of the physiological and behavioral responses of humans. This kind of uncertainty is, itself, routine and accepted.

There are two additional classes of activities performed by physicians that require definition; these are "nonvalidated practices" and "practice for the benefit of others." These are less familiar terms than "research" and "practice." For reasons I shall present, some of the ethical norms and procedures designed for research might, in some situations, be applicable to these classes of activities.

NONVALIDATED PRACTICES

Early in the course of its deliberations, the Commission defined a class of activities as "innovative therapy":

> Uncertainties may be introduced by the application of novel procedures as, for example, when deviations from common practice in drug administration or in surgical, medical, or behavioral therapies are tried in the course of rendering treatment. These activities may be designated innovative therapy, but they do not constitute research unless formally structured as a research project. . . . There is concern that innovative therapies are being applied in an unsupervised way, as part of

Robert J. Levine, *Ethics and Regulation of Clinical Research*, 2nd edition (Baltimore: Urban and Schwarzenberg, 1986), 3–10.

practice. It is our recommendation that significant innovations in therapy should be incorporated into a research project in order to establish their safety and efficacy while retaining the therapeutic objectives.

In the context of the Commission's deliberations, it is clear that diagnostic and prophylactic maneuvers are included under this rubric. Thus, a more descriptive title for this class of activities is "innovative practices." Subsequently, it has become clear that novelty is not the attribute that defines these practices; rather, it is the lack of suitable validation of the safety [or] efficacy of the practice. Therefore, the best designation for this class of activities is "nonvalidated practices." A practice might be nonvalidated because it is new; i.e., it has not been tested sufficiently often or sufficiently well to permit a satisfactory prediction of its safety or efficacy in a patient population. It is equally common for a practice to merit the designation "nonvalidated" because in the course of its use in the practice of medicine there arises some legitimate cause to question previously held assumptions about its safety or efficacy. It might be that the practice was never validated adequately in the first place (e.g., implantation of the internal mammary artery for the treatment of coronary artery disease or treatment of gastric ulcers with antacids) or because a question has been raised of a previously unknown serious toxicity (e.g., renal failure with some sulfa drugs). At the time of the first substantial challenge to the validity of an accepted practice modality, the proposition that subsequent use of that modality should be considered nonvalidated should be taken seriously. For purposes of ethical justification, all nonvalidated practices may be considered similarly. As the Commission has suggested for innovative therapy, these practices *should* be conducted in the context of a research project designed to test their safety or efficacy or both; however, the research should not interfere with the basic therapeutic (or diagnostic or prophylactic) objectives.

[T]he ethical norms and procedures that apply to nonvalidated practices are complex. Use of a modality that has been classified as a nonvalidated practice is justified according to the norms of practice. However, the research designed to develop information about the safety and efficacy of the practice is conducted according to the norms of research.

The term used by the FDA [Food and Drug Administration—eds.] for regulated test articles (e.g., drugs and medical devices) that have not yet been approved for marketing is "investigational." Because I find this term acceptable, when discussing test articles I shall often use the terms "investigational" and "nonvalidated" interchangeably.

In the routine practice of medicine, many therapeutic modalities have not been validated in the strict sense. For example, many drugs and devices approved for use by the FDA are prescribed for uses that are not listed on the FDA-approved package label. This does not mean that all such uses must be made the object of a formal study designed to establish safety and efficacy. At Yale, for example, formal studies that must be reviewed and approved by the IRB [institutional review board—eds.] are required when they are mandated by FDA regulations. In general, this means that the industrial sponsor of an approved drug intends to collect data to support addition of the new indication to the FDA-approved label.

In situations in which the regulations do not give clear guidance, Yale's policy is in accord with the Commission's conclusion on this point. If a drug or other therapeutic modality is to be studied systematically according to a formal plan with the aim of developing generalizable knowledge about the drug, then the physician is required to prepare a protocol for review by the IRB. The status of the proposed use of the drug as approved or nonapproved by the FDA is immaterial. We require, for example, IRB approval of plans to conduct a randomized clinical trial designed to compare the safety and efficacy of two drugs even when both drugs are being administered according to the advice provided on the FDA-approved package label.

Physicians who propose to use drugs or other therapeutic modalities in ways that differ substantially from their use in customary medical practice are encouraged—and occasionally required—to develop a protocol designed to show that the drug is truly safe and effective for the new indication or in the new dosage schedule. In such cases, it is necessary to exercise judgment as one determines whether the degree of departure from the standards of customary medical practice is sufficient to impose the requirement for IRB review. This is not accomplished by comparing the physician's plans with the FDA-approved package label. If so, it would be necessary for the IRB to review approximately 80% of all prescriptions written by pediatricians.

FDA CLASSIFICATION OF DRUG STUDIES

FDA regulations refer to various phases of drug studies. Phases II and III conform to the definition of nonvalidated practices. In general, Phase I studies do not, because the purpose of drug administration is to develop information on drug toxicities, metabolism, and dynamics rather than to enhance the well-being of an individual patient or client. Although the recipients of drugs in Phases II and III are always patients for whom the drug is intended to provide a therapeutic effect, in Phase I they are most commonly "normals." When Phase I studies are performed using patients for whom a therapeutic effect is intended, as in the development of most cancer chemotherapeutic agents, they may at times also be considered nonvalidated practices. In Phase IV, the drugs may be either validated or nonvalidated, as in cases in which marketed drugs are being tested for safety and efficacy for new indications or new populations, such as children.

Phase I Clinical Pharmacology is intended to include the initial introduction of a drug into [humans]. It may be in the usual "normal" volunteer subjects to determine levels of toxicity and, when appropriate, pharmacologic effect and be followed by early dose-ranging studies in patients for safety and, in some cases, for early evidence of effectiveness.

Alternatively, with some new drugs, for ethical or scientific considerations, the initial introduction into [humans] is more properly done in selected patients. When normal volunteers are the initial recipients of a drug, the very early trials in patients which follow are also considered part of Phase I.

Drug dynamic and metabolic studies, in whichever stage of investigation they are performed, are considered to be Phase I clinical pharmacologic studies. While some, such as absorption studies, are performed in the early stages, others, such as efforts to identify metabolites, may not be performed until later in the investigations.

Phase II Clinical Investigation consists of controlled clinical trials designed to demonstrate effectiveness and relative safety. Normally, these are performed on closely monitored patients of limited number.

Phase III Clinical Trials are the expanded controlled and uncontrolled trials. These are performed after effectiveness has been basically established, at least to a certain degree, and are intended to gather additional evidence of effectiveness for specific indications and more precise definition of drug-related adverse effects.

Phase IV Postmarketing Clinical Trials are of several types:

1. Additional studies to elucidate the incidence of adverse reactions, to explore a specific pharmacologic effect, or to obtain more information of a circumscribed nature.

2. Large scale, long-term studies to determine the effect of a drug on morbidity and mortality.

3. Additional clinical trials similar to those in Phase III, to supplement premarketing data where it has been deemed in the public interest to release a drug prior to acquisition of all data which would ordinarily be obtained before marketing.

4. Clinical trials in a patient population not adequately studied in the premarketing phase, e.g., children.

5. Clinical trials for an indication for which it is presumed that the drug, once available, will be used.

PRACTICE FOR THE BENEFIT OF OTHERS

As we examine the universe of professional activities of physicians, we find that there is one set that does not conform to the definitions of practice, research, or nonvalidated practice. It departs from the definition of practice only in that it is not ". . . designed solely to enhance the well-being of an individual." However, it does meet ". . . the customary standard for routine and accepted practice . . ." in that it has ". . . a reasonable expectation of success." In addition, the purpose of this activity is not ". . . to develop or contribute to generalizable knowledge." Thus, it does not conform to the definitions of either research or nonvalidated practice. Practice for the benefit of others is a class of activities in which interventions or procedures are applied to one individual with the expectation that they will (or could) enhance the well-being or convenience of one or many others.

Although practices for the benefit of others may yield direct health-related benefits to the individuals on whom they are performed, this is not necessarily the case. For example, one activity in this class, the donation of an organ (e.g., kidney) or tissue (e.g., blood), brings no direct health benefit to the donor; in this case, the beneficiary is a single other person who may or may not be related to the donor. In some activities, the beneficiary may be society generally as well as the individual patient (e.g., vaccination), while in others the only beneficiary may be society (e.g., quarantine). At times individuals are called upon to undergo psychosurgery, behavior modification, psychotherapy, or psychochemotherapy so as to be less potentially harmful to others; this is particularly problematic when the individual is offered the "free choice" between the sick role and the criminal role. In some cases the beneficiaries may include succeeding generations, as when persons are called upon to undergo sterilization because they are considered genetically defective or otherwise incompetent to be parents. There are also situations in which one beneficiary of therapy may be an institution; there may be serious disputes over the extent to which the purpose of therapy is to provide administrative convenience to the institution, e.g., heavy tranquilization of disruptive patients in a mental institution or treatment of hyper-kinetic schoolchildren with various stimulant and depressive drugs.

Although practice for the benefit of others is clearly a subset of practice, it has one important attribute in common with research: persons are called upon to assume various burdens for the benefit of others. Therefore, it seems appropriate to apply some of the ethical norms and procedures designed for research to this class of activities.

OTHER DEFINITIONS

[T]he term "physician" will be used to refer to a professional who is performing the practice of medicine; his or her client will be referred to as a "patient." An "investigator" is an individual who is performing research; the investigator may or may not be a physician. The individual upon whom the investigator performs research will be called "subject"; the terms "volunteer," "participant," and "respondent" will be used as synonyms. At times, more complex constructions will be required. For example, in the conduct of research designed to prove the safety and efficacy of a nonvalidated practice, various roles might be performed by such individuals as "physician-investigators" and "patient-subjects."

Department of Health and Human Services regulations provide this definition (Section 46.102(f)):

> "Human subject" means a living individual about whom an investigator (whether professional or student) conducting research obtains (1) data through intervention or interaction with the individual, or (2) identifiable private information.

[...]

UNACCEPTABLE TERMINOLOGY

There are some terms that are commonly used in the discussion of the ethics and regulation of research that [should be avoided]. These are "therapeutic research," "nontherapeutic research," and "experimentation." [...]

It is not clear to me when the distinction between therapeutic and nontherapeutic research began to be made in discussions of the ethics and regulation of research. The Nuremberg Code draws no such distinction. The original Declaration of Helsinki distinguishes nontherapeutic clinical research from clinical research combined with professional care. In the 1975 revision of this Declaration, "medical research combined with professional care" is designated "clinical research," while "nontherapeutic biomedical research" is also called "nonclinical biomedical research."

The problem with the distinction between therapeutic and nontherapeutic research is, quite simply, that it is illogical. All ethical codes, regulations, and commentaries relying on this distinction have, therefore, contained serious errors. This is exemplified by placing a principle of the Declaration of Helsinki developed for clinical research (II.6) in immediate proximity with one developed for nonclinical research (III.2).

> II.6. The doctor can combine medical research with professional care, the objective being the acquisition of new medical knowl-

edge, only to the extent that medical research is justified by its potential diagnostic or therapeutic value for the patient.

> III.2. The subjects should be volunteers—either healthy persons or patients for whom the experimental design is not related to the patient's illness.

This classification has several unfortunate and unintended consequences. First, many types of research cannot be defined as either therapeutic or nontherapeutic. Consider, for example, the placebo-controlled, double-blind drug trial. Certainly, the administration of a placebo for research purposes is not "... justified by its potential diagnostic or therapeutic value for the patient." Therefore, according to the Declaration of Helsinki, this is nontherapeutic, and those who receive the placebo must be "... either healthy persons or patients for whom the experimental design is not related to the patient's illness." This, of course, makes no sense. Another unfortunate consequence is that a strict interpretation of the Declaration of Helsinki would lead us to the conclusion that all rational research designed to explore the pathogenesis of a disease is to be forbidden. Because it cannot be justified as prescribed in Principle II.6, it must be considered nontherapeutic and therefore can be done only on healthy persons or patients not having the disease one wishes to investigate. Again, this makes no sense.

In recognition of these sorts of problems, the Commission abandoned the concepts of therapeutic and nontherapeutic research. Instead of "nontherapeutic research," the Commission simply refers to "research" which is, by definition, something other than therapeutic. More cumbersome language is employed by the Commission to convey the meaning intended most commonly by those who had used the expression "therapeutic research." For example, in *Research Involving Prisoners,* Recommendation 2 states in part, "Research on practices, both innovative and accepted, which have the intent and reasonable probability of improving the health or well-being of the individual may be conducted. . . ." The same concept is reflected in Recommendation 3 of *Research Involving Children.* It is made clear that the risks and benefits of therapeutic maneuvers are to be analyzed similarly, notwithstanding the status of the maneuver as either nonvalidated or standard (accepted). "The relation of benefit to risks ... (should be) at least as favorable to the subjects as that presented by any . . ." available alternative. The risks of research maneuvers (designed to benefit the collective) are perceived differently. If they are "... greater than those normally encountered (by children) in their daily lives or in routine medical or psychological examinations ..." review at a national level may be required.

It is worth underscoring the point that risks and benefits of therapeutic maneuvers are to be assessed similarly notwithstanding their status as either nonvalidated or standard. This point is particularly important in understanding the requirement of a null hypothesis in the ethical justification of an RCT. Investigators who propose to begin an RCT must be able to defend a claim that there is no scientifically valid reason to predict that either of the two or more therapies to be compared will prove superior. In many RCTs, a new therapy (nonvalidated practice) is compared with an established standard therapy. Thus, what is called for is a formal claim of therapeutic equivalency between a nonvalidated modality and an accepted standard. This is consistent with the Commission's recommendations. [...]

A third term that [should be avoided] is "experimentation." Experimentation is commonly and incorrectly used as a synonym for research. Although some experimentation is research, much of it is not. "Experiment" means to test something or to try something out. In another sense, an experiment is a tentative procedure, especially one adopted with uncertainty as to whether it will bring about the desired purposes or results. As noted earlier, much of the practice of diagnosis and therapy is experimental in nature. One tries out a drug to see if it brings about the desired result. If it does not, one either increases the dose, changes to another therapy, or adds a new therapeutic modality to the first drug. All of this experimentation is done in the interests of enhancing the well-being of the patient.

When experimentation is conducted for the purpose of developing generalizable knowledge, it is regarded as research. One of the problems presented by much research designed to determine the safety and efficacy of drugs is that this activity is much less experimental than the practice of medicine. It must, in general, conform to the specifications of a protocol. Thus, the individualized dosage adjustments and changes in therapeutic modalities are less likely to occur in the context of a clinical trial than they are in the practice of medicine. This deprivation of the experimentation ordinarily done to enhance the well-being of a patient is one of the burdens imposed on the patient-subject [in] a clinical trial. [...]

12   Demarcating Research and Treatment: A Systematic Approach for the Analysis of the Ethics of Clinical Research

Benjamin Freedman, Abraham Fuks, and Charles Weijer

The correct description of an action is critical for ethical evaluation. A kiss may be just a kiss; but, depending upon the context in which bestowed, it may also be a mark of affection, the fulfillment of a contract for services, or as in the Godfather saga, the pronouncement of the death penalty.

The same is true of medical acts; their morally relevant context as well as physical effects must be specified to arrive at a proper ethical evaluation. Not all venipunctures are ethically equal. Most are for the subject's own benefit. Some are for the benefit of others, as when a patient's blood is tested for HIV on behalf of a worried health care worker who was exposed to that person's blood. Some done without consent are assaults. This paper is concerned with a

Benjamin Freedman, Abraham Fuks, and Charles Weijer, "Demarcating Research and Treatment: A Systematic Approach for the Analysis of the Ethics of Clinical Research," *Clinical Research* 40 (1992): 653–60.

protocol that raised one question of this type. When is a blood test or any clinical intervention judged as therapy and when as research? And what ethical difference does this make?

[...] There remains an important difference between projects considered research by the United States Food and Drug Administration but not under regulations of the DHHS [Department of Health and Human Services—eds.]. Some organizations believe research to be distinctly characterized by its design, others by its intention, others by its use of novel agents or techniques. This literature shares one view in common: Research must be distinguished from therapy on a project, regimen, or protocol basis. The bundle of medical observations and interventions which a person shall undergo is classified as a whole as therapeutic, research, or—a much-criticized third category—"therapeutic research."

[T]his paper will proceed upon an alternative basis. Rather than ask whether the study as a whole is research or therapy, we will ask which of its interventions are grounded in research and which in therapy, and will describe why that is important. We call this task of intra-trial analysis the demarcation of therapeutic and research interventions. We will describe the manner and implications of demarcation in ways we believe to be consistent with the intent (if not in all respects the letter) of the United States' regulations on research with human subjects. We believe that our approach affords a better understanding of the task of ethical review that may contribute to clearer deliberations as well as more justifiable—and more uniform in the case of multicenter trials—conclusions.

The following proposal submitted by Dr. L to an institutional review board (IRB) precipitated our examination of the general question of research demarcation:

> A major side effect (in some cases approaching the limiting toxicity) of chemotherapy is peripheral neuropathy. A new substance, compound S, has been shown in animal tests to have a protective effect on the peripheral nervous system when exposed to neurotoxic drugs. In Phase I studies on normal volunteers, compound S has not demonstrated any toxic side effects at the amount extrapolated to be of potential therapeutic benefit.
>
> With funding from the drug company producing compound S, Dr. L has designed a placebo-controlled trial of its safety and efficacy at preventing peripheral neuropathy in patients receiving neurotoxic chemotherapy. Subjects are women who have experienced a recurrence of ovarian cancer. They will be treated aggressively with a multidrug regimen of high and accelerated doses of chemotherapy (including nonexperimental potentially neurotoxic drugs), followed by autologous bone-marrow transplantation (ABMT). Matched subpopulations will receive at the time of intravenous chemotherapy additional infusions of either placebo or compound S. The incidence and severity of peripheral neuropathy will be measured by clinical observation, responses to a brief questionnaire, and by a sensory test using a vibrating instrument applied to the extremities.
>
> The protocol Dr. L devises includes a complex form, six pages in length, for patient information and consent, including, for example, 15 progressively more dire side effects of chemotherapy, and a detailed discussion of risks and benefits of salvage autologous bone marrow transplant.

But how much of Dr. L's proposal is in fact research and what are the risks and benefits associated with that research? Treatment by multidrug chemotherapy is standard for this patient population. Dr. L's use of salvage ABMT following high and accelerated doses of chemotherapy represents his own clinical approach, one shared by a respectable (and growing) minority of his colleagues. Arguably, all of these elements of his proposal should be considered clinical treatment rather than research. The specific research interventions are to all current knowledge innocuous: The addition of an infusion via a preplaced intravenous catheter of either saline or a substance with no anticipated side effects and a few minutes spent trying to feel whether a rod applied to the feet or hands is vibrating. The measurement of peripheral neuropathy by recorded clinical observation and response to a questionnaire represents good, perhaps unaccustomedly-careful, clinical practice. The consent form to this research proposal as described in narrow terms would be less than a single page long.

DEMARCATING RESEARCH INTERVENTIONS: TWO STAGES OF REVIEW

That therapeutic and research interventions need to be demarcated in the ethical analysis of clinical studies underlies several comments made by the Belmont Commission [see the Belmont Report, included in this volume—eds.] and the interpreters of the United States' regulations adopted following that Commission's recommendations. These speak of the need to distinguish which procedures are "purely investigational," which parts of the activities "are research and which are practice," and to analyze the "various components of a research protocol" to discern which procedures "are designed solely to benefit society. . . ." However, there remains practical uncertainty in attempting to apply the distinction. How do we define therapy in demarcating interventions? Do we treat nonvalidated therapies as research or as therapeutic maneuvers? Most fundamentally: Is research intention or therapeutic grounding the basic factor? In logically partitioning therapy and research, do we define therapy as the negation of research, or vice versa?

For the purposes of ethical review by IRBs, the demarcation of research must be done by a process of exclusion begun by defining therapy. Ordinary therapeutic practice is managed within the health provider–patient relationship however dangerous the intervention or ambiguous the indication. The doctrines of patient consent to care and of professional autonomy are intended to ensure that the intervention in question is the product of joint deliberation and agreement between patient and doctor—moreover, of sole agreement between them. No outsiders need be consulted. (Irrelevant in this theoretical context, though often controlling in the real world, is the significance of this freedom to contract in the absence of secure funding for care.) Any third-party involvement will come retrospectively. The doctor-patient interaction may be reviewed and criticized after the fact by a hospital committee, council of peers, court, or others.

To settle the matter of "jurisdiction" in the legal and ethical senses, the IRB must begin by demarcating off the therapeutic elements contained within a protocol. The IRB has no authority to interfere with those elements; the provision of treatment within the physician-patient relationship is constitutionally protected within the right of privacy or otherwise.

What maneuvers are included under the therapeutic category? The answer is clear when there exists a single standard treatment for a condition. However, the law does not insist upon a model of "one disease–one treatment" in judging whether an intervention is therapeutic. A degree of professional discretion is allowed; interventions may be accepted by all average, reasonable practitioners, or merely by a "respectable minority" of practitioners. In either case, attempts by an IRB to interfere with physician-patient choice exceed its authority. Think of the previous example of Dr. L. Because his therapeutic approach is so aggressive, some members of the research committee may privately object to it; but to do so *as a research committee* would pervert that committee's role and unjustly interfere with the physician's clinical discretion and the patient's autonomy. Dr. L's therapeutic approach is not the single standard form of treatment, but falls within the acceptable range of standard treatments; it is not malpractice, nor does it approach malpractice.

If a physician's customary interventions are therapeutic, does it follow that all noncustomary interventions must be demarcated as research? It is a common feature of many research studies that the major deviations from standard practice they involve are unaccustomedly-close and frequent diagnostic interventions, e.g., more blood tests than usual, added x-rays, questionnaires, doctor visits. These appear, therefore, to be demarcated research maneuvers. Their associated risks appear to be incremental added to the ordinary risks of disease and of treatment. As demarcated research risks these appear to be the specific target of regulatory attention: "In evaluating risks and benefits, the IRB should consider only those risks and benefits that may result from the research (as distinguished from risks and benefits of therapies subjects would receive even if not participating in the research)."

Closer examination suggests that some noncustomary interventions nevertheless have substantial therapeutic intention and justification. Ordinary diagnostic practice is not optimal practice, but represents a sometimes uneasy compromise between ideal medicine and reality, economic and otherwise. Cancer investigators, for example, commonly feel that their practice on protocols is better for patients than standard practice. Far from their additional blood tests representing an overall incremental research risk to subjects, they represent incremental benefit: Neutropenia will be picked up earlier and drug doses adjusted accordingly, for example. (We assume for the sake of argument that the belief that added tests are beneficial can be validated.)

Because therapy has a privileged legal and ethical status, insulated from control by third parties (such as IRBs), demarcation must take it as basic. The principle is: Each intervention within the research study that has a therapeutic justification is treatment; all others required by the study are demarcated research maneuvers. Accordingly, we can distinguish between all treatment risks and those risks associated with demarcated research maneuvers. The sum of these latter risks constitutes the incremental research risk of the study.

Nonvalidated treatments fall outside of the realm of physician discretion and are the frequent focus of a clinical study: new chemical compounds or biological agents, new combinations of treatments or adjuvant treatments. A nonvalidated treatment may be tested in a clinical trial alone (e.g., in a Phase I pharmacokinetic or toxicity study), or in a study controlled by one or more other arms of treatment or placebo. How are the risks associated with nonvalidated treatments ethically evaluated? Are these treatment risks or research risks?

Because the U.S. regulations in principle allow informed adults to be the subjects of risky research that promises great scientific benefit, these regulations had no need to distinguish between treatment and research risks. However, the regulations are strict regarding research on children. A low ceiling of research risks was imposed to differentiate them from risks of treatment. Accordingly, [the regulations] understand the risks of nonvalidated, experimental arms of trials to be treatment risks. However, unlike standard treatment which is beyond the authority of IRBs, nonvalidated therapies must be closely evaluated by committees. The regulations require that the IRB be satisfied that "the relation of the anticipated benefit" of the nonvalidated arm of the trial "is at least as favorable to the subjects as that presented by available alternative approaches" that are standard treatment practices.

In our view, the ethics of trials need not distinguish between children and adults in this way. The commonly accepted ethical requirement that controlled clinical trials begin with an honest null hypothesis means that participation in a clinical trial must not systematically enroll subjects in a form of treatment known to be inferior. This requirement has been interpreted and expanded by one of us as requiring a showing that the nonvalidated therapy is in a state of clinical equipoise with all alternative regimens of treatment on and off the trial. [See Freedman, "Equipoise and the Ethics of Clinical Research," in this volume—eds.]

The IRB is charged with determining that all arms of the trial satisfy the clinical equipoise condition. In so doing it has not unlawfully interfered with the treatment autonomy of physician and patient, for by definition the nonvalidated arm has not been accepted as within the range of standard treatments by the medical community—nor will it until the satisfactory conclusion of a well-designed clinical study.

The committee's determination that all arms on (and off) a study are in clinical equipoise may rest upon a balancing of a variety of factors, each of which is important to the therapeutic index associated with a treatment. These factors may include short- and long-term efficacy, side effects, and even ancillary factors such as patient compliance or ease of administration. For a nonvalidated intervention to be in equipoise with a standard treatment arm, its associated expectation of risk and benefit must be roughly equivalent to those of treatments commonly used in clinical practice (or placebo if no treatment is commonly accepted). This overall risk-benefit equivalency does not require strict numeric equality. For example: In testing new versus old chemotherapy, those undergoing the new form of treatment may require more frequent blood tests because of uncertainty about how swiftly reversible side effects may develop. The two treatments are nonetheless in a state of equipoise because of warranted hope that the new form of treatment is a more effective anticancer agent than the old. Although in one sense the risks associated with these added blood tests are caused by participation in research, because the two treatments are in equipoise they are nonetheless treatment risks.

The ethical evaluation of "mixed" studies, as Levine had termed them, that include a treatment and a research component, is therefore accomplished in two stages. In the first stage, the treatment risk-benefit ratios of the nonvalidated treatment and of standard treatment are assessed and must be found to satisfy the requirement of clinical equipoise. In the second stage, an evaluation of any demarcated research risks is done; [these are] the risks of all interventions done that carry with them no therapeutic warrant for the subject. To be acceptable, demarcated research interventions must be minimized; that is, every effort consistent with the scientific validity of the trial must be taken to eliminate or reduce them. The regulations further state that demarcated interventions must bear an acceptable risk-benefit ratio. In this case, although the risk is faced by subjects, the "benefit" will come in the form of enhanced scientific knowledge that is itself unlikely to help these subjects. The phrase "risk-benefit ratio" is therefore misleading in this context. The requirement would be more accurately phrased as involving a "risk-knowledge" ratio. In addition, the requirement that research upon children not expose them to risks that exceed a minor increase over minimal risk would be understood as referring to the sum of incremental risks associated with demarcated research interventions, rather than to the treatment risks of either standard or nonvalidated therapeutic arms. [Table omitted—eds.]

These two stages of evaluation are fundamentally discontinuous because benefit to the subject, as in the evaluation of treatment risks, is not comparable to the scientific contribution of research. A deficiency in one stage of the analysis cannot be rectified by reference to the other stage. For example, an inappropriately-high level of incremental research risk cannot be justified by claiming that the subjects are still receiving a net benefit associated with an extraordinarily good experimental treatment. Were that experimental treatment known to be that good, the requirement that the trial arms be in clinical equipoise would be violated and all patients would need to be offered it as clinical treatment. Similarly, an experimental treatment thought *a priori* to be inferior to the control arm cannot be justified by loading the research plans with the incidental and unconnected benefits often afforded in clinical research settings: added patient-physician contact, access to superior medical facilities. A fair evaluation of a non-validated treatment's ratio of hoped-for benefit to feared risk must be made on that treatment itself, just as a restaurant serving obnoxious meatloaf does not improve its bill of fare by promising a free bottle of ketchup with every purchase.

FORMS OF RESEARCH AND THE NORMATIVE DIFFERENCES RESEARCH ENTAILS

We can consider the logical universe of studies to be comprised of three disjoint sets: Studies each of whose interventions is demarcated research; those with a mixture of clinical and research interventions; and those involving only clinical interventions. This division serves as a useful framework for considering some of the special ethical requirements imposed upon clinical studies.

The first category consists of studies we will call pure (or fully demarcated) research done on normal healthy volunteers as in studies of normal physiology or in Phase I pharmaceutical trials. Since everything to be done to these subjects is demarcated research, all risks are accounted into the research budget as incremental research risks without countervailing therapeutic benefit. The second category consists of those controlled or uncontrolled studies of new treatments which we call "mixed" studies. These involve some combination of therapeutic and demarcated research interventions. They require the two stages of ethical analysis of their associated risks that were described previously.

The third category is comprised of studies that do not involve demarcated research interventions. Consider a research study organized by a group practice in pediatrics of whom some use antibiotic A for a common infection while others use B. Patients will be assigned to A or B. After some interval their computer records will be checked to see if any important differences appear. [. . .] When testing head to head the efficacy of two treatments that fall within the range of standard practice, as judged by an endpoint examined in standard practice as well, the design of the study may achieve generalizable knowledge while its methods do not go beyond those employed therapeutically. Because nothing will be done to subjects without therapeutic justification, we will call these pure treatment studies. It is important to note that they may be as scientifically valid and valuable a form of research as pure or mixed studies.

As discussed previously, research is subject to prospective third-party control while therapy is reviewed retrospectively. The terms of the research bargain to be struck must be reviewed and approved by a committee before the investigator approaches a prospective subject. It is this need for antecedent committee approval (rather than simply antecedent consent by the subject) that most sharply sets research aside from ordinary practice. (Incidentally, this requirement serves as the strongest incentive to avoid the research label and thereby circumvent "bureaucratic interference.")

It is obvious that prior review by [an] IRB is needed in the case of pure research or mixed studies. In both cases, investigators must show that the incremental risk associated with demarcated research interventions has been minimized and bears an acceptable risk-knowledge ratio. In addition, the committee must be satisfied in the case of mixed studies that all arms of the trial satisfy clinical equipoise. But why should prior review of pure treatment studies be required inasmuch as nothing will be done to subjects without therapeutic justification? Would not the imposing of prior review in these cases be an unjustified interference in physician discretion and patient autonomy?

In general, prior review of research studies is motivated by the divergence of goals of investigators and subjects, and in the sequelae of this divergence—repeated historical instances of scandal in which subjects were misused in the name of medical science. In the research context, persons may need protection from the zeal of investigators pursuing their own scientific agendas. The investigator labors under a potentially conflicting set of responsibilities even when examining alternate therapeutic modalities of putative direct benefit to the subjects. This gives rise to an index of suspicion attaching to any alteration of his or her routine clinical practice that has been generated by research considerations.

Although the use of either antibiotic is common in the group practice, children are treated by physicians, not by the group. Some members of the practice use A, some B; perhaps some alternate from time to time. But none alternate continually to achieve a quasi-random distribution. Each enrolling physician is altering clinical practice—albeit in a minor way—on behalf of achieving generalizable knowledge, which is a goal that goes beyond the clinical care of the patient. The prior review of this study is triggered by the potential for conflict of interest grounded in the stereotyped alteration of the practice of participating physicians on behalf of achieving generalizable knowledge.

A second dimension of ethical difference between research and therapy is consent. It is agreed that the minimal information requirements for a valid consent to research exceed those of therapy, and that exceptions to the need for consent available for therapy (under emergency conditions and "therapeutic privilege") are invalid as exceptions to the need for consent to research. The lengthy DHHS list of disclosures required for consent to research are more formal and comprehensive than that which clinicians associate with informed consent.

It is clear that consent to demarcated research interventions in pure or mixed research studies must be judged according to the full rigor of the regulations. Also, in spite of a finding of equipoise, the context of uncertainty surrounding nonvalidated treatments would similarly require a careful, research-oriented consent process. But what of cases of randomized research assignment in pure treatment studies? And what of interventions that will be provided as standard therapy to all trial participants?

Consent to random assignment in a pure research study is illustrated by this antibiotic study. Were patients (and/or parents) not to be told of the study, unbeknownst to them a patient who would otherwise have received A will receive B, or vice versa. Even though A and B are in clinical equipoise, that reflects only their rough equivalence and is consistent with different profiles of side effects associated with each that might matter to the patient. Thus, in general, the fact of the study, the quasi-randomization process, and the different implications of the drugs involved should be disclosed. Arguably, however, those subjects who would have received A outside of the trial, and who did in fact receive A within the trial, have not had their care influenced by inclusion; hence, they are consenting to a clinical intervention. (This view underlies Marvin Zelen's proposed "pre-randomization" of consent for subjects in trials.)

What of consent to interventions provided as standard therapy to all trial participants? This issue is posed in the trial with which we began: Dr. L's study of compound S as prophylaxis for peripheral neuropathy in chemotherapy patients. All participants in this trial were being treated by chemotherapy and autologous bone marrow transplantation. In this and similar cases, we believe that consent to such treatment interventions should be governed by the norms of consent to treatment, and exempted from the panoply of formalities that the regulations require of consent to research interventions. We would understand the clinical treatment of these women by chemotherapy and ABMT not as part of the research, but as simply the occasion for research. The case is relevantly similar to the following study: A group of patients undergoing chemotherapy will be weighed twice daily for two weeks to track their progressive weight loss. Although this research depends upon the fact that the subjects are receiving chemotherapy, it would be absurd to require that subjects receive detailed information about their chemotherapy as part of informed consent to this research. In the same manner, the consent of Dr. L's patients to chemotherapy and ABMT should be understood as a requirement of consent to treatment, not research; the consent to research should only deal with the implications of random assignment to compound S or placebo; the consent form should be a single page in length. We believe the practice of those committees that require information about these components to be included within the research consent form, according to the same standards and specificity as are sought of demarcated research maneuvers, or nonvalidated or randomized therapeutic interventions, reflects an overly conservative reading of ambiguous regulations.

Does it really make any difference whether consent to these common interventions is subject to norms of consent to treatment or research? In one sense, no; the significance of the ethical (rather than regulatory or legal) difference between consent to treatment and to research is easily exaggerated. While the law and regulation of consent to research is more formal than that governing treatment, law and regulation only state the minimum norms. The scrupulous, perplexed physician does not ask what is the minimum information he or she must impart to patients or subjects, but rather how much information it is desirable to impart. It has been accepted therefore that the information to be provided to a patient or a subject are similar: What will a decision to accept or reject the offer (of treatment or research) mean to me? How will it affect my fate? What doors will be opened, which foreclosed? In our case, Dr. L's patients will require disclosure of relevant facts about their disease, the proposed treatments, and alternatives that are available (even if disfavorable in Dr. L's judgment), as a clinical obligation of medical ethics in roughly the same degree of detail that would be required for research.

From the point of view of the amount of information that must be conveyed, it may not matter whether the prevailing norms are therapy or research. From the point of view of procedure, however, the distinction can make a big difference in determining the authority and work-load of IRBs. In addition, we believe that it is misleading and confusing to bundle consent to common treatment interventions together with research interventions in a single package. By doing so, Dr. L's patients may be led to understand that their participation in the proposed research involves risks up to and including death, as is stated with respect to the side effects of aggressive chemotherapy. They may on that basis decline to participate in research, choosing instead a therapeutic regimen. But the dread risks are concomitant to therapy itself, not the research component. A patient who understood that might well have enrolled in the study.

Even accepting as a matter of principle our above point, some members of research committees who are skeptical about the adequacy of clinical consent might wish that information about all interventions should be included in a single document under research norms. Whether or not this skepticism is justified, action upon it is not an IRB prerogative. If the information and consent procedures associated with clinical maneuvers are indeed less than adequate, this speaks to an ethical lapse; but surely not to a breach of the norms governing research as such.

CONCLUSION

A number of questions remain for future investigation. We have noted the claim by researchers that some demarcated research interventions (e.g., added blood tests) result in net benefit for rather than risk to subjects. If true, this claim needs examination because it would have important implications for the ethical review of research.

We believe that several changes in the consent process as presented here may both aid subject understanding and increase subject accrual. These changes include an explicit demarcation of research and treatment interventions; separation of treatment risks from incremental research risks; and provisions for separately dealing with those therapeutic interventions offered in common to all of the research subjects. Our belief that these changes will yield the suggested benefits must be empirically examined.

Studies of the process of research review by IRBs may also be of interest. The authors' experience suggests that relatively few clinical research studies pose a high incremental risk associated with fully demarcated interventions. Moreover, arguments about "risk" at the other stage of evaluation, considering clinical equipoise, are more accurately framed as issues of uncertainty. This impression should be compared with the experiences of others and should be explored if the implications are valid.

In the context of Dr. L's proposal, this analysis was essential to focusing IRB evaluation and suggesting changes in the informed consent process. The chief benefit of this paper, however, would lie in its furnishing research agencies, members of IRBs, investigators, and subjects themselves with a common and accurate language to use in discussing the ethics of research. Only then can fruitful debate proceed and progressive consensus be achieved.

Section Two

The Ethics of Randomized Clinical Trials

Clinical Equipoise

---

13   Of Mice but Not Men

Problems of the Randomized Clinical Trial

SAMUEL HELLMAN AND DEBORAH S. HELLMAN

As medicine has become increasingly scientific and less accepting of unsupported opinion or proof by anecdote, the randomized controlled clinical trial has become the standard technique for changing diagnostic or therapeutic methods. The use of this technique creates an ethical dilemma. Researchers participating in such studies are required to modify their ethical commitments to individual patients and do serious damage to the concept of the physician as a practicing, empathetic professional who is primarily concerned with each patient as an individual. Researchers using a randomized clinical trial can be described as physician-scientists, a term that expresses the tension between the two roles. The physician, by entering into a relationship with an individual patient, assumes certain obligations, including the commitment always to act in the patient's best interests. As Leon Kass has rightly maintained, "[T]he physician must produce unswervingly the virtues of loyalty and fidelity to his patient." Though the ethical requirements of this relationship have been modified by legal obligations to report wounds of a suspicious nature and certain infectious diseases, these obligations in no way conflict with the central ethical obligation to act in the best interests of the patient medically. Instead, certain nonmedical interests of the patient are preempted by other social concerns.

The role of the scientist is quite different. The clinical scientist is concerned with answering questions—i.e., determining the validity of formally constructed hypotheses. Such scientific information, it is presumed, will benefit humanity in general. The clinical scientist's role has been well described by Dr. Anthony Fauci, director of the National Institute of Allergy and Infectious Diseases, who states the goals of the randomized clinical trial in these words: "It's not to deliver therapy. It's to answer a scientific question so that the drug can be available for everybody once you've established safety and efficacy." The demands of such a study can conflict in a number of ways with the physician's duty to minister to patients. The study may create a false dichotomy in the physician's opinions; according to the premise of the randomized clinical trial, the physician may only know or not know whether a proposed course of treatment represents an improvement; no middle position is permitted. What the physician thinks, suspects, believes, or has a hunch about is assigned to the "not knowing" category, because knowing is defined on the basis of an arbitrary but accepted statistical test performed in a randomized clinical trial. Thus, little credence is given to information gained beforehand in other ways or to information accrued during the trial but without the required statistical degree of assurance that a difference is not due to chance. The randomized clinical trial also prevents the treatment technique from being modified on the basis of the growing knowledge of the physicians during their participation in the trial. Moreover, it limits access to the data as they are collected until specific milestones are achieved. This prevents physicians from profiting not only from their individual experience, but also from the collective experience of the other participants.

The randomized clinical trial requires doctors to act simultaneously as physicians and as scientists. This puts them in a difficult and sometimes untenable ethical position. The conflicting moral demands arising from the use of the randomized clinical trial reflect the classic conflict

Samuel Hellman and Deborah S. Hellman, "Of Mice but Not Men: Problems of the Randomized Clinical Trial," *New England Journal of Medicine* 324 (1991): 1585–89.

between rights-based moral theories and utilitarian ones. The first of these, which depend on the moral theory of Immanuel Kant (and seen more recently in neo-Kantian philosophers, such as John Rawls), asserts that human beings, by virtue of their unique capacity for rational thought, are bearers of dignity. As such, they ought not to be treated merely as means to an end; rather, they must always be treated as ends in themselves. Utilitarianism, by contrast, defines what is right as the greatest good for the greatest number—that is, as social utility. This view, articulated by Jeremy Bentham and John Stuart Mill, requires that pleasures (understood broadly, to include such pleasures as health and well-being) and pains be added together. The morally correct act is the act that produces the most pleasure and the least pain overall.

A classic objection to the utilitarian position is that according to that theory, the distribution of pleasures and pains is of no moral consequence. This element of the theory severely restricts physicians from being utilitarians, or at least from following the theory's dictates. Physicians must care very deeply about the distribution of pain and pleasure, for they have entered into a relationship with one or a number of individual patients. They cannot be indifferent to whether it is these patients or others that suffer for the general benefit of society. Even though society might gain from the suffering of a few, and even though the doctor might believe that such a benefit is worth a given patient's suffering (i.e., that utilitarianism is right in the particular case), the ethical obligation created by the covenant between doctor and patient requires the doctor to see the interests of the individual patient as primary and compelling. In essence, the doctor-patient relationship requires doctors to see their patients as bearers of rights who cannot be merely used for the greater good of humanity.

As Fauci has suggested, the randomized clinical trial routinely asks physicians to sacrifice the interests of their particular patients for the sake of the study and that of the information that it will make available for the benefit of society. This practice is ethically problematic. Consider first the initial formulation of a trial. In particular, consider the case of a disease for which there is no satisfactory therapy— for example, advanced cancer or AIDS. A new agent that promises more effectiveness is the subject of the study. The control group must be given either an unsatisfactory treatment or a placebo. Even though the therapeutic value of the new agent is unproved, if physicians think that it has promise, are they acting in the best interests of their patients in allowing them to be randomly assigned to the control group? Is persisting in such an assignment consistent with the specific commitments taken on in the doctor-patient relationship? As a result of interactions with patients with AIDS and their advocates, Merigan recently suggested modifications in the design of clinical trials that attempt to deal with the unsatisfactory treatment given to the control

group. The view of such activists has been expressed by Rebecca Pringle Smith of Community Research Initiative in New York: "Even if you have a supply of compliant martyrs, trials must have some ethical validity."

If the physician has no opinion about whether the new treatment is acceptable, then random assignment is ethically acceptable, but such lack of enthusiasm for the new treatment does not augur well for either the patient or the study. Alternatively, the treatment may show promise of beneficial results but also present a risk of undesirable complications. When the physician believes that the severity and likelihood of harm and good are evenly balanced, randomization may be ethically acceptable. If the physician has no preference for either treatment (is in a state of equipoise), then randomization is acceptable. If, however, he or she believes that the new treatment may be either more or less successful or more or less toxic, the use of randomization is not consistent with fidelity to the patient.

The argument usually used to justify randomization is that it provides, in essence, a critique of the usefulness of the physician's beliefs and opinions, those that have not yet been validated by a randomized clinical trial. As the argument goes, these not-yet-validated beliefs are as likely to be wrong as right. Although physicians are ethically required to provide their patients with the best available treatment, there simply is no best treatment yet known.

The reply to this argument takes two forms. First, and most important, even if this view of the reliability of a physician's opinions is accurate, the ethical constraints of an individual doctor's relationship with a particular patient require the doctor to provide individual care. Although physicians must take pains to make clear the speculative nature of their views, they cannot withhold these views from the patient. The patient asks from the doctor both knowledge and judgment. The relationship established between them rightfully allows patients to ask for the judgment of their particular physicians, not merely that of the medical profession in general. Second, it may not be true, in fact, that the not-yet-validated beliefs of physicians are as likely to be wrong as right. The greater certainty obtained with a randomized clinical trial is beneficial, but that does not mean that a lesser degree of certainty is without value. Physicians can acquire knowledge through methods other than the randomized clinical trial. Such knowledge, acquired over time and less formally than is required in a randomized clinical trial, may be of great value to the patient.

Even if it is ethically acceptable to begin a study, one often forms an opinion during its course—especially in studies that are impossible to conduct in a truly doubleblinded fashion—that makes it ethically problematic to continue. The inability to remain blinded usually occurs in studies of cancer or AIDS, for example, because the therapy is associated by nature with serious side effects. Trials attempt to restrict the physician's access to the data in order to prevent such unblinding. Such restrictions should make physicians eschew the trial, since their ability to act in the patient's best interests will be limited. Even supporters of randomized clinical trials, such as Merigan, agree that interim findings should be presented to patients to ensure that no one receives what seems an inferior treatment. Once physicians have formed a view about the new treatment, can they continue randomization? If random assignment is stopped, the study may be lost and the participation of the previous patients wasted. However, if physicians continue the randomization when they have a definite opinion about the efficacy of the experimental drug, they are not acting in accordance with the requirements of the doctor-patient relationship. Furthermore, as their opinion becomes more firm, stopping the randomization may not be enough. Physicians may be ethically required to treat the patients formerly placed in the control group with the therapy that now seems probably effective. To do so would be faithful to the obligations created by the doctor-patient relationship, but it would destroy the study.

To resolve this dilemma, one might suggest that the patient has abrogated the rights implicit in a doctor-patient relationship by signing an informed-consent form. We argue that such rights cannot be waived or abrogated. They are inalienable. The right to be treated as an individual deserving the physician's best judgment and care, rather than to be used as a means to determine the best treatment for others, is inherent in every person. This right, based on the concept of dignity, cannot be waived. What of altruism, then? Is it not the patient's right to make a sacrifice for the general good? This question must be considered from both positions—that of the patient and that of the physician. Although patients may decide to waive this right, it is not consistent with the role of a physician to ask that they do so. In asking, the doctor acts as a scientist instead. The physician's role here is to propose what he or she believes is best medically for the specific patient, not to suggest participation in a study from which the patient cannot gain. Because the opportunity to help future patients is of potential value to a patient, some would say physicians should not deny it. Although this point has merit, it offers so many opportunities for abuse that we are extremely uncomfortable about accepting it. The responsibilities of physicians are much clearer; they are to minister to the current patient.

Moreover, even if patients could waive this right, it is questionable whether those with terminal illness would be truly able to give voluntary informed consent. Such patients are extremely dependent on both their physicians and the health care system. Aware of this dependence, physicians must not ask for consent, for in such cases the very asking breaches the doctor-patient relationship. Anxious to please their physicians, patients may have difficulty refusing to participate in the trial the physicians describe. The patients may perceive their refusal as damaging to the relationship,

whether or not it is so. Such perceptions of coercion affect the decision. Informed-consent forms are difficult to understand, especially for patients under the stress of serious illness for which there is no satisfactory treatment. The forms are usually lengthy, somewhat legalistic, complicated, and confusing, and they hardly bespeak the compassion expected of the medical profession. It is important to remember that those who have studied the doctor-patient relationship have emphasized its empathetic nature.

> [The] relationship between doctor and patient partakes of a peculiar intimacy. It presupposes on the part of the physician not only knowledge of his fellow men but sympathy.... This aspect of the practice of medicine has been designated as the art; yet I wonder whether it should not, most properly, be called the essence.

How is such a view of the relationship consonant with random assignment and informed consent? The Physician's Oath of the WMA affirms the primacy of the deontologic view of patient's rights: "Concern for the interests of the subject must always prevail over the interests of science and society."

Furthermore, a single study is often not considered sufficient. Before a new form of therapy is generally accepted, confirmatory trials must be conducted. How can one conduct such trials ethically unless one is convinced that the first trial was in error? The ethical problems we have discussed are only exacerbated when a completed randomized clinical trial indicates that a given treatment is preferable. Even if the physician believes the initial trial was in error, the physician must indicate to the patient the full results of that trial.

The most common reply to the ethical arguments has been that the alternative is to return to the physician's intuition, to anecdotes, or to both as the basis of medical opinion. We all accept the dangers of such a practice. The argument states that we must therefore accept randomized, controlled clinical trials regardless of their ethical problems because of the great social benefit they make possible, and we salve our conscience with the knowledge that informed consent has been given. This returns us to the conflict between patients' rights and social utility. Some would argue that this tension can be resolved by placing a relative value on each. If the patient's right that is being compromised is not a fundamental right and the social gain is very great, then the study might be justified. When the right is fundamental, however, no amount of social gain, or almost none, will justify its sacrifice. Consider, for example, the experiments on humans done by physicians under the Nazi regime. All would agree that these are unacceptable regardless of the value of the scientific information gained. Some people go so far as to say that no use should be made of the results of those experiments because of the clearly unethical manner in which the data were collected. This extreme example may not seem relevant, but we believe that in its hyperbole it clarifies the fallacy of a utilitarian approach to the physician's relationship with the patient. To consider the utilitarian gain is consistent neither with the physician's role nor with the patient's rights.

It is fallacious to suggest that only the randomized clinical trial can provide valid information or that all information acquired by this technique is valid. Such experimental methods are intended to reduce error and bias and therefore reduce the uncertainty of the result. Uncertainty cannot be eliminated, however. The scientific method is based on increasing probabilities and increasingly refined approximations of truth. Although the randomized clinical trial contributes to these ends, it is neither unique nor perfect. Other techniques may also be useful.

Randomized trials often place physicians in the ethically intolerable position of choosing between the good of the patient and that of society. We urge that such situations be avoided and that other techniques of acquiring clinical information be adopted. For example, concerning trials of treatment for AIDS, Byar et al. have said that "some traditional approaches to the clinical-trials process may be unnecessarily rigid and unsuitable for this disease." In this case, AIDS is not what is so different; rather, the difference is in the presence of AIDS activists, articulate spokespersons for the ethical problems created by the application of the randomized clinical trial to terminal illnesses. Such arguments are equally applicable to advanced cancer and other serious illnesses. Byar et al. agree that there are even circumstances in which uncontrolled clinical trials may be justified: when the prognosis is uniformly poor, and when there is a reasonable expectation of benefit without excessive toxicity. These conditions are usually found in clinical trials of advanced cancer.

The purpose of the randomized clinical trial is to avoid the problems of observer bias and patient selection. It seems to us that techniques might be developed to deal with these issues in other ways. Randomized clinical trials deal with them in a cumbersome and heavy-handed manner, by requiring large numbers of patients in the hope that random assignment will balance the heterogeneous distribution of patients into the different groups. By observing known characteristics of patients, such as age and sex, and distributing them equally between groups, it is thought that unknown factors important in determining outcomes will also be distributed equally. Surely, other techniques can be developed to deal with both observer bias and patient selection. Prospective studies without randomization, but with the evaluation of patients by uninvolved third parties, should remove observer bias. [. . .] Prospective matched-pair analysis, in which patients are treated in a manner consistent with their physician's views, ought to help ensure equivalence between the groups and thus mitigate the effect of patient selection, at least with regard to known covariates. With regard to unknown covariates, the security would rest, as in randomized trials, in the enrollment of large numbers of patients and in confirmatory studies. This method would not pose ethical difficulties, since patients would receive the treatment recommended by their physician. They would be included in the study by independent observers matching patients with respect to known characteristics, a process that would not affect patient care and that could be performed independently any number of times.

This brief discussion of alternatives to randomized clinical trials is sketchy and incomplete. We wish only to point out that there may be satisfactory alternatives, not to describe and evaluate them completely. Even if randomized clinical trials were much better than any alternative, however, the ethical dilemmas they present may put their use at variance with the primary obligations of the physician. In this regard, Angell cautions, "If this commitment to the patient is attenuated, even for so good a cause as benefits to future patients, the implicit assumptions of the doctor-patient relationship are violated." The risk of such attenuation by the randomized trial is great. The AIDS activists have brought this dramatically to the attention of the academic medical community. Techniques appropriate to the laboratory may not be applicable to humans. We must develop and use alternative methods for acquiring clinical knowledge.

14   Equipoise and the Ethics of Clinical Research

Benjamin Freedman

There is widespread agreement that ethics requires that each clinical trial begin with an honest null hypothesis. In the simplest model, testing a new treatment B on a defined patient population P for which the current accepted treatment is A, it is necessary that the clinical investigator be in a state of genuine uncertainty regarding the comparative merits of treatments A and B for population P. If a physician knows that these treatments are not equivalent, ethics requires that the superior treatment be recommended. Following Fried, I call this state of uncertainty about the relative merits of A and B "equipoise."

Equipoise is an ethically necessary condition in all cases of clinical research. In trials with several arms, equipoise must exist between all arms of the trial; otherwise the trial design should be modified to exclude the inferior treatment. If equipoise is disturbed during the course of a trial, the trial may need to be terminated and all subjects previously enrolled (as well as other patients within the relevant population) may have to be offered the superior treatment. It has been rigorously argued that a trial with a placebo is ethical only in investigating conditions for which there is no known treatment; this argument reflects a special application of the requirement for equipoise. Although equipoise has commonly been discussed in the special context of the ethics of randomized clinical trials, it is important to recognize it as an ethical condition of all controlled clinical trials, whether or not they are randomized, placebo-controlled, or blinded.

The recent increase in attention to the ethics of research with human subjects has highlighted problems associated with equipoise. Yet, as I shall attempt to show, contemporary literature, if anything, minimizes those difficulties. Moreover, there is evidence that concern on the part of investigators about failure to satisfy the requirements for equipoise can doom a trial as a result of the consequent failure to enroll a sufficient number of subjects.

The solutions that have been offered to date fail to resolve these problems in a way that would permit clinical trials to proceed. This paper argues that these problems are predicated on a faulty concept of equipoise itself. An alternative understanding of equipoise as an ethical requirement of clinical trials is proposed, and its implications are explored.

Many of the problems raised by the requirement for equipoise are familiar. Shaw and Chalmers have written that a clinician who "knows, or has good reason to believe," that one arm of the trial is superior may not ethically participate. But the reasoning or preliminary results that prompt the trial (and that may themselves be ethically mandatory) may jolt the investigator (if not his or her colleagues) out of equipoise before the trial begins. Even if the investigator is undecided between A and B in terms of gross measures such as mortality and morbidity, equipoise may be disturbed because evident differences in the quality of life (as in the case of two surgical approaches) tip the balance. In either case, in saying "we do not know" whether A or B is better, the investigator means "no controlled study has yet had results that reach statistical significance."

Late in the study—when P values are between 0.05 and 0.06—the moral issue of equipoise is most readily apparent, but the same problem arises when the earliest comparative results are analyzed. Within the closed statistical universe of the clinical trial, each result that demonstrates a difference between the arms of the trial contributes exactly as much to the statistical conclusion that a difference exists as does any other. The contribution of the last pair of cases in the trial is no greater than that of the first. If, therefore, equipoise is a condition that reflects equivalent evidence for alternative hypotheses, it is jeopardized by the first pair of cases as much as by the last. The investigator who is concerned about the ethics of recruitment after the penultimate pair must logically be concerned after the first pair as well.

Finally, these issues are more than a philosopher's nightmare. Considerable interest has been generated by a paper in which Taylor et al. describe the termination of a trial of alternative treatments for breast cancer. The trial foundered on the problem of patient recruitment, and the investigators trace much of the difficulty in enrolling patients to the fact that the investigators were not in a state of equipoise regarding the arms of the trial. With the increase in concern about the ethics of research and with the increasing presence of this topic in the curricula of medical and graduate schools, instances of the type that Taylor and her colleagues describe are likely to become more common. The requirement for equipoise thus poses a practical threat to clinical research.

———

Benjamin Freedman, "Equipoise and the Ethics of Clinical Research," *New England Journal of Medicine* 317 (1987): 141–45.

RESPONSES TO THE PROBLEMS OF EQUIPOISE

The problems described above apply to a broad class of clinical trials, at all stages of their development. Their resolution will need to be similarly comprehensive. However, the solutions that have so far been proposed address a portion of the difficulties, at best, and cannot be considered fully satisfactory.

Chalmers' approach to problems at the onset of a trial is to recommend that randomization begin with the very first subject. If there are no preliminary, uncontrolled data in support of the experimental treatment B, equipoise regarding treatments A and B for the patient population P is not disturbed. There are several difficulties with this approach. Practically speaking, it is often necessary to establish details of administration, dosage, and so on, before a controlled trial begins, by means of uncontrolled trials in human subjects. In addition, as I have argued above, equipoise from the investigator's point of view is likely to be disturbed when the hypothesis is being formulated and a protocol is being prepared. It is then, before any subjects have been enrolled, that the information that the investigator has assembled makes the experimental treatment appear to be a reasonable gamble. Apart from these problems, initial randomization will not, as Chalmers recognizes, address disturbances of equipoise that occur in the course of a trial.

Data-monitoring committees have been proposed as a solution to problems arising in the course of the trial. Such committees, operating independently of the investigators, are the only bodies with information concerning the trial's ongoing results. Since this knowledge is not available to the investigators, their equipoise is not disturbed. Although committees are useful in keeping the conduct of a trial free of bias, they cannot resolve the investigators' ethical difficulties. A clinician is not merely obliged to treat a patient on the basis of the information that he or she currently has, but is also required to discover information that would be relevant to treatment decisions. If interim results would disturb equipoise, the investigators are obliged to gather and use that information. Their agreement to remain in ignorance of preliminary results would, by definition, be an unethical agreement, just as a failure to call up the laboratory to find out a patient's test results is unethical. Moreover, the use of a monitoring committee does not solve problems of equipoise that arise before and at the beginning of a trial.

Recognizing the broad problems with equipoise, three authors have proposed radical solutions. All three think that there is an irresolvable conflict between the requirements that a patient be offered the best treatment known (the principle underlying the requirement for equipoise) and the conduct of clinical trials; they therefore suggest that the "best treatment" requirement be weakened.

Schafer has argued that the concept of equipoise, and the associated notion of the best medical treatment, depends on the judgment of patients rather than of clinical investigators. Although the equipoise of an investigator may be disturbed if he or she favors B over A, the ultimate choice of treatment is the patient's. Because the patient's values may restore equipoise, Schafer argues, it is ethical for the investigator to proceed with a trial when the patient consents. Schafer's strategy is directed toward trials that test treatments with known and divergent side effects and will probably not be useful in trials conducted to test efficacy or unknown side effects. This approach, moreover, confuses the ethics of competent medical practice with those of consent. If we assume that the investigator is a competent clinician, by saying that the investigator is out of equipoise, we have by Schafer's account said that in the investigator's professional judgment one treatment is therapeutically inferior—for that patient, in that condition, given the quality of life that can be achieved. Even if a patient would consent to an inferior treatment, it seems to me a violation of competent medical practice, and hence of ethics, to make the offer. Of course, complex issues may arise when a patient refuses what the physician considers the best treatment and demands instead an inferior treatment. Without settling that problem, however, we can reject Schafer's position. For Schafer claims that in order to continue to conduct clinical trials, it is ethical for the physician to offer (not merely accede to) inferior treatment.

Meier suggests that "most of us would be quite willing to forego a modest expected gain in the general interest of learning something of value." He argues that we accept risks in everyday life to achieve a variety of benefits, including convenience and economy. In the same way, Meier states, it is acceptable to enroll subjects in clinical trials even though they may not receive the best treatment throughout the course of the trial. Schafer suggests an essentially similar approach. According to this view, continued progress in medical knowledge through clinical trials requires an explicit abandonment of the doctor's fully patient-centered ethic.

These proposals seem to be frank counsels of desperation. They resolve the ethical problems of equipoise by abandoning the need for equipoise. In any event, would their approach allow clinical trials to be conducted? I think this may fairly be doubted. Although many people are presumably altruistic enough to forgo the best medical treatment in the interest of the progress of science, many are not. The numbers and proportions required to sustain the statistical validity of trial results suggest that in the absence of overwhelming altruism, the enrollment of satisfactory numbers of patients will not be possible. In particular, very ill patients, toward whom many of the most important clinical trials are directed, may be disinclined to be altruistic. Finally, as the study by Taylor et al. reminds us, the problems of equipoise trouble investigators as well as patients. Even if patients are prepared to dispense with the best treatment, their physicians, for reasons of ethics and professionalism, may well not be willing to do so.

Marquis has suggested a third approach. "Perhaps what is needed is an ethics that will justify the conscription of subjects for medical research," he has written. "Nothing less seems to justify present practice." Yet, although conscription might enable us to continue present practice, it would scarcely justify it. Moreover, the conscription of physician investigators, as well as subjects, would be necessary, because, as has been repeatedly argued, the problems of equipoise are as disturbing to clinicians as they are to subjects. Is any less radical and more plausible approach possible?

THEORETICAL EQUIPOISE VERSUS CLINICAL EQUIPOISE

The problems of equipoise examined above arise from a particular understanding of that concept, which I will term "theoretical equipoise." It is an understanding that is both conceptually odd and ethically irrelevant. Theoretical equipoise exists when, overall, the evidence on behalf of two alternative treatment regimens is exactly balanced. This evidence may be derived from a variety of sources, including data from the literature, uncontrolled experience, considerations of basic science and fundamental physiologic processes, and perhaps a "gut feeling" or "instinct" resulting from (or superimposed on) other considerations. The problems examined above arise from the principle that if theoretical equipoise is disturbed, the physician has, in Schafer's words, a "treatment preference"—let us say, favoring experimental treatment B. A trial testing A against B requires that some patients be enrolled in violation of this treatment preference.

Theoretical equipoise is overwhelmingly fragile; that is, it is disturbed by a slight accretion of evidence favoring one arm of the trial. In Chalmers' view, equipoise is disturbed when the odds that A will be more successful than B are anything other than 50 percent. It is therefore necessary to randomize treatment assignments beginning with the very first patient, lest equipoise be disturbed. We may say that theoretical equipoise is balanced on a knife's edge.

Theoretical equipoise is most appropriate to onedimensional hypotheses and causes us to think in those terms. The null hypothesis must be sufficiently simple and "clean" to be finely balanced: Will A or B be superior in reducing mortality or shrinking tumors or lowering fevers in population P? Clinical choice is commonly more complex. The choice of A or B depends on some combination of effectiveness, consistency, minimal or relievable side effects, and other factors. On close examination, for example, it sometimes appears that even trials that purport to test a single hypothesis in fact involve a more complicated, portmanteau measure—e.g., the "therapeutic index" of A versus B. The formulation of the conditions of theoretical equipoise for such complex, multidimensional clinical hypotheses is tantamount to the formulation of a rigorous calculus of apples and oranges.

Theoretical equipoise is also highly sensitive to the vagaries of the investigator's attention and perception. Because of its fragility, theoretical equipoise is disturbed as soon as the investigator perceives a difference between the alternatives—whether or not any genuine difference exists. Prescott writes, for example, "It will be common at some stage in most trials for the survival curves to show visually different survivals," short of significance but "sufficient to raise ethical difficulties for the participants." A visual difference, however, is purely an artifact of the research methods employed: When and by what means data are assembled and analyzed and what scale is adopted for the graphic presentation of data. Similarly, it is common for researchers to employ interval scales for phenomena that are recognized to be continuous in nature—e.g., five-point scales of pain or stages of tumor progression. These interval scales, which represent an arbitrary distortion of the available evidence to simplify research, may magnify the differences actually found, with a resulting disturbance of theoretical equipoise.

Finally, as described by several authors, theoretical equipoise is personal and idiosyncratic. It is disturbed when the clinician has, in Schafer's words, what "might even be labeled a bias or a hunch," a preference of a "merely intuitive nature." The investigator who ignores such a hunch, by failing to advise the patient that because of it the investigator prefers B to A or by recommending A (or a chance of random assignment to A) to the patient, has violated the requirement for equipoise and its companion requirement to recommend the best medical treatment.

The problems with this concept of equipoise should be evident. To understand the alternative, preferable interpretation of equipoise, we need to recall the basic reason for conducting clinical trials: There is a current or imminent conflict in the clinical community over what treatment is preferred for patients in a defined population P. The standard treatment is A, but some evidence suggests that B will be superior (because of its effectiveness or its reduction of undesirable side effects, or for some other reason). (In the rare case when the first evidence of a novel therapy's superiority would be entirely convincing to the clinical community, equipoise is already disturbed.) Or there is a split in the clinical community, with some clinicians favoring A and others favoring B. Each side recognizes that the opposing side has evidence to support its position, yet each still thinks that overall its own view is correct. There exists (or, in the case of a novel therapy, there may soon exist) an honest, professional disagreement among expert clinicians about the preferred treatment. A clinical trial is instituted with the aim of resolving this dispute.

At this point, a state of "clinical equipoise" exists. There is no consensus within the expert clinical community about the comparative merits of the alternatives to be tested. We may state the formal conditions under which such a trial would be ethical as follows: at the start of the trial, there must be a state of clinical equipoise regarding the merits of the regimens to be tested, and the trial must be designed in such a way as to make it reasonable to expect that, if it is successfully concluded, clinical equipoise will be disturbed. In other words, the results of a successful clinical trial should be convincing enough to resolve the dispute among clinicians.

A state of clinical equipoise is consistent with a decided treatment preference on the part of the investigators. They must simply recognize that their less-favored treatment is preferred by colleagues whom they consider to be responsible and competent. Even if the interim results favor the preference of the investigators, treatment B, clinical equipoise persists as long as those results are too weak to influence the judgment of the community of clinicians, because of limited sample size, unresolved possibilities of side effects, or other factors. (This judgment can necessarily be made only by those who know the interim results—whether a data-monitoring committee or the investigators.)

At the point when the accumulated evidence in favor of B is so strong that the committee or investigators believe no open-minded clinician informed of the results would still favor A, clinical equipoise has been disturbed. This may occur well short of the original schedule for the termination of the trial, for unexpected reasons. (Therapeutic effects or side effects may be much stronger than anticipated, for example, or a definable subgroup within population P may be recognized for which the results demonstrably disturb clinical equipoise.) Because of the arbitrary character of human judgment and persuasion, some ethical problems regarding the termination of a trial will remain. Clinical equipoise will confine these problems to unusual or extreme cases, however, and will allow us to cast persistent problems in the proper terms. For example, in the face of a strong established trend, must we continue the trial because of others' blind fealty to an arbitrary statistical benchmark?

Clearly, clinical equipoise is a far weaker—and more common—condition than theoretical equipoise. Is it ethical to conduct a trial on the basis of clinical equipoise, when theoretical equipoise is disturbed? Or, as Schafer and oth- ers have argued, is doing so a violation of the physician's obligation to provide patients with the best medical treatment? Let us assume that the investigators have a decided preference for B but wish to conduct a trial on the grounds that clinical (not theoretical) equipoise exists. The ethics committee asks the investigators whether, if they or members of their families were within population P, they would not want to be treated with their preference, B? An affirmative answer is often thought to be fatal to the prospects for such a trial, yet the investigators answer in the affirmative. Would a trial satisfying this weaker form of equipoise be ethical?

I believe that it clearly is ethical. As Fried has emphasized, competent (hence, ethical) medicine is social rather than individual in nature. Progress in medicine relies on progressive consensus within the medical and research communities. The ethics of medical practice grants no ethical or normative meaning to a treatment preference, however powerful, that is based on a hunch or on anything less than evidence publicly presented and convincing to the clinical community. Persons are licensed as physicians after they demonstrate the acquisition of this professionally validated knowledge, not after they reveal a superior capacity for guessing. Normative judgments of their behavior—e.g., malpractice actions—rely on a comparison with what is done by the community of medical practitioners. Failure to follow a "treatment preference" not shared by this community and not based on information that would convince it could not be the basis for an allegation of legal or ethical malpractice. As Fried states: "[T]he conception of what is good medicine is the product of a professional consensus." By definition, in a state of clinical equipoise, "good medicine" finds the choice between A and B indifferent.

In contrast to theoretical equipoise, clinical equipoise is robust. The ethical difficulties at the beginning and end of a trial are therefore largely alleviated. There remain difficulties about consent, but these too may be diminished. Instead of emphasizing the lack of evidence favoring one arm over another that is required by theoretical equipoise, clinical equipoise places the emphasis on informing the patient of the honest disagreement among expert clinicians. The fact that the investigator has a "treatment preference," if he or she does, could be disclosed; indeed, if the preference is a decided one, and based on something more than a hunch, it could be ethically mandatory to disclose it. At the same time, it would be emphasized that this preference is not shared by others. It is likely to be a matter of chance that the patient is being seen by a clinician with a preference for B over A, rather than by an equally competent clinician with the opposite preference.

Clinical equipoise does not depend on concealing relevant information from researchers and subjects, as does the use of independent data-monitoring committees. Rather, it allows investigators, in informing subjects, to distinguish appropriately among validated knowledge accepted by the clinical community, data on treatments that are promising but are not (or, for novel therapies, would not be) generally convincing, and mere hunches. Should informed patients decline to participate because they have chosen a specific clinician and trust his or her judgment—over and above the consensus in the professional community—that is no more than the patient's right. We do not conscript patients to serve as subjects in clinical trials.

THE IMPLICATIONS OF CLINICAL EQUIPOISE

The theory of clinical equipoise has been formulated as an alternative to some current views on the ethics of human research. At the same time, it corresponds closely to a pre-analytic concept held by many in the research and regulatory communities. Clinical equipoise serves, then, as a rational formulation of the approach of many toward research ethics; it does not so much change things as explain why they are the way they are.

Nevertheless, the precision afforded by the theory of clinical equipoise does help to clarify or reformulate some aspects of research ethics; I will mention only two.

First, there is a recurrent debate about the ethical propriety of conducting clinical trials of discredited treatments, such as Laetrile. Often, substantial political pressure to conduct such tests is brought to bear by adherents of quack therapies. The theory of clinical equipoise suggests that when there is no support for a treatment regimen within the expert clinical community, the first ethical requirement of a trial—clinical equipoise—is lacking; it would therefore be unethical to conduct such a trial.

Second, Feinstein has criticized the tendency of clinical investigators to narrow excessively the conditions and hypotheses of a trial in order to ensure the validity of its results. This "fastidious" approach purchases scientific manageability at the expense of an inability to apply the results to the "messy" conditions of clinical practice. The theory of clinical equipoise adds some strength to this criticism. Overly "fastidious" trials, designed to resolve some theoretical question, fail to satisfy the second ethical requirement of clinical research, since the special conditions of the trial will render it useless for influencing clinical decisions, even if it is successfully completed.

The most important result of the concept of clinical equipoise, however, might be to relieve the current crisis of confidence in the ethics of clinical trials. Equipoise, properly understood, remains an ethical condition for clinical trials. It is consistent with much current practice. Clinicians and philosophers alike have been premature in calling for desperate measures to resolve problems of equipoise.

---

15   Randomized Controlled Trials

Lessons from ECMO

Robert D. Truog

Extracorporeal membrane oxygenation (ECMO) is a technique for providing prolonged cardiopulmonary bypass to patients with potentially reversible pulmonary and/or cardiac failure. During ECMO therapy venous blood is drained from the right atrium, pumped through a membrane oxygenator, then infused into the aorta. [Figure omitted—eds.] In the early 1980s, pediatricians were using ECMO increasingly for treatment of neonatal respiratory failure despite the lack of a convincing randomized controlled trial (RCT) demonstrating its superiority over conventional therapy. In response to calls for a scientific evaluation of this new technique, O'Rourke and colleagues at Harvard University undertook and published the Harvard Neonatal ECMO Trial, an RCT comparing ECMO against conventional therapy. The study was provocative both for the statistical design it employed and for the ethical questions it raised. The debate that ensued over these issues culminated in a rare reprimand of the hospital's Institutional Review Board from the National Institutes of Heatlh.

Now ECMO is accepted widely for the treatment of neonatal respiratory failure, and several centers are administering this therapy to older children. However, since respiratory failure in pediatric patients differs pathophysiologically from that in neonates, many clinicians insist that

Robert D. Truog, "Randomized Controlled Trials: Lessons from ECMO," *Clinical Research* 40 (1992): 519–27.

ECMO must be evaluated in this older patient population with an RCT. A planning committee has been organized to undertake a multi-institutional evaluation of pediatric ECMO against conventional therapy. The purpose of this paper is to critique the methods of the Harvard Neonatal ECMO Trial and to make recommendations concerning the design of the proposed Pediatric ECMO Trial.

THE HISTORY OF ECMO

When initially developed in the 1950s, cardiopulmonary bypass could sustain patients for no more than several hours during surgical procedures. The development of the membrane oxygenator in the 1950s, however, made prolonged cardiopulmonary bypass a possibility. Following reports of several successes with this new technology, the National Heart, Lung, and Blood Institute sponsored a multi-institutional RCT comparing ECMO against standard therapy in adults with acute respiratory failure. Few patients survived in either treatment group, and interest in ECMO waned.

Robert Bartlett, one of the collaborators in this initial study, hypothesized that ECMO might be more effective in treating neonatal respiratory failure. Whereas the adults treated with ECMO may have already developed irreversible pulmonary failure, respiratory insufficiency in neonates is associated often with a reversible condition of persistent pulmonary hypertension of the newborn (PPHN). While often acutely life-threatening, this condition generally resolves over several days. PPHN can be associated with various causes of respiratory failure, such as meconium aspiration syndrome, pneumonia, sepsis, hyaline membrane disease, or congenital diaphragmatic hernia.

Bartlett initially used ECMO to treat 16 critically ill infants, and reported 6 survivors. Encouraged by these initial results, Bartlett continued to develop the technology. By 1980 he achieved 75 percent survival in patients judged to have a 95 percent mortality when managed with conventional therapy. However, many remained skeptical about the effectiveness of ECMO in the absence of an RCT. Bartlett realized the need for a rigorous comparison of ECMO against standard therapy, but was concerned about denying some patients a therapy he viewed as potentially life-saving. He therefore conducted an RCT that employed a form of adaptive randomization based on a "play-the-winner" design. This strategy altered the randomization weightings after each patient so that the next patient would be more likely to receive the therapy that was proving more successful. The only patient who received conventional therapy died; all 11 patients who received ECMO survived. The study was criticized by clinicians and statisticians alike as inadequate to demonstrate conclusively the superiority of ECMO over conventional therapy.

THE HARVARD NEONATAL ECMO TRIAL

As demand increased for a more conventional evaluation of ECMO in neonates, the Children's Hospital in Boston found itself in a uniquely well-suited position to perform such a study. Most of the critically ill neonates at that hospital were cared for in the Neonatal Intensive Care Unit [ICU], but those with surgical problems (e.g., congenital diaphragmatic hernia) were treated in the Multidisciplinary ICU. Physicians in the Multidisciplinary ICU had been intrigued with ECMO for some time; in fact, they had used ECMO to treat several newborns with congenital diaphragmatic hernia. Physicians in the Neonatal ICU, on the other hand, were skeptical about both the effectiveness of ECMO and its side effects, and refused to administer ECMO in the absence of a convincing RCT. This situation represented an ideal example of "clinical equipoise," with proponents of both the standard and the experimental therapy willing to cooperate in conducting the trial. In addition, by admitting all of the patients who received ECMO to the Multidisciplinary ICU and all of the patients who received conventional therapy to the Neonatal ICU, physicians were allowed to deliver the therapy that they believed to be superior. Finally, the Multidisciplinary ICU physicians and staff already had experience using ECMO for infants with congenital diaphragmatic hernia, so they were beyond the steep portion of their "learning curve." Infants with congenital diaphragmatic hernia were not included in the ECMO trial, since the pathogenesis and course of their disease differs markedly from those with nonsurgical causes of PPHN. Since infants with nonsurgical causes of PPHN had never been offered ECMO at Children's Hospital prior to the trial, these infants were not being denied a therapy that would have been previously available to them. In other words, initiation of the study did not limit the treatment options available to patients with nonsurgical PPHN.

The investigators identified those PPHN patients at high risk of death with a retrospective review of all PPHN patients admitted over a two-year period prior to the study. Physiologic indices that predicted an 85 percent mortality during this period were adopted as entrance criteria for the prospective study.

The study designed by O'Rourke and colleagues was innovative on two counts. First, like the Bartlett study, it employed an adaptive randomization approach. In Phase I of the study, infants were assigned to either ECMO or conventional therapy with 50:50 randomization. Phase I continued until there were 4 deaths in one of the treatment arms. After the fourth death in one arm, Phase II was begun. During Phase II, all of the infants were assigned to the more successful treatment arm until a fourth death occurred in that arm, or until the number of survivors reached statistical significance.

The results were as follows: During Phase I, 9 patients were assigned to ECMO and all survived. Ten patients received conventional therapy; 6 survived and 4 died. With the fourth death in the conventional arm, Phase II began. An additional 20 patients were enrolled to receive ECMO; 19 survived and 1 died. At this point ECMO was judged to be statistically superior to conventional therapy.

The second innovative feature of the study was the use of randomized consent. Zelen had described this approach several years earlier. It had been used in many chemotherapy trials as well as in the Bartlett study. In this design, the investigators seek and obtain consent only from those patients who are randomized to the experimental group. These patients are informed of the risks of the experimental therapy, and if they refuse to participate in the study they receive the standard therapy. In the Neonatal ECMO Trial, none of the parents of the 29 newborns randomized to the experimental arm refused ECMO. Patients who were randomized to the control arm were not informed of their inclusion in the study. In Zelen's view, since these patients received the best available standard therapy, they were not research subjects.

Both of the innovative features of the Harvard Neonatal ECMO Trial were subsequently criticized. The decision of the investigators to employ adaptive randomization was faulted by some as being too conservative and by others as not being conservative enough. Some asserted that it was unethical to randomize at all; others claimed that the study lost all validity by aborting randomization after Phase I. Taken together, perhaps these extreme claims support the conclusion that this strategy was an effective compromise between the desire to deliver compassionate care and the need to perform good science. Randomized consent, the other innovative feature, eventually proved to be even more ethically problematic. In view of the upcoming Pediatric ECMO trial, this approach needs careful scrutiny. [...]

RANDOMIZED CONTROLLED TRIALS AND POTENTIALLY LIFE-SAVING THERAPIES

The most important reason for adopting randomized consent in the Harvard Neonatal ECMO Trial was because it created the illusion that there was not a conflict in the patient-physician relationship. Randomized consent allowed the parents of the children in the control group to believe that their physicians were considering only their child's best interest in determining therapy. It allowed the physicians and staff to rationalize their actions by appeal to "clinical equipoise." The investigators adopted randomized consent as a compromise solution for dealing with the unacceptable conflict between their role as scientific investigators and their role as clinicians.

Schafer articulated this conflict clearly: "In his traditional role of healer, the physician's commitment is exclusively to his patient. By contrast, in his modern role of scientific investigator, the physician engaged in medical research or experimentation has a commitment to promote the acquisition of scientific knowledge." Randomization creates a conflict because determining therapy by "a flip of the coin" appears to violate the physician's pledge to administer what the physician believes to be the best therapy.

Some claim that this ethical conflict can be resolved. First, physicians should only prescribe treatments that are known to be effective. A physician's personal judgment about the effectiveness of a particular therapy does not obligate the physician to recommend that therapy if that judgment is not shared by the medical community at large. In other words, physicians need not claim to be in a state of personal equipoise regarding the effectiveness of alternative therapies, provided a sufficient degree of uncertainty exists within the medical community as a whole. Freedman refers to this latter state of equipoise as "clinical equipoise." Second, the only way to document the effectiveness of an experimental therapy is with an RCT. On this view, physicians should have no ethical difficulty enrolling patients into RCTs even when they have a personal belief that one of the therapies is superior.

This attempt to resolve the conflict between the roles of the healer and the scientific investigator is inadequate, however. First, patients do not expect physicians to only employ therapies that have been scientifically proven. Patients ask physicians to make recommendations based upon the totality of the physician's knowledge, judgment, and experience. No clinical decisions are free of uncertainty, so patients expect their physicians to make the best recommendations possible, all things considered. In the unusual case where a physician is entirely undecided about the best therapeutic choice, randomization could be considered an ethical option. However, this would be an exceptionally fragile situation, since any additional information could bias the physician toward one alternative or the other. Furthermore, even if the physician was in a state of equipoise, the patient may have preferences based upon the nature of the side effects or the patient's attitude toward risk. This level of uncertainty on the part of both the physician and the patient would clearly be so rare as to be practically irrelevant.

Furthermore, even clinical equipoise will inevitably deteriorate as experimental evidence accumulates during the course of a study in favor of one therapy over another. The choice of .05 as the cutoff for statistical significance is essentially arbitrary, and often requires continuation of clinical trials beyond the point at which the investigators are convinced of the eventual outcome. This may have been the case during the Harvard Neonatal ECMO Trial. Clinical equipoise must have been strained as deaths accumulated in the conventional arm while all of the ECMO patients were surviving.

Furthermore, the claim that the only way to demonstrate the effectiveness of an experimental therapy is with an RCT greatly exaggerates the importance of RCTs to medical progress. Though RCTs are unquestionably the best method for evaluating new therapies when they are practically feasible and do not entail serious ethical conflicts, they are not the only valid approach. The assertion that without RCTs we are doomed to decision-making based on guesswork and intuition is a gross overstatement. As Charles Fried noted, "[T]he claims for the RCT have been greatly, indeed preposterously overstated. The truth of the matter is that the RCT is one of many ways of generating information, of validating hypotheses. The proponents of the RCT, however, have elevated what is in theory a frequent (though by no means universal) advantage of degree into a gulf as sharp as that between the kosher and the non-kosher."

Indeed, very few of the daily decisions made by physicians in the care of their patients are based upon the results of an RCT. There has never been an RCT demonstrating the effectiveness of an appendectomy for appendicitis, or of penicillin for pneumococcal pneumonia. The tobacco industry's defense of their product is based on the absence of RCTs linking it to lung cancer, but few doubt the causal connection. "We should not proceed on the fallacious assumption that where there is no randomization, there is no truth."

The conflict between the roles of scientist and physician in conducting an RCT in many ways mirrors the conflict between the two major schools of thought in moral philosophy, consequentialism and deontology. Consequentialism, as its name implies, evaluates an action solely on its consequences. The best action is that which produces the best outcome, all things considered. Deontological approaches, on the other hand, view some actions as inherently wrong, regardless of their consequences. A consequentialist view of RCTs would likely take the position of the "scientist," and hold that since a valid trial will be of benefit to many patients in the future, the requirements of the trial should take precedence over the constraints of the patient-physician relationship.

Consequentialists could also appeal to fairness as a justification for randomized trials. Fairness demands that present patients should not benefit at the expense of future patients. Present patients have benefited from the RCTs of the past. Unless present patients also participate in RCTs, then future patients will be at a disadvantage. Fairness demands that each generation should contribute its "fair share."

A deontological approach to RCTs, on the other hand, would see them as always unethical under the traditional view of the patient-physician relationship. No matter how great the gains to society as a whole, physicians must recommend only therapies in which they personally believe. Some have suggested modifying this stand by asserting that patients can relieve physicians of this constraint through the process of informed consent. Patients consenting to an RCT would understand that their physician would no longer be operating under the traditional ethic with regard to the study. This suggestion is problematic, however. While acknowledging that individuals are free to make voluntary sacrifices to promote the common good, physicians should not be in the position of requesting such sacrifices. Critically ill patients and their families are extremely vulnerable and are frequently eager to please their physicians and conform to the expectations of the medical staff. On the deontological view, appropriate safeguards should prevent patients from being allowed to consent for RCTs.

In this analysis of the debate over RCTs, the two main schools of thought in moral philosophy are instructive because they indicate that the differences are fundamental and unlikely to be easily resolved. Just as neither a consequentialist nor a deontological morality has been found to be suitable for all circumstances, neither is one viewpoint on RCTs applicable to all situations.

When should we consider alternatives to RCTs? When are the ethical obligations that emerge from the traditional view of the patient-physician relationship powerful enough to override the need for performing the most rigorous and efficient studies possible? Some argue that deontologic considerations make RCTs unethical in all cases. This was the stand taken by the World Medical Association in the Declaration of Helsinki: "Concern for the interests of the subject must always prevail over the interests of science and society." This position overstates the issue, however. The great majority of RCTs are conducted without any objections from either the research subjects or the clinicians over the ethical conflicts that are theoretically present. Few criticize the RCT that seeks to identify the best antibiotic for treating acute otitis media or the best antacid for peptic ulcer disease. While these trials entail the same ethical conflicts as those involving potentially life-saving therapies, the goal of quickly reaching a scientifically rigorous conclusion is more important. The value of these studies to the well-being of society as a whole overrides the small potential for harm to the patient-physician relationship.

When the therapies under investigation are potentially life-saving, however, the balance shifts. Critically ill patients are extraordinarily dependent upon their physicians. In routine health matters many patients view their physicians as simply a provider of service, and negotiate as they would with a mechanic or plumber. However, when patients become critically ill, the relationship often becomes more intimate. The nature of the association shifts from contractual to fiduciary. In this setting, patients must be convinced that their physician is entirely devoted to pursuing their best interest, without any conflict of loyalty. The possibility that the physician may be balancing the needs of the critically ill patient against the needs of society is unthinkable for most patients and physicians alike. The AIDS epidemic dramatically illustrates these points. Patients with AIDS have vocally protested their participation in RCTs of potentially life-saving medications. In considering these objections, some conclude that AIDS presents unique features that are not suitable for conventional clinical trials. The unique feature about AIDS is not the disease, however; it is the articulate and strident activists who persistently make their case against RCTs. The problem is not new, only the awareness is new. The problem exists for all RCTs that involve potentially life-saving therapies, whether medications for AIDS or ECMO for neonatal respiratory failure.

Potentially life-saving therapies cannot always be differentiated from less critical interventions, however. Whether an intervention is potentially life-saving is a matter of degree, and must be defined over a spectrum. When is the pursuit of rigorous and efficient science justified, and when must this give way to the dictates of the patient-physician relationship? Clearly no definitive answer can be given, and many cases will be borderline. The existence of gray does not prevent us from differentiating white from black, however. The Harvard Neonatal ECMO Trial, for example, typifies a situation where any form of RCT placed an unbearable strain upon the traditional role of the physician. In this case, the decision to use a randomized consent design could be seen as a symptom of this problem. Randomized consent was invoked to mollify the conflict the investigators felt over their competing roles as physicians and scientists. The need to resort to this strategy should have been a powerful clue that there were serious ethical problems with the underlying study design.

RANDOMIZED CONTROLLED TRIALS AND RAPIDLY DEVELOPING TECHNOLOGIES

In addition to being a potentially life-saving therapy, ECMO is also a rapidly developing technology. For example, since the Harvard Neonatal ECMO Trial was completed many institutions have switched from the initial practice of withdrawing blood from the internal jugular vein and returning it to the carotid artery (veno-arterial ECMO) to a technique that uses the internal jugular vein for both withdrawing and returning (veno-venous ECMO). In addition, newborns who are still treated with veno-arterial ECMO now often have their carotid arteries repaired rather than ligated when the ECMO cannulae are removed. ECMO circuits which do not require the use of

anticoagulation are being developed. Some or all of these developments may significantly reduce the risks of ECMO, making it more favorable in comparison to conventional therapy. Driven at least in part by a desire to avoid the risks associated with the use of ECMO, many innovations have occurred in the administration of conventional therapy as well. Since completion of the Harvard Neonatal ECMO Trial, clinicians have reported success with high-frequency ventilation, negative-pressure ventilation, and surfactant therapy. When both the experimental and conventional therapies are rapidly evolving, at least two additional ethical issues arise.

The first relates to a problem inherent in the requirements of RCTs. Since RCTs demand that the interventional techniques be kept relatively constant during the trial, and since most trials require several years to complete, the technology offered to patients toward the end of the trial may be different and potentially inferior to that offered to concurrent patients treated outside of the trial. Patients who are "on protocol" may not benefit from innovations introduced during the period of the study. Since conventional therapy must also be kept constant during the study, patients in the control arm will likewise not benefit from advances that have occurred during the period of the trial. Toward the end of the trial, investigators cannot truthfully claim that the patients receiving the experimental therapy are being treated with state-of-the-art technology, nor can they claim that the control patients are receiving the best standard therapy. Again, there is a conflict between the patient's expectations of the physician and the scientist's desire to conduct a valid study. In addition, the trial itself may retard the development of new technologies, since during the trial the investigators are forbidden to alter the technology in significant ways. RCTs impose a moratorium on the development of new technologies among these institutions involved in the study.

The second problem relates to the relevance of the study. Perhaps the most fundamental ethical requirement of clinical trials is that they have the potential to generate useful knowledge. When technologies are developing rapidly, however, the trial may conclude with a comparison of two therapeutic approaches that have both become obsolete over the course of the study. Over the six and half years required by both the retrospective and prospective components of the Harvard Neonatal ECMO Trial, for example, the mortality of conventionally treated infants fell from 80 percent to perhaps as little as 10 percent. Clearly the 80 percent mortality assumed by the investigators in designing the trial had become a seriously misleading assumption. By the time it was completed, therefore, the Harvard Neonatal ECMO Trial was of diminished relevance in helping clinicians choose between ECMO and conventional therapy.

RECOMMENDATIONS FOR
A PEDIATRIC ECMO TRIAL

The ethical dilemmas raised by the proposed Pediatric ECMO Trial are very similar to those that plagued the Harvard Neonatal ECMO Trial. A Pediatric ECMO study will face all the problems that attend to studies involving both potentially life-saving therapies and rapidly developing technologies. The ideal study design would both preserve the essence of the traditional patient-physician relationship and provide results that are reflective of up-to-date modifications in both experimental and standard therapies. For the reasons discussed above, an RCT would fail on both counts. First, while an RCT could certainly be designed that did not depend upon randomized consent, this would be treating the symptoms without correcting the more fundamental problem with the RCT. An RCT that utilized the traditional consent process would merely make both physicians and patients alike more acutely aware of the conflicts involved. In decisions as momentous as whether to institute ECMO in a critically ill child, the child's parents must have no doubts about the undivided loyalty of the physician to their child's care. Second, the rapid pace of developments in ECMO and other alternative approaches to the management of respiratory failure threaten to make the results of an RCT obsolete even before such a trial could be completed.

As an alternative to an RCT, I propose a prospective observational study of ECMO in the pediatric population. Clinicians caring for children with cardiorespiratory failure would treat their patients with the therapy or combination of therapies they believe to be most efficacious. The study would not impose any restrictions in the choices physicians make on behalf of their patients. All institutions participating in the trial would forward data relative to the patient's condition, prognosis, and hospital course to a central registry. Significant alterations in therapeutic approach or technique would be noted as well. Data of the effectiveness of different interventions in patients with particular diagnoses and severity of illness would be periodically analyzed. Algorithms would be devised to assess the outcomes of patients matched for clinical similarity. The investigators would not expect to achieve the degree of statistical significance demanded from a randomized trial, but would utilize the database to extract trends in effectiveness and safety. The study would never be "completed" in the usual sense, but would continue to generate information on the current effectiveness of a variety of approaches to cardiorespiratory failure. Rather than arriving at a definitive "answer" at one point in time, this approach would indicate trends that would continually provide successive approximations to the best answer at the present point in time.

The most obvious objection to this proposal is that it is simply not as scientifically valid as an RCT. This objection is founded on the belief that only RCTs can provide definitive answers to clinical questions. Clearly, however, even RCTs are never definitive; they can never provide certainty. All information has a price, and "you get what you pay for." At least two prominent statisticians, Professors Donald Berry and Richard Royall, have argued that comprehensive prospective databases can and should be used instead of RCTs in evaluating potentially life-saving therapies. They affirm that the difference between a prospective observational study and an RCT is not the difference between good and bad or true and false; it is merely the difference between varying degrees of confidence.

Could a prospective observational study have made the Harvard Neonatal ECMO Trial unnecessary? A review of 715 newborns treated with ECMO published in 1988 demonstrated an 81 percent survival with ECMO and indicated that ECMO was statistically superior to any other treatment with a survival rate less than 78.4 percent. If this ECMO registry had been supplemented with data from infants receiving conventional therapy, it is likely that valid conclusions could have been reached without the need for an RCT. Indeed, statistician Berry believes that even without a concurrent database of conventionally treated neonates, these results from the National ECMO database were more convincing evidence of ECMO's effectiveness than the results of the subsequent randomized trial. Furthermore, a concurrent database of both ECMO and conventionally managed neonates would have indicated a more accurate assessment of mortality from conventional ventilation, and would have yielded a more relevant comparison of the effectiveness of ECMO against conventional therapy.

A prospective observational study would be an innovative attempt to find methods of analysis that are both scientifically valid and ethically sensitive. This study would require courage on the part of the investigators, granting agencies, and journal editors, since it would be breaking new ground in challenging the unquestioned superiority of RCTs. Statisticians would have to develop new methodologies and investigators would have to consider new ways of evaluating uncertainty. Similar demands have been put forward for the evaluation of new drugs in the treatment of AIDS and creative investigators are responding. A prospective observational study of ECMO in the pediatric population will provide the best balance between the need for maintaining the traditional values of the patient-physician relationship and the need to determine the best therapy for these critically ill children.

Section Three

The Role of Placebos in Clinical Research

16   The Continuing Unethical Use of Placebo Controls

KENNETH J. ROTHMAN AND KARIN B. MICHELS

Is it ethical to use a placebo? The answer to this question will depend, I suggest, upon whether there is already available an orthodox treatment of proved or accepted value. If there is such an orthodox treatment the question will hardly arise, for the doctor will wish to know whether a new treatment is more, or less, effective than the old, not that it is more effective than nothing.

—A. Bradford Hill

Unaccountably, in these times of raised ethical consciousness, placebo treatments are still commonly used in medical research in circumstances in which their use is unethical. We refer not to the deceptive use of placebo, but to studies in which patients are informed that they may receive a placebo and then give their consent. Even so, such studies are unethical if patients are assigned a placebo instead of a therapy effective in treating their condition. Here we examine why this ethical breach persists and suggest ways to reduce it.

THE ETHICS OF PLACEBO CONTROLS

The Nuremberg Code, "the cornerstone of modern human experimentation ethics," was formulated shortly after World War II in response to Nazi atrocities. The World Health Organization adopted a version of the code in 1964 as the Declaration of Helsinki. The declaration elevates concern for the health and rights of individual patients in a study over concern for society, for future patients, or for science. "In any medical study," it asserts, "every patient—including those of a control group, if any—should be assured of the best proven diagnostic and therapeutic

Kenneth J. Rothman and Karin B. Michels, "The Continuing Unethical Use of Placebo Controls," *New England Journal of Medicine* 331 (1994): 394–98.

method." This statement effectively proscribes the use of a placebo as control when a "proven" therapeutic method exists. The declaration also directs that a study that violates its precepts should not be accepted for publication.

Nevertheless, studies that breach this provision of the Declaration of Helsinki are still commonly conducted, with the full knowledge of regulatory agencies and institutional review boards. Although some are published in peer-reviewed medical journals, the declaration notwithstanding, many trials that are conducted in order to gain regulatory approval for new drugs or devices never reach libraries. Thus, there is no straightforward way to estimate how many trials are undertaken that involve the unethical use of placebos.

Below are a few examples from among those that have actually been published. Some of these examples might be challenged by specialists in the disciplines involved, who might argue that the use of placebo was justifiable in the case under discussion. In the aggregate, however, the examples indicate that patients in trials are often denied "best proven" treatments.

Ivermectin Trial

In 1985 a group of investigators reported the efficacy of ivermectin to treat onchocerciasis, or river blindness. The investigators assigned some of the study participants to placebo when, according to the investigators themselves, the drug diethylcarbamazine had been "the standard therapy . . . for over three decades." The study participants were illiterate Liberian seamen, some of whom indicated their "informed consent" by thumbprint.

Rheumatoid Arthritis Trials

In recent years there have been numerous placebo-controlled trials of secondary treatments for rheumatoid arthritis. In many of these trials, some enduring for years, all the patients were assigned to receive a primary therapy, such as a nonsteroidal anti-inflammatory agent, and were then randomly assigned to receive either a new secondary treatment or a placebo in addition. New placebo trials of secondary treatments for arthritis continue to be proposed and conducted, even though many such trials have shown various secondary treatments to be more effective than placebo. Participants who receive placebo in these studies are at risk for serious and irreversible degenerative changes that can, to some extent, be prevented.

Antidepressant-Drug Trials

A 1992 report of a randomized trial of treatment for major depression began with the statement "Effective antidepressant compounds have been available for over 30 years." Nevertheless, the investigators in that study assigned half the seriously depressed patients in the trial to receive placebo and the other half to receive paroxetine. Placebo controls are commonplace in trials of antidepressant drugs, despite the availability of therapies whose success is acknowledged.

Ondansetron Trials

Considerable advances have been made in controlling chemotherapy-induced emesis [nausea and vomiting—eds.] in recent years. Several drugs are available for use singly or in combination: they include metoclopramide, phenothiazines, substituted benzamides, corticosteroids, and benzodiazepines. Nevertheless, when a new agent, ondansetron, was tested, it was compared with placebo in several trials. (The use of placebo was criticized in an editorial accompanying the published report of one of the trials.)

Trials of Drugs for Congestive Heart Failure

Angiotensin-converting-enzyme inhibitors are accepted as a standard treatment for congestive heart failure. Although a number of these drugs have been approved, new ones, as well as other drugs for congestive heart failure, are commonly evaluated against placebo.

Antihypertensive-Drug Trials

Trials of new drugs for mild-to-moderate hypertension typically use placebo controls, despite the established efficacy of many agents in treating mild-to-moderate hypertension. For example, in the introduction to a "dose-ranging" study of the calcium antagonist verapamil, verapamil was described as "an effective antihypertensive drug, which is dose dependent, superior to placebo, comparable to or more effective than propranolol, and comparable with nifedipine." Despite these assertions, the investigators assigned some patients in the study to receive placebo.

PLACEBO CONTROLS AND DRUG APPROVAL

In the United States, many drug studies are conducted to meet the requirements of the Food and Drug Administration (FDA) so that the drug can be marketed. The Code of Federal Regulations under which the FDA operates is ambiguous about the acceptability of placebo controls. In one place it suggests that they should be avoided: "The test drug is compared with known effective therapy; for example, where the condition treated is such that administration of placebo or no treatment would be contrary to the interest of the patient." The regulations go on, however, to suggest including both placebo controls and active-treatment controls in a study: "An active treatment study may include additional treatment groups, however, such as a placebo control...."

In practice, FDA officials consider placebo controls the "gold standard." Agency guidelines specify the study designs required to obtain approval for new drugs. Placebo controls are, in effect, required for disorders of moderate severity and pain, even when an alternative treatment is available. For example, in its "Guidelines for the Clinical Evaluation of Anti-Inflammatory and Antirheumatic Drugs," the FDA demands the inclusion of a placebo group when new-drug applications are submitted for fixed-dose combinations of nonsteroidal anti-inflammatory drugs (NSAIDs) with codeine: "The combination must be shown to be superior to each component and the NSAID must be superior to placebo in order for the study to be persuasive." For the clinical evaluation of disease-modifying antirheumatic drugs (DMARDs), placebo controls also appear necessary: "In order to develop the body of information necessary for approval of a DMARD, studies using the following different control groups should generally be conducted: Comparison of the drug with a placebo...."

In at least one instance, the FDA refused to approve a new drug, a beta-blocker for use in angina pectoris, even though the application showed that the new drug had an effect similar to that of propranolol, an already approved drug. The application was rejected because the drug had not been tested against placebo, even though a placebo-controlled trial would have violated the Declaration of Helsinki.

IS THERE A SCIENTIFIC RATIONALE FOR PLACEBOS?

The FDA is not alone in pushing for placebo controls. For example, a recent textbook on clinical drug trials advocates using them because "if a new drug has only been compared to an active control (without a placebo-controlled trial), this is not a convincing proof of efficacy (even if equivalence can be demonstrated)." Without justification, such statements confer on placebo control a stature that ranks it with double blinding and randomization as a hallmark of good science.

The randomized, controlled trial is well recognized as the most desirable type of study in which to evaluate a new treatment. This recognition acknowledges the essential role of comparison and the importance of randomization in enhancing the comparability of two or more treatment groups. Using a placebo for comparison controls for the psychological effects of receiving some treatment and also permits blinding. No scientific principle, however, requires the comparison in a trial to involve a placebo instead of, or in addition to, an active treatment. Why, then, are placebo controls considered important? Three arguments have been advanced, none of which withstands scrutiny.

Establishing a Reference Point

By allowing the investigator to determine whether a new treatment is better than nothing (beyond the psychological benefits of treatment), a placebo control offers a clear benchmark. After all, even if a new treatment is worse than an existing one, it may still be "effective" in that it is better than no treatment. On the other hand, as Hill pointed out in 1963, the essential medical question at issue is how the new treatment compares with the old one, not whether the new treatment is better than nothing.

Avoiding Difficult Decisions about Comparison Treatments

Determining whether one treatment is better than another is not always a straightforward matter. Beyond the question of efficacy, one can and should take into account unintended effects, interactions, costs, routes of administration, and other factors. Thus, it may appear simplistic to demand that the best proven treatment be chosen as the standard for comparison, if "best proven" refers only to efficacy. For some patients there may be advantages to a treatment that is inferior to a current standard with regard to efficacy but better with respect to cost or quality of life. For example, the adverse effects of some accepted treatments might offset the therapeutic benefits for some patients sufficiently that a placebo control would be ethically justified. This reasoning involves a complex decision that should be defended in submitted research proposals and published reports. It is not justifiable, however, to assign placebo controls simply to avoid the complex decision of which treatment should be used as a standard. Investigators are ethically obliged to make such decisions.

Bolstering Statistical Significance

One FDA scientist contends that placebo-controlled trials are superior to studies using an active treatment as the control because it is much easier to demonstrate a statistically significant effect in the former case. The FDA relies heavily on statistical significance in judging the efficacy of new drugs. Despite its popularity, however, this tool is not a good one for measuring efficacy. The significance of an association depends on two characteristics—the strength of the association and its statistical variability. A weak effect can be "significant" if there is little statistical variability in its measurement, whereas a strong effect may not be "significant" if there is substantial variability in its measurement. Of the two characteristics, only the strength of the effect should be fundamental to the decision about approval of the drug. Ideally, statistical variability should be reduced nearly to zero when the magnitude of a drug effect is assessed, so that random error does not influence the assessment.

Unfortunately, the main way to reduce statistical variability is to conduct large studies, which are expensive. Statistical significance, on the other hand, can be obtained even in small studies, if the effect estimate is strong enough. When a placebo control is used instead of an effective treatment, the effect of a new drug appears large and may be statistically significant even in a small study. The scientific benefit, however, is illusory. Because the study is small, the measurement of the effect is subject to considerable statistical error. Thus, the actual size of the effect, even when a new drug is compared with placebo, remains obscure, and the study does not address the question of the effectiveness of the new treatment as compared with currently accepted treatments.

The small placebo-controlled studies fostered by the FDA benefit drug companies, which can more easily obtain approval of an inferior drug by comparing it with placebo than they can by testing it against a serious competitor. Smaller studies are also cheaper. Unfortunately, the costs saved by the drug company are borne by patients, who receive placebos instead of effective treatments, and by the public at large, which is supplied with a drug of undetermined efficacy.

There is no sound scientific basis for these arguments on behalf of placebo controls. Furthermore, regardless of any apparent merit these arguments have, scientific considerations should not take precedence over ethical ones, even if the use of active controls requires more difficult decisions about study design, more costly studies, and more complicated analyses.

ETHICAL COUNTERARGUMENTS

Two ethical arguments are sometimes advanced to justify the use of placebos when effective therapies exist. First, one can argue that withholding an accepted treatment may not lead to serious harm. For example, treating pain or nausea with a placebo may cause no long-term adverse effects, and the patient can call attention to any treatment failure or even choose to drop out of the study. Nevertheless, although withholding an accepted treatment may occasionally seem innocuous, allowing investigators to do so runs counter to the ethical principle that every patient, including those in a control group, should receive either the best available treatment or a new treatment thought to be as good or better. Instead, it concedes to individual investigators and to institutional review boards the right to determine how much discomfort or temporary disability patients should endure for the purpose of research. Ethical codes in medical experimentation have been developed expressly to shield patients from such vulnerability.

The second justification offered is that of informed consent. This argument says that if patients are fully informed about the risks of entering a trial and still agree to participate, there is no reason to prevent them from doing so. The ethical burden is passed directly to the patients. Informed consent is always desirable, but investigators should not put patients in a position in which their health and well-being could be compromised, even if the patients agree. There are several reasons. Despite the best efforts to inform patients, they will rarely if ever be as well informed about their treatment options as their physicians. Moreover, even informed patients may not be disinterested enough to decide rationally whether it is tolerable to be deprived of an accepted treatment. Finally, patients are given the choice of participating in a trial or not, but they are given no choice about which treatments will be studied. It may be more desirable to a patient to be a part of the trial than to decline to participate, but it might have been preferable to be in a different trial that did not have a placebo arm.

RECOMMENDATIONS

Placebo is likely to continue to be used in place of an effective control until all parties to such studies are held strictly accountable for the ethical conduct of the research. We recognize that in some situations an accepted treatment may not be better than placebo for a given indication and that arguments can be made to justify the use of placebo instead of an existing treatment. The burden of justification, however, should fall not on critics but on those responsible for the research, including investigators, regulatory agencies, research sponsors, institutional review boards, and journal editors. All these parties should adhere to the precept that patients ought not to face unnecessary pain or disease on account of a medical experiment, and they should question the ethical legitimacy of using placebos in any experiment. Investigators should be routinely required by regulatory agencies, institutional review boards, and funding agencies to justify in writing the use of placebos in any study that uses them. This explanation should be part of all proposals, protocols, and published papers. Editors should be vigilant about questioning the use of placebos in experiments involving humans; regardless of assertions authors make about institutional review, editors should always require authors to justify in their manuscripts any use of placebo controls.

The change needed most is the enforcement of ethical guidelines at regulatory agencies, such as the FDA, which review research that may never be published. The FDA should conduct an ethical review of every study submitted to it. Any study proposing to use placebos in place of effective treatments without making a persuasive ethical justification should be disapproved. Studies involving unethical use of placebos should be ignored in the drug-approval process. Above all, scientific imperatives should never be weighed against established ethical canons.

---

17 Placebo-Controlled Trials and the Logic of Clinical Purpose

Benjamin Freedman

The exercise of human intelligence ramifies in numerous and diverse ways. Nevertheless, as applied in theory or practice, in work or play, directed toward life or toward

Benjamin Freedman, "Placebo-Controlled Trials and the Logic of Clinical Purpose," *IRB: A Review of Human Subjects Research* 12, no. 6 (1990): 1–6.

death, each manifestation shares a common underlying method: organized comparison. Whether deriving equations in mathematics, or developing progressions of chords in jazz, or, in business, studying the impact of advertisements upon defined populations, reason is at bottom engaged in the single process of comparison, the delineation of sameness and difference.

Medicine partakes of this commonality of method, and has come to grant greatest credence to those propositions established by the cleanest possible comparison: the controlled clinical trial that methodically examines sameness and difference in outcome across cohorts. All of the diverse strategies introduced to reduce bias (e.g., stratification and randomization) in fact simply aim to ensure the precision of comparison.

In pursuing the strategy of organized comparison, however, a prior question must be posed: For what purpose is comparison sought? Many of the controversies concerning the design of clinical trials can be best understood as grounded in the two distinct purposes an investigator may have in mind: on the one hand, achieving a biologist's understanding of the human organism; on the other, healing and ameliorating conditions experienced by suffering patients.

This paper addresses one specific ramification of this fundamental issue of clinical trials: the use of a placebo instead of an active treatment control group in investigating therapeutic agents. In many cases, when standard treatment has been clearly validated as beneficent, there is no question that it, not placebo, must serve as the control. In many other cases involving treatments of dubious efficacy (especially if they also carry known serious side effects), all agree that placebo must be used as the control. The field of battle for the controversy I am speaking of is of course the large grey zone in between.

Although the arguments of the two camps have commonly proceeded upon the belief that this is a case of the conflicting demands of science (ordinarily favoring the use of placebo) and ethics (arguing on behalf of active treatment controls), a number of other profound scientific and philosophical issues are relevant to the choice as well. [...] I shall describe an approach to the choice of appropriate control groups that reflects a view of trials on human subjects as being logically based in and ethically justified by their reflection of, and contribution to, clinical practice.

Consider, as one example, the following case within the grey zone. Imagine that theoretical considerations and animal studies support a trial in humans of a new drug for chronic idiopathic urticaria (itchy hives of unknown cause). There exists a current standard pattern of treatment for this condition, involving a staged approach of mild antihistamines followed, if necessary, by H_2 receptor antagonists (drugs that block the other main site that picks up histamines). What is the appropriate control group for an efficacy trial of the new drug?

The investigator argues that the standard approach to chronic idiopathic urticaria has never been convincingly shown superior to placebo in any well-controlled study. On that basis, he proposes testing the new drug against placebo. On the other side, the research committee argues that though the standard regimen is admittedly not a fully satisfactory treatment, it is widely believed to be effective (and superior to placebo). No good controlled trial of this regimen has been conducted that shows the contrary, i.e., that failed to disconfirm the null hypothesis that standard treatment is no better than placebo. (Had such a trial been done, we would be out of the grey zone.) Under the current circumstances, proving that the new drug is more effective than placebo might be of scientific interest but would still be devoid of clinical value, for a placebo-controlled trial will not address the clinician's question: Is this new drug better than my current practice? The appropriate control from this point of view is the standard regimen.

Given the very large number of "standard" medical and surgical interventions that have never been validated in well-controlled circumstances, the above case is paradigmatic of a problem of substantial intrinsic importance. But the dispute points to an even broader *conceptual* issue: Where is the burden of proof to be placed? The investigator finds that nonvalidated clinical practice bears no weight; the research committee, perhaps believing that departures from standard practice, validated or not, are considered by law to be malpractice, thinks such departures need to be justified. How has the literature on research design and ethics addressed this sort of choice between placebo versus active treatment controls? And more to the point: How *ought* the choice be made?

CURRENT VIEWS ON PLACEBOS

Current views on placebo-controlled studies commonly imply that in the above example, because standard treatment has not been rigorously validated, the investigator is correct to want to use a placebo control. The practicalities involved in satisfying drug regulators, particularly the United States Food and Drug Administration (FDA), undoubtedly influence investigators in this preference for placebo controls. Even under the title "Placebo Controls Are Not Always Necessary," for example, one FDA regulator writes "... it is well to state that in almost all plans for the study of the effectiveness of a new drug, it is desirable to include some placebo-controlled studies unless it is considered unethical to do so." Explaining the FDA stance, Temple has stated that the use of standard treatment as control should generally be restricted to those cases in which that treatment has regularly [*sic!*] been shown superior to placebo in well-controlled trials.

The preference for placebo appears to rest upon common agreement regarding several propositions:

• The randomized, double-blind, placebo-controlled trial is the scientific gold standard for all drug evaluation.

• Standard treatment controls are a poor second to placebo, from a scientific and economic point of view.

- Ethical considerations intrude, however, preventing the use of this gold standard in all instances.
- Some form of balance must be struck between science and ethics to resolve this dilemma.

An examination of two statements on the use of placebo controls in clinical research prepared by professional associations shows how this dilemma is commonly resolved. A relatively early and very influential statement on the ethical use of placebos was included within a thoughtful review of the ethics of research issued by a committee of the American Academy of Pediatrics. [...] They write,

> The conditions under which the use of placebos is ethical in drug research in children include (1) when there is no commonly accepted therapy for the condition and the agent under study is the first one that may modify the course of the disease process; (2) when the commonly used therapy for the condition is of questionable or low efficacy; (3) when the commonly used therapy for the condition carries with it a high frequency of unacceptable side effects; (4) when the incidence and severity of undesirable side effects produced by adding a new treatment to an established regimen are uncertain; (5) when the disease process is characterized by frequent, spontaneous exacerbations and remissions.

This stance was referred to and followed, with some elaboration, by clinical investigators in gastroenterology. [...] The American College of Gastroenterology's position paper states,

> There are at least three principal circumstances in which inclusion of placebo groups in randomized clinical trials should present no ethical problem. The first category comprises those situations in which a standard therapy is for one reason or another unavailable, ineffective, inappropriate, or of unproven efficacy. The second category consists of conditions in which placebo is in and of itself relatively effective therapy. And the third category includes cases in which even the ongoing disease process has little if any adverse impact on the patient's overall health.

A number of problems are raised by these statements. First, they fail to distinguish between those instances in which the use of a placebo control is scientifically necessary and those in which it is ethically justifiable. For example, the pediatrician's insistence upon placebo controls with respect to conditions involving spontaneous exacerbations and remissions is surely a point driven by the scientific need to use a placebo as a "control for time," to avoid the error of

attributing a spontaneous variation in the course of an illness to the specific effect of the drug under study.

Second, they fail to distinguish between instances in which use of a placebo control is ethically justified from those in which it is considered excusable. The last condition noted by the gastroenterologists' statement—allowing placebo for those conditions in which a lack of treatment "will have little or any adverse effect upon the patient's health"—is particularly troubling for having failed to spell out who gets to say what shall count as an adverse effect. In our case of mild, chronic urticaria, practitioners may be inclined to see the untreated condition as not at all urgent, but simply as uncomfortable and, perhaps, unsightly. From the patient's point of view, the mere fact that he or she made an appointment with a doctor indicates distress with the condition and hope that it will be treated expeditiously.

Third, by treating separately considerations that need to be considered globally, the statements introduce needless complication and, possibly, error. The net therapeutic advantage of a treatment will be the term used to refer to the compendious measure of a treatment's attractiveness. This measure considers the treatment's direct impact upon the event causing the disease and specific benefit with respect to a patient's short- and long-term prognosis, symptomatology, and functioning, discounted by the treatment's detrimental side effects. In addition, such ancillary factors as providing a uniform dose of a bioavailable drug and ease of administration are properly included within the calculation of the net therapeutic advantage. [...]

From the point of view of the expert clinical community, it is always the compendious measure of a drug's net therapeutic advantage that determines that drug's attractiveness *vis-à-vis* alternative treatments. An antibiotic that is attractive because of its specific microbial action may be less favored because of its toxic side effects, or because it can only be administered intravenously under constant medical monitoring. Only if, taking all these factors into account, the community is undecided between alternatives, can they be said to be fit competing arms within a randomized clinical trial. Ideally, the successful conclusion of the trial will determine one arm to have a superior net therapeutic advantage *vis-à-vis* competitors; but more commonly, the trial will yield a judgment on a measure that may be used as a surrogate for net therapeutic advantage, or provide the preliminary information necessary for preparing such a trial.

As applied to a trial of drug d versus placebo p, therefore, we could say generally that the trial is ethical provided current consensus has not decided that the net therapeutic advantage associated with d is better than that of p. Under the common (but somewhat inaccurate) assumption made by designers of trials, that the net therapeutic advantage of placebo itself is nil, this condition reduced further to the belief that the net therapeutic advantage associated with the drug is itself entirely likely to prove to be nil. This may be because the drug's likely toxicity may be so great as to balance off its benefits, or because the drug is likely to be as useless in specific effect as it is benign in side effect. Whenever parsing a drug's net therapeutic advantage, it is important to keep in mind the dynamic balance these elements involve.

Rather than state that a placebo-controlled trial of d is justified if and only if the net therapeutic advantage of the drug under investigation is nil, however, the statements noted above by organizations of investigators rely upon elements entering into the computation of the net therapeutic advantage such as efficacy and toxicity. If we are to take these statements at their word, therefore, a number of problems become immediately evident. We are told that when an "agent under study is the first one" promising success, a placebo control may be used. Few would agree, however, if: the condition were one of uniform mortality or extensive morbidity; there is a strong theoretical case, and promising animal results, on behalf of the treatment d; and if d has been used for many years on humans for other indications, with few if any side effects. These circumstances indicate a priori a positive net therapeutic advantage associated with d, which would therefore need to be verified without the use of a placebo control. By the same token, many proven effective treatments produce a high or even uniform "frequency of unacceptable side effects," but a placebo control would be rejected because the course of the disease process that the treatment is known to control is more unacceptable yet.

These points, however, only succeed in somewhat narrowing the scope of judgment and discretion required in considering placebo controls. A more fundamental critique is needed if a clinically rational approach to the justification of the use of placebo controls is to be successfully sketched.

THE BASIS OF PLACEBO BIAS

The bias on behalf of placebo, and against standard treatment, comprises several components. Numerous confounding factors arising in standard treatment controls that otherwise would need to be controlled for are avoided: factors like drug form and formulation, time/dose relationships, side effects encountered, and drug synergism. Consequently, it is thought that in "studies smaller than those with active controls, one can ascertain the effectiveness of a new drug early in the process and thereafter not have to worry about whether one is dealing with a useful drug." Above all, a placebo control for d will give a clean indication of d's specific effects on the condition under study. By the simple stratagem of blind control with placebo (to provide a benchmark of nil net therapeutic advantage), systematic differences between the control and experimental group can be accounted to the specific effect of d.

These advantages would, however, be substantially vitiated in the light of finding that placebos share the confounding characteristics of standard treatment, and especially if placebos do not themselves bear a nil net therapeutic advantage. But just those points have been established by the past several decades' investigation of placebos and the placebo effect.

We will assume, as research does itself, that the placebo administered is an inert substance indistinguishable from the active drug d under study. [...]

Given that the study has provided a genuine placebo, the weight of research on the placebo effect indicates that the assumptions underlying the belief that placebos, unlike standard treatment, yield a zero baseline comparison of nil therapeutic benefit are mistaken. It is unnecessary to rehearse the very extensive evidence that placebo provides a positive rather than nil net therapeutic advantage for a broad class of conditions. That fact, if granted, leaves placebo benefit undisturbed as a useful basis for comparison of drug effect. But this will now have to be understood as yielding a relative rather than an absolute measure. Since the benefit of placebo is not zero, drug effectiveness is being measured upon an ordinal, rather than a cardinal scale.

Much less familiar is the evidence research provides that the profile of placebo effectiveness partakes of the same complexities bedeviling pharmaceutically active preparations. Expressing the spirit of contemporary placebo research, one investigator writes:

> The placebo effect should be considered as a potent therapeutic intervention in its own right, rather than merely a nuisance variable. The placebo can be understood as if it were another active (pharmacological) agent whose positive (and sometimes negative) effects can be independently evaluated, and whose mode of action is worthy of independent investigation.

Many clinicians have felt that placebo injections have a stronger effect on patients than do tablets, and this belief in placebo variation is borne out in research that indicates, for example, that capsules commonly elicit a more powerful placebo response than do tablets, and even that depending upon the condition the color of the placebo may be a factor—red placebo stimulants stimulate better than blue ones! Just like drugs, moreover, placebos have demonstrable peak effects that degrade over time, as well as carryover and cumulative effects; and placebos produce their own toxicities and side effects.

In each case, there arises of course a problem in attributing causation. Are we to say, for example, that the side effect experienced is caused by the placebo, or by the patient's expecting to experience side effects flagged in the consent form, or to the medical context of administration, or some combination of these? The question of causality need not be resolved for our purposes, though, for the fact remains that the same questions arise for the administration of the experimental drug, or for the active treatment control. The precise point is that within the clinical trial, all of these confounding factors are held constant and influence the attribution of results in interpreting any arm, including placebo. The trend of the research, over and above the established results, suggests that over time the concept of the monolithic placebo will be further eroded, giving rise to new questions for researchers. For example, should a placebo-controlled trial of an active agent wait for the results of trials that establish whether pink capsules or red tablets are the *most effective* placebo for the condition in question?

The nature of the placebo effect, in other words, undermines the assumption that placebo controls provide the ideally clean benchmark for testing a drug's effectiveness. A further complication is generated when we consider the possible *mechanism artifact* underlying the placebo effect (over and above subject and investigator artifacts). If, for example, placebo effectiveness is mediated by a patient's perception that his complaint is being addressed as a serious medical ailment, his response might be bolstered as a function of the vigorousness—even onerousness—of the treatment provided. This would validate the practitioner's impression that injections are more powerful placebos than pills. The very presence of iatrogenic pain and symptom-irrelevant side effects may enhance the placebo effect. Acting in accordance with this model mechanism of placebo, for example, Friedman used atropine to study against amitriptyline as an active placebo that mimics side effects like dryness of mouth.

In an effort to correct these factors, a number of stratagems have been proposed. Ross and Buckalew have argued that trials commonly need four cohorts, receiving active drug, placebo, smuggled drugs (active drugs administered without the cohort's knowledge), and no treatment whatsoever. More recently, Kirsh and Weixel, in a fascinating discussion of systematic, and somewhat paradoxical divergences between the responses of subjects to substances administered under a consented double-blind condition versus those given deceptively (i.e., having been told they will receive an active drug), have suggested that

> experimental designs that more closely
> mimic real life drug use should be used in
> testing drug effectiveness. Specifically, in
> order to elicit comparable expectancies for
> altered responding, experimental drugs and
> placebos should be administered with subjects in both conditions led to believe that
> they are receiving the active drug. Subjects'
> consent can be obtained following provision
> of the information that depending on group

assignment, they may or may not be receiving the experimental drug. After consent has been obtained, subjects are informed or misinformed about the group to which they have been assigned, and they are debriefed at the conclusion of data collection.

These approaches face obvious ethical drawbacks. The ethics of placebo-controlled research had been consensually resolved when understood as a practice based upon concealment rather than deception: Subjects were not *misinformed* regarding the activity of the drug they were taking, but rather, knowing that the study was one of drug versus placebo, agreed to remain ignorant of their cohort assignment. But these approaches, if adopted, would require that investigators ethically regress to reliance upon deception. Furthermore, these and similar approaches are likely to be self-defeating as a *practical* matter. By requiring additional "placeboid" cohorts to control for the multifarious functions of placebo, the original advantages of simplicity, speed, and economics attributed to placebo-controlled research are lost.

What concern underlies these gimmicks? I suggest that clinical researchers have been seduced by a scientistic paradigm of inquiry, inappropriately modeled upon physics, within which the experiment must be designed to eliminate perturbing factors. The exposition by the philosopher of science, Adolf Grünbaum, provides one clear example of this error. Grünbaum distinguishes between what he calls the characteristic factors of a drug, F, and its "incidental" characteristics, C, that may commonly or even universally accompany the drug but are nonetheless not essential to it or its action. (As an extreme example for the sake of clarity, Grünbaum says that although digoxin is always swallowed with water, the water is merely incidental to the drug.) Among those incidental characteristics of a drug are expectancy and the other sources of the placebo effect, and in Grünbaum's understanding of placebo research, "by subtracting the therapeutic gains [caused by expectancy from those caused by F, characteristic factors of the drug] . . . investigators can obtain the sought-after measure of the incremental remedial potency of the characteristic factors" in the treatment under study.

I think this conception of the purpose of placebo-controlled studies is widely shared by investigators, as when Dollery writes that "scientists who are interested in the *specific* properties of drugs must design their experiments to *minimize the effect of these extraneous factors* upon their conclusions." (Emphases added.) The stratagems discussed above evolved in the service of the view that sees clinical research as directed toward theoretical clarification of a drug's activity, rather than improvement of clinical practice; toward the generation of information about drugs, not treatment; toward understanding, rather than toward healing.

It is simple enough to see what is wrong with this view. The scientist is interested, to use Dollery's terms, in distinguishing specific properties from extraneous factors; but from the clinician's point of view, if these other factors are commonly or even universally present there is no point to distinguishing them. A theoretical physicist can deal in the abstract with isolated systems, hermetically sealed from perturbation; he may need to distinguish characteristic factors F from incidentals C. But a clinician's purposes are different. The clinician will treat the patient as the patient is found, in the messiness of life rather than the ordered world of the laboratory. Characteristic factors should not be analytically separated from incidentals for at least two reasons: the therapeutic intent behind clinical practice; and the synergism and reciprocal causation characteristic of biological systems. In other words, if F and C always come together, and have reciprocal rather than separate, additive interactions, their discrete activity is not even of notional importance to science in the service of healing, rather than of understanding.

Separate examples of these two reasons, therapeutic intent and reciprocal interaction, may be given. A biologist may have some interest, to take Grünbaum's example, in distinguishing the effects of digoxin, or inhaled beclomethasone, from the perturbing factor of the accompanying sip of water. The clinician is not [interested]; the speed with which digoxin without water will induce esophageal irritation, or beconase without water causes thrush, is quite beside the therapeutic point, provided the patient is instructed always to take the medicine with water.

An example of reciprocal causal interaction may be drawn from a study by Penick and Hinkle, testing phenmetrazine against placebo as an appetite suppressant. When subjects were provided these without being told that the investigators believe the drug will cause suppression of appetite, the effects of the two were indistinguishable. However, when this information was provided with both, phenmetrazine was significantly more effective than placebo in suppressing appetite. One plausible way of interpreting these results is that expectancy effects act synergistically with pharmacologic activity, suggesting that an analytic effort at separating the two is misguided.

For science in the service of healing rather than understanding, what is important is the compendious effect of a treatment as it will be applied, its net therapeutic advantage, as compared with alternatives. It is that clinical perspective that needs to be preserved in developing a methodical approach to placebo controls.

A CLINICAL APPROACH TO PLACEBO CONTROLS

What, then, is the proper role for placebo controls in clinical trials? An ethical controlled trial, apart from needing to be both valid and valuable, requires the satisfaction of two premises: First, that each arm of the trial is in clinical equipoise, i.e., there exists or there is in prospect a controversy among the community of expert clinicians concerning the relative therapeutic merits of each treatment within the trial—including placebo—if the study includes a placebo control. Second, the design of the trial must warrant confidence that its successful completion will show which of the competitors is superior, thereby *disturbing* this state of equipoise, and influencing clinical practice accordingly. Even when rejected, the treatment shown inferior will be relegated to a secondary status in practice, e.g., as a fallback drug for those not responding to (the newly established) "standard treatment."

Both requirements crucially depend upon a developed concept of the relative net therapeutic advantage associated with alternative treatments, a *portmanteau* measure including all the elements that contribute to the acceptance of a drug within clinical practice. And both requirements, as ethical premises, are grounded in the normative nature of clinical practice, the view that a patient is ethically entitled to expect treatment from his or her physician—an entitlement that cannot be sacrificed to scientific curiosity. This viewpoint involves the opposite of placebo bias, for now *deviations* from clinical practice must be the exception, requiring specific justification.

Apart from the very rare case in which a new treatment warrants the expectation of an overwhelmingly positive net therapeutic advantage (e.g., a promising new treatment for a heretofore lethal illness), it remains true, however, even from this perspective, that placebo controls are justified (and in fact necessary) in testing treatments falling within five broad classes of cases:

1. Conditions that have no standard therapy at all.

2. Conditions whose standard therapy has been shown to be no better than placebo.

3. Conditions whose standard treatment is placebo.

4. Conditions whose standard therapy has been called into question by new evidence warranting doubt concerning its presumed net therapeutic advantage.

5. Conditions whose validated optimal treatment is not made freely available to patients, because of cost constraints or otherwise.

The first two classes are self-explanatory. The third class, in a sense a subset of the second, accounts for the peculiar fact that accepted clinical practice for conditions like depression involve an initial trial of placebo that will be continued for as long as placebo remains effective. The fourth class involves those treatments that have fallen under suspicion because of previously unsuspected side effects, because of new information garnered about the disease process in question, or otherwise. An interesting subset of this class would occur when a reasonable concern arises that *all* of a drug's therapeutic benefit is a mechanism artifact, grounded in what were thought to be side effects of the drug in question. (Friedman may have thought amitriptyline *only* works because of expectancy enhanced by side effects.) In that case, it would be clinically reasonable to investigate and control for this mechanism artifact, on the grounds that there are safer ways of producing this effect. The active placebo would then have a favorable net therapeutic advantage. Still, this circumstance is rare. Much more common is the suspicion that *a portion* of the drug's effectiveness is artifactual in this way. But a biologist's artifact is a clinician's mechanism of action, and there is no reason to control for a mechanism artifact that is only partly (and quite possible synergistically) responsible for benefit.

The last class is likely to be the least familiar, yet its justification gets to the root of ethical considerations underlying clinical trials. Consider an unusually expensive, newly introduced treatment whose marginal relative effectiveness is beyond question, like erythropoietin (EPO) for the treatment of anemia associated with chronic hemodialysis. While relative effectiveness has been shown, a government insurer or other third-party payer will not fund this drug unless its absolute benefit is shown to surpass a given threshold. A drug company is interested in sponsoring a trial of EPO specifically for this purpose and will supply EPO (or identical matched placebo) to study participants. Is such a trial ethical? *Ex hypothesi*, within this scenario patients are not *entitled* to this drug, pending a positive outcome to the proposed trial. Withholding EPO from the placebo cohort therefore does not violate their right to treatment, and may consequently be ethically justified.

(A caveat: I believe the principle may only be applied when background conditions of justice prevail within the health care system in question. If, to the contrary, the health care system established no entitlement to even a minimal level of care, the principle must not be misappropriated on behalf of justifying placebo-controlled trials of standard antibiotics upon the poor, on grounds that the poor would not otherwise be entitled to receive this treatment.)

In brief, I have been arguing that placebo controls may ethically be employed when they contribute to practice what I have called science in the service of healing, and not otherwise. The common assumption that standard treatment controls are a poor second to placebos, the gold standard of clinical trials, should be questioned; and the grounding for this assumption—the desire to achieve a clean biological analysis of the specific effect of a drug, uncontaminated by patient, investigator, or mechanism artifacts—should be rejected.

The philosophy underlying this approach may be illustrated by a parable. A skilled, successful, and pious physician became troubled. He was uncertain whether his success was due to his skill or some other factor. He prays for his patients, and urges them to repent; perhaps his religious devotion is the cause of his success. Perhaps God is the cause of his patients' improvement; perhaps the Devil, urging him to complacency. He thought perhaps to resolve his worry by performing an experiment, for example, he would omit praying on behalf of one group of his patients; but then he feared this would be a sin, and endanger his patient's life. Troubled, he approached a rabbi with his doubts; and the rabbi told him not to worry over the cause of the physician's success. Quoting Paracelsus, the rabbi said, "It matters not whether it be God or the Devil, Angels or unclean Spirits cure him, so that he be eased." The doctor then responded, "But Rabbi, shall we trust this source?! Paracelsus was accused of heresy, even of magic and sorcery!" And the rabbi beamed and said, "Yes, that is exactly my point."

18 Placebo-Controlled Trials and Active-Control Trials in the Evaluation of New Treatments, Part 1

Ethical and Scientific Issues

Robert Temple and Susan S. Ellenberg

[...]

THE ETHICS OF PLACEBO CONTROLS

The Declaration of Helsinki

The Declaration of Helsinki is an international document that describes ethical principles for clinical investigation. Those who contend that placebo controls are unethical whenever known effective therapy exists for a condition usually cite the following sentence in the Declaration as support for that position: "In any medical study, every patient—including those of a control group, if any—should be assured of the best proven diagnostic and therapeutic method."

We believe that an interpretation of this sentence as barring placebo controls whenever an effective treatment exists is untenable. First, the requirement that all patients receive the "best proven diagnostic and therapeutic method" would bar not only placebo-controlled trials but also active-control and historically controlled trials. When effective treatment exists, the patient receiving the investigational treatment instead of the established therapy is clearly not getting the best proven treatment.

Second, it does not seem reasonable to consider as equivalent all failures to use known effective therapy. Historically, concerns about placebo use have usually arisen in the context of serious illness. There is universal agreement that use of placebo or otherwise untreated controls is almost always unethical when therapy shown to improve survival or decrease serious morbidity is available. But in cases in which the treatment does not affect the patient's long-term health, an ethical imperative to use existing therapy is not plausible. Can it be, for example, that because topical minoxidil or oral finasteride can grow hair, a placebo-controlled trial of a new remedy for baldness is unethical? Is it really unethical to use placebos in short-term studies of drugs for allergic rhinitis, insomnia, anxiety, dermatoses, heartburn, or headaches in fully informed patients? We do not believe that there is a reasonable basis for arguing that such studies and many other placebo-controlled studies of symptom relief are unethical and that an informed patient cannot properly be asked to participate in them.

Third, there is good reason to doubt that the cited phrase was intended to discourage placebo-controlled trials. The phrase under discussion was not part of the original 1964 Declaration but was added in 1975 to reinforce the idea that the physician-patient relationship "must be respected just as it would be in a purely therapeutic situation not involving research objectives." In the explanation accompanying the 1975 change, the issue of placebo-controlled trials was not even mentioned. The American Medical Association, the World Health Organization, and the Council for International Organizations of Medical Sciences have rejected the position that the Declaration uniformly bars placebo-controlled trials when proven therapy is available.

Informed Consent in Placebo-Controlled Trials

Patients asked to participate in a placebo-controlled trial must be informed of the existence of any effective therapy, must be able to explore the consequences of deferring such therapy with the investigator, and must provide fully informed consent. Concern about whether consent to participate in trials is as informed as we would like to believe is valid, but these concerns apply as much to the patient's decision to forgo known effective treatment and risk exposure to a potentially ineffective or even harmful new agent in an active-control trial as to a decision to accept possible persistence of symptoms in a placebo-controlled trial. Thus, this problem is not unique to placebo-controlled trials.

For the above reasons, we conclude that placebo-controlled trials may be ethically conducted even when effective therapy exists, as long as patients will not be harmed by participation and are fully informed about their alternatives. Although in many cases application of this standard will be fairly straightforward, in others it will not, and there may be debate about the consequences of deferring treatment.

Robert Temple and Susan S. Ellenberg, "Placebo-Controlled Trials and Active-Control Trials in the Evaluation of New Treatments, Part 1: Ethical and Scientific Issues," *Annals of Internal Medicine* 133 (2000): 455–63.

ASSESSMENT OF EFFECTIVENESS WITH ACTIVE-CONTROL TRIALS

Clinical trials that, because of deficiencies in study design or conduct, are unlikely to provide scientifically valid and clinically meaningful results raise their own ethical concerns. The remainder of this paper will address the inability of commonly proposed alternatives to placebo-controlled trials to evaluate the effectiveness of new treatments in many medical settings.

Active-Control Equivalence Trials (Noninferiority Trials)

The ability to conduct a placebo-controlled trial ethically in a given situation does not necessarily mean that placebo-controlled trials should be carried out when effective therapy exists. Patients and physicians might still prefer a trial in which every participant is given an active treatment. What remains to be examined is why placebo-controlled trials (or, more generally, trials intended to show an advantage of one treatment over another) are frequently needed to demonstrate the effectiveness of new treatments and often cannot be replaced by active-control trials showing that a new drug is equivalent or noninferior to a known effective agent. The limitations of active-control equivalence trials (ACETs) that are intended to show the effectiveness of a new drug have long been recognized and are well described but are perhaps not as widely appreciated as they should be. [...]

The Fundamental Problem: Need for Assay Sensitivity

There are two distinct ways to show that a new therapy is effective. One can show that the new therapy is superior to a control treatment, or one can show that the new therapy is equivalent to or not worse by some defined amount than a known effective treatment. Each method can be valid, but each requires entirely different inferential approaches. A well-designed study that shows superiority of a treatment to a control (placebo or active therapy) provides strong evidence of the effectiveness of the new treatment, limited only by the statistical uncertainty of the result. No information external to the trial is needed to support the conclusion of effectiveness. In contrast, a study that successfully shows "equivalence"—that is, little difference between a new drug and known active treatment—does not by itself demonstrate that the new treatment is effective. "Equivalence" could mean that the treatments were both effective in the study, but it could also mean that both treatments were ineffective in the study. To conclude from an ACET that a new treatment is effective on the basis of its similarity to the active control, one must make the critical (and untestable within the study) assumption that the active control had an effect in that particular study. In other words, one must assume that if a placebo group had been included, the placebo would have been inferior to the active control. Support for this assumption must come from sources external to the trial. Although it might appear reasonable to expect a known active agent to be superior to placebo in any given appropriately designed trial, experience has shown that this is not the case for many types of drugs.

The ability of a study to distinguish between active and inactive treatments is termed *assay sensitivity*. If assay sensitivity cannot be assumed, then even if the new and standard treatments appear virtually identical and the confidence interval for their comparison is exquisitely narrow, the study cannot demonstrate effectiveness of the new drug. (Note that in practice, ACETs are not designed simply to show lack of a statistically significant difference between treatments. Rather, such trials are designed to show noninferiority—that the new treatment is not inferior to the control by more than a specified margin. [...])

The best evidence that an active drug would have an effect superior to that of placebo in a given study would be a series of trials of similar design in which the active drug has reliably outperformed placebo. The ACET thus requires information external to the trial (the information about past placebo-controlled studies of the active control) to interpret the results. In this respect, an ACET is similar to a historically controlled trial. In some settings, such as highly responsive cancers, most infectious diseases, and some cardiovascular conditions, such external information is available and ACETs can and do provide a valid and reliable basis for evaluating new treatments. In many cases, however, the historically based assumption of assay sensitivity cannot be made; for many types of effective drugs, studies of apparently adequate size and design do not regularly distinguish drugs from placebo. More than 20 years ago, Lasagna described this difficulty particularly well (reflecting long recognition of the problem among analgesiologists):

> ... a comparison between new drug and standard ... is convincing only when the new remedy is superior to standard treatment. If it is inferior, or even indistinguishable from a standard remedy, the results are not readily interpretable. In the absence of placebo controls, one does not know if the "inferior" new medicine has any efficacy at all, and "equivalent" performance may reflect simply a patient population that cannot distinguish between two active treatments that differ considerably from each other, or between active drug and placebo. Certain clinical conditions, such as serious depressive states, are

notoriously difficult to evaluate because of the delay in drug effects and the high rate of spontaneous improvement, and even known remedies are not readily distinguished from placebo in controlled trials.

The problem is well recognized in studies of antidepressant drugs. In practice, many such studies include three arms—new drug, active control, and placebo—to provide clear evidence of effectiveness (new drug vs. placebo) and an internal standard (active control vs. placebo). This design allows a clear distinction (particularly valuable to a drug manufacturer) between a *drug* that does not work (the standard agent is superior to placebo but the new drug is not) and a *study* that does not work (neither the standard drug nor the new drug is superior to placebo). [...]

A recently published overview by Tramer and coworkers of studies of ondansetron, a widely used and very effective antiemetic, provides a further example of this phenomenon. Although the totality of data clearly supports the efficacy of this agent, many placebo-ondansetron comparisons show no effect of the drug. It is notable that the incidence of nausea and vomiting varied greatly among the trials and in some cases was so low that it precluded any demonstration of efficacy. In a placebo-controlled study of an antiemetic, a low rate of nausea and vomiting in the placebo group would lead to a negative outcome—the drug could not appear superior to placebo, and the trial could not provide evidence of effectiveness. In contrast, an ACET (new drug vs. ondansetron) with a low rate of nausea and vomiting in both arms would not be unambiguously interpretable. If one assumed that the low rate in the active-control group reflected the known ability of ondansetron to reduce a rate of nausea and vomiting that would have been high in the absence of treatment, one would conclude that the new drug was also effective. But the article by Tramer and coworkers shows that such an assumption cannot be supported in many situations. Clearly, if many placebo-controlled studies of ondansetron showed no effect, a trial showing "equivalence" of a new agent to ondansetron could not be considered reliable evidence that the new agent was effective, unless one could identify a treatment setting (for example, a setting defined by the chemotherapy administered) in which ondansetron was regularly distinguishable from placebo. [...]

STUDYING RELATIVE EFFECTIVENESS

In some cases, a study may be intended to evaluate the comparative effectiveness of two known active treatments. In that case, too, the presence of assay sensitivity is essential to interpretation of the trial. If one cannot be confident that the trial could have distinguished active drug from placebo, one cannot be confident that it could have distinguished a more effective drug from a less effective drug. A three-arm study (new drug, placebo, and active control) is optimal because it can (1) assess assay sensitivity and, if assay sensitivity is confirmed, (2) measure the effect of the new drug and (3) compare the effects of the two active treatments. [...]

REGULATORY STATUS OF STUDY DESIGNS

Critics of placebo-controlled trials have often attributed their use to FDA practices that favor the smallest possible trials, seek to assess absolute efficacy, and ignore what they consider the more important clinical questions of how a new drug compares with standard therapy. Although a broad range of trial designs can be used to demonstrate the effectiveness of a new drug, regulations describing adequate and well-controlled studies have since 1985 indicated concerns about the interpretation of ACETs, reflecting views expressed since the 1950s by numerous clinical and statistical researchers. Thus, where assay sensitivity cannot be established for an ACET, trials that show a difference between treatments (a placebo-controlled trial is only one such example) would be needed to demonstrate effectiveness. The basis for this requirement is not a preference for small trials (although efficiency is not a trivial matter) nor indifference to comparisons (although under law, a drug need not be superior to or even as good as other therapy to be approved), but rather the fundamental need for evidence of assay sensitivity to interpret an ACET as showing effectiveness of a new drug.

CONCLUSIONS

Placebo controls are clearly inappropriate for conditions in which delay or omission of available treatments would increase mortality or irreversible morbidity in the population to be studied. For conditions in which forgoing therapy imposes no important risk, however, the participation of patients in placebo-controlled trials seems appropriate and ethical, as long as patients are fully informed. Arguments to the contrary are not based on established ethical principles but rather rely on a literal reading of one passage in the Declaration of Helsinki that would also preclude the conduct of active-control trials, and even historically controlled trials, whenever effective treatment exists. It seems inconceivable that the authors of the 1975 revision intended such an outcome, and nothing in their explanation of the revision suggests they did. We therefore believe this interpretation is untenable.

If ACETs were always adequate substitutes for placebo-controlled trials, the ethical issue might not arise. Unfortunately, ACETs are often uninformative. They can neither demonstrate the effectiveness of a new agent nor provide a valid comparison to control therapy unless assay sensitivity can be assured, which often cannot be accomplished without inclusion of a concurrent placebo group. [...]

[Table and figure omitted—eds.]

19   The Ethics of Placebo-Controlled Trials

A Middle Ground

EZEKIEL J. EMANUEL AND FRANKLIN G. MILLER

The first placebo-controlled trial was probably conducted in 1931, when sanocrysin was compared with distilled water for the treatment of tuberculosis. Ever since then, placebo-controlled trials have been controversial, especially when patients randomly assigned to receive placebo have forgone effective treatments. Recently, the debate has become polarized. One view, dubbed "placebo orthodoxy" by its opponents, is that methodologic considerations make placebo-controlled trials necessary. The other view, which might be called "active-control orthodoxy," is that placebo orthodoxy sacrifices ethics and the rights and welfare of patients to presumed scientific rigor. The latest revision of the Declaration of Helsinki, although controversial, embraces the active-control orthodoxy. Both views discount the ethical and methodologic complexities of clinical research. In this essay, we argue that placebo-controlled trials are permissible when proven therapies exist, but only if certain ethical and methodologic criteria are met.

PLACEBO ORTHODOXY

Advocates of placebo-controlled studies argue that it is ethical to conduct such trials even in the case of medical conditions for which there are interventions known to be effective, because of the methodologic limitations of trials in which active treatment is used as the control. Sometimes therapies that are known to be effective are no better than placebo in particular trials because of variable responses to drugs in particular populations, unpredictable and small effects, and high rates of spontaneous improvement in patients. Consequently, without a placebo group to ensure validity, the finding that there is no difference between the investigational and standard treatments can be misleading or uninterpretable. New treatments that are no better than existing treatments may still be clinically valuable if they have fewer side effects or are more effective for particular subgroups of patients. However, no drug should be approved for use in patients unless it is clearly superior to placebo or no treatment. Despite the methodologic rigor of placebo-

controlled trials, commentators acknowledge that they are unethical in some circumstances, especially when withholding an effective treatment might be life-threatening or might cause serious morbidity.

There are serious problems with placebo orthodoxy. First, in our opinion, the criteria for ethical use of placebo controls are never precisely stated. In a recent review, for instance, Temple and Ellenberg claimed that the use of placebo controls is ethical if the research participants who receive placebo will experience "no permanent adverse consequence," if there is a risk of "only temporary discomforts," or if they "will not be harmed." We think that these formulations are not equivalent. Since patients may be harmed by temporary but reversible conditions, the criterion of no harm would exclude many placebo-controlled trials that meet the criterion of no permanent adverse consequence.

Second, the criteria permit intolerable suffering on the part of study participants. This point is illustrated by trials of the antinausea medication ondansetron. In 1981, research demonstrated clinically and statistically significant differences between metoclopramide and placebo for the treatment of vomiting induced by chemotherapy. In the early 1990s, placebo-controlled trials of ondansetron for chemotherapy-induced vomiting, some of which involved patients who had not previously received chemotherapy, were reported. These trials were unethical. Although vomiting induced by chemotherapy, especially with highly emetic drugs such as cisplatin, is not life-threatening and does not cause irreversible disability, it causes serious, avoidable harm that is more than mere discomfort. Indeed, the need for better antiemetic medication had been justified in the first place by the argument that "uncontrolled nausea and vomiting [from chemotherapy] frequently results in poor nutritional intake, metabolic derangements, deterioration of physical and mental condition, as well as the possible rejection of potentially beneficial treatment." Even in 1990, patients receiving the chemotherapeutic drugs evaluated in the ondansetron trials were routinely given antiemetic prophylaxis. Other trials conducted at the time used active controls.

Finally, the proponents of placebo controls seem to focus on physical harm. In arguing for placebo-controlled trials of antidepressants, Temple and Ellenberg suggest that the only relevant harm is depression-induced suicide.

Ezekiel J. Emanuel and Franklin G. Miller, "The Ethics of Placebo-Controlled Trials: A Middle Ground," *New England Journal of Medicine* 345 (2001): 915–19.

140   THE ETHICS OF CLINICAL TRIAL DESIGN

Psychological and social harms caused by depression—such as mental anguish, loss of employment, and disruption of relationships—are either not considered or dismissed. Yet psychological and social harms are invoked to justify the value of the research. This is contradictory. In evaluating the risk-benefit ratio, psychological and social harms must be addressed.

ACTIVE-CONTROL ORTHODOXY

Because of these problems, commentators have attacked placebo orthodoxy as unethical. Proponents of active controls contend that whenever an effective intervention for a condition exists, it must be used in the control group. Furthermore, they argue that placebo controls are inappropriate because the clinically relevant question is not whether a new drug is better than nothing but whether it is better than standard treatments. To justify this approach, they cite the Declaration of Helsinki, the most recent version of which states, "The benefits, risks, burdens, and effectiveness of a new method should be tested against those of the best current prophylactic, diagnostic, and therapeutic methods. This does not exclude the use of placebo, or no treatment, in studies where no proven prophylactic, diagnostic, and therapeutic methods exists." Advocates of active controls criticize placebo orthodoxy for placing the demands of science ahead of the rights and well-being of study participants.

Active-control orthodoxy also has several problems. First, the dichotomy between rigorous science and ethical protections is false. Scientific validity constitutes a fundamental ethical protection. Scientifically invalid research cannot be ethical no matter how favorable the risk-benefit ratio for study participants. If placebo controls are necessary or desirable for scientific reasons, that constitutes an ethical reason to use them, although it may not be a sufficient reason.

Second, in some cases, the harm and discomfort associated with the use of placebo controls are non-existent or are so small that there can be no reasonable ethical requirement for new treatments to be tested only against standard treatments. Who could persuasively argue that for trials involving conditions such as baldness or some types of headaches, it is unethical to withhold effective treatments from some study participants and give them placebo instead? There is no meaningful harm that stringent ethicists should worry about in letting a person who has given informed consent continue to suffer temporarily from a headache or untreated baldness as part of a clinical trial. Some critics of placebo controls contend that such trials are unethical because physicians owe medical care to patients who are seeking treatment for these ailments. This argument conflates clinical research with clinical care. Clinicians frequently do not treat such ailments and patients often forgo treatment, indicating that there can be no ethical necessity to provide it. The absolute prohibition against the use of placebo controls in every case in which an effective treatment exists is too broad; the magnitude of harm likely to be caused by using placebo must be part of the ethical consideration.

Third, opponents of placebo-controlled trials pay insufficient attention to the power of the placebo response. Substantial proportions of patients receiving placebo have measurable and clinically meaningful improvements—for example, 30 to 50 percent of patients with depression and 30 to 80 percent of those with chronic stable angina. A recent meta-analysis of randomized clinical trials with both placebo and no-treatment groups found little evidence of the therapeutic benefits of placebo over no treatment. However, the patients given no treatment received clinical attention that may have contributed to observed improvements. This clinical attention may account for the placebo effect. Placebo-controlled trials in which patients receive potentially therapeutic clinical attention test whether an investigational treatment is better than this attention, not whether it is better than nothing.

Most important, trials with active controls may expose more patients to harm than placebo-controlled trials. Equivalence trials, which evaluate the hypothesis that one drug is equivalent to another, typically require larger samples to achieve sufficient power, because the delta, or difference between the rates of response to the two drugs, is likely to be smaller than that between the rates of response to an investigational treatment and placebo. Consider an equivalence trial in which an investigational drug is compared with a standard drug that is known to have a 60 percent response rate. With a delta of 10 percent (if they were equivalent, the difference between the standard and investigational drugs would be less than 10 percent) and a one-sided statistical test to show equivalence, each group must contain 297 participants. Conversely, if a placebo is hypothesized to have a 30 percent response rate and the investigational drug a 60 percent response rate, then only 48 participants are needed in each group.

With the sample required for the equivalence trial—larger by a factor of six than the sample required for the placebo-controlled trial—many more subjects will be exposed to an investigational drug that may be ineffective or even more toxic than the standard drug. Moreover, if it turns out that the rate of response to the investigational drug is 53 percent—still within the 10 percent range for equivalence—more participants will actually be harmed by not receiving the standard treatment than if a placebo-controlled trial were conducted instead. That is, in an equivalence trial of an investigational drug with a response rate of 53 percent, there will be 21 more subjects without a response in the group of 297 receiving the investigational drug than in the group of 297 receiving the standard drug with a known response rate of 60 percent. Then, there will be 19 more subjects without a response in the group of 96 patients participating in the trial than if all 96 patients had received the standard drug. Indeed, the lower the rate of response to the investigational drug, the larger the number of participants in an equivalence trial who will be exposed to the harms associated with nonresponse. It is therefore simplistic to argue that placebo-controlled trials involving conditions for which the existing interventions are only partly effective necessarily sacrifice the well-being of patients.

A MIDDLE GROUND

For clinical research to be ethical, it must fulfill several universal requirements. Among other requirements, it must be scientifically valid and must minimize the risks to which the research participants are exposed. When these requirements conflict, advocates of placebo controls opt for maintaining scientific validity, whereas advocates of active controls opt for minimizing risks. We believe these absolute positions are neither tenable nor defensible.

There is a middle ground. First, both sides agree that certain placebo-controlled trials are clearly unethical. If effective, life-saving, or at least life-prolonging treatment is available, and if patients assigned to receive placebo would be substantially more likely to suffer serious harm than those assigned to receive the investigational drug, a placebo-controlled trial should be prohibited. The efficacy of streptokinase in reducing morbidity and mortality after myocardial infarction made it unethical to conduct placebo-controlled trials of tissue plasminogen activator.

Second, advocates of active controls should agree that for ailments that are not serious, if there is only a minimal chance that patients randomly assigned to receive placebo will suffer harm or even severe discomfort, the use of placebo controls is ethical. A placebo-controlled trial of a new treatment for allergic rhinitis would be ethical because the moderate discomfort associated with allergic rhinitis typically does not impair health or cause severe discomfort. Indeed, the risks associated with such trials are no greater than those deemed acceptable in natural-history and epidemiologic studies in which blood samples are obtained solely for research purposes and in pharmacokinetic studies in which medications are administered to healthy volunteers and blood samples obtained from them even though there is no prospect of a benefit to the study participants.

The disagreements center on whether it is ethical to use placebo controls when there is a treatment known to be effective and there is some potential for harm to participants receiving placebo. In this context, it is important to recognize that placebo-controlled trials and those in which active treatment is used as the control frequently have distinct objectives, and each type of trial may have a role in a sequential approach to evaluating new interventions. Whenever the risks of research with placebos are similar to the risks in these other types of studies, the use of placebo should be ethically justifiable. Placebo-controlled trials are often deemed important to determine the efficacy of a new treatment and to facilitate the design of larger trials in which the new treatment is compared with standard interventions. In addition, a trial comparing standard and new interventions may include a placebo group for internal validity when high placebo-response rates are anticipated. However, proponents of active controls deem even those initial efficacy and three-group trials unethical when effective standard therapies exist. Placebo-controlled trials of treatments for angina and depression have been the focus of this disagreement, as have short-term trials designed to establish the efficacy of new treatments for asthma and hypertension before large, randomized trials are conducted to compare the new intervention with standard therapies.

When effective treatments exist, there must be compelling methodologic reasons to conduct a placebo-controlled trial. Proving that a new treatment has sufficient efficacy before large-scale equivalence trials are conducted is such a reason, whereas conducting a scientifically valid study with a smaller sample is not. A placebo-controlled trial has a sound scientific rationale if the following criteria are met: there is a high placebo-response rate; the condition is typically characterized by a waxing-and-waning course, frequent spontaneous remissions, or both; and existing therapies are only partly effective or have very serious side effects; or the low frequency of the condition means that an equivalence trial would have to be so large that it would reasonably prevent adequate enrollment and completion of the study.

If these methodologic criteria are met, then the risk of using a placebo control should be evaluated according to several criteria. Research participants in the placebo group should not be substantially more likely than those in the active-treatment group to die; to have irreversible morbidity or disability or to suffer other harm; to suffer reversible but serious harm; or to experience severe discomfort. There is no way of removing qualifying words such as "serious" or "severe" from these criteria, since ethical evaluation necessarily calls for contextualized judgments. Just as courts are empowered to make contextualized judgments about the standard of a separation between church and state, federal regulations empower institutional review boards to determine the levels of risk and severity of harm associated with research.

Although placebo-controlled trials that meet these methodologic and ethical criteria may be justifiable even though the participants forgo therapies known to be effective, they remain worrisome because of the potential to cause suffering. Consequently, standard precautions must be scrupulously implemented for these trials. When such a trial is proposed, the institutional review board must ensure that the following safeguards are instituted to minimize harm: participants at increased risk of harm from nonresponse are excluded; the placebo period is limited to the minimum required for scientific validity; subjects will be carefully monitored, with inpatient observation when appropriate; rescue medications will be administered if serious symptoms develop; and there are explicit and specific criteria for the withdrawal of subjects who have adverse events. In addition, as part of the informed-consent process, the investigators must clearly disclose the rationale for using placebo, explain that subjects who are randomly assigned to the placebo group will not receive standard effective treatments, and state the risks associated with forgoing such treatments. The protocol should include provisions to ensure optimal treatment for participants who withdraw early or who remain symptomatic at the conclusion of the trial.

A CASE EXAMPLE

Chronic stable angina can cause substantial functional impairment and suffering. It is associated with a placebo-response rate of 30 to 80 percent. Patients with chronic stable angina typically have fluctuating courses with spontaneous remissions, and for some patients, current therapies are partly effective at best. The long history of positive findings from open trials of cardiovascular treatments that have subsequently been disproved by blinded, placebo-controlled trials—including ligation of the internal mammary artery for angina, chelation for claudication, encainide and flecainide for arrhythmias, and most recently, laser systems that create holes in cardiac tissue—provides good scientific reasons for conducing placebo-controlled trials of treatments for chronic angina.

Even if it is methodologically sound, a placebo-controlled trial of a new treatment for chronic angina should satisfy the ethical criteria for an acceptable level of risk—that is, participation in the trial would not cause death, irreversible disability, reversible but serious harm, or severe discomfort. There is no evidence that medical management of chronic angina prolongs survival. Furthermore, a comprehensive review of double-blind, placebo-controlled, randomized trials of treatment for chronic angina showed that the risk of adverse events did not differ significantly between the drug and placebo groups. The authors concluded that "withholding active treatment does not increase the risk of serious cardiac events." Nonetheless, patients at high risk for myocardial infarction and other cardiac events should be excluded from such trials, nitroglycerin should be provided for breakthrough anginal pain, and the period of treatment with placebo should be brief, usually less than 10 weeks. Patients should be contacted frequently to ensure careful monitoring of their condition, and those whose symptoms exceed an explicit threshold should be with-drawn from the trial. The informed-consent process must make it clear to patients that their angina may worsen and that they are free to withdraw from the trial at any time.

CONCLUSIONS

Placebo-controlled trials are caught in a battle between two orthodoxies. One is that placebo should be used as a control unless there is an increased risk of death or irreversible morbidity associated with its use. The other view is that if an effective therapy exists, the use of a placebo should be prohibited. These two positions are both absolute and indefensible. We propose a middle ground in which placebo-controlled trials are permitted but only when the methodologic reasons for their use are compelling, a strict ethical evaluation has made it clear that patients who receive placebo will not be subject to serious harm, and provisions have been made to minimize the risks associated with the receipt of placebo. This framework provides a basis for deliberation in difficult cases, with the recognition that reasonable people might make divergent judgments in a particular case.

Section Four

The Ethics of Phase I Research

20   On the Nature and Ethics of Phase I Clinical Trials of Cancer Chemotherapies

MORTIMER B. LIPSETT

Physicians and members of the public understand that each new drug must, at some point, be given to humans for the first time without confident knowledge of its effects and toxic potential. Although the ethics and constraints necessary for this testing have been discussed widely, there has been little attention given specifically to the first trials of new cancer chemotherapeutic agents (phase I trials). However, new cancer chemotherapeutic agents cannot be treated simply as new drugs; their toxic effects are often so much greater than those of other drugs that the clinical investigator must weigh many conflicting arguments to justify the trial. Referring physicians, in their role as advisors, are often called on to explain the trials and to counsel patients who may enter them. Thus, they should have full appreciation of the nature and ethics of such trials.

A phase I clinical trial in patients with cancer does not appear unexpectedly from the universe of possible trials. Rather, it is one decision point in a long trial of experimentation and testing. The decision network of the National Cancer Institute (NCI) examines each aspect of the chemistry, biochemistry, pharmacology, toxicity, and therapeutic potential of each new drug in animal systems before recommending the agent for clinical trial. Only one agent in the 1,000 to 2,000 that enter the screening procedure ever reaches the point of a phase I clinical trial, and the effort to reach this decision takes several years and some millions of dollars. As part of its mission, the NCI continually strives to shorten the process by using better animal models, *in vitro* testing systems, and computer simulations of drug action and kinetics; thus, there is an increasingly selective entry of new drugs. How extensive preclinical testing should be is a matter of judgment about which informed physicians and pharmacologists may disagree. It is

certain, however, that the decisions are never made casually but rather that they represent the consensus of experienced scientists and physicians.

It is important to state explicitly the purposes of phase I clinical trials. First, there is always therapeutic intent. The drugs entering phase I trials have been shown to cause tumor regression in *in vitro* systems and in at least one experimental animal tumor model. Second, a dosage scheme must be worked out, starting at low doses of the agent and gradually escalating the dose to reach either toxic levels or therapeutic effect. This study in pharmacology is essential, since drug disposition and elimination in any experimental animal may not predict these processes in man. Finally, the common toxic effects of the drug must be appreciated. These will be observed during the process of escalating the dose. The physician needs to know whether toxic reactions are predictable, tolerable, and reversible. Until the ideal chemotherapeutic drug appears (i.e., having high therapeutic efficacy and few toxic effects), it is necessary to give enough of any drug to find the maximum tolerated dose before concluding that the drug has been adequately tested. This process may include altering dosage schedules or ways of administering the drug.

The aims of the phase I trial define, in large part, the type of patient who is eligible for the trial. Thus, the patient must have extensive metastatic disease but must still have a reasonable life expectancy, since otherwise there would be no therapeutic potential and no opportunity to establish maximum tolerated dose and toxic effects. The patients must have exhausted all other therapeutic modalities that offered the possibility of success. The type of cancer need not be specified, since promising agents must be tried in patients with a wide variety of cancers. The history of chemotherapy is replete with examples of chemotherapeutic agents that were ineffective for some cancers but surprisingly effective in others. The success of cisplatin in the treatment of testicular cancer is such an example. It was not predictable from either theoretical considerations

Mortimer B. Lipsett, "On the Nature and Ethics of Phase I Clinical Trials of Cancer Chemotherapies," *JAMA* 248 (1982): 941–42.

or results of animal experiments; rather, it was first demonstrated in a clinical trial. There should be little controversy about these statements, although some critics of phase I trials have maintained that there is no therapeutic intent. This misstatement should be rebutted vigorously by the physician; an agent selected for a phase I trial is selected on the basis of its therapeutic potential.

The larger questions about the ethics of phase I clinical trials of cancer chemotherapies have not been discussed in depth. Two ethical problems are present: First, is this phase I trial an example of the sacrifice of the individual for the good of society? Second, do patients with far-advanced cancer constitute a vulnerable class of patients, and, as such, do they warrant special protection?

The dimensions of the first question are broad and have been discussed sporadically during the past two centuries and intensively since World War II. The question is philosophical in nature, and the answers are conditioned by the prevailing morals of society. It is clear that in certain circumstances we mandate individual sacrifice for the good of society. For example, the citizen drafted into the armed services may have to risk his life without prospect of immediate personal gain, although, even here, remote personal gain, such as preservation of home, family, and way of life, can be invoked.

Although this social contract has been generally accepted, as we move away from defense of the nation, considerations change. A foundation stone of our moral and legal framework is autonomy—the right to personal inviolability, control of one's person, and the exercise of free will in taking risks. The applicability of this concept to medical research has been reaffirmed on many occasions in law and moral precept since the promulgation of the Nuremberg Code. In medical research, the imperative for sacrifice is not present, nor is it part of the social contract today. One need only recall the horrors of medical experimentation during World War II to appreciate the brutal extension of the utilitarian philosophy of the sacrifice of the individual for a societal purpose.

The physician working with patients in phase I clinical trials follows the precepts of the Nuremberg Code and its successor, the Declaration of Helsinki, and the many subsequent modifications. The essentials of these codes are embodied in the regulations of the Department of Health and Human Services that prescribe a reasonable standard of behavior for physicians working in clinical investigation or using new drugs under the aegis of the Food and Drug Administration. At the beginning, each proposal must be reviewed by an institutional review board (IRB). These boards, composed of physicians, other members of the health care profession, and nonscientists, consider the research and "justify its decision that these risks are so outweighed by the sum of the benefit to the subject and the importance of knowledge to be gained as to warrant the Board's decision to *permit* the subject to accept the risks." In practice, this means that no single physician is entrusted with the responsibility of subjecting a patient involved in clinical research to an unacceptable risk.

The written consent document prepared for the patient must include an explanation of the study and a description of risks, benefits, and alternative therapies. However, a signed consent document is only one step in the process of obtaining informed consent. The conduct of this process must also meet the requirement that the autonomy of the patient be respected. In practice, this means that the patient and physician discuss the purpose and methods of the trial and its risks and benefits and that at the end the patient understands as completely as possible.

It may be helpful to know how these trials are actually presented to the patient. At the Clinical Center, the research hospital of the National Institutes of Health, [. . .] the patient is told that the chief purpose of the study is to find an effective dose of the drug. The expected toxic effects are discussed, and the hope of a favorable effect stated. Implicit in this explanation is the conviction of the physician that there is a chance of remission of disease. The patients, with advice from family or friends, evaluate risks and benefits and make their own decisions. The risks, including death, are often clear, but the benefits are frequently undefined. There is the benefit of hope, for "the miserable have no other medicine but only hope." There is the benefit of participation in a trial that could help others—a powerful incentive to some during the last months of life. There are also the very practical benefits of care and hospitalization, often with reduced financial demands on patient and family, that can be part of the participation in a phase I clinical trial. These last benefits may be potent inducements to participation in phase I clinical trials and can thereby make the patient more vulnerable to any importuning by the clinical investigator for participation in the research.

The President's Commission for the Study of Ethical Problems in Medicine and Biomedical and Behavioral Research developed and extended the concept of the vulnerable subject in medical research. Children, prisoners, and the mentally disabled were defined as vulnerable because a variety of constraints and inducements effectively removed their capacity to function autonomously. Similarly, patients with advanced cancer are faced with inducements that may sway their judgment of the risk-benefit ratio. Should such patients be treated as vulnerable research subjects necessitating extraordinary supervision by third parties?

Every patient entering any therapeutic trial is vulnerable to a certain extent by virtue of the disease and the "unique" opportunity to receive an agent that has the promise of being better than other available therapies. Another element that may constrain the exercise of free will and mature judgment is the aura that surrounds many academic referral centers where phase I trials are carried out. Vulnerability to constraints and inducements varies through a spectrum from the most severely compromised, such as children, prisoners, and the mentally disabled, to patients with relatively mild illnesses. Patients with far-advanced cancer fall between these extremes.

The morals of our society impel us to involve these patients in clinical research, since we are committed to the cure and amelioration of disease. However, we must find ways to ensure that vulnerable patients are protected and that they retain the rights of autonomy. This can be accomplished by painstaking consultation and preparation. In the case of patients with far-advanced cancer, the involvement of family or friends, the peer judgment inherent in the academic clinical research setting, and the judgment

of the IRBs are, in my view, generally sufficient safeguards for this class of vulnerable patients. However, each center that conducts phase I clinical trials should be prepared to use third-party consultation in the consent process when the investigator or the IRB has reason to believe that the situation of the clinical trial is such that there is greater vulnerability than normal.

Thus, we can conclude that phase I clinical trials of new cancer chemotherapies are ethical and necessary. They offer the patient benefits commensurate with risks. Clinical investigators must maintain their vigilance in carrying out the process of informed consent. When this is done honestly, sympathetically, and knowledgeably, the phase I clinical trial in cancer chemotherapy takes its place in medical research as an indispensable aspect of our quest for improving human life.

---

21   The Changing Landscape of Human Experimentation

Nuremberg, Helsinki, and Beyond

GEORGE J. ANNAS

[...A]lthough the concept of vulnerable populations has been recognized, there are no international research guidelines that provide special rules or protections for the terminally ill, and there are no specific rules for research on terminal illnesses such as cancer and AIDS. We have witnessed a general trend away from the Nuremberg Code toward considering the protection of *either* rights (consent) or welfare (prior peer review) sufficient for human subject protection. With regard to research on terminal illnesses such as AIDS and cancer in the developed countries, this usually means that the research will be seen as therapy, and patients (subjects) who have the disease will be expected to protect themselves through the mechanism of informed consent. In developing countries, on the other hand, research on AIDS may be characterized as "community-based," and prior ethical review seen as sufficient protection for the rights and welfare of community members. In both cases the primary justification for research on terminal illnesses is the same: desperation in the face of death.

RESEARCH ON DYING PATIENTS: AIDS AND CANCER

Perhaps the primary reason that existing national and international research guidelines have little practical relevance for individuals with terminal illnesses is that the terminal diagnosis itself determines both what researchers and physicians deem "reasonable," and what the subjects (patients) themselves find acceptable—even desirable. Many researchers themselves fear death, and believe that terminally ill patients really can't be hurt (they are "going to die anyway") and therefore have "nothing to lose." Prior peer review of protocols under such circumstances becomes pro forma and provides no meaningful protections for subjects. Likewise, terminally ill patients who are told that medicine has "nothing to offer" them have come to view experimental protocols as treatment. Therefore, instead of being suspicious of experimentation, patients may *demand* access to experimental interventions as their right. Under such circumstances informed consent alone provides no meaningful protection.

Psychiatrist Jay Katz has noted that when medicine seems impotent to fight the claims of nature, "all kinds of senseless interventions are tried in an unconscious effort to cure the incurable magically through a 'wonder drug,' a novel surgical procedure, or a penetrating psychological interpretation." Although physicians often justify such inter-

George J. Annas, "The Changing Landscape of Human Experimentation: Nuremberg, Helsinki, and Beyond," *Health Matrix* 2 (1992): 119–40.

ventions as simply being responsive to patient needs, "they may turn out to be a projection of their own needs onto patients." Similarly, transplant surgeon Francis Moore has observed of transplant experiments based on the "desperate remedies" rationale: "There must be some likelihood of success before the desperate remedy becomes more than a desperate search for an opportunity to try a new procedure awaiting trial." AIDS activist Rebecca Pringle Smith put it similarly, "Even if you have a supply of compliant martyrs, trials must have some ethical validity."

Susan Sontag has noted that cancer and AIDS have become linked as perhaps the two most feared ways to die in the developed world. In her words, "AIDS, like cancer, leads to a hard death. . . . The most terrifying illnesses are those perceived not just as lethal but as dehumanizing, literally so." And although philosopher Michel Foucault was not speaking of the medicalization of death by cancer and AIDS, he could have been when he chronicled how the power of government over life and death has shifted in the past two centuries. "Now it is over life, throughout its unfolding, that power establishes its domination; death is power's limit, the moment that escapes it. . . ." In human experimentation on the terminally ill we have Foucault's vision of public power played out in private: researchers take charge of the bodies of the dying in an attempt to take charge of the patients' lives and prevent their own personal deaths, and death itself.

The Nazi doctors' chief defense at Nuremberg was that experimentation was necessary to support the war effort. Now combating disease has itself become a "war," as we speak of a "war on cancer" and a "war on AIDS." And in that war, patients, especially terminally ill patients, are conscripted as soldiers. As [a] former editor of the *New England Journal of Medicine,* Franz Ingelfinger, put it: "[T]he thumb screws of coercion are most relentlessly applied" to "the most used and useful of all experimental subjects, the patient with disease." But as Sontag reminds us, war metaphors are dangerous in disease because they encourage authoritarianism, overmobilization, and stigmatization. In her words:

> No, it is not desirable for medicine, any more
> than for war, to be "total." Neither is the crisis
> created by AIDS a "total" anything. We are
> not being invaded. The body is not a battle-
> field. The ill are neither unavoidable casual-
> ties nor the enemy. We—medicine, society—
> are not authorized to fight back by any means
> whatever. . . .

Cancer

In the early 1980s the President's Commission for the Study of Ethical Problems in Medicine and [Biomedical and]

Behavioral Research attempted to get agreement on categorizing Phase 1 drug studies with anti-cancer agents. Are they research or therapy? Federal Food and Drug Administration (FDA) regulations state that Phase 1 studies are intended to have no therapeutic content, but are to determine "toxicity, metabolism, absorption, elimination, and other pharmacological action, preferred route of administration, and safe dosage range." Nonetheless, National Cancer Institute (NCI) researchers insisted that Phase 1 cancer studies, using cancer patients as subjects, should be described as therapeutic. The Assistant Secretary of the Department of Health and Human Services (DHHS) wrote to Congress in 1981:

> Notwithstanding the fact that some individu-
> als within HHS may not concur, the official
> position of the Department, including NCI,
> NIH, and FDA, is to regard Phase 1 trials of
> anti-cancer drugs as *potentially* therapeutic.
> The often small, but real possibility of benefit
> must be weighed against the nearly 100 per-
> cent probability of death if experimental
> therapy is not attempted for the advanced
> cancer patients who participate in Phase 1
> studies.

The President's Commission never received a better answer to its inquiry, and this answer is not helpful. In a sick person, virtually any intervention, even a placebo, can be described as "potentially therapeutic," and once this misleading label is applied, the nonbeneficial Phase 1 study is de facto eliminated and transformed into "experimental therapy." Any distinction between experimentation and therapy is lost. Under these circumstances the President's Commission could only bow weakly to informed consent: "It is important that patients who are asked to participate in tests of new anti-cancer drugs are not misled about the likelihood (or remoteness) of any therapeutic benefit they might derive from such participation."

American oncologists use so many approved drugs for unapproved uses that it seems fair to conclude that for most cancers there are no standard treatments, and sound scientific studies are needed. A 1990 survey, for example, found that fully one-third of all the drugs used on cancer patients are of unproven safety and efficacy for the purpose for which they are given; and unapproved use is even more prevalent for malignancies that have metastasized than for earlier cancers. Unapproved chemotherapy for patients being treated with palliative intent is twice the rate for curative intent, indicating an appropriately higher degree of risk-taking for quality of life enhancement. Oncologist Charles Moertel, commenting on the study, noted that the major beneficiaries of such an approach to cancer treatment are the "appointment book of the oncologist" and "the pharmaceutical companies and their stock-holders." In short, business ethics seem to be supplanting medical ethics. As to the argument that oncologists are just responding to the demand of dying patients, Moertel responded: "This argument abandons the scientific basis for medical practice and could just as well be used to justify quackery. Also, one wonders how many patients with advanced pancreatic cancer, for example, would really demand cytotoxic drugs if the sheer futility of such therapy was honestly explained."

If we accept patient demand as sufficient justification to mistreat them, it is a short step to say that the patient should have the right to demand to be killed by his physician. In fact, this very argument was made in early 1992 in the *New England Journal of Medicine,* where another oncologist noted that cancer chemotherapy, while it can prolong life, often makes the patient's dying "unbearable." He went on to argue that, "since we physicians brought the patient [subject] to the state she is in, we cannot abandon her by saying that euthanasia violates the purpose of our profession." The use of killing as "damage control" for a physician-created harm to patients is chilling. It is far better to avoid the harm than to use it to justify killing. The quest to master terminal illness may, however, make killing by physicians seem reasonable.

The "desperate remedies" rationale used to justify experimentation on the terminally ill is seriously flawed. There are fates worse than death, and many Americans have written living wills and health care proxies to *prevent* their lives from being prolonged under certain circumstances. Likewise, the horrible and prolonged deaths of Barney Clark and William Schroder on the permanent artificial heart insured the end of all further experiments with the Jarvik 7. Although the device can obviously prolong life, it cannot do so at an acceptable level of quality. The conclusion is clear: dying patients are real people, not objects, who value quality over quantity of life, and cannot be legally or ethically used simply as a means to an end. Individuals do have a right to refuse *any* treatment or experiment. But respecting patient autonomy does *not* require that we accept demands for mistreatment, experimentation, torture, or whatever the dying might want, anymore than we must accede to demands for illegal (but effective) drugs like heroin and LSD, unlicensed practitioners, or a physician-induced death.

Closely related to the difficulty of distinguishing research from treatment is distinguishing the role of the researcher from the role of the physician when these two conflicting roles are merged in one person. For example, in a 1992 article on cancer and AIDS research two prominent commentators seem to assume that "cancer researchers" are properly seen as doctors providing "treatment" to "patients." Little attention has been paid to the researcher's inherent conflict of interest. It is unlikely that patients can ever draw the distinction between physician and researcher, because most simply do not believe that their physician would either knowingly do something harmful to them, or would knowingly use them simply as a means for their own ends. Cancer researchers, however, know better. James F. Holland, for example, has said simply, "Patients have to be subsidiaries of the trial. . . . I'm not interested in holding patients' hands. I'm interested in curing cancer. . . . Every patient becomes a piece of scientific data." As candid as Holland is, it seems almost certain that his patients come to him for a cure, and look upon him as their physician—not as simply a researcher. In such a circumstance, the Helsinki Declaration's theoretical division between therapeutic and non-therapeutic research is meaningless.

Finally, we should emphasize that which has generally been marginalized: most studies on the terminally ill, including cancer and AIDS clinical trials, are funded by private drug companies that have tremendous financial stakes in their success. Clinical investigators may even "own equity interest in the company that produces the product or may serve as paid consultants and scientific advisers," roles that at least call their objectivity into question. Medical ethics is being eroded by a new commercialism in medicine. This fact has led most leading medical journals in the United States to require financial disclosure prior to publication of research results. However, neither IRBs nor individual subjects are routinely informed of the financial aspects of proposed clinical trials, even though the finances often create major potential conflicts of interest among the sponsor, the researcher, and the patient-subject.

One need not search far for examples. In early February, 1992, the stock of U.S. Bioscience lost $550 million in value in one day after the FDA review panel refused to recommend approval of its drug, Ethyl (a drug said to protect healthy cells from the toxic effects of cancer chemotherapy). One week later another United States biotechnology company lost half of its value in one day when a clinical trial of one of its cancer drugs was halted because of adverse effects on the subjects. Financing may be *the* major change in clinical trials over the past two decades, and this change has not been mirrored in research regulations. New research findings are often reported first on the financial pages of newspapers, and only later in the medical literature. It thus came as little surprise in March 1992, when Dow Corning openly declared that its decision to discontinue the manufacture of silicone breast implants was made strictly on "the basis of business." [. . .]

THE SPECIAL PROBLEMS OF TERMINALLY ILL RESEARCH SUBJECTS

Because the voluntary and understanding nature of consent of the terminally ill subject is compromised, and because this population is especially subject to exploitation by researchers who are often unrealistically optimistic in their expectations and believe their subjects cannot be harmed, adoption of the following additional safeguards is suggested. The primary goals of these safeguards should be to protect the quality of life of conscious patients, and to protect the unconscious from being used simply as objects for the end of others.

Proposed Regulations Governing Research on Terminally Ill Patients

1. For the purpose of these regulations a "terminally ill patient" is one whose death is reasonably expected to occur within six months even if currently accepted and available medical treatment is used.

2. In addition to all other legal and ethical requirements for the approval of a research protocol by national and local scientific and ethical review boards (including IRBs), research in which terminally ill patients participate as research subjects shall be approved only if the review board specifically finds that:

   (a) The research, if it carries any risk, has the intent and *reasonable probability* (based on scientific data) of improving the health or well-being of the subject, or of significantly increasing the subject's length of life without significantly decreasing its quality;

   (b) There is no *a priori* reason to believe that the research intervention will significantly decrease the subject's quality of life because of suffering, pain, or indignity attributable to the research; and,

   (c) Written informed consent will be required of all research participants over the age of sixteen in research involving any risk, and such consent may be solicited only by a physician acting as a *patient rights advocate* who is appointed by the review committee, is independent of the research, and whose duty it is to fully and objectively inform the potential subject of all reasonably foreseeable risks and benefits inherent in the research protocol. The patient rights advocate will also be empowered to monitor the actual research itself.

3. The vote on and basis for each of the findings in subpart 2 shall be set forth in writing by the review board, and be available to all potential subjects and the public.

4. All research protocols (including the financial arrangements between the sponsor and the researcher) involving terminally ill subjects shall be available to the public, and the meetings of the scientific and ethical review boards on these protocols shall be open to the public.

The major features of this proposal are worth emphasizing. The first is that so-called non-therapeutic research may not be performed on terminally ill patients at all unless there is no risk to the patient. Nor may "potentially," or "hopefully," or "possibly" therapeutic research be performed—the research must have "the intent and *reasonable probability* (based on scientific data) of improving the health or well-being of the subject. . . ." The fact that there is no treatment for the condition does *not* make any intervention "therapeutic" or even "probably" therapeutic. Phase 1 cancer drug research, for example, may not be performed on terminally ill subjects under these guidelines because there is no reasonable probability that it will benefit the subjects. Second, for subjects over the age of sixteen, only the subjects themselves are permitted to give consent for any research that involves any risk. Unless the condition is unique to children, no experimentation should be done on children until it has been demonstrated to meet the "reasonable probability" standard in adults. Proxy consent is acceptable only for *no* risk research (such as observation and monitoring studies, blood sampling, and research involving comatose patients). Third, the researcher is disqualified from obtaining the subject's consent. This task must be performed by an independent physician acting as a patient rights advocate, and whose primary obligation is to protect the rights and welfare of the potential research subject. Finally, the protocols, their financing, votes on them, and meetings concerning them, shall be open to the public.

These steps should help to protect both the rights and welfare of the terminally ill. Changes in codes and procedures alone, however, will not be sufficient to clarify societal goals for research and the practice of medicine, to define the meaning of progress, or to delineate the appropriate content of the practice of medicine. Resolving these central questions requires a recognition on the part of both society and medical practitioners that immortality is not a reasonable goal for medicine or humanity, that there are fates worse than death, and that quality of life is more important than quantity of life.

We can harm the terminally ill by treating them as objects with nothing to lose. They are our most vulnerable population, and need much more protection than they are currently afforded. It will take reality-based care for the dying, rather than fantasy-based experiments on the dying, to reclaim medicine's commitment in The Declaration of Geneva: "The health of my patient will be my first consideration."

Part IV

The Ethics of Research Participant Recruitment

Clinical research would not be possible without the willingness and generosity of those persons who serve as human participants. The search for knowledge useful to understanding and improving human health requires the study of humans and creates serious ethical quandaries. Regardless of the purpose or design of any specific project, those conducting research with human participants also always have responsibilities to the participants themselves. Since the purpose of clinical research is to generate useful knowledge and not necessarily to directly benefit participants though it does not preclude this, it is critical that participants be duly respected and protected from possible exploitation and harm in the conduct of research.

Fundamental to the avoidance of exploitation and to a demonstration of respect for research participants is focusing care and attention on the selection, recruitment, and enrollment of groups and individuals in research. Who should be included as participants in research? Are some individuals or groups more vulnerable to harm or exploitation than others? How should participants be recruited and enrolled?

Historical examples abound of studies in which participants were selected because they were convenient or were compromised in some way.[1] As articulated in the Belmont Report and in the U.S. federal regulations governing research with human participants (45 CFR 46)—both included in Part II of this volume—those who carry out research should be committed to a notion of justice that requires fairness in the selection of participants for research and in the distribution of the benefits and burdens of research.

People should be selected for participation in research in order to ensure good science, while at the same time ensuring that the burdens and potential benefits of research participation are equitably distributed. Therefore, after identifying those best able to answer the clinical research question, an account must be taken of how the particular benefits and bur-

dens of a research study will affect the proposed participants. There is great variation in the possibility of therapeutic benefit offered to individuals through research participation; some studies, such as Phase I drug studies with healthy volunteers, offer no direct benefit at all. The range of possible risks and the vulnerability of individuals or groups to risk vary considerably. It is ethically justifiable to exclude those at greater risk of injury. For example, if headaches and renal toxicity are among the potential risks of a particular investigational drug, those with a history of renal insufficiency or migraine headaches may be more vulnerable to these risks than others without such a history and may be excluded. After careful consideration of the scientific question, along with the risks and potential benefits that the particular study poses, participants are identified, recruited, and enrolled according to appropriate eligibility criteria.

Ethical strategies for recruitment should take into account various influences on individuals' ability to understand the research protocol, as well as their willingness to participate, and the appropriate measures should be employed to protect against "undue influence." The writings in Part IV address the complex issues of who should be invited to participate in research and how one should think about the equitable distribution of research burdens and potential benefits, and they discuss one form of potentially undue influence on research participation, namely, the payment of participants.

SECTION ONE. JUSTIFICATIONS FOR THE RECRUITMENT OF RESEARCH PARTICIPANTS

Hans Jonas considers possible philosophical justifications for participant recruitment. Jonas claims that exploitation in research is a problem not so much because we use people as means, as this happens all the time in the social context, but rather because research makes the person involved a passive thing—as he puts it, "a mere token, a sample merely to be acted upon." Securing someone's consent to participate in research, however, does not alone alleviate this problem. According to Jonas, medical progress through clinical research is an optional social goal, thus neither part of the social contract nor necessary for society's survival. Put differently, human experimentation is an "extraordinary" means of serving the common good. As such, it lies between the extremes of a collective emergency, such as war, in which the sacrifice of individual rights may be required, and the normal transactions of the social contract, in which individual interests are balanced with those of others and of society more generally.

According to Jonas, the enrollment of participants in research is similar to conscription. Since consent, although required, does not adequately resolve the ethical problems involved, how one solicits participation and enrolls participants is critical. He argues that participants should first be sought from among the most highly motivated, most educated, and least captive members of the community, such as researchers themselves and other members of the scientific community. Members of such groups have the highest degree of personal or professional identification with the research project and, he thinks, the greatest comprehension and freedom of choice. Such persons are at the top of what Jonas calls a "descending order of permissibility"; enrollment of others in a research study should be done with increasing hesitation as one goes down the list.

Jonas also recognizes that a crucial part of the justification for enrolling participants is a "worthy" research objective; therefore, a prime duty of the research community is to ensure that "this sacred source [participants] is never abused for frivolous ends." As Jonas puts it: "For a less than adequate cause, not even the freest, unsolicited offer should be accepted." Because *patients* can often be vulnerable, Jonas argues for the application of the same "descending order of permissibility" to the selection of patients as research participants; that is, those with the most motivation, information, and absence of external pressures should be asked to participate first.

David Heyd explores three possible answers to the question "Why should one take part in medical experimentation?" He considers and rejects answers based on rational choice or prudence because the best choice for an individual—that is, the choice with the most "therapeutic" benefit or value to him or her—is most often *individualized* care provided through a personal physician rather than participation in research. Heyd then considers and rejects the view based on a notion of justice or a social contract, that one has an obligation to participate in research. The social justice view contends that because one is, or may soon be, a beneficiary of past medical research, one thereby incurs an obligation to pay one's fair share for that research. Because medical research is often an intergenerational enterprise and, as Heyd argues, there can be no coherent intergenerational social contract, the use of social contract views to ground an obligation to participate in medical research fails. He concludes that participation in research is best thought of as an act of supererogation, or "Good Samaritanism." In participating in research, Heyd believes one is going beyond the call of duty. In doing so, research participants thereby demonstrate their virtue, nobility of character, and solidarity with humanity. The fact that research participants are "supererogatory volunteers" implies that researchers and physicians incur heavy responsibilities not to violate their trust.

SECTION TWO. ACCESS TO RESEARCH

Infamous examples of research gone awry, many of which are described in Part I, led to the characterization of medical research as a "risky" enterprise and to an emphasis on the protection of vulnerable persons from the burdens of research. The 1980s, at least partially due to the vocal activism of advocates for those with acquired immune deficiency syndrome (AIDS) and breast cancer, witnessed a shift in attitudes about research participation.[2] Rather than viewing research as a burden from which people should be protected, many began to clamor for access to clinical research and to experimental drugs. Some saw participation in research not only as beneficial, but as *essential* to their medical care and their chances for survival. There emerged more of an emphasis on the equitable distribution of the potential benefits rather than the burdens of participation in research.[3] Exclusion of certain groups, originally intended to protect the vulnerable, was decried as an injustice.[4] This was not only because exclusion denied individual participants access to the potential benefits of participation, but because it often denied entire groups of people, such as women,[5] access to the benefits of research results that could be safely applied in clinical practice.

Rebecca Dresser discusses the ubiquitous exclusion of women from medical research. Dresser's claim is that because most medical research has been carried out on men, especially white men, the research results thereby generated cannot rightly inform the clinical care of women or minorities. Biological and treatment response differences may well make it inappropriate to generalize research findings from one racial, ethnic, or gender group to another. Dresser finds that the justifications given for this "ethical blindspot" are inadequate. As she argues, those who claim a need for simple and clean data are simply assuming that the "model human" is the white male. Moreover, arguments for the exclusion of women based on the need to protect fetuses or potential fetuses must be counterbalanced against the harms of denying women the potential benefits of research participation. Dresser recommends that institutional review boards (IRBs) consider far more carefully the proposed composition of study cohorts to ensure that they are representative of affected populations. As a result of critiques such as Dresser's, inclusion of women and minorities is currently a requirement for all studies funded by the National Institutes of Health (NIH).[6]

Charles Weijer and Robert A. Crouch critically examine the scientific and ethical bases for the recent NIH guidelines regarding the inclusion of women and minorities in clinical research. They argue for the inclusion of women and minorities in clinical research based upon Freedman's concept of clinical equipoise. Given that there is a legitimate scientific justification for research that produces generalizable data, they argue that a proper understanding of clinical equipoise—the idea that trials should be designed such that there is a reasonable probability that disputes within the medical community will be resolved upon completion of the study—implies that adequate numbers of women, as well as members of minority groups and other biologically important subgroups, should be included in clinical research. Without adequate inclusion, they argue, the community of medical practitioners will remain unconvinced as to the comparative merits of, say, two interventions in a specific population of persons who suffer from the condition in question.

Charles Weijer and Abraham Fuks look at the other side of the coin, namely, the duty to exclude certain research participants. They argue that clinical investigators have a duty to screen for, and exclude, potential research participants who may be unduly vul-

nerable to the risks of a particular trial. This requires careful attention to the determination of and adherence to eligibility criteria that are chosen for both scientific and ethical reasons. In addition, Weijer and Fuks argue that there is a need for "clinical judgment ... the necessary lens through which eligibility criteria are viewed, because no set of eligibility criteria alone can protect people from harm." They claim that the obligation of researchers to minimize risks in research includes the moral and legal obligation to screen and exclude those who are unduly vulnerable, as well as to create special measures to ensure the safety of vulnerable individuals in the "unusual circumstance" of their inclusion. Since, as in the case of informed consent, the function of screening and excluding the vulnerable is separable from the duty to do so, Weijer and Fuks suggest that this function may be delegated and recommend that investigators be asked to sign a statement to attest to the fulfillment of this duty.

SECTION THREE. PAYMENT TO RESEARCH PARTICIPANTS

Once participants are identified and appropriate inclusion and exclusion criteria are specified, strategies are put into place to recruit and enroll participants in the research. One controversial strategy for facilitating recruitment is the offer of payment or other incentives for research participation. Although payment may serve as a straightforward reimbursement for expenses or as compensation for the time and effort of those who participate, money may also serve as an incentive. The extent to which money is an acceptable incentive, and under what circumstances it might be an undue incentive, have been the subject of some debate.[7]

Neal Dickert and Christine Grady recognize the prevalence of paying people for their research participation and describe three models for such payment: a market model, a wage payment model, and a reimbursement model. They argue that the wage payment model is the most ethically appropriate because it recognizes the contribution that participants make while minimizing the potential for undue inducement and the possibility of competition between studies. They suggest that this model applies to both patients and healthy participants alike, and may possibly serve to reduce the "therapeutic misconception" that makes patient-participants particularly vulnerable.

Trudo Lemmens and Carl Elliott argue that research studies with healthy volunteers are best understood as a kind of labor relation. They claim that we should be more worried about exploitation of healthy participants by not offering fair compensation than about undue inducement by offering too much. They suggest that current regulations and guidelines, as well as arguments by bioethicists about paying participants, actually increase the possibility of exploiting healthy participants by denying them a fair wage and the legal resources available to others in high-risk jobs. However, Lemmens and Elliott make a distinction between healthy volunteers and patients, and argue that because patients are more vulnerable than healthy volunteers, "importing commercial considerations" by paying patient-participants would only increase the risk of exploitation.

Conversely, Paul McNeill argues that *neither* patients nor healthy volunteers should be paid for research participation. In his view, participation in research is unlike other types of work because work-related risks are usually predictable and small, whereas research exposes people to risks of harm, some of which are unknown in advance. McNeill agrees with Hans Jonas that medical progress is optional, meaning that the results of research are not necessary to society in the same way that other work may be. Because risks in research cannot be eliminated, participants should not be induced by money to disregard or downplay these risks. Furthermore, since payment is likely to increase "the inequity of research conducted on the impecunious for the benefit of the well off," he concludes that payment should be prohibited, although reimbursement for expenses may be ethically permitted.

1. Jonathan D. Moreno, "Convenient and Captive Populations," in *Beyond Consent*, ed. Jeffrey P. Kahn, Anna C. Mastroianni, and Jeremy Sugarman (New York: Oxford University Press, 1998), 111–30 (included in Part VI, Section Three, of this volume); Susan E. Lederer, *Subjected to Science: Human Experimentation in America before the Second World War* (Baltimore: Johns Hopkins University Press, 1995).

2. Rebecca Dresser, *When Science Offers Salvation* (New York: Oxford University Press, 2001); Steven Epstein, *Impure Science* (Berkeley: University of California Press, 1996); Barron H. Lerner, *The Breast Cancer Wars* (New York: Oxford University Press, 2002).

3. Charles Weijer, "Evolving Ethical Issues in the Selection of Subjects for Clinical Research," *Cambridge Quarterly of Healthcare Ethics* 6 (1996): 334–45.

4. Carol Levine, "Has AIDS Changed the Ethics of Human Subjects Research?" *Journal of Law, Medicine, and Health Care* 16 (1988): 167–73; Carol Levine, Nancy Neveloff Dubler, and Robert J. Levine, "Building a New Consensus: Ethical Principles and Policies for Clinical Research on HIV/AIDS," *IRB: A Review of Human Subjects Research* 13, nos. 1–2 (1991): 1–17; Harold Edgar and David J. Rothman, "New Rules for New Drugs: The Challenge of AIDS to the Regulatory Process," *Milbank Quarterly* 68, Suppl. 1 (1990): 111–42.

5. Vanessa Merton, "The Exclusion of Pregnant, Pregnable, and Once-Pregnant People (a.k.a. Women) from Biomedical Research," *American Journal of Law & Medicine* 19 (1993): 369–451.

6. NIH Guidelines on the Inclusion of Women and Minorities as Subjects in Clinical Research (1994, updated 2001), available online at grants1.nih.gov/grants/funding/women_min/guidelines_amended_10_2001.htm.

7. *American Journal of Bioethics* 1, no. 2 (Spring 2001).

Section One

Justifications for the Recruitment of Research Participants

---

22   Philosophical Reflections on Experimenting with Human Subjects

HANS JONAS

[...]

I. THE PECULIARITY OF HUMAN EXPERIMENTATION

Experimentation was originally sanctioned by natural science. There it is performed on inanimate objects, and this raises no moral problems. But as soon as animate, feeling beings become the subjects of experiment, as they do in the life sciences and especially in medical research, this innocence of the search for knowledge is lost and questions of conscience arise. [...] One profound difference between the human experiment and the physical [...] is this: The physical experiment employs small-scale, artificially devised substitutes for that about which knowledge is to be obtained, and the experimenter extrapolates from these models and simulated conditions to nature at large. Something deputizes for the "real thing"—balls rolling down an inclined plane for sun and planets, electric discharges from a condenser for real lightning, and so on. For the most part, no such substitution is possible in the biological sphere. We must operate on the original itself, the real thing in the fullest sense, and perhaps affect it irreversibly. [...] Up to a point, animals may fulfill the proxy role of the classical physical experiment. But in the end man himself must furnish knowledge about himself, and the comfortable separation of noncommittal experiment and definitive action vanishes. [...] Human experimentation for whatever purpose is always *also* a responsible, nonexperimental definitive dealing with the subject himself. And not even the noblest purpose abrogates the obligations this involves.

This is the root of the problem with which we are faced:

Hans Jonas, "Philosophical Reflections on Experimenting with Human Subjects," *Dædalus* 98 (1969): 219–47.

Can both that purpose and this obligation be satisfied? If not, what would be a just compromise? [...] On principle, it is felt, human beings *ought not* to be dealt with in that way (the "guinea pig" protest); on the other hand, such dealings are increasingly urged on us by considerations, in turn appealing to principle, that claim to override those objections. [...] We must justify the infringement of a primary inviolability, which needs no justification itself; and the justification of its infringement must be by values and needs of a dignity commensurate with those to be sacrificed.

Before going any further, we should give some more articulate voice to the resistance we feel against a merely utilitarian view of the matter. It has to do with a peculiarity of human experimentation quite independent of the question of possible injury to the subject. What is wrong with making a person an experimental subject is not so much that we make him thereby a means (which happens in social contexts of all kinds), as that we make him a thing—a passive thing merely to be acted on [...].

These compensations of personhood are denied to the subject of experimentation, who is acted upon for an extraneous end without being engaged in a real relation where he would be the counterpoint to the other or to circumstance. Mere "consent" (mostly amounting to no more than permission) does not right this reification. Only genuine authenticity of volunteering can possibly redeem the condition of "thinghood" to which the subject submits. [...]

II. "INDIVIDUAL VERSUS SOCIETY" AS THE CONCEPTUAL FRAMEWORK

The setting for the conflict most consistently invoked in the literature is the polarity of individual versus society—the possible tension between the individual good and the common good, between private and public welfare. [...] In terms of rights, we let some of the basic rights of the individual be overruled by the acknowledged rights of society—as a matter of right and moral justness and not of mere force or dire necessity (much as such necessity may be adduced in defense of that right). But in making that concession, we require a careful clarification of what the needs, interests, and rights of society are, for society—as distinct from any plurality of individuals—is an abstract and, as such, is subject to our definition, while the individual is the primary concrete, prior to all definition, and his basic good is more or less known. Thus the unknown in our problem is the so-called common or public good and its potentially superior claims, to which the individual good must or might sometimes be sacrificed, in circumstances that in turn must also be counted among the unknowns of our question. [...]

"Consent," however, is the other most consistently emphasized and examined concept in discussions of this issue. This attention betrays a feeling that the "social" angle is not fully satisfactory. If society has a right, its exercise is not contingent on volunteering. On the other hand, if volunteering is fully genuine, no public right to the volunteered act need be construed. [...] But the awareness of the many ambiguities besetting the "consent" actually available and used in medical research prompts recourse to the idea of a public right conceived independently of (and valid prior to) consent; and, vice versa, the awareness of the problematic nature of such a right makes even its advocates still insist on the idea of consent with all its ambiguities: an uneasy situation either way.

Nor does it help much to replace the language of "rights" by that of "interests" and then argue the sheer cumulative weight of the interests of the many over against those of the few or the single individual. "Interests" range all the way from the most marginal and optional to the most vital and imperative, and only those sanctioned by particular importance and merit will be admitted to count in such a calculus—which simply brings us back to the question of right or moral claim. Moreover, the appeal to numbers is dangerous. Is the number of those afflicted with a particular disease great enough to warrant violating the interests of the non-afflicted? Since the number of the latter is usually so much greater, the argument can actually turn around to the contention that the cumulative weight of interest is on *their* side. [...]

III. THE SACRIFICIAL THEME

Yet we must face the somber truth that the *ultima ratio* of communal life is and has always been the compulsory, vicarious sacrifice of individual lives. [...] One of the fellowship of men had to die so that all could live, the earth be fertile, the cycle of nature renewed. [...]

But in moments of national danger we still send the flower of our young manhood to offer their lives for the continued life of the community, and if it is a just war, we see them go forth as consecrated and strangely ennobled by a sacrificial role. Nor do we make their going forth depend on their own will and consent, much as we may desire and foster these. We conscript them according to law. We conscript the best and feel morally disturbed if the draft, either by design or in effect, works so that mainly the disadvantaged, socially less useful, more expendable, make up those whose lives are to buy ours. No rational persuasion of the pragmatic necessity here at work can do away with the feeling, a mixture of gratitude and guilt, that the sphere of the sacred is touched with the vicarious offering of life for life. [...] But a troubled conscience compels us, the undeserving beneficiaries, to ask: Who is to be martyred? In the service of what cause and by whose choice?

Not for a moment do I wish to suggest that medical experimentation on human subjects, sick or healthy, is to be likened to primeval human sacrifices. Yet something sacrificial is involved in the selective abrogation of personal inviolability and the ritualized exposure to gratuitous risk of health and life, justified by a presumed greater, social good. [...]

IV. THE "SOCIAL CONTRACT" THEME

[...T]he "social contract," [...] premised on the primacy of the individual, was designed to supply a rationale for the *limitation* of individual freedom and power required for the existence of the body politic, whose existence in turn is for the benefit of the individuals. The principle of these limitations is that their *general* observance profits all, and that therefore the individual observer, assuring this general observance for his part, profits by it himself. I observe property rights because their general observance assures my own; I observe traffic rules because their general observance assures my own safety; and so on. The obligations here are mutual and general; no one is singled out for special sacrifice. Moreover, for the most part, *qua* limitations of my liberty, the laws thus deducible from the hypothetical "social contract" enjoin me from certain actions rather than obligate me to positive actions (as did the laws of feudal society). Even where the latter is the case, as in the duty to pay taxes, the rationale is that I am myself a beneficiary of the services financed through these payments. [. . .] Thus, by some stretch, such contributions can still be subsumed under the principle of enlightened self-interest. But no complete abrogation of self-interest at any time is in the terms of the social contract, and so pure sacrifice falls outside it. Under the putative terms of the contract alone, I cannot be required to die for the public good. [...]

But in time of war our society itself supersedes the nice balance of the social contract with an almost absolute precedence of public necessities over individual rights. In this and similar emergencies, the sacrosanctity of the individual is abrogated, and what for all practical purposes amounts to a near-totalitarian, quasi-communist state of affairs is *temporarily* permitted to prevail. In such situations, the community is conceded the right to make calls on its members, or certain of its members, entirely different in magnitude and kind from the calls normally allowed. It is deemed right that a part of the population bears a disproportionate burden of risk of a disproportionate gravity; and it is deemed right that the rest of the community accepts this sacrifice, whether voluntary or enforced, and reaps its benefits—difficult as we find it to justify this acceptance and this benefit by any normal ethical categories. We justify it transethically, as it were, by the supreme collective emergency, formalized, for example, by the declaration of a state of war.

Medical experimentation on human subjects falls somewhere between this overpowering case and the normal transactions of the social contract. On the one hand, no comparable extreme issue of social survival is (by and large) at stake. And no comparable extreme sacrifice or foreseeable risk is (by and large) asked. On the other hand, what is asked goes decidedly beyond, even runs counter to, what it is otherwise deemed fair to let the individual sign over of his person to the benefit of the "common good." Indeed, our sensitivity to the kind of intrusion and use involved is such that only an end of transcendent value or overriding urgency can make it arguable and possibly acceptable in our eyes.

V. HEALTH AS A PUBLIC GOOD

The cause invoked is health and, in its more critical aspect, life itself—clearly superlative goods that the physician serves directly by curing and the researcher indirectly by the knowledge gained through his experiments. There is no question about the good served nor about the evil fought—disease and premature death. But a good to whom and an evil to whom? Here the issue tends to become somewhat clouded. In the attempt to give experimentation the proper dignity (on the problematic view that a value becomes greater by being "social" instead of merely individual), the health in question or the disease in question is somehow predicated on the social whole, as if it were society that, in the persons of its members, enjoyed the one and suffered the other. [...]

VI. WHAT SOCIETY CAN AFFORD

[...] What is it that *society* can or cannot afford—leaving aside for the moment the question of what it has a *right* to? It surely can afford to lose members through death; more than that, it is built on the balance of death and birth decreed by the order of life. [...] The specific question seems to be whether society can afford to let some people die

whose death might be deferred by particular means if these were authorized by society. [...] If cancer, heart disease, and other organic, non-contagious ills, especially those tending to strike the old more than the young, continue to exact their toll at the normal rate of incidence (including the toll of private anguish and misery), society can go on flourishing in every way.

Here, by contrast, are some examples of what, in sober truth, society cannot afford. It cannot afford to let an epidemic rage unchecked; a persistent excess of deaths over births, but neither—we must add—too great an excess of births over deaths; too low an average life expectancy even if demographically balanced by fertility, but neither too great a longevity with the necessitated correlative dearth of youth in the social body; a debilitating state of general health; and things of this kind. These are plain cases where the whole condition of society is critically affected, and the public interest can make its imperative claims. [...]

[...] Society, in a subtler sense, cannot "afford" a single miscarriage of justice, a single inequity in the dispensation of its laws, the violation of the rights of even the tiniest minority, because these undermine the moral basis on which society's existence rests. Nor can it, for a similar reason, afford the absence or atrophy in its midst of compassion and of the effort to alleviate suffering [...] one form of which is the effort to conquer disease. [...] And in short, society cannot afford the absence among its members of *virtue* with its readiness for sacrifice beyond defined duty [...] it must protect this most precious capital from abuse.

For what objectives connected with the medico-biological sphere should this reserve be drawn upon—for example, in the form of accepting, soliciting, perhaps even imposing the submission of human subjects to experimentation? We postulate that this must be not just a worthy cause, [...] but a cause qualifying for transcendent social sanction. Here one thinks first of those cases critically affecting the whole condition, present and future, of the community we have illustrated. Something equivalent to what in the political sphere is called "clear and present danger" may be invoked and a state of emergency proclaimed, thereby suspending certain otherwise inviolable prohibitions and taboos. We may observe that averting a disaster always carries greater weight than promoting a good. Extraordinary danger excuses extraordinary means. This covers human experimentation, which we would like to count, as far as possible, among the extraordinary rather than the ordinary means of serving the common good under public auspices. [...]

VII. SOCIETY AND THE CAUSE OF PROGRESS

Much weaker is the case where it is a matter not of saving but of improving society. Much of medical research falls into this category. As stated before, a permanent death rate from heart failure or cancer does not threaten society. So long as certain statistical ratios are maintained, the incidence of disease and of disease-induced mortality is not (in the strict sense) a "social" misfortune. I hasten to add that it is not therefore less of a human misfortune, . . . [b]ut it is misleading to equate the fundamentally human response to it with what is owed to society: it is owed by man to man—and is thereby owed by society to the individuals as soon as the adequate ministering to these concerns outgrows (as it progressively does) the scope of private spontaneity and is made a public mandate. It is thus that society assumes responsibility for medical care, research, old age, and innumerable other things not originally of the public realm (in the original "social contract"), and they become duties toward "society" (rather than directly toward one's fellow man) by the fact that they are socially operated.

Indeed, we expect from organized society no longer mere protection against harm and the securing of the conditions of our preservation, but active and constant improvement in all the domains of life: the waging of the battle against nature, the enhancement of the human estate—in short, the promotion of progress. This is an expansive goal, one far surpassing the disaster norm of our previous reflections. It lacks the urgency of the latter, but has the nobility of the free, forward thrust. [. . .] The more optional goal of pushing forward is also more exacting. We have this syndrome: Progress is by our choosing an acknowledged interest of society, in which we have a stake in various degrees; science is a necessary instrument of progress; research is a necessary instrument of science; and in medical science experimentation on human subjects is a necessary instrument of research. Therefore, human experimentation has come to be a societal interest.

The destination of research is essentially melioristic. It does not serve the preservation of the existing good from which I profit myself and to which I am obligated. Unless the present state is intolerable, the melioristic goal is in a sense gratuitous, and this not only from the vantage point of the present. Our descendants have a right to be left an unplundered planet; they do not have a right to new miracle cures. [. . .]

VIII.   THE MELIORISTIC GOAL, MEDICAL RESEARCH, AND INDIVIDUAL DUTY

Nowhere is the melioristic goal more inherent than in medicine. [. . .] Gratuitous we called it (outside disaster conditions) as a social goal, but noble at the same time. Both the nobility and the gratuitousness must influence the manner in which self-sacrifice for it is elicited, and even its free offer accepted. Freedom is certainly the first condition to be observed here. The surrender of one's body to medical experimentation is entirely outside the enforceable "social contract."

Or can it be construed to fall within its terms—namely, as repayment for benefits from past experimentation that I have enjoyed myself? But I am indebted for these benefits not to society, but to the past "martyrs," to whom society is indebted itself, and society has no right to call in my personal debt by way of adding new to its own. Moreover, gratitude is not an enforceable social obligation; it anyway does not mean that I must emulate the deed. Most of all, if it was wrong to exact such sacrifice in the first place, it does not become right to exact it again with the plea of the profit it has brought me. If, however, it was not exacted, but entirely free, as it ought to have been, then it should remain so, and its precedence must not be used as a social pressure on others for doing the same under the sign of duty.

What about the moral law as such a transcendent motivation of conduct? It goes considerably beyond the public law of the social contract. The latter, we saw, is founded on the rule of enlightened self-interest: *Do ut des*—I give so that I be given to. The law of individual conscience asks more. Under the Golden Rule, for example, I am required to give as I wish to be given to under like circumstances, but not in order that I be given to and not in expectation of return. Reciprocity, essential to the social law, is not a condition of the moral law. [. . .]

IX.   MORAL LAW AND TRANSMORAL DEDICATION

Can I, then, be called upon to offer myself for medical experimentation in the name of the moral law? *Prima facie*, the Golden Rule seems to apply. I should wish, were I dying of a disease, that enough volunteers in the past had provided enough knowledge through the gift of their bodies that I could now be saved. I should wish, were I desperately in need of a transplant, that the dying patient next door had agreed to a definition of death by which his organs would become available to me in the freshest possible condition. I surely should also wish, were I drowning, that somebody would risk his life, even sacrifice his life, for mine.

But the last example reminds us that only the negative form of the Golden Rule ("Do not do unto others what you do not want done unto yourself") is fully prescriptive. The positive form ("Do unto others as you would wish them to do unto you"), in whose compass our issue falls, points into an infinite, open horizon where prescriptive force soon ceases. We may well say of somebody that he ought to have come to the succor of B, to have shared with him in his need, and the like. But we may not say that he ought to have given his life for him. To have done so would be praiseworthy; not to have done so is not blameworthy. It cannot be asked of him; if he fails to do so, he reneges on no duty. But *he* may say of himself, and only he, that he ought to have given his life. *This* "ought" is strictly between him and himself, or between him and God; no outside party—fellow man or society—can appropriate its voice. [...]

We must, in other words, distinguish between moral obligation and the much larger sphere of moral value. [...] The ethical dimension far exceeds that of the moral law and reaches into the sublime solitude of dedication and ultimate commitment, away from all reckoning and rule—in short, into the sphere of the *holy.* From there alone can the offer of self-sacrifice genuinely spring, and this—its source—must be honored religiously. How? The first duty here falling on the research community, when it enlists and uses this source, is the safeguarding of true authenticity and spontaneity.

X. THE "CONSCRIPTION" OF CONSENT

But here we must realize that the mere issue of the appeal, the calling for volunteers, with the moral and social pressures it inevitably generates, amounts even under the most meticulous rules of consent to a sort of *conscripting.* And some soliciting is necessarily involved. [...] And this is why "consent," surely a non-negotiable minimum requirement, is not the full answer to the problem. Granting then that soliciting and therefore some degree of conscripting are part of the situation, who may conscript and who may be conscripted? Or less harshly expressed: Who should issue appeals and to whom?

The naturally qualified issuer of the appeal is the research scientist himself, collectively the main carrier of the impulse and the only one with the technical competence to judge. But his being very much an interested party (with vested interests, indeed, not purely in the public good, but in the scientific enterprise as such, in "his" project, and even in his career) makes him also suspect. [...]

XI. SELF-RECRUITMENT
OF THE COMMUNITY

To whom should the appeal be addressed? The natural issuer of the call is also the first natural addressee: the physician-researcher himself and the scientific confraternity at large. With such a coincidence—indeed, the noble tradition with which the whole business of human experimentation started—almost all of the associated legal, ethical, and metaphysical problems vanish. If it is full, autonomous identification of the subject with the purpose that is required for the dignifying of his serving as a subject—here it is; if strongest motivation—here it is; if fullest understanding—here it is; if freest decision—here it is; if greatest integration with the person's total, chosen pursuit—here it is. With the fact of self-solicitation the

issue of consent in all its insoluble equivocality is bypassed *per se.* Not even the condition that the particular purpose be truly important and the project reasonably promising, which must hold in any solicitation of others, need be satisfied here. By himself, the scientist is free to obey his obsession, to play his hunch, to wager on chance, to follow the lure of ambition. [...]

It would be the ideal, but is not a real solution, to keep the issue of human experimentation within the research community itself. Neither in numbers nor in variety of material would its potential suffice for the many-pronged, systematic, continual attack on disease into which the lonely exploits of the early investigators have grown. Statistical requirements alone make their voracious demands; and were it not for what I have called the essentially "gratuitous" nature of the whole enterprise of progress, [...] the simplest answer would be to keep the whole population enrolled, and let the lot, or an equivalent of draft boards, decide which of each category will at any one time be called up for "service." It is not difficult to picture societies with whose philosophy this would be consonant. We are agreed that ours is not one such and should not become one. The specter of it is indeed among the threatening utopias on our own horizon from which we should recoil, and of whose advent by imperceptible steps we must beware. [...]

XII. "IDENTIFICATION" AS THE
PRINCIPLE OF RECRUITMENT IN GENERAL

If the properties we adduced as the particular qualifications of the members of the scientific fraternity itself are taken as general criteria of selection, then one should look for additional subjects where a maximum of identification, understanding, and spontaneity can be expected—that is, among the most highly motivated, the most highly educated, and the least "captive" members of the community. From this naturally scarce resource, a descending order of permissibility leads to greater abundance and ease of supply, whose use should become proportionately more hesitant as the exculpating criteria are relaxed. An inversion of normal "market" behavior is demanded here—namely, to accept the lowest quotation last (and excused only by the greatest pressure of need); to pay the highest price first.

The ruling principle in our considerations is that the "wrong" of reification can only be made "right" by such authentic identification with the cause that it is the subject's as well as the researcher's cause—whereby his role in its service is not just permitted by him, but *willed.* That sovereign will of his which embraces the end as his own restores his personhood to the otherwise depersonalizing context. [...] The following, for instance, may be responsive to the "call" we are discussing: compassion with human suffering, zeal for humanity, reverence to the Golden Rule, enthusiasm for progress, homage to the cause of knowledge, even longing for sacrificial justification [. . .]. On all these, I say, it is defensible and right to draw when the research objective is worthy enough; and it is a prime duty of the research community [. . .] to see that this sacred source is never abused for frivolous ends. [. . .]

XIII. THE RULE OF THE "DESCENDING ORDER" AND ITS COUNTER-UTILITY SENSE

[. . .] The combined attribute of motivation and information, plus the absence of external pressures, tends to be socially so circumscribed that strict adherence to the rule might numerically starve the research process. This is why I spoke of a descending order of permissibility, which is itself permissive, but where the realization that it is a *descending* order is not without pragmatic import. [. . .] I merely indicate the principle of the order of preference: The poorer in knowledge, motivation, and freedom of decision (and that, alas, means the more readily available in terms of numbers and possible manipulation), the more sparingly and indeed reluctantly should the reservoir be used, and the more compelling must therefore become the countervailing justification.

Let us note that this is the opposite of a social utility standard, the reverse of the order by "availability and expendability": The most valuable and scarcest, the least expendable elements of the social organism, are to be the first candidates for risk and sacrifice. [. . .] It is also the opposite of what the day-to-day interests of research clamor for, and for the scientific community to honor it will mean that it will have to fight a strong temptation to go by routine to the readiest sources of supply—the suggestible, the ignorant, the dependent, the "captive" in various senses. [. . .]

XIV. EXPERIMENTATION ON PATIENTS

So far we have been speaking on the tacit assumption that the subjects of experimentation are recruited from among the healthy. To the question "Who is conscriptable?" the spontaneous answer is: Least and last of all the sick—the most available of all as they are under treatment and observation anyway. That the afflicted should not be called upon to bear additional burden and risk, that they are society's special trust and the physician's trust in particular—these are elementary responses of our moral sense. Yet the very destination of medical research, the conquest of disease, requires at the crucial stage trial and verification on precisely the sufferers from the disease, and their total exemption would defeat the purpose itself. In acknowledging this inescapable necessity, we enter the most sensitive area of the whole complex, the one most keenly felt and most searchingly discussed by the practitioners themselves. No wonder, it touches the heart of the doctor-patient relation, putting its most solemn obligations to the test. [. . .]

A. *The Fundamental Privilege of the Sick*

In the course of treatment, the physician is obligated to the patient and to no one else. He is not the agent of society, nor of the interests of medical science, nor of the patient's family, nor of his co-sufferers, or future sufferers from the same disease. The patient alone counts when he is under the physician's care. By the simple law of bilateral contract [. . .], the physician is bound not to let any other interest interfere with that of the patient in being cured. [. . .]

B. *The Principle of "Identification" Applied to Patients*

On the whole, the same principles would seem to hold here as are found to hold with "normal subjects": Motivation, identification, understanding on the part of the subject. But it is clear that these conditions are peculiarly difficult to satisfy with regard to a patient. His physical state, psychic preoccupation, dependent relation to the doctor, the submissive attitude induced by treatment—everything connected with his condition and situation makes the sick person inherently less of a sovereign person than the healthy one. [A]ll the factors that make the patient, as a category, particularly accessible and welcome for experimentation at the same time compromise the quality of the responding affirmation that must morally redeem the making use of them. [. . .]

Still, [. . .] there is scope among patients for observing the rule of the "descending order of permissibility" that we have laid down for normal subjects [. . .]. By the principle of this order, those patients who most identify with and are cognizant of the cause of research—members of the medical profession (who after all are sometimes patients themselves)—come first; the highly motivated and educated, also least dependent, among the lay patients come next; and so on down the line. An added consideration here is seriousness of condition, which again operates in inverse proportion. Here the profession must fight the tempting sophistry that the hopeless case is expendable (because in prospect already expended) and therefore especially usable; and generally the attitude that the poorer the chances of the patient the more justifiable his recruitment for experimentation (other than for his own benefit). The opposite is true. [. . .]

XVII. CONCLUSION

[. . .] Let us not forget that progress is an optional goal, not an unconditional commitment, and that its tempo in particular, compulsive as it may become, has nothing sacred about it. Let us also remember that a slower progress in the conquest of disease would not threaten society, grievous as it is to those who have to deplore that their particular disease be not yet conquered, but that society would indeed be threatened by the erosion of those moral values whose loss, possibly caused by too ruthless a pursuit of scientific progress, would make its most dazzling triumphs not worth having. [...]

23   Experimentation on Trial

Why Should One Take Part in Medical Research?

David Heyd

THE ETHICAL BASIS OF EXPERIMENTATION ON HUMAN SUBJECTS

[...] Experimental research on human subjects obviously raises ethical questions which do not arise in other fields of scientific investigation. Like "pharmakon," the word "subject" is typically ambiguous, denoting both the being which is passively "subjected" to the experimental procedure and the person who is the putative beneficiary of the procedure as well as the active maker of the choice to take part in it. Paradoxically, as we shall see, the more sophisticated research protocols become in their methodology, the more difficult it is to justify them ethically. [...]

The issue of medical experimentation on human subjects is particularly sensitive, since there is a tension between the high esteem in which we hold the experimental method characterizing modern science and the deep suspicion with which we view any attempt to use human beings for purposes other than their own individual welfare. We are aware that the achievements of modern medicine are mostly the result of experimental methods, but we can never forget the widespread abuse of human beings by either maliciously driven "researchers" or by well-meaning but over-zealous scientists. [...]

There are two levels on which the issue of the ethics of experimentation can be discussed: the general moral basis for the practice of experimenting with human beings and the particular conditions which should be satisfied for the practice to be considered morally acceptable. The vast majority of writings on the subject belong to the second level. [...] I am going to [...] concentrate on the relatively neglected topics pertaining to the first, more general level,

David Heyd, "Experimentation on Trial: Why Should One Take Part in Medical Research?" *Jahrbuch für Recht und Ethik* [Annual Review of Law and Ethics] 4 (1996): 189–204.

namely the ethical basis of the practice of experimenting with human beings.

This topic can be approached from two perspectives: from the point of view of society and the medical profession or from that of the individual subject. The former consists of the attempt to justify experimentation as a social good or as a means to promote public health or as a necessary condition for the advancement of knowledge. [...] But medical experimentation is a subject in which the gap between what is rational and good for the collective and what is rational and good for the individual is markedly wide, since the stakes are high for both parties.

I propose to discuss the individual-oriented issue, namely why should one take part in medical experiments, in three stages or levels:

I.   Rationality: does one have good self-regarding reasons to subject oneself to medical experimentation?

II. Justice: does one have a duty or an obligation to take part in experimental medical research?

III. Virtue: ought one to contribute to the long-term attempt to promote medical knowledge and the overall health of human beings?

The three questions are ordered in a hierarchical way: prudence, moral duty, and supererogation; or, in terms of three alternative bases of moral theory: rational choice, social contract, and value; or, in other words, what is worthwhile for me, what I owe to others, and the best way in which I can serve a human ideal. From the point of view of motivation, the subject is driven on the first level by egoistic concern, on the second by the demands of duty and obligation, and on the third by the free choice to volunteer. These are three distinct grounds for expecting people to take part in medical trials, in which the second is built on the failure of the first, and the third is advanced as an admission of the shortcomings of the second. In other words, I propose to show that the appeal to self-regarding reasons cannot suffice to serve as a justification of medical experimentation, and that the morally-based reasons of justice and fairness cannot play this justificatory role either. This will lead us to view the individual's involvement, at least in some medical experiments, as a matter of Good Samaritanism.

I. Rational Choice

Prudential reasons are methodologically superior to moral reasons. Their force is usually less controversial and their motivational effectiveness more direct. Thus, the attempt to justify the recruitment of human subjects to medical experiments on the basis of the potential benefit to *them* is particularly attractive. But of course there are different levels of rationality, from the most direct short-term egoistic benefit to the highly abstract long-term probabilistically supported expected utility.

Every individual has a deep interest in getting the best medical treatment possible. But the best treatment a doctor can offer is based on long experience, that is on a haphazard or systematic series of cases from which conclusions as to the effectiveness of the treatment are drawn. [E]very patient has an interest in participating in the process of experimentation. [. . .] It is the most basic kind of experiment which is designed purely with the individual patient in his unique condition in mind. This is the most primitive kind of experiment from the point of view of scientific rationality, but the easiest to justify as rational from the point of view of the subject. [. . .]

[However,] the randomized controlled trial (RCT) [. . .] has become the privileged and most reliable means of attaining new knowledge in many fields of medical research. Randomization of the grouping of human subjects neutralizes all sorts of interfering, "irrelevant" variables, which have in the past distorted scientific results. [. . .] But both randomization and blindness [i.e., double-blind design—eds.] open a significant gap between the patient's direct interest in getting the best treatment for her condition and the overall potential of advancing medical knowledge.

The individual rational chooser is left with a dilemma: should he opt for the traditional experience-based trials of his individual doctor, or rather for the double-blind RCT. The former, personalized method is superior in its therapeutic potential since it is sensitive to the particular conditions of the individual patient and promises an immediate effect for the individual. On the other hand, only the latter, impersonal method of the RCT can be expected to yield the rationally supported breakthrough in the treatment of disease. The situation is reminiscent of the Prisoner's Dilemma, in which two principles of rationality conflict with each other. I have good reasons for preferring a treatment based on a "trial" specifically designed for my particular condition; but this is a rational choice only if *others*, by taking part in impersonalized, randomized trials, contribute to general medical knowledge, including that of my own doctor. Thus, if everybody opted for the same personalized treatment, as I do, there would be no advance in medical competence, which would make the choice ultimately irrational also from the point of view of the individual chooser.

One way to overcome this paradox of rationality is to narrow the gap between the two principles of rationality by allowing for *therapeutic* experimentation only. If I take part in an experiment which seeks a new drug for the condition from which I am suffering, it is true that I cannot be guaranteed the best treatment which suits my individual case (which might even be already known to the doctor), but I still stand to benefit personally from the research in the longer run. Provided that certain restrictions are placed on the research protocol so as to ensure that I do not risk my health to an unreasonable degree, it could be easily conceived that a rational chooser has good reason to take part in such an experiment. [. . .]

As in other Prisoner's Dilemma situations, there are ways in which the prudential reasoning of the individual can be regulated through the manipulation of the conditions under which the choice is made. Thus, society may resort to negative incentives (such as sanctions for not participating), or to positive incentives (such as monetary compensation or early release from prison). These are means which in the past have proved very effective in recruiting subjects for experiments, but like direct deception, or physical enforcement, are considered morally unacceptable by any enlightened society today. A possibly less repugnant proposal is to let the patient choose between a "research hospital" and a "non-research institution." The former would offer a better, more up-to-date treatment, but the patient would be committed to take some part in new research. These examples serve to show that rational choice cannot be defined in a context-neutral way. The conditions under which the choice is made by the individual are constitutive of its "rationality"; that is to say, if we wish to justify medical experimentation in terms of its rationality for the subject, we must specify certain conditions of autonomy characterizing the subject making the choice. But the basic criticism of some of these "solutions" refers to the *unfairness* of the conditions themselves.

II. Justice and Fairness

There is a long tradition starting with Hobbes which tries to articulate the conditions for rational choice in terms of the ultimate rationality of all the parties concerned. This is the beginning of the idea of the social contract, in which individuals construct a political system which radically constrains their individual freedom to exercise their choices so as to achieve overall benefits. This approach could be translated in the present context to imply that the sovereign (state) is given absolute power to compel individuals to participate in medical experiments in every case in which this can be shown to contribute to an overall promotion of health. Now, such a system would be far from absurd, since it would force individuals out of a situation in which no one is willing to risk oneself in an experiment, leading to the stagnation of medical science which would be bad for everybody.

Furthermore, the rationality of such a system consists in its impartiality. In a Rawlsian version of such a contract, no one would know in advance the chances of being closer to the giving or to the receiving end. The scheme seems to be fair in the sense that it contains the elements of a lottery in which people have equal chances overall. Healthy people are summoned to take part in control groups; ill people are called to take part in research done on the disease from which they are suffering; and no one knows in advance whether she will be healthy or ill. Thus, the artificially induced randomness of the selection of subjects in RCT complements the natural lottery which distinguishes between the ill and the healthy. Furthermore, the fact that modern experimentation is randomized makes the distribution of risks and benefits fair, since participants are not only given an equal chance to belong to either of the randomized groups, but there is absolutely no trace of favoritism or bias in the selection. No one is singled out for the experiment except for the *group* of the ill patients who are usually the scientifically eligible subjects, and even this apparent bias is compensated for by including healthy subjects in control groups.

This approach may provide a way out of the dilemma of "equipoise" or what has been referred to as the "null hypothesis." If the two competing hypotheses to be tested in an experiment (e.g., alternative drugs or methods of surgery) are not equally supported by the existing evidence, how can the doctor justify using a randomized method in which half of his patients are going to get a treatment which is in his own opinion less than the optimal? One condition for making an experiment morally acceptable is that even though individual doctors may have a preference for one of the alternatives, others might have the opposite preference, or in other words there is no "standard" treatment or accepted practice. In such a case even from the point of view of the patient, the fact that she is consulting one doctor rather than another makes it a matter of "luck" that she gets one treatment rather than another. And if that is the case, the "luck" involved in taking part in a scientifically randomized protocol is no less rational than accepting the subjective preference of one's own doctor. [. . .]

The difficulties in the rational choice approach to the justification of experimentation lead to the idea of a social contract based on the extra-rational notion of fairness. The idea in a nutshell is that being a beneficiary of past medical research, one is under an obligation to give "one's share" by taking part in further studies. The process of medical advance is understood as an ongoing enterprise which is necessarily based on cooperation. Cooperation is a framework for a social interaction in which gaining without contributing is considered *unfair,* taking a free ride. There is nothing irrational in taking advantage in such an unfair way, but it is nevertheless morally wrong. In Rawlsian terms, the obligation to take part in experimentation is derived not from the long-term overall expectation of a personal gain, but from the choice behind a "veil of ignorance" to establish a system of cooperation in which people will invest time, forgo comfort, or even risk their health so as to guarantee a fairly distributed collective effort to promote public health.

There are, however, theoretical problems in applying the contractarian justification to the issue of experimentation, which is an enterprise that crosses generations. The point is that standard systems of cooperation, that is contracts, refer to individuals existing roughly at the same time. In other words, contracts are based on the principle of *mutuality,* or the mutual dependence of the parties to the contract. Cooperation is rational only between people who stand to lose from uncooperative behavior. Now, much of medical experimentation is long-term, that is, its benefits can be expected to be reaped only by people not yet born. Unlike military service, in which soldiers and those whose lives and property they defend exist simultaneously and where a fair division of labor can be devised, future generations are dependent on our present willingness to take part in medical experiments, but not vice versa. Thus, from the point of view of prudential rationality, we can lose nothing by benefiting from the fruits of past medical progress without giving anything of our own to later generations. And from the point of view of fairness, it is logically hard to describe us as *owing* anything to anyone: our ancestors who did us good by taking part in experiments could be the object of our duty of mutual benefit, but they are not around anymore; and to those whom we are able to benefit, the next generation, we owe nothing, since they have not benefited us in any way. Enforcing a vaccination program, even if individuals run a certain degree of risk, may be justified in contractarian terms of fairness in a way which does not apply to the apparently similar case of experimentation.

We are thus left with an extended notion of a transgenerational contract, which at least metaphorically tries to view humanity in its history as a community. John Rawls's analogy to families and family lines is an attempt to make this historically defined community more intuitive. But unlike our commitment to our own children and grandchildren, even in circumstances in which the condition of mutuality is not satisfied, we have no analogous motivation to take part in experiments whose beneficiaries are by definition completely unknown to us. In any case, describing our refusal to give our share to medical research may be described as "unfair" only if we are entitled to assume that our ancestors' condition for benefiting us was that we do the same for our descendants. This is usually not the case and hence hardly a reason grounded in justice that warrants risking our health for the sake of future people.

But of course there are experiments which yield more immediate results and from which present people may benefit. Do these fall into the framework of a social contract? Almost all ethicists believe that experimentation is not analogous to military service or to taxation, that is, to systems of fair distribution of burdens from which the whole community benefits. Experiments are more risky and invasive of our privacy than paying taxes and their goal is less existentially urgent than that of military defense; it seems therefore that no social contract can justify enforcing participation in them as in the two other cases. But this distinction between the two kinds of contribution to the public good may change in the future, particularly since medical experiments are becoming so crucial for the progress of medicine and the promotion of public health.

However, there is one general principle of fairness which cannot be doubted: the wider the group of potential beneficiaries of the experiment, the more difficult it is to justify the expectation to take part in it in terms of fairness. Thus, the narrowest group is the individual himself; when I stand to benefit directly from an experimental procedure, the expectation that I take part in it is fair. The next group is that of people suffering from the syndrome studied by the investigator. Beyond their medical eligibility, it is accordingly fair to recruit people suffering from migraines to test a new drug for headaches, since they stand to benefit from the new discovery more than other people. Finally, we may consider all contemporary people, who stand a chance to gain something from new medication for diseases which they one day might contract. Here the mutuality condition is satisfied only in a very remote and abstract way, and hence society tends not to impose a duty to take part in experimentation. As for future people, by definition, they can only be beneficiaries but not participants in present medical research, and hence our relations with them cannot be a matter of justice at all.

III. Virtue and Solidarity

We have so far shown the serious difficulties in justifying experimentation in terms of either rational choice or of duties of justice. This does not mean that there is no way to justify compelling people to take part in medical research on the basis of the overall good or utility which could arise. But recall that we are restricting our discussion to the point of view of the individual and her reasons, putting aside the

otherwise legitimate perspective of the policy-maker or legislator. It should again be emphasized that typically liberal principles (such as the right of an individual over his body and privacy) call for special protection of individuals from the otherwise legitimate concern for the promotion of public good and health. The almost sanctimonious condition of informed consent in the recruitment of subjects for experiments typically indicates that primacy of the point of view of the individual over general utilitarian considerations. Such consent is never called for in the case of other serious invasions by the guardians of the collective interest into the life of the individual, as in military conscription or the financing of public projects through taxation. Consent in the case of taxation and military conscription is given in the indirect, collective way of the democratic process. Participation in medical experiments, however, cannot be enforced through majority vote.

What reason, then, does an individual have to enter a medical experiment? To help us move to the third stage of the analysis, consider as an analogy the traditional system of blood donation: the entire medical demand for blood being supplied by voluntary donations from individuals who with no incentive (such as money or a family insurance for blood) come every year to the blood bank to contribute that fluid which is precious for the recipient but almost costless to the donor. Their act is highly valuable though typically non-obligatory. It is what is referred to in ethical theory as an act of *supererogation*. [. . .]

Now, taking part in a medical experiment is obviously a different case. It involves a much higher risk to the subject and a much lower certainty of benefit to the (unidentifiable) recipient. But it shares with blood donation the altruistic motive, free giving with no expectation of return, an unenforced contribution to the welfare of others. The particular value of volunteering to subject oneself to a medical trial lies in its being completely beyond the call of duty, that is, beyond the legitimate moral requirements of justice and fairness. Volunteering is optional not only from the legal point of view, but equally from the moral perspective. This implies that medical researchers cannot blame or morally criticize individuals for refusing to take part in experimental procedures. The answer to the question why take part in a medical experiment is simply "Good Samaritanism," [. . .] that is to say, an act which is neither legally enforced nor morally required.

Among supererogatory actions, there are those motivated by a particular concern for a particular individual or a group of individuals. This category includes the act of a soldier who volunteers to sacrifice his life in order to save those of his friends or a ruler's act of pardoning a criminal. But there are supererogatory actions which are partly or completely anonymous, that is, there is no personal relationship between the donor and the donee [. . .]. [W]e can say that both blood donation and participation in medical experiments are supererogatory acts of the purest kind, since they are not motivated by any personal or class interest.

What then is the motive behind these acts of supreme charity? One possible answer is solidarity. By taking part in an ongoing enterprise such as medical progress, people express their solidarity with their society or indeed with humanity at large. Another possible altruistic motive is identification with the medical profession. Individuals who are not themselves scientists but subscribe to the general ideal of scientific advance, can partake in the process of the growth of knowledge by being part of the experimental adventure. [...]

In his classical article on the ethics of experimentation on human subjects, Hans Jonas proposes a view which is close to the supererogatory model of free giving, though still containing some elements of a moral requirement. Jonas seems to argue that there is no justification for placing anyone under a *duty* to take part in an experiment, since no advancement of medical knowledge (unless it is vital for saving the life of the whole society in emergency situations such as plagues) justifies putting at risk the life and health of individuals; on the other hand, he is aware of the high value of such progress, and of the special duty it imposes primarily on the community of researchers. He is thus led to treat the call to take part in experimentation as *noblesse oblige,* a particular "duty" derived from the privileged status of a certain class in society. Its basis is typically religious, and Jonas explicitly identifies the realm beyond the call of duty as that of the *holy.*

This is a typically elitist approach, which on the one hand tends to impose a quasi-moral duty on a small number of "interested" parties, yet not only exempts all others from the duty to participate, but even excludes them altogether from the opportunity to volunteer, on the grounds of the risk of being exploited or of having the wrong kind of motivation. The ignorant, the poor, the sick, and the young are all "captive" groups, which usually should not be permitted to take part in the otherwise noble enterprise of the advancement of knowledge and the contribution to the health of future people. This is a highly restrictive view of autonomy, in which only the idealistically motivated reasons are allowed to play a role in human choice.

However, the purely supererogatory approach to experimentation and that based on the "duties of the chosen few" share the view that through voluntary participation in this worthy but risky enterprise individuals express their *virtue,* their particularly noble traits of character, their solidarity with humanity at large. One significant implication of such a view is that it lays a particularly heavy responsibility on the scientist and researcher; it is based on *trust.* Relations founded on supererogatory volunteering are less controlled by rules and conditions than relations based on commercial interests or principles of distributive justice. In

medical experimentation the subject has virtually no way to know when she is exploited, and she is dependent on the protection of the ethical committees that assess the validity of the experiment. Worse, the committees themselves are dependent to a large extent on the conscientiousness of the experimenters who are expected to apply the conditions of the experiment faithfully. A violation of the trust of the volunteer is destructive of the likelihood of the future cooperation of well-motivated subjects.

Replacing the expression "experimentation *on* human subjects" with the idea of "experimentation *with* human subjects" is the epitome of the supererogatory model of the justification of medical research. It treats research as a cooperative enterprise in which the role of the subject undergoing the experiment is no less active than that of the experimenter, despite the unbridgeable gap in skill and expertise. It forms certain bonds of partnership between the two parties. This implies primarily that the group of scientists should be the first to volunteer (whenever possible) to undergo the experiment, thus serving both as role models and as personal guarantors for the patients' trust. But, contrary to Jonas, it seems that within a democratic idea of human autonomy, there is no justification to restrict volunteering to the "elite," and that the very opportunity for *all* members of society to take part in a voluntary venture expresses the equal respect which a liberal society wishes to accord to everyone in it. [...]

CONCLUSION

The ethical basis of experimentation on human subjects has been examined in this article under three alternative models: rational choice (prudence), justice and fairness (social contract), and supererogatory giving (charity). [...]

It seems, then, that different contexts give rise to different grounds for expecting people to subject themselves to medical research. There are cases in which self-interest plays a dominant role; there are others in which a reconstruction of a hypothetical contract might serve to justify a distribution of the burden of experimentation for the good of everybody; there are, however, situations in which only an altruistic motive, a concern for unidentified future people or a wish to promote the abstract value of the advancement of knowledge, can account for the act of volunteering.

But we remain with one main philosophical problem which is of a second-order epistemological kind: how do we know to which of these categories a particular experimental situation belongs? This is not a simple empirical problem. It is a conceptual difficulty, since we have a chance of knowing the answer only after the experiment has taken place and yielded results. The prudential benefit of a research project can be only assessed post hoc, as can its benefits to contemporary people who live under the conditions of mutuality. This problem adds to the superiority of the last, supererogatory model. But as with blood donations, the model of charity, despite its clear moral attraction, is highly precarious: it works only if enough people are moved to volunteer of their own accord. Once the voluntary system is eroded, society has no alternative but to resort to undesirable economic incentives or even to partly coercive measures, lest medical progress stop altogether.

But while in cases like blood supply (or care for the poor) commercialization involves "only" the abandonment of noble moral ideals, subjecting medical experimentation (like the supply of live organs) to the forces of the market may directly lead to the violation of the most basic human rights and dignity.

Section Two

Access to Research

24   Wanted: Single, White Male for Medical Research

<small>Rebecca Dresser</small>

In June 1990, the General Accounting Office revealed that despite a 1986 federal policy to the contrary, women continued to be seriously underrepresented in biomedical research study populations. According to the National Institutes of Health (NIH), this practice "has resulted in significant gaps in [our] knowledge" of diseases that affect both men and women. In short, many of the important human health data generated by the modern biomedical research revolution are data about men.

The failure to include women in research populations is ubiquitous. An NIH-sponsored study showing that heart attacks were reduced when subjects took one aspirin every other day was conducted on men, and the relationship between low cholesterol diets and cardiovascular disease has been almost exclusively studied in men. Yet coronary heart disease is the leading cause of death in women. Similarly, the first twenty years of a major federal study on health and aging included only men. Yet two-thirds of the elderly population are women. The recent announcement that aspirin can help prevent migraine headaches is based on data from males only, even though women suffer from migraines up to three times as often as men.

The list goes on: Studies on AIDS treatment frequently omit women, the fastest growing infected population. An investigation of the possible relationship between caffeine

and heart disease involved 45,589 male research subjects. Most amazing is the pilot project on the impact of obesity on breast and uterine cancer conducted—you guessed it—solely on men. Moreover, the customary research subject not only is male, but is a white male. African-Americans, Latinos, and other racial and ethnic groups have typically been excluded from studies, again in spite of a formal NIH guideline encouraging the inclusion of such groups in study populations. Children and elderly persons also have received short shrift, particularly in the testing of new drugs. And in basic research, even female rats are frequently excluded as research subjects!

The physiology of women and men differs in ways that can affect how disease and treatment manifest themselves. Beyond the obviously sex-linked diseases such as uterine and prostate cancer, there is evidence that heart disease, AIDS, depression, and numerous other ostensibly "gender-neutral" conditions are expressed differently in women and men. A similar situation exists among different racial and ethnic groups. Lupus, for example, reportedly affects one in 750 women generally, but its incidence is one in 245 among African-American women and one in 500 among Latinas. Such differences make it inappropriate simply to generalize findings based on one gender or racial group to all human beings. As a result of the past over-representation of white men in research populations, physicians now frequently lack adequate evidence on whether women and people of color will be helped, harmed, or not affected at all by numerous therapies now endorsed as promoting "human health." [...]

Rebecca Dresser, "Wanted: Single, White Male for Medical Research," *Hastings Center Report* 22, no. 1 (1992): 24–29.

ALLEGED JUSTIFICATIONS FOR THE EXCLUSIONARY PRACTICE

Some scientists and officials have explained that there often is "scientific" justification for studying only white males. Clean, simple data are needed for studies; the more alike the subjects, the more any variation can be attributed to the experimental intervention. Including women would "complicate" a study due to the hormone changes of the menstrual cycle. I have two responses to this claim. First, even if it is scientifically justifiable to study humans who have a similar physiology, why study white men? Perhaps the choice of racial group can be supported by its dominant proportion in the U.S. population, but not so for the choice of gender. In this country, women are numerically in the majority. Why then the choice of the minority white male? Why is it female, but not male, hormones that "complicate" research? Second, focusing on one type of human physiology reduces the generalizability of the experimental data. Although there is probably a place for such narrowly focused projects, why have they so rarely been conducted on anyone but white men? Again, what accounts for the relative infrequency of studies on homogeneous populations of other kinds of people?

One can also challenge the notion that a study conducted on physiologically close subjects is usually the "best" scientific approach. Such a judgment divorces the concept of scientific merit from its broader context. A project may be designed with the greatest of scientific elegance, but if the data it produces have little value to society, it is not necessarily a meritorious project. Merit, at least in the context of government funding decisions, is tied to a proposal's promise of benefit to society. If NIH's goal is to award support to the projects most likely to advance our knowledge of important human health concerns, it would seem that white-male-only clinical investigations of widespread conditions such as coronary artery disease and aging would have less merit than studies that provided data with broader applicability. In fact, the latest NIH directive explicitly instructs its scientific reviewers to consider inclusion of women and minorities in study populations when they evaluate a proposal's scientific merit.

Two other explanations have been offered for the practice of excluding women from study populations. One is concern for the condition of women who could become pregnant while enrolled as research subjects. Threats of miscarriage, birth defects, and so forth are cited as justifications for omitting women. Exclusion is appropriate, it is alleged, to protect potentially pregnant women and their potential children. The Department of Health and Human Services (DHHS) regulations governing human subjects research sets special conditions on research involving fetuses and pregnant women, and the Food and Drug Administration (FDA) guidelines for clinical evaluation of drugs restricts but does not ban participation of "women of childbearing potential" in clinical trials. Certainly caution is warranted here. But is maternal-fetal protection always a valid reason for failing to include female subjects?

Our nation has a long history of excluding women from various activities on grounds that participation would harm the "weaker sex," and thus often denying women the significant benefits of participation. Likewise, the failure to conduct biomedical research on women denies them the benefits of research. The vast majority of women who are not pregnant cannot with sufficient confidence take advantage of numerous health recommendations that have emerged from men-only research studies. In the name of *potential* protection of *potentially* pregnant women and their fetuses, all women have lost opportunities to improve and extend their lives.

Complete exclusion of women subjects is an unnecessarily blunt instrument to accomplish the goal of maternal-fetal protection. The exclusionary approach, as Carol Levine notes, "assumes that all women are alike, that all women are sexually active, and that all are unreliable in their contraceptive practices." To the contrary, as one physician pointed out, "Most female cardiac patients are not planning to get pregnant." Neither are the women likely to be subjects in an aging study!

If a study poses a legitimate threat to the potential offspring of women participants, two options come to mind. One is simply to exclude fertile women of reproductive age. Again, however, this seems overbroad; indeed, this is the approach the Supreme Court recently struck down in *Johnson Controls* as violating federal law prohibiting sex discrimination in the workplace. It would be better to adopt a more nuanced approach. In her recent article on the underrepresentation of women in HIV/AIDS research, for example, Levine endorses a three-tiered categorization system to address the problem. Many, perhaps most, human studies fail to pose a foreseeable risk to future children. The unknown and unforeseeable teratogenic risk that accompanies practically any physiological intervention fails to justify excluding fertile women from studies in this category. Similarly, women should have the opportunity to enroll in studies that present known risks to future children, but also have the potential for significantly benefiting the research participants. In these two categories of research, adequate disclosure of the risks and potential benefits of research participation, together with the availability of highly reliable contraceptives and abortion, would give women a reasonable choice regarding whether to accept the risks of participating. The possibility that a few women might become pregnant, might choose against abortion, and might have a child who is harmed by exposure to an experimental intervention is too small to justify the current exclusionary practices. The risk of tort liability in such cases is also small. Women who consent to the risk of harm to potential offspring and who decide against abortion when they become unexpectedly pregnant would be unlikely to recover damages. Any injured children might themselves have a claim, however. Perhaps some form of legislative immunity is needed here. But it should be recognized that the current approach also fails to protect health professionals and drug manufacturers against liability. The present practice merely moves the source of the claims to the damaged future children of women patients who receive drugs and other treatments in the clinical setting.

A third research category is more complicated, however. Levine argues that sexually active fertile women should be excluded from studies that present both a known significant risk to potential offspring and minimal or unknown benefit to women subjects, because parents have a moral responsibility to make reasonable efforts to protect their future children's health and the knowledge sought from such studies is obtainable through other means. Given the ever-present danger of contraceptive failure, the misunderstandings "informed" subjects may have about a protocol's risks and potential benefits, and the possibility that subjects' awareness or appreciation of their exposure to risk could decline over time, it is better to conduct such studies on other groups, Levine contends. If early results reveal a possible substantial benefit for women participants, she suggests that the intervention could be made available to individual women off-protocol.

This would be appropriate, in my view, as long as the same approach is applied to sexually active fertile men. Researchers have been extremely concerned about reproductive risks to women, while largely neglecting the reproductive risks research participation may pose to men. There is growing evidence that many substances may be damaging to sperm, thereby creating the possibility of birth defects in offspring. The emphasis on reproductive hazards to women thus is an unjustifiably narrow means of protecting children's health. If society deems the health of potential future children to justify the blanket exclusion of fertile women from certain research protocols, the exclusion should cover *all* fertile subjects whose offspring could be endangered, not just female ones. Furthermore, men's lengthier reproductive capacity could lead to their exclusion from risky studies for many more years than women.

The final rationale for women's exclusion from study populations involves alleged recruitment difficulties. For example, researchers in the aspirin and heart disease study claimed that they wanted to include women, but were unable to find enough potential subjects to do so. Their study population was physicians over age forty, they explained, and women comprised only 10 percent of this group. Moreover, according to one NIH official, it was doubtful that a sufficient number of women would be "interested in participating and be content to go through the hassle of taking a placebo." In other heart disease studies, researchers

have asserted that they could not locate enough women with the condition. Although this is partly due to the lower overall incidence and later development of this disease among women, it turns out that another factor is the medical community's failure to recognize serious heart disease in women.

Blaming the scarcity of potential women subjects for the exclusionary practice is unacceptable. In effect, this adds insult to injury by building on past bias to justify its perpetuation in a different realm. The traditional exclusion of women from the medical profession is the source of the small number of middle-aged women physicians. Health stereotypes about women—"women just don't get heart disease"; "women somaticize their emotional problems"— are one source of physicians' failure to recognize heart disease in women. As one physician put it,

> If a fifty-year-old man goes to the doctor
> complaining of chest pains, the next day he
> will be on a treadmill taking a stress test. If a
> fifty-year-old woman goes to the doctor and
> complains of chest pains, she will be told to
> go home and rest.

When heart disease studies exclude women, they only reinforce physicians' misplaced assumptions. And why was it assumed that women would be less interested than men in "go[ing] through the hassle of taking a placebo"? Women who were adequately informed of their risk of heart disease would have as much incentive as men to participate in the study.

Biomedical research studies should be designed to surmount the alleged difficulties in recruiting women. If enough female physicians are not available, why not study female nurses, or some other reasonably accessible group of women? [...] If scientists conducting heart disease research are afraid that physicians will not refer enough women patients, then extra recruiting measures should be taken to ensure that they do. Research costs may go up, but the benefits of including women subjects are worth the expense.

WHAT'S WRONG WITH EXCLUSION

The current disparity between the health information we have about white males and the information we have about women and people of color contravenes basic ethical principles governing human experimentation. Most clearly violated is the principle of beneficence, which holds that biomedical research should be designed to maximize benefit and minimize harm. Proposals promising to advance knowledge of important human health and welfare concerns should receive funding priority. Awarding support to studies on white males withholds research benefits from other groups of people and possibly exposes such people to risk when they and their physicians follow recommendations based on data from white male subjects. When diseases disproportionately affecting women and people of color are given low funding priority, knowledge that could alter current ineffective or detrimental routine medical care is never produced.

The harm produced by the exclusionary practices is not easily dismissed. Simple extrapolation from white males to everyone else can be dangerous. One study, for example, found that due to physiological differences, African-Americans given the "normal" dose of lithium (established in trials on white men) frequently experienced toxic reactions, heightening their already high risk of renal failure. Similarly, the male-only studies of heart disease and cholesterol led the American Heart Association to recommend a diet that could actually exacerbate the risk of heart disease for women. Oral contraceptives can cause excessive cholesterol levels, yet it has not been systematically demonstrated that the cholesterol-lowering medication proven effective in men works when taken in conjunction with oral contraceptives. The current lack of knowledge on the connection between diet and breast cancer denies women a potential opportunity to protect themselves against a frequently lethal disease that strikes one in nine women. Antiseizure and antidepressant drugs may require different doses over the menstrual cycle to achieve their desired effect, and the failure to calibrate asthma medication to this cycle may contribute to the existing premenstrual rise in asthma deaths.

Scientists and policymakers must recognize that the choice is not whether to protect women and people of color from research risks. Instead, the choice is whether to expose some consenting members of these groups to risk in the closely monitored research setting, or to expose many more of them to risk in the clinical setting without these safeguards, which is the result of the current approach.

The present situation is also unjust. The justice principle mandates fair distribution of the benefits and burdens of biomedical research. But instead, taxpayers excluded from study populations have been charged for research without the assurance that they will share in any health benefits it might produce. Historically disadvantaged groups have subsidized health benefits for the more privileged, while being denied similar benefits for themselves.

The modern response to past injustice in the selection of human subjects may have contributed to the current imbalance in study populations. Ethical codes governing experimentation on human subjects arose primarily in reaction to the horrors of the Nazi experiments, the Tuskegee syphilis study, and other research on vulnerable populations that exposed uninformed and unconsenting persons to extreme harm for the benefit of the better off. Hence, the overall reform goal was to eliminate such practices. This may have led to the notion that white middle- and upper-class men were the best people to bear the burdens of research participation. But these burdens have now been substantially reduced, while participation offers significant benefit to the members of other racial and ethnic groups. A move perhaps designed to protect disadvantaged groups has simply shifted potential harm away from research subjects and imposed it on people in the community who may be receiving inappropriate health information and medical treatment.

"Tuskegee fallout" probably has contributed in an additional way to the present underrepresentation of people of color in study populations. In light of past scandals, some members of disadvantaged communities are justifiably suspicious of the research establishment's motivation in seeking their participation as subjects. But this product of past abuses ought not excuse the current underrepresentation. People of color also continue to experience a disproportionate share of economic, health care, and other deprivation that creates barriers to their research participation. Today's researchers face the task of educating these communities on the positive dimensions of research participation. Special support services may be necessary to facilitate the participation of those who wish to serve as subjects, including child care and transportation assistance. Furthermore, society has an obligation to ensure that members of these communities actually have access to any health care benefits produced by the research in which they participate.

THE HIDDEN ROOTS OF EXCLUSION

How did white males come to be the prototype of the human research subject? Like the pronoun "he," it was taken for granted that the white male subject stood for all of us. In her examination of how the law treats differences among people, Martha Minow suggests some reasons for this. As individuals, she points out, we are all different from everyone else in countless ways. In society, however, certain differences are deemed relevant to how people are regarded. The choice of which differences "matter" inevitably reflects and reinforces existing social structures, and normality and abnormality are determined by the most powerful social group's (usually unstated) point of reference. Accordingly, "women are different in relation to the unstated male norm. Blacks, Mormons, Jews, and Arabs are different in relation to the unstated white Christian norm." Members of the dominant group making decisions in reliance on this norm may discount or be oblivious to the influence of their particular perspective. To the contrary, they see themselves as "objective," and the existing social structure as "normal."

It is easy to see this process at work in the research setting. NIH officials and biomedical researchers have, consciously or unconsciously, defined the white male as the normal, representative human being. From this perspective, the goal of advancing human health can be achieved by studying the white male human model. Physical differences between males and females, or between whites and people of color, are unacknowledged or irrelevant in this world view. Including women and people of color would simply complicate the work, thus making it more difficult and costly, which would detract from the researchers' mission of improving human health and welfare. According to this world view, "special money" must be raised to study women and people of color, so that the "regular money" can be reserved for "normal" research.

Perhaps there was also a more insidious influence on the decisions about study populations. At least some scientists and government officials might have believed it was not important even to find out whether data from studies on white males applied to women and people of color. We cannot dismiss the possibility that the exclusionary practice reflected implicit social worth judgments on who ought to have priority in obtaining the fruits of biomedical research. An emphasis on the economic costs of human disease could also have inadvertently contributed to the view that research should focus on the "normal" economic contributor, that is the young or middle-aged white male.

In attempting to trace the origins of the exclusionary practice, we must consider as well the identity of the major players in the research establishment. Science has been and to some extent still is largely populated by white males. [...] A white male–dominated group will assess the nation's biomedical research priorities from a particular vantage point. Decisions by such a group could intentionally or inadvertently undervalue the health concerns of "outsiders." When one researcher asked investigators about the exclusion of African-Americans from clinical trials, many responded that they simply had "never thought about" the matter. [...]

An overly simplistic concept of equality might also have helped to create homogeneous study populations. In many social contexts, advancing the ideal of equality requires decision-makers to disregard gender, racial, and ethnic differences among people. If all human beings have equal moral value, then in some sense they are identical and interchangeable. If all people are identical, then it might appear that any human subject could adequately represent the general human population. In this framework, it would be unnecessary to recruit research subjects according to their gender, race, or ethnicity; the white male subject could stand for everyone. Gender, racial, and ethnic differences that affect health and disease must, however, be recognized if women and people of color are to have truly equal access to the health benefits of biomedical research.

REMEDYING THE SITUATION: THE DOWNSIDE

Even though there are compelling reasons to conduct research on the possible health effects of gender, race, and ethnicity, one must also acknowledge that adverse consequences could flow from such research. Studies of women and particular racial and ethnic groups could indicate that these populations are more susceptible to conditions that reinforce group stereotypes. Thus, for example, research suggesting that monthly hormone fluctuations make women more prone than men to depression and other emotional disturbances could become potent ammunition for those seeking to exclude women from important policy positions. Certain evidence indicating significant physiological differences between men and women could trigger controversy similar to that surrounding Carol Gilligan's work on gender differences in psychological and moral development, which some feminists see as strengthening the traditional picture of women as nurturing, sacrificing, and passive. When gender, racial, and ethnic differences are characterized as "natural," they may be deemed impervious to change. The role of environment in shaping human physiology and behavior can be ignored, thus reducing the pressure to minimize the environmental sources of difference.

Moreover, as Gilligan reminds us, our culture "hasn't been able to represent difference without hierarchy." There is a danger that studies finding gender, racial, and ethnic health differences will be used to support unjust discrimination against historically excluded groups. The employment and other discrimination experienced by African-Americans carrying sickle-cell trait is just one example of this pattern. Meanwhile, the potential value of certain health differences found in these groups could be ignored. For instance, women's relative physical endurance and longevity are differences that could justify a female-dominated workforce in at least some settings. Yet this biological advantage has had virtually no influence on employment policy; instead, policies tend to focus on pregnancy and family-related "problems" of employing women.

THE LESSONS OF EXCLUSION

The revelations of gender and other biases in the study of human health reminds us of how far we are from fully escaping the discriminatory legacies of the past. Much of our current social structure still embodies, albeit often inadvertently, the idea that the white man is the best to represent all people. Yet in many significant respects, he is not. Biomedical research must respond to this reality.

The immediate task for scientists and government officials involves revamping study design and reordering funding priorities to remedy past exclusionary practices. The NIH and other funding agencies should back up their paper policies with concrete implementation measures, including the added financial expenditures that may be necessary to ensure more representative study populations. There is also a need for more carefully reasoned policies governing the inclusion of women—and men—of reproductive potential in clinical research. Institutional review boards ought to consider explicitly the composition of proposed study populations in determining whether the selection of subjects is equitable. But the remedies also extend beyond this realm. One task is to continue and to redouble the effort to reduce the disproportionate representation of white men in important scientific and policy positions. Diversity among powerful decisionmakers is one of the best methods to guard against conscious as well as unconscious discriminatory practices.

Second is the challenge to use the emerging knowledge about biological differences for the benefit of historically disadvantaged groups. Perhaps we have come far enough to recognize such differences without transforming them into tools for maintaining the traditional social hierarchy. Particular biological characteristics of women and members of nonwhite racial and ethnic groups must not be viewed through the narrow prism of the status quo, which too frequently labels "difference" as "problem." From a wider perspective, the contributions of people who are "different" can in some cases be "better." Moreover, sometimes, as Martha Minow has noted, it is the system that should adjust to embrace the difference. The goal is to move beyond the restrictive traditional patterns of labeling difference toward a richer, more expansive view. [...]

---

25 Why Should We Include Women and Minorities in Randomized Controlled Trials?

CHARLES WEIJER AND ROBERT A. CROUCH

THE EXCLUSION OF WOMEN AND MINORITIES FROM CLINICAL TRIALS

Ethical issues in the selection of subjects for participation in clinical research have evolved over the last 30 years. [...] In the 1990s, a new issue has engendered considerable debate among ethicists, scientists, and regulators, namely, the applicability of research results to women and members of racial and ethnic minority groups.

Rebecca Dresser touched off the debate with an article in which she claimed that "the failure to include women in research populations is ubiquitous." [...] Quantifying the representation of women and minorities in clinical trials has proven difficult due to the lack of a centralized registry and incomplete reporting in trial communications. Despite these obstacles, the report of the Institute of Medicine's Committee on the Ethical and Legal Issues Relating to the Inclusion of Women in Clinical Studies (hereafter the IOM Report) concludes: "Although the committee was unable to establish that gender inequity existed in the whole of past clinical research, it was able to find evidence relevant to this issue in two areas of disease research: AIDS and heart disease. In both fields, there is some evidence of studies that either exclude women altogether or include them in num-

Charles Weijer and Robert A. Crouch, "Why Should We Include Women and Minorities in Randomized Controlled Trials?" *Journal of Clinical Ethics* 10 (1999): 100–106.

bers too small to yield meaningful information about their treatment...."

A variety of harms may ensue from the failure to include adequate numbers of women and members of minority groups in clinical trials. Women and minorities may be exposed to ineffective treatments, unexpected side-effects may occur, and delays may ensue in the diagnosis and treatment of disease. Indeed, there is evidence that women suffering from heart disease have incurred some of these harms. Women with heart disease are less likely to receive diagnostic and therapeutic procedures than men with equivalent disease. Furthermore, heart disease tends to be more advanced in women by the time they receive surgery and, perhaps as a result, women have a higher operative mortality rate for coronary artery bypass.

NIH GUIDELINES

[...] In 1993 the Food and Drug Administration removed barriers to the inclusion of women of "childbearing potential" in early-stage clinical trials and encouraged, but stopped short of requiring, the representative inclusion of women in clinical trials. Perhaps the most important policy statement, however, is the National Institutes of Health Guidelines on the Inclusion of Women and Minorities as Subjects in Clinical Research (hereafter, the NIH Guidelines) issued in March of 1994. The NIH Guidelines outline a wide range of new responsibilities for clinical researchers funded by the NIH and for institutional review boards (IRBs). All NIH-funded clinical research must now include representative numbers of women and members of racial or ethnic minority groups. Furthermore, phase III randomized controlled trials (RCTs), trials designed to change clinical practice, must ensure that the efficacy of new treatments in women and racial and ethnic minority groups is proven adequately. [...]

SCIENTIFIC AND ETHICAL JUSTIFICATIONS FOR THE NIH GUIDELINES

A variety of valid scientific and ethical justifications have been marshaled in support of the NIH Guidelines. Scientific justifications have focused on the issue of generalizability, that is, the applicability of study results to the target population of patients in clinical practice. "To whom are the results of research applicable?" is a question that trial designers, clinical researchers, and practitioners must constantly confront. If biologically relevant subgroups of patients have not been included in a clinical trial, it is inappropriate to generalize study results to such excluded groups. Accordingly, the issue of scientific generalizability is the prime motivating factor expressed in the NIH Guidelines:

> Since a primary aim of research is to provide scientific evidence leading to a change in health policy or a standard of care, it is imperative to determine whether the intervention or therapy being studied affects women or men or members of minority groups and their subpopulations differently. To this end, the guidelines published here are intended to ensure that all future NIH-supported biomedical and behavioral research involving human subjects will be carried out in a manner sufficient to elicit information about individuals of both genders and the diverse racial and ethnic groups and, in the case of clinical trials, to examine differential effects on such groups.

Ethical justifications of the NIH Guidelines complement and strengthen the scientific basis of the policy. The ethical principle of justice requires that the burdens and benefits of research participation be distributed equitably. The systematic exclusion of women and minorities is unjust because it does not allow excluded groups to share in the benefits of research, including knowledge regarding optimal medical treatment:

> In the most general sense, the failure to match study groups with target user groups can cause the unstudied or understudied group to receive no medical treatment, ineffective medical treatment, or even harmful

treatment. . . . Under the distributive paradigm, what steps might be required to remedy the injustice of excluding women from clinical studies? The minimum measure required is the appropriate inclusion of women in future clinical studies. . . .

Thus, an appeal to distributive justice [as the IOM Report does in the above quote] provides an argument for the representative inclusion of women in clinical studies.

While justice-based approaches have convincingly defended the representative inclusion of women and minorities in clinical research, important aspects of the NIH Guidelines remain without an explicit moral justification. Specifically, justice theorists have been silent on important questions: Must the efficacy of all new treatments be proven separately (for example, in trials or subgroups with high statistical power) for women and racial or ethnic minorities? If not for all new treatments, then which ones? Wholeheartedly supporting the importance of the NIH Guidelines, we seek to provide a moral justification for the aspects of the guidelines relating to subgroup analysis. Thereby, we hope to bolster the moral imperative for trial designers, researchers, and IRBs to implement the NIH Guidelines fully. It is our thesis that the justification of these aspects of the document does not lie with an appeal to justice, but rather Freedman's notion of clinical equipoise, one component of the ethical principle of beneficence.

SETTING UP THE MORAL PROBLEM

Our ethical analysis, then, must address the question: How many subjects from a given subgroup need to be included in a trial in order to provide a sound basis for the treatment's generalizability to clinical practice? We take it as uncontroversial that if no subjects from a group defined by some factor of potential biological (or clinical) importance are included in a trial, no valid inference can be made regarding the treatment's efficacy to that group. But is the inclusion of a representative proportion of individuals from a given group in a trial a sufficient basis to conclude that the treatment is proven effective in—for example, can be generalized to—that group? Or must we prove the effectiveness of a treatment for *each* group by means of a formal demonstration of a statistically and clinically significant difference in favor of the study treatment?

One attempt at a solution to this problem might begin by considering the plausibility of the following premise: A trial large enough to allow for a separate and sufficiently powerful comparison for each group of biological or clinical interest is to be preferred over a smaller trial designed to determine the overall effect. Indeed, this claim is consistent with the text of the original NIH Revitalization Act of 1993 (P.L. 103-43)—the act of Congress leading to the NIH

Guidelines—which required large clinical trials, studies powerful enough to prove treatments effective separately for men and women, in nearly all cases. [...] This approach was explicitly rejected by the authors of the IOM Report and implicitly eschewed by the authors of the NIH Guidelines. While the authors of the IOM Report argue against the approach on scientific and pragmatic grounds, no principled ethical rationale opposing it is forthcoming. What principled ethical objection might be voiced to such a universal requirement?

Prior to answering this question, one must first recognize the profound practical problems that such a requirement presents. Depending on the number of groups of biological or clinical interest, studies that are designed to detect treatment differences in clinically relevant subgroups will be much larger indeed than those designed to show an overall effect. Consider the example given by Yusuf et al.: Suppose one is planning an RCT to examine the effect of β-blockers on post–myocardial infarction mortality. The expected mortality in the control group is approximately 10 percent and the expected mortality in the experimental arm is 7.5 percent (a relative mortality reduction of 25 percent). If power is set at 90 percent and two-sided significance level at 0.01, then just under 4,000 subjects will be required in each of the two study arms, for a total of about 8,000 subjects. Suppose now that we wish to examine the effect of the treatment separately in two groups, anterior infarctions and inferior infarctions. Holding all else constant, the trial will now require 16,000 subjects. Of course, there may be many other groups of interest—women versus men, older versus younger, class of cardiovascular disability (four classes)—and the sample size of the trial will increase proportional to the product (in this case, $2 \times 2 \times 4$) of the number of categories of interest. Clearly, as acknowledged by the authors of the IOM Report, the feasibility of this approach to trials is questionable—a single trial may consume all the resources that a funding agency has available.

But there is an even more vexing problem with this approach and it is of an ethical rather than a purely pragmatic or scientific nature. If we assume that the treatment effect is constant across the groups of interest (and that accrual to each of the groups is uniform), then an analysis for average effect will reach statistical significance long before the comparisons in the individual groups. This will leave the investigators in the uncomfortable position of "knowing" that *on average* the experimental treatment is superior to the control treatment, and yet being forced to continue the trial to allow this effect to be proven—or not—in each of the subgroups. As such, continuing the trial in this circumstance seems to violate the Declaration of Helsinki. [...]

Underlying this dilemma is a basic question of medical epistemology [...] that gets at the heart of the ethical permissibility of clinical research: When has a treatment been *proven* effective? When ought/must we stop a trial?

One approach to this problem is to examine the conditions that must exist *ab initio* for a trial to be ethical; if and when, during the conduct of the trial, these conditions no longer obtain, the trial must then be stopped.

THE LENS OF CLINICAL EQUIPOISE

It is widely accepted that at the beginning of an RCT comparing two or more treatments, an honest null hypothesis must exist. In other words, uncertainty must exist as to the comparative merits of the treatments being tested in the trial. Some authors have argued that this means that the treatments in a trial must be precisely balanced—a state referred to as "theoretical equipoise"—that is, no empirical grounding for a preference for one treatment over another in a trial can exist. As Freedman has correctly pointed out, however, this understanding of equipoise is all-too-fragile: the fate of a single patient in an RCT could throw the balance in favor of one treatment or the other, thus requiring that the trial be stopped. Freedman has persuasively argued for a different, and more robust, conception of equipoise termed "clinical equipoise." Clinical equipoise exists when there is an honest, professional disagreement in the community of expert clinicians as to the preferred treatment. Thus, an RCT is ethically permissible if the following conditions obtain:

> At the start of the trial, there must be a state of clinical equipoise regarding the merits of the regimens to be tested, and the trial must be designed in such a way as to make it reasonable to expect that, if it is successfully concluded, clinical equipoise will be disturbed. In other words, the results of a successful trial should be convincing enough to resolve the dispute among clinicians.

If the yardstick of a successful and ethical RCT is its ability to settle dispute with regard to treatment preference among expert clinicians, then the need for an overall demonstration of the superiority of one agent over another versus the demonstration of superiority in a set of clinically relevant subgroups will depend on the skepticism in the expert community with regard to the universal applicability of the treatments to a patient population. Since medical practice is evidence-based, this skepticism will largely be a function of the existence of evidence (or substantial theoretical considerations) that one or more of the treatments is likely to have substantially different effects in one or more subgroups. In the absence of strong evidence for such a differential therapeutic effect, we would contend, the demonstration of the superiority of one treatment in the aggregate is likely to be sufficient to resolve the disagreement among expert practitioners. Since, at this point, clinical equipoise is disturbed, the conditions for the ethical permissibility of the trial have been altered and, hence, the trial must be stopped. One treatment is now (at least *in potentio*) held by expert practitioners to be superior, and therefore, continuing to enroll subjects to the other treatment arms would be unacceptable since they would be deprived of the "best proven . . . therapeutic methods."

If, on the other hand, strong evidence exists that a subgroup of the patient population may respond substantially differently from the rest of the population—perhaps the group is thought to be more likely to suffer serious adverse effects, or, for some reason, is thought less likely to benefit from the treatment—the RCT ought to be designed to be sufficiently powerful to convincingly answer the question for each of the groups in question. The demonstration of an advantage for one treatment in the aggregate is, in this case, not likely to sway practice; thus, the trial ought to be continued in these groups until the question is answered for these groups. Since, at this point in the trial (that is, when only proof for an average effect exists), clinical equipoise has not been disturbed, no patient is disadvantaged in terms of his or her medical treatment by the trial's continuation. Indeed, since it is a characteristic of an ethical trial that the "results of a successful trial should be convincing enough to resolve the dispute," it would be unethical to stop the trial prematurely.

What is the proper place for subgroup analyses in the first of these two scenarios, that is, when no strong evidence exists *a priori* for a differing effect in different groups? A number of excellent reviews of the use and interpretation of subgroup analyses in those trials designed around the investigation of an aggregate effect have recently appeared and bring to light several important points. The first is that the average effect across subgroups is the most reliable indicator of the effect of a treatment. Thus, if the overall result of the trial is negative, subgroup analyses are to be discouraged. Conversely, if the overall result of a trial is positive, that is, the experimental treatment is shown (overall) to be superior to the standard treatment, the absence of a statistically significant effect in some subgroups should not be interpreted as a lack of efficacy in those subgroups, but rather, as an indication that these statistical comparisons are likely to be substantially underpowered. Returning to our example of the β-blocker trial with 8,000 subjects enrolled, if the true effect of the treatment is a 25 percent mortality reduction, and this is true for the subgroups of anterior and inferior myocardial infarctions, an analysis done separately for each of the two subgroups will only have a power of 56 percent. Thus, assuming that the subgroup analyses are independent of each other, there is only a 31 percent chance that both subgroup analyses will conclude that the treatment is effective. Thus, when no prior convincing evidence exists for a differential therapeutic effect in subgroups, subgroup analyses should be understood as being useful for generating hypotheses for future study, but never for confirming *ad hoc*, exploratory hypotheses.

An analysis of the problem through the lens of clinical equipoise provides us with moral clarity with regard to the question of "adequate proof" for new treatments for women and members of minority groups. Thus, aspects of the NIH Guidelines pertaining to subgroup analysis are given not only a firm *scientific* grounding, but an *ethical* justification as well. That scientific and ethical analyses lead to an identical solution will, perhaps to some, seem surprising. There are at least two reasons for the identity of outcomes in this case: First, although the argumentation presented in the NIH Guidelines refers only to generalizability of research findings, the authors of the NIH Guidelines invoke the notion of "clinical equipoise" in another publication and it may be that their analysis was guided, at least in part, by it.

Second, and most importantly, clinical equipoise frames the ethical preconditions of clinical research as an issue in medical epistemology. The patient's right to good medical treatment is rooted in the physician-patient relationship; and what constitutes "good treatment" is defined by practice accepted by the community of expert practitioners. As Freedman notes, the ethical and normative meaning of a treatment preference for a patient population should not be based on "anything less than evidence publicly presented and convincing to the clinical community." Thus, equipoise maps out an overlapping area of ethical and scientific concern.

The importance of this realization for the scope of inquiry in the ethics of research can scarcely be overstated. Research ethicists have long worked at the fringes of science, concerning themselves with matters of "pure" ethical interest, for example, informed consent, or defining the limits of permissible scientific endeavor, for example, risk-benefit analysis. In requiring that *ab initio* "the results of a successful trial should be convincing enough to resolve the dispute among clinicians," clinical equipoise implies that aspects of the design of clinical trials are matters of ethical concern. Questions typically regarded as solely within the domain of science are now open to ethical analysis: What question will be asked? What will be tested? Who will be tested? How many will be tested? To whom will the results apply? When will the test be complete? Thus, clinical equipoise, fully and properly understood, requires that ethicists engage scientists in a dialogue as to the nature of good science.

In this article we have addressed but one of these questions, namely, To whom will the results apply? Clinical equipoise prescribes how a study ought to be designed in accord with the evidence that exists at the beginning of a trial as to the likelihood of clinically relevant differences in treatment effect among subgroups. In the absence of strong evidence (or substantial theoretical grounds) for a differential effect, a trial designed to demonstrate an aggregate effect ought to be mounted and recruitment should attempt to ensure that the study population mirrors the target population. The proper role of *post hoc* subgroup analyses in this case is hypothesis generating, that is, a substantial difference in treatment effect in a subgroup ought to generate further study. If, however, strong evidence does exist that a different response to treatment is likely in differing groups, then the trial must be designed to demonstrate efficacy separately in each of the relevant groups. Difficult questions remain at the interface of compensatory justice and clinical equipoise. For example, in the context of a disease affecting both genders, may a study including only women be mounted on the justification that women have historically been excluded from the study of this particular disease? Further work ought to explore this important area.

FURTHER CONSEQUENCES

While our analysis provides a firmer ethical foundation for the NIH Guidelines as written, it also suggests that the scope of the guidelines be expanded. First, the arguments we lay out support the inclusion of all biologically important subgroups and not just women and minority groups. Other groups have been excluded from important lines of clinical investigation and the NIH Guidelines fail to capture this problem. For example, the elderly have long been excluded from cancer RCTs despite the fact that they carry the largest share of the burden of the disease. This practice has led to a serious lack of information regarding the proper treatment of older persons with cancer and puts older persons with cancer at risk of under-treatment. Our analysis suggests that trial designers, researchers, and IRBs should be concerned about the proper inclusion and data analysis of any biologically important subgroup.

Second, the force of the ethical argument carries implications for all human subject research, not merely that which is funded by the NIH. We realize, of course, that the stipulation in the NIH Guidelines regarding funding source is a matter of jurisdiction. Nonetheless, it is our belief that both clinical trialists who design and implement RCTs, and IRBs who regulate such trials, could profitably adopt the approach outlined in the NIH Guidelines.

---

26   The Duty to Exclude

Excluding People at Undue Risk from Research

CHARLES WEIJER AND ABRAHAM FUKS

DEATH IN WINNIPEG

In 1989, a 34-year-old woman with severe asthma was recruited to a clinical trial explicitly designed for mild to moderate asthmatic patients. As the trial initiated with a 1-week placebo washout, she was immediately deprived of the theophylline preparation upon which she depended. Within 12 [hours] of the first placebo dose, the day after beginning the trial, she died in status asthmaticus. How is it that someone so vulnerable to the particular risks of this trial could be enrolled? Could the trial have been designed so as to avert such an event?

To answer these questions, we offer a hypothesis and a proposal. The trial was designed as a "double-blind, placebo-controlled, cross-over comparison of Volmax

Charles Weijer and Abraham Fuks, "The Duty to Exclude: Excluding People at Undue Risk from Research," *Clinical and Investigative Medicine* 17 (1994): 115–22.

(Salbutamol controlled release) tablets and Theo-Dur (Theophylline sustained release) tablets in the control of nocturnal asthma." Patients with severe asthma (brittle asthmatics; those requiring maintenance high dose steroids; and those who had intensive care admissions) were *implicitly* excluded by the following inclusion criterion for the protocol: "Patients must be diagnosed as having mild to moderate reversible airways obstruction (FEV_1 [forced expiratory volume in 1 second] 60–80% of predicted value) with nocturnal symptoms."

The patient in question was described by her own physician as a "severe asthmatic." How is it, then, that this woman was accrued to this trial? It is not uncommon for patients who are ineligible for a particular trial to be accrued. In other instances, eligibility criteria require the subjective interpretation of the clinician. Examples of this include "severe asthmatic" or "life expectancy of 10 years." In this instance, we speculate that this woman was included in the trial because her FEV_1 was within the limits required by the inclusion criterion. In clinical medicine, the FEV$_1$ alone is an inadequate measure for the determination of asthma severity. This determination will depend primarily on the patient's history. What medications does the patient take? How frequent are the attacks? Have steroids been required for long periods? Has intensive care admission for mechanical ventilation been required? It seems that, in this instance, these questions may not have been asked.

The response at this juncture is immediate, and *prima facie* reasonable. The eligibility criteria should have been more explicit so as to exclude this patient. However, could any finite list of eligibility criteria exclude all patients at undue risk? We think not. Ultimately, especially in the oncologic setting, many important determinations, such as performance status, life expectancy, and tolerance of experimental therapies, rest upon the judgment of the clinician. Factors such as these are often listed as eligibility criteria but, by their very nature, require clinical interpretation; clinical judgment is the necessary lens though which these criteria are viewed. In addition, there will be potential subjects for a trial whose specific risk factors cannot be foreseen and, hence, are not captured by the eligibility criteria of the trial. [...] Short of the absurd exclusion of all persons from participation, no set of eligibility criteria can offer protection to such vulnerable subjects. Hence, we must turn to the clinical judgment of the investigator to achieve this end.

Exigencies of science certainly demand that the clinical investigator adhere to the inclusion and exclusion criteria set forth, particularly in multi-centre trials. The clinical investigator has, however, a more fundamental and overriding obligation to the individual research subject, namely, the duty to protect. Although fatalities of the type described above are rare in clinical trials, serious side effects, such as grade IV toxicities and idiosyncratic reactions, are not infrequent across the scope of therapeutic and non-therapeutic clinical trials. There are relatively few empirical studies examining harm to research subjects. From this work, it would seem that therapeutic trials present a greater risk of harm to subjects than non-therapeutic trials. Arnold studied the incidence of harm due to research in a series of 3,772 research subjects: 2,573 enrolled in phase I trials, and 1,199 enrolled in phase II–IV trials. In his study, all 6 deaths and 36 of the 41 adverse clinical events requiring hospitalization occurred among the phase II–IV trial participants. Provocatively, of the 57 injuries resulting in death or permanent injury in Cardon's survey of 133,000 research subjects, the majority were related to cancer chemotherapy. (Cardon's survey may have underestimated the true incidence of research harm, as it depended on the recollection of the investigator during a telephone interview.)

Given the importance of this problem, we would like to examine the ethical and legal underpinnings of the duty of the clinical investigator to protect research subjects. We will further suggest that this duty ought to be reinforced by having the clinical investigator sign a statement to the effect that his or her duty has been responsibly discharged for each patient accrued to a clinical trial. [...]

THE DUTY TO EXCLUDE VULNERABLE PATIENTS

The clinical investigator, as either a named investigator in a single-institution study or as a cooperative group-registered investigator in a multi-centre study, has a clear scientific obligation to adhere to the eligibility criteria of a clinical trial protocol. We believe that the investigator has a responsibility to protect research subjects that goes beyond adherence to the inclusion and exclusion criteria. The clinical investigator's duty to protect research subjects from harm derives clearly from the principle of non-maleficence. This principle entails that not only must investigators not harm subjects, they must also protect them from undue risk of being harmed. The obligation to protect research subjects from harm is clearly expressed in several canonical codes of research ethics. A clear statement occurs in the *United States* v. *Karl Brandt* (commonly referred to as the Nuremberg Code): "No experiment should be conducted where there is an *a priori* reason to believe that death or disabling injury will occur. . . ." This requirement is reflected in the code of ethics of the Canadian Medical Association as follows: "An ethical physician . . . will ensure that, before initiating clinical research involving humans . . . the individuals are unlikely to suffer any harm." [...]

The moral axiom to protect research subjects from harm applies both to subjects as members of a group and to subjects as individuals. [...] As a group, then, research subjects may not be exposed to research that is inherently very risky either to an individual or to that group. For example, it would neither be permissible to give healthy subjects potentially fatal toxic substances nor to subject patients with advanced cardiac disease to a protocol that required extreme exertion. As an individual, a research subject may not be exposed to research which is inherently very risky for him or her. For example, it would not be permissible to recruit a cardiac patient with concurrent asthma to a trial involving a β-blocker. It would be similarly impermissible to expose a post–myocardial infarction patient to the risks of a trial that included ASA [i.e., aspirin—eds.] if that person were known to have an idiopathic hypersensitivity to that drug.

The clinical world is, naturally enough, not so black and white. There are patients for whom the added risk of a particular trial is merely suspected. There are also clinical situations where the benefits of the trial for the patient outweigh minor increments of added risk. In such circumstances the following applies (again, *United States* v. *Karl*

Brandt): "Proper preparations should be made and adequate facilities provided to protect the experimental subject against *even remote possibilities* of injury, disability, or death [emphasis added]." This implies taking extra precautions for patients who may be minimally more vulnerable to the risks of a trial. For example, if a patient with a minimal cardiac history is included in a drug trial, cardiac monitoring may be appropriate even when this is above and beyond the requirements of the protocol *per se.*

Other canons of research ethics have included these obligations more generally under an obligation to minimize risk to subjects. The Department of Health and Human Services Regulations, for example, require that "risks to subjects are minimized . . . [and that] risks to subjects are reasonable in relation to anticipated benefits, if any, to subjects and [to] the importance of the knowledge that may reasonably be expected to result." Following this line, Levine states that "[e]thical codes and regulations require not only that risks be justified by being in a favorable relationship to hoped-for benefits but also that they be minimized. . . . Prescreening tests may be done to identify prospective subjects who ought to be excluded because they are vulnerable to injury." With reasoning parallel to our own, an obligation to minimize risk to research subjects is taken to entail an obligation to screen (and exclude) unduly vulnerable patients. Levine continues:

> In consideration of harm, is there any means by which individuals who are most susceptible to harm might be identified? If so, will these means be used and will those individuals either be excluded from the research or informed that they are especially vulnerable? For example, in planning research designed to test the effects of strenuous exercise in normal humans, one would ordinarily plan to perform various screening tests to identify individuals with coronary artery disease in order to exclude them.

In our prefatory example, this would require that patients unduly susceptible to the risks of a placebo washout period be screened for and excluded. In this and many other clinical settings, a straight-forward history and physical examination may be a sufficient additional "test." In other situations, further investigation, such as an electrocardiogram, may be required. In the assessment of a potential subject's vulnerability to harm, the clinician investigator must not forget the primary care physician as a source of invaluable information. At the very least, research protocols that may have an impact on a chronic condition of the patient, or that involve a modification of treatment for that chronic condition, demand that the prudent clinical investigator be in contact with the primary care physician.

The irreplaceable nature of clinical judgment is perhaps best illustrated by multi-agent chemotherapeutic regimens in which subjects must be deemed able to *tolerate* the experimental intervention of the trial. Aggressive multi-agent therapy in an otherwise fatal condition, e.g. acute leukemia, may entail a significant on-trial morbidity and mortality. Such a clinical trial may be justified, in that the risk-benefit ratio for the class of acute leukemia patients is deemed acceptable. The physician must nonetheless review the risk-benefit calculus for each individual prospective research subject. Some patients, whether due to organ compromise or to general frailty, may be unduly susceptible to the risks of such a trial. These patients should be excluded from trial participation by the clinical investigator and treated by some other perhaps more tolerable modality off-trial.

So then, a number of sources require that vulnerable subjects be identified and excluded whenever possible. In the (what we take to be unusual) event that such patients are included in a trial, the onus is on the clinical investigator to take special measures to ensure the safety of that *individual* subject. Having examined the ethical underpinnings of this duty, let us now turn to its legal aspects.

THE OBLIGATION TO EXCLUDE
VULNERABLE PATIENTS AND THE LAW

North American jurisprudence pertaining to clinical research is limited. In only 2 instances have subjects of nontherapeutic research sued for damages, *Halushka* v. *University of Saskatchewan* and *Weiss* v. *Solomon*, both Canadian legal cases. While *Halushka* centered on issues of consent, *Weiss* is directly relevant here.

Julius Weiss was a 62-year-old male who underwent an operation for cataracts in 1981. After the surgery, his surgeon recommended that he speak to another physician, a clinical investigator, about participating in a clinical trial testing the ability of indomethacin drops to reduce retinal edema following cataract surgery. This was to be assessed via a series of fluorescein angiograms. Seconds after being injected with fluorescein dye, Mr. Weiss had a cardiac arrest and died. The family brought forward a suit claiming in part "that Weiss, who had a long (but asymptomatic) history of hypertropic cardiomyopathy, should have been excluded from the clinical trial; failing that, he should have been informed of the rare risk of cardiac arrest resulting from a fluorescein injection, a risk they claimed to be enhanced for those with Weiss' heart ailment." The judgment was found for the plaintiffs on all counts. Several aspects of the judgment bear direct relevance to our discussion.

First, the judge clearly recognized the obligation of the clinical investigator (and the hospital via the research ethics board [REB; this is equivalent to the American institutional review board or IRB]) to protect research subjects. "While the language of the judgment does not make the bases of liability completely clear, Judge De Blois implies that the investigator and the hospital (in the person of its research committee) bore equivalent responsibilities in both these areas, and that both fell short of that required standard." This obligation to protect patients is, in the judgment, taken to entail an obligation to screen potential subjects and exclude those at undue risk. Indeed, "[w]here a research protocol exposes a subject to significant risk or where previous health conditions will increase the risk for any subject, an effective screening program would appear to be required." For failing to screen and exclude Mr. Weiss, the clinical investigator and the hospital were held liable.

Second, the referring physician, Dr. Solomon, was not held to be liable. "The . . . [referring] physician's participation in the research was limited to describing the study to Weiss in cursory fashion and suggesting that he volunteer for the trial. The . . . [referring] physician was therefore held not to have played a determining role in the research or in the subject's decision to participate." This aspect of the judgment clearly places the responsibility for protection of patients with the clinical investigator. This seems eminently sensible, as it is the clinical investigator who is most familiar with the trial, who questions and examines the patient, and who ultimately decides whether the patient is eligible for the trial or not. [. . .]

We have thus laid both the moral duty and the legal obligation to exclude vulnerable patients squarely at the feet of the clinical investigator. Have we not, however, by this, arrived at the untenable position of requiring an investigator in a large trial to see every patient individually? In small trials this may indeed be advisable. It would seem, though, that such a requirement would fetter larger trials. Can this apparent *reductio* be circumvented without losing the impact of the moral duty to protect research subjects?

DELEGABILITY

[. . .] As the duty to exclude unduly vulnerable patients is similar to the duty to obtain informed consent (it is enforced on an individual basis), an argument may be made for suggesting the permissibility of a similar division of labor between duty and function. The result of this would be that the duty to exclude vulnerable patients would remain that of the clinical investigator. Particularly with larger trials though, it would be allowable for the clinical investigator to appoint another physician or a clinical trials nurse to perform the function of screening and exclusion. It would remain the clinical investigator's duty to oversee this function and monitor its quality. Part of this function would be to ensure that the person or persons chosen to carry it out have sufficient expertise to do so competently. The qualifications required for negotiating informed consent are not identical with those required for screening subjects. (The definition of these qualifications might be useful to REBs and investigators, and may represent a fruitful area for further research.) In the event that a research subject was accrued to a trial inappropriately, the clinical investigator would remain liable. For this reason, especially in smaller trials, it may well be prudent for the clinical investigator to carry out the tasks of screening and exclusion personally. [. . .]

RECOMMENDATION

[. . .] Both a mechanism and a precedent for reinforcing the obligations of clinical investigators come from the types of statements that investigators currently sign in the conduct of clinical research. Just as the obligation to obtain consent functions on a patient-by-patient basis, so does the obligation to exclude the unduly vulnerable patient. In order to emphasize and make explicit the obligation of the clinical investigator to exclude unduly vulnerable research subjects, we recommend that he or she be required to sign a statement, appended to each consent form, that this obligation has been properly discharged. If the patient was reviewed by an appropriately qualified delegate, then the delegate would sign the statement.

The pertinent aspects of the statement would include attestation that (1) the relevant facts regarding the potential subject have been reviewed, and (2) that based on these facts and the clinical judgment of the investigator, the patient is deemed not to be at undue risk from participation in the research. Such a statement may be quite brief, we believe, and may read as follows:

> I, [name of clinical investigator], have reviewed the patient's relevant historical data, physical findings, and laboratory data and, in my clinical judgment, his or her participation in this research study will not place him or her at undue risk.

Whether such a statement is signed or not, the fact remains that the clinical investigator is both morally and legally obliged to exclude vulnerable patients. Requiring the investigator to sign such a statement for each recruited research subject will remind the investigator of this obligation and reinforce its necessity. The statement would in no case diminish the legal responsibility of investigators; indeed, it may even serve to enhance it by rendering it more explicit. [. . .]

Section Three

Payment of Research Participants

27   What's the Price of a Research Subject?

Approaches to Payment for Research Participation

Neal Dickert and Christine Grady

Successful clinical research depends on the ability to recruit research subjects. Tension between the need to recruit subjects and the obligation to offer them certain types of protection has made recruitment a persistent ethical challenge. One important and difficult issue involves whom investigators should enroll in research studies. A different but equally crucial issue concerns the types of inducement investigators should use to recruit subjects.

For decades, many investigators have paid subjects for participating in research studies, and this practice remains one of the most controversial methods of recruitment. Despite discussions over many years, ethical issues about payment remain unresolved. The predominant concern expressed is that payment of subjects might represent "undue inducement," by leading to a decrease in either the voluntariness or the understanding with which subjects agree to participate. A second concern is that the payment of subjects may result in economically disadvantaged populations' bearing an unduly large share of the risks and burdens of research participation. Many people also worry that the use of money as a recruitment tool will lead to putting subjects at risk who do not care about or support the goals of the study. Finally, some believe that the payment of subjects violates the ethical norms of the investigator-subject relationship by turning it into a commercial relationship. This worry is particularly apparent when subjects are very ill.

Although some argue that the payment of subjects is never ethical, this practice has long been an integral part of the recruitment of research participants. In fact, the payment of subjects is likely to become even more pervasive as the need to recruit grows along with the capacity for tech-

Neal Dickert and Christine Grady, "What's the Price of a Research Subject? Approaches to Payment for Research Participation," *New England Journal of Medicine* 341 (1999): 198–203.

nological discovery and the level of commercial funding for clinical research. The frequency of payment may also increase in response to requirements for greater inclusion of women, minorities, and children in research studies. As this practice becomes more frequent, it is essential to recognize that payment can be made in various ways, some of which are more ethically acceptable than others.

No consensus has emerged on when and in what manner it is ethical to pay subjects. Although federal regulations and guidelines call attention to some of the moral issues that payment raises, they offer little substantive guidance for clinical investigators, institutional review boards, or contract research organizations on how to pay subjects ethically. The federal "Common Rule" never mentions the payment of subjects, and the guidelines of the Office for Protection from Research Risks [OPRR, now the Office for Human Research Protections or OHRP—eds.] and the Food and Drug Administration (FDA) merely reflect the controversy over how to approach payment. For instance, FDA information sheets offer seemingly contradictory advice, suggesting that payment should be viewed as a "recruitment incentive" while simultaneously requiring institutional review boards to ensure that payment is not "unduly influential."

PAYING PATIENTS OR HEALTHY SUBJECTS

Most of the literature on the payment of subjects reflects the common perception that only healthy subjects—those who do not have the condition under study—are paid for their participation in clinical research. It is true that patients are rarely or never paid in some types of research, such as clinical trials of cancer chemotherapy. However, listings and advertisements of ongoing clinical trials are evidence that patients with such diseases as asthma and human immunodeficiency virus infection are frequently paid for participating in clinical research.

The ethical argument against the payment of patients rests on one or both of the following premises: patients are particularly vulnerable, and patients are deriving medical benefit in a way that healthy subjects are not. The special vulnerability of patients is most often attributed to two factors: the inability of patients to distinguish clinical care from research, often called the "therapeutic misconception," and a perceived difference in power between patients and investigators, especially when an investigator is both the clinician and the researcher. In the absence of empirical data, however, it is not clear how payment exploits either source of vulnerability. Because patients typically pay for their clinical care, it seems plausible that paying patients for participating in research may, in fact, reduce the therapeutic misconception by distinguishing the procedures that are undertaken purely for research purposes from those that are performed as part of clinical care. Paying patients may also help to minimize the power differential by making participation seem less like a "favor" the patient is being asked to do for the physician-investigator.

The second premise—that patients are deriving benefit—also fails to justify an absolute prohibition against paying patients. After all, many studies enrolling patients offer little or no prospect of direct benefit. In fact, some of these studies also involve healthy subjects who are paid to participate. For example, a researcher may use positron-emission tomography to study the differences in brain function between patients with obsessive-compulsive disorder and healthy controls. In cases in which neither patients nor healthy subjects would receive any immediate or direct benefit from the procedure, not paying patients while paying healthy subjects appears to violate the principle of justice, which demands that cases be treated alike. In studies that offer potential benefits, such as many phase 3 studies, there may be no reason to pay patients, but it is not clear why it would be unethical to do so simply because they may benefit from participating.

There is no inherent reason to treat patients and healthy subjects differently with respect to payment. Therefore, our analysis of payment generally applies to both types of participants.

THREE MODELS OF PAYMENT

In this article, we evaluate three models of payment: the market model, the wage-payment model, and the reimbursement model. Careful consideration of these models will help in choosing the most ethical approach. Other types of "payment," such as free medical services, do raise many of the same considerations, but this discussion refers only to payments in cash. Because cash payments are so pervasive and influential, and because they are more fungible than other forms of inducement, a careful analysis of their use is important.

The Market Model

The market model is grounded in traditional libertarian theory. The principle of supply and demand determines whether and how much subjects should be paid for participating in a given study at a specific site. When research is arduous or risky and offers little or no prospect of direct benefit to subjects, there is little apparent reason for a person to participate. This model allows money to be the reason. For example, money may be an incentive for a healthy person to participate in a study of natural patterns of sleep, or in a phase 1 pharmacokinetic study of a treatment for a disease the person does not have. Similarly, it may be an incentive for a patient to participate in a nontherapeutic "challenge study" to examine the pathophysiologic features of a particular condition.

Use of the market model would probably result in high payment for participation in studies that offer subjects no prospect of direct benefit, but involve risky or uncomfortable procedures. Payment may also be high when investigators want to recruit subjects very quickly, or when few people are eligible to participate. In addition, the market model sanctions the use of large completion bonuses and other incentives to encourage compliance with the protocol. After all, the value of a subject's participation is often dependent on the subject's completion of the study. The market model would, however, suggest that there be little or no payment when people are eager to enroll in a study, as may be the case for studies involving such agents as trastuzumab (Herceptin) and antiangiogenesis factors for the treatment of cancer.

The Wage-Payment Model

The wage-payment model operates on the notion that participation in research requires little skill but does require time, effort, and the endurance of undesirable or uncomfortable procedures. This model adopts the egalitarian position that subjects performing similar functions should be paid similarly. Participating in research is similar to many other forms of unskilled labor in that it requires little skill or training, may involve some risk, and often involves relatively little "labor." The wage-payment model thus involves the payment of subjects on a scale commensurate with that of other unskilled but essential jobs. Application of the wage-payment model would lead to the payment of a fairly low, standardized hourly wage, augmented by increases for particularly uncomfortable or burdensome procedures. The payment of completion bonuses is also consistent with this model; however, they should not constitute a large proportion of the payment, because this model bases payment primarily on the time subjects spend "working" (i.e., participating in the research).

The wage-payment model is not entirely distinct from

the market model, but there are two fundamental differences between them. First, in the wage-payment model, payment is set according to the unskilled-labor market rather than the supply of persons eligible for participation. Second, the wage-payment model requires standardization, both among different protocols and between research and other forms of unskilled labor.

The Reimbursement Model

According to the reimbursement model, payment is provided simply to cover subjects' expenses. This model reflects a different form of egalitarianism, and it is based on the view that research participation should not require financial sacrifice but should be "revenue neutral" for participants. One application of this model would involve reimbursing subjects only for expenditures such as travel, meals, and parking. Alternatively, use of this model could involve reimbursing subjects for their time away from work at whatever rate the subjects are typically paid in addition to reimbursement for expenses. With either version, each subject would be paid according to his or her own expenses.

The reimbursement model differs from both of the other models in three important ways. First, it precludes subjects' making a profit. Second, it does not use money to compensate for nonfinancial "expenses," such as effort or discomfort. Third, payment does not depend on any market, either for research participation or for unskilled labor.

APPLYING THE MODELS TO A CASE

Delineating the practical implications of each model is crucial; people who appear to agree in theory often use different models in determining payment for a particular study, resulting in widely divergent payment practices. Consider a study testing the effect of a protease inhibitor on the bioavailability of a narcotic pain medication. The subjects are healthy persons, and the study requires them to take the protease inhibitor daily for 12 days and to come to the clinic eight times. For two of the visits, the subjects must remain at the clinic all day. Overall, the study takes 29 hours and involves a screening examination, administration of the pain medication with serial blood collections, and follow-up. This protocol offers no direct benefit, involves the discomfort of serial blood collection, and requires taking medications that may cause diarrhea, nausea, or other side effects.

The three models would lead to very different payments for participation in this study. True application of the market model would depend on the current market. On the basis of amounts commonly offered today, it is reasonable to estimate that subjects might be paid $25 an hour, $200 for taking the medications, and a $200 completion bonus, leading to a total payment of $1,125. The wage-payment model would lead to payment of about $10 per hour, just below the 1998 total national average for non-farm production workers, as well as $50 for the inconvenience of taking the drug for two weeks and $50 for the more invasive serial blood collection. Total payment would be $390. One formulation of the reimbursement model would involve payment only for travel, meals, and parking expenses. If parking cost $3 per hour, lunch cost $6 for each of the two days the subject was required to remain at the clinic all day, and the subject traveled 40 miles round trip and was reimbursed at $0.30 per mile, total payment would be $195. Alternatively, in addition to reimbursement for their expenses, subjects could also be paid their regular wages for 29 hours. A professor might then be paid $50 per hour for a total of $1,645. Yet a student who worked outside of class for $7 per hour would receive $398. Applying the three models to this case illustrates that different models can lead to large variations in the amount paid to subjects for participating in the same study.

ADVANTAGES AND DISADVANTAGES OF EACH MODEL

The market model has four potential advantages. First, it is likely to ensure a sufficient number of subjects in the time frame in which they are needed. Similarly, large completion bonuses are likely to ensure that the subjects complete the study. A third advantage is that the market model may allow subjects to make money while making a socially beneficial contribution. Finally, this model is likely to reduce or eliminate the financial sacrifice of participation. The latter two advantages depend, of course, on the study's popularity, because this model will lead to little or no payment for participation in studies in which many subjects are eager to enroll without being paid.

Conversely, there are several possible disadvantages. One potential problem is that payment may be so high that all other factors become irrelevant to subjects' decisions to participate or to remain in research studies. Whether escalating payment can really compromise voluntariness is controversial. But, it may be ethically problematic to commercialize research participation by "hiring" subjects who are motivated only by profit or to offer very high payments to economically vulnerable groups. In addition, large total payments and completion bonuses may provide an incentive for the subject not to explore carefully the risks and benefits of the research or to conceal important health information in order to become or remain eligible for the study and thus receive payment. Finally, the market model is likely to lead to situations in which researchers are competing with each other for subjects on the basis of the amount they pay their subjects.

There are five potential advantages of the wage-payment model. First, the possibility of undue inducement or exploitation is lessened if subjects have other options for earning similar amounts of money. Second, this model would lead to the standardization of payment among studies, lessening interstudy competition based on payment and potentially creating an incentive for investigators to minimize risks to subjects. The wage-payment model reduces the financial sacrifice of participation for subjects. In addition, the wages offered by similarly risky unskilled jobs serve as a lower limit on the amount offered for paid studies. Finally, the wage-payment model allows people to be paid for work that is valuable to society.

This model may be less likely than the market model to yield a sufficient number of subjects in the desired time frame. The wage-payment model could also make paid studies attractive primarily to people with low incomes, particularly because it might involve financial sacrifice for wealthier participants. Finally, treating the subject's role as an unskilled job may be seen as inappropriately commercializing participation in research.

The reimbursement model has four potential advantages. By prohibiting monetary inducement, it not only alleviates any concern about undue inducement, but it also presents no incentive to conceal information or remain uninformed about risks and benefits. Furthermore, the reimbursement model does not preferentially induce vulnerable populations to participate. Finally, this model lessens the financial sacrifice of research participation to some degree.

The most obvious disadvantage of the reimbursement model is that it may yield an insufficient number of subjects within the desired time frame. After all, in the current climate of commercialization, it provides no incentive to participate, and it will actually require financial sacrifice for almost all subjects if time away from work is not reimbursed. The only people who would not incur additional expenses if their time were not reimbursed would be those who are already hospitalized or who are unemployed. On the other hand, if time as well as other expenses are accounted for, different people will be paid unequally for the same contribution to research, a disparity that seems unfair. The latter formulation is also likely to lead to either exorbitant costs or the targeting of low-income people in order to avoid paying higher participation costs.

THE MODEL OF CHOICE: WAGE PAYMENT

We recommend the adoption of the wage-payment model for three principal reasons. First, the wage-payment model greatly reduces the common worry about undue inducement. Because most potential subjects are likely to have other options for earning similar amounts of money, they will presumably choose participation in research when they prefer it to other options for earning an unskilled-labor wage. Given the prevalent view that subjects should to some extent support the goals of research, money should not be the only factor influencing participation. Although money may be a motivating factor in subjects' decisions, it will not have such a predominant role as to negate the influence of other considerations. Because this concern is especially important when a study is very risky, not allowing payment to escalate according to risk constitutes a crucial safeguard.

Second, standardization among studies is extremely valuable for several reasons. The minimization of competition for subjects on the basis of payment will help to contain the cost of research. Standardization also averts the creation of barriers to the success of less well funded studies and the encouragement of research on potentially lucrative drugs over equally important research on disease mechanisms and rarer diseases. Because the level of funding of a research study often correlates most closely with the commercial potential of the drug or device under study and not necessarily with its quality or social value, it is important to adopt practices that do not favor only well-funded studies. Standardized payment schedules will also be extraordinarily helpful to institutional review boards and investigators as a means of determining payments. Furthermore, not altering payments on the basis of risk creates an incentive for investigators to minimize risks in order to recruit subjects effectively.

Third, because payment is based on the contribution subjects make, the wage-payment model adheres to a basic assumption of the principle of justice: that similar people should be treated similarly. This feature represents a great advantage over the reimbursement model, according to which already well-paid subjects would be paid more than those with lower incomes enrolled in the same study. It is also an advantage over the market model, which would allow site-specific markets to lead to very different levels of payment at different sites in multi-center studies.

The disadvantages of the market model are too serious for it to be the best approach. The chances that money would overshadow such factors as risk would be greatest in the studies with the greatest risks. Even for people who believe that subjects need no protection from monetary influence, there are important reasons to reject the market model. Its likely effect on which studies are conducted and on the cost of research is profound. In addition, the potential effect of large completion bonuses on subjects' willingness to report side effects or withdraw from studies is problematic. Such an effect could compromise the validity of study data, thereby placing future patients and subjects at risk.

The reimbursement model is too restrictive, unfair, and unworkable. The mere payment of expenses incurred without reimbursement for time spent would no doubt hamper recruitment. Although reimbursement for these expenses may be incorporated into some versions of the wage-payment model, such reimbursement on its own would still entail considerable financial sacrifice for most participants. Alternatively, paying subjects the equivalent of their salaries for the time they spend participating appears unjust and will either drive up the cost of research or lead to the selection of only low-income people.

CONCLUSIONS

We believe that the wage-payment model represents the most ethical approach to paying research subjects, and we think it is an approach that can be successfully implemented through several key steps. To ensure local standardization of payment, research institutions and institutional review boards should develop specific policies or guidelines outlining how investigators should determine in which cases and in what manner to pay subjects who enroll in their studies. We also encourage the FDA and the Office for Protection from Research Risks to publish guidelines suggesting this model of payment, so that there will be more national standardization of payment practices. Finally, we encourage pharmaceutical and biotechnology companies to develop industry standards conforming to the wage-payment model.

Although we recommend the broad implementation of this model, it is important to emphasize that further investigation of the payment of research subjects is critical, given the current lack of data. Four types of research will be particularly helpful in refining this model. First, it is crucial to evaluate the extent to which the cognitive, social, and physical status of potential subjects should alter decisions about payment for research participation. Second, there is a need for empirical research to determine the ways in which offers of money affect the quality of subjects' informed consent. Third, it is important to study whether payment leads to the recruitment of a disproportionate number of poor subjects. Finally, there is a need for data on the importance of payment with respect to successful recruitment; little is known about the effect of different amounts or methods of payment on recruitment efforts.

For the present, the wage-payment model, coupled with a commitment to rigorous research, will most effectively balance the increasing need for human research subjects with adequate protection of the subjects who make such research possible.

[Table omitted—eds.]

---

28   Justice for the Professional Guinea Pig

TRUDO LEMMENS AND CARL ELLIOTT

Six news items:

In a Scottish study healthy volunteers are paid £600 to drink orange juice laced with pesticides.

In the United States the Environmental Protection Agency (EPA) announces that it will be considering guidelines to allow pesticide testing in humans. In accordance with the Food Quality Protection Act of 1996, the EPA must review 9,000 pesticides currently on the market to ensure that they meet new safety standards.

Researchers at the National Institutes of Mental Health (NIMH) and elsewhere pay healthy subjects $100 to take a hallucinogenic drug called ketamine. Ketamine is ordi-

narily used as an animal tranquilizer, but it has also gained notoriety as a street drug. Because of the alleged use of ketamine for date rape, several states have made possession of it a felony. The purpose of the NIMH studies is to induce a temporary psychotic state. Researchers argue that the studies may offer new insights into the treatment of schizophrenia.

Opposition parties in Canadian Parliament raise questions about the collaboration of the army in vaccination trials to protect soldiers against chemical agents during the Gulf War. A contract is revealed showing that a private contract research organization (CRO) has conducted these trials on healthy volunteers, offering Can$1400 for participation. The consent form raises the spectrum of a host of potential side effects, "including death."

VanTx, a CRO operating in Basel, Switzerland, and with subsidiaries in many different countries, recruited research subjects from Estonia, Poland, Macedonia, Slovakia, Peru,

Trudo Lemmens and Carl Elliott, "Justice for the Professional Guinea Pig," *American Journal of Bioethics* 1, no. 2 (2001): 51–53.

and Ecuador to participate in Phase I and II drug trials. All subjects are paid for their participation. Some are flown in from outside Switzerland. Others are asylum seekers.

A Philadelphia 'zine for human research subjects called *Guinea Pig Zero* publishes "report cards" on a number of research laboratories. Bob Helms, its publisher, gives high marks to several laboratories but criticizes others severely. He writes of incompetent venipuncturists, surly doctors and nurses, last-minute cancellations, and a patient in one study who "emerged with $7,000 in his pocket and his mind on planet Zork." *Harper's Magazine* reprints several of *Guinea Pig Zero*'s report cards. Both *Harper's* and *Guinea Pig Zero* are promptly sued by one of the criticized institutions. *Harper's* prints an apology and a retraction.

Should we be worried that healthy people are being paid to enroll in research studies? Bioethicists cannot decide and so the issue has dropped into a regulatory vacuum. U.S. and Canadian regulations and guidelines frown on paying research subjects, but they do not prohibit it. They allow researchers to pay subjects, but discourage them from paying very much, lest subjects be "unduly influenced" or "coerced" into enrolling in a study against their better judgment. Some guidelines or statutes suggest that "compensation for loss and inconvenience is acceptable," but other payment is not (for example, see the Québec Civil Code Article 25 (2)). Given this sort of waffling, it is no wonder that institutional review boards (IRBs) are baffled. How much are researchers allowed to pay a research subject undergoing a bronchoscopy? How much for a simple blood drawing? What is it worth to go without sleep for 36 hours, or to be exposed to malaria, or to try an experimental antipsychotic drug?

In the world that regulatory bodies have created, healthy subjects take part in studies because of the money, yet researchers have to pretend that the subjects are motivated by something other than money. Research subjects cannot negotiate payment, since payment is not supposed to be the focus of the transaction. Local research ethics boards are expected not to determine what is fair, but what is "undue inducement." Even worse, they must determine this on a case-by-case basis. Thus, if the research population is very poor, IRBs can plausibly conclude that payment must be kept very low, so as not to unduly induce subjects into enrolling. But if the research population is wealthy, subjects can be paid much more.

If you are a hammer everything looks like a nail; and if you are a North American bioethicist, everything looks like a problem of informed consent. But the matter of paying healthy subjects to enroll in research studies is not merely a problem of informed consent. It is a problem of exploitation. Like it or not, research on healthy subjects has become a commercial transaction. Volunteers generally take part in research studies not for humanitarian motives, but for the money. The studies they take part in are often funded or conducted by pharmaceutical companies or other large corporate bodies. In many cities these protocols take place in CROs—for-profit bodies often set up solely for the purpose of conducting research, mostly on healthy volunteers. Unlike patients, healthy volunteers have no personal stake in the illnesses to which the research might be applied. They typically volunteer in response to advertisements in the newspapers or on the Internet.

It is time to stop pretending that the relationship between for-profit, multibillion-dollar corporate entities and healthy volunteers is the same as the relationship between an academic physician-investigator and sick patients. We have argued [elsewhere] that research studies on healthy subjects—unlike research on sick patients—are best characterized as a kind of labor relation. If regulatory bodies realized this, they would be in a far better position to protect these subjects from exploitation. Labor-type legislation could give research agencies the clout of occupational health and safety agencies by giving them the power to conduct inspections and ensure that "working" conditions are safe. Collective negotiations and unionization could give research participants a stronger voice in arguing for good working conditions. Research participants could negotiate standards of payment based on the level of discomfort they are asked to undergo, the number and types of procedures, the duration of the studies, and other factors. As with worker compensation schemes, research sponsors could offer appropriate compensation schemes to provide some form of financial security in case participants are harmed in research studies.

Are there dangers to this kind of shift? Yes, absolutely. The most serious danger is that the payment argument could be hijacked to defend even more commercialization of the research enterprise and even more exploitation of vulnerable subjects. Research participants could be placed at even greater risk of exploitation if limitations on payment are simply lifted without significant regulatory overhaul. *Guinea Pig Zero* notwithstanding, research participants are not yet organized sufficiently to obtain better working relations through negotiations and labor pressure tactics. And since participating in research studies currently does not count as "employment," research participants do not even qualify for the resources and protection provided by labor legislation. When research subjects from Eastern Europe and South America were brought to Switzerland, their only goal was to make money. Yet their work did not fall under any category of labor. Immigration and labor authorities did not deal with the issue as a matter of immigration law. Occupational health and safety regulations did not protect the research participants, nor did employment regulations. Thus the issue was left in the hands of Swiss health authorities, who acted only after the media became involved in the case.

It would also be a mistake to force all research partici- pants, sick and healthy, into the same regulatory box. Dickert and Grady have argued in the *New England Journal of Medicine* that "[t]here is no inherent reason to treat pa- tients and healthy subjects differently with respect to pay- ment." But patients are in situations fundamentally differ- ent from those of healthy volunteers. Often they are vulnerable because of their illnesses. They are frequently asked to accept significant risks by forgoing standard treat- ment and accepting experimental treatment. They may have a sense of obligation toward the physician-investigator or to an institution that has provided them with care in the past. To import commercial considerations into this al- ready fragile relationship would be to court the risk of se- rious exploitation.

There are other dangers in introducing payment with- out significant regulatory changes. First, if market mecha- nisms are introduced without well-constructed limita- tions, noncommercial research sponsors could find themselves facing problems recruiting study participants. Second, efforts to compensate participants fairly according to local market standards may be undermined as research moves beyond national borders. Third, payment could cre- ate problems with subject selection and the generalizability of research findings by attracting a limited, unrepresenta- tive population of participants. However, this risk may be minimal in many clinical trials involving healthy volun- teers, which are often of little scientific value and are con- ducted simply to fulfill regulatory testing requirements for "me-too" drugs.

The current regulatory system is even more danger- ous. Ethical guidelines and regulations ought to protect healthy research subjects from exploitation. But instead, the current regulatory scheme prohibits subjects from re- ceiving a fair wage and denies them the legal resources available to other high-risk workers. As the lawsuit against *Guinea Pig Zero* showed, research participants are virtually powerless in their dealings with the multibillion-dollar bio- medical research industry. Labor legislation, in contrast, would reflect the recognition that healthy research subjects volunteer because they are in financial need, and that fi- nancial need is the locus of their vulnerability.

---

29   Paying People to Participate in Research

Why Not?

PAUL MCNEILL

[... Martin] Wilkinson and [Andrew] Moore argue that it is inconsistent to allow people to volunteer for research but to deny them the right to be paid for the same research. Essentially they contend that researchers want to pay sub- jects so as to get enough subjects for their research and sub- jects are happy to accept a financial reward. The result is that both are better off and no-one is worse off. One of the ar- guments they consider (and reject) is that inducement may invalidate informed consent especially when the research subjects are poor. They appeal, however, to the analogy of work, where it is normally accepted that poor people may be induced by financial rewards to accept work that other people might not accept, in order to show that there is no good argument against withholding inducement from poor people to consent to taking part in research. Such a decision can still be an autonomous decision. They also reject the ar-

Paul McNeill, "Paying People to Participate in Research: Why Not?" *Bioethics* 11 (1997): 390–96.

gument that inducement may be coercive. To the contrary, it is paternalistic to withhold financial inducements from people for participating in research.

Wilkinson and Moore consider whether the offering of inducement is in itself exploitative. They conclude that even if exploitation is conceded, it is not in itself a persua- sive argument against offering inducement. The fact that someone cannot pay for necessities, such as medical treat- ment for their children, may be injust. However it is not ap- palling to offer such a person an inducement to participate in research. The researchers are not responsible for the poverty of those people consenting to take part in the re- search and the money they offer alleviates that poverty, even if only to a small extent.

EXPERIMENTATION AND WORK

Wilkinson and Moore equate payment for participating in experiments on human beings with ordinary work relationships. For example, in the same way that any of us might choose to work for a doctor as a receptionist and accept payment for it, we should also be free to accept payment from the same doctor for offering our bodies as an experimental field in a trial of new drugs. I simply disagree on the ground that the two are not equivalent and that work is not an appropriate analogy for participating in research.

My main point relates to the risk that is inherent in any experiment on human beings. Work is not normally a risky practice. The risks of being harmed in our work are usually known in advance and can be minimized by adopting safe practices. The situation is not comparable to research. By definition, research, which involves experimentation on human subjects, exposes these human subjects to risks of harm and those risks cannot be known in advance. If the outcome was known to be safe, prior to the experiment, then it would not be an experiment by definition. The authors have not taken sufficient account of this essential element in the debate: That experimenting on human subjects exposes them to unknown risks of harm.

At one point the authors refer to "risky work" which they say "few seek to prohibit." At first blush this appears to counter the view I have just put. However, it is not the case that few seek to prohibit risky work. In general dangerous work is prohibited. Any dangerous work that is accepted must be justified by some greater need. Risky work is work that must be undertaken for society to maintain other highly valued advantages. Furthermore, whilst we may accept work that is risky (where it is justified in this way), most believe that every effort should be taken to minimize the risks inherent in the work. This is not simply a matter of individual autonomy. Society has an important protective role here.

It is open to debate whether the advantages of allowing dangerous work are worth the risks involved for a few individuals. This is the debate that surfaces when someone is harmed. Few would agree that monetary payments justify the work when it would be possible to reduce the risks. It is conceded that, in spite of all efforts to reduce risks, some dangerous work still remains to be done. Although it is reasonable to pay people more money for taking on those risks, this obviously does not mean that payment itself justifies the work. The issue of whether dangerous work is acceptable needs to be considered carefully. Is this work something that society really needs? Even if some dangerous work (such as fire-fighting) is necessary, it does not follow that experimenting on human beings can be similarly justified.

In essence my argument is that the analogy with dangerous or risky work does not apply to research because the results of experiments are not necessary to society in the way in which some dangerous work may be. The justification for research is always in terms of progress: some added benefit to society in the form of new knowledge, a new treatment or a new and potentially better response to a problem. As Jonas has said, "Let us not forget that progress is an optional goal." There is no necessity about seeking new knowledge or finding "new miracle cures." Furthermore, even when some benefit is indicated as a possibility, it is not clear that an experiment will result in a benefit to society sufficient to justify the risks.

INDUCEMENT TO ACCEPT RISK

The authors fail to give sufficient emphasis to the risk that is inherent in human experimentation. They refer to the story that I told in my book *The Ethics and Politics of Human Experimentation*. My daughter was considering volunteering for drug trials in the United Kingdom during her travels and, yes it is true, I sent her money rather than have her accept the inducement of money to participate in drug trials. My reason however was not, as the authors assume, because her consent was invalidated by any inducement to take part in the research. The reason I sent her money was because I did not want her to be exposed to the obvious risk of ingesting a chemical substance with unknown effects. I am particularly concerned about the use of healthy "volunteers" in Phase I trials of drugs which aim to find the "safe dosage" of drugs (potentially poisonous substances) in a human body. My concern is not whether her consent was invalidated by the inducement. My concern was that the inducement, of a considerable sum of money, would expose my daughter to additional and unnecessary risks. There was no possibility, that without financial inducement, she would have exposed herself to those risks. In fact she did not take part in the drug trial once she knew that I was to send her the money she needed. Whilst I acknowledge that this may have been an effective ploy on her part (given her knowledge of my views) this does not detract from the point I am making and the point that Wilkinson and Moore have failed to adequately address: that financial inducement to participate in research exposes people to risks that they may not otherwise accept. Added to this is the reality (even in the absence of inducement) that research subjects are often in a poor position, and a relatively powerless position, to adequately assess the risks when asked to volunteer for research.

It is the element of risk of harm that is particularly problematic in research. How can we ensure that the research will not harm the person participating in it? This is the main issue in research review and why independent review by committee is needed. The need is based on the recognition that researchers are not always capable of putting the interests of their subjects ahead of their research objectives.

PATERNALISM

The authors have "general ethical worries" with the "legitimacy of paternalism." Yet committee review is inherently paternalistic. It is a form of paternalism (or parentalism) well justified by the continuing evidence of abuse of human beings by researchers. The primary role of a committee is to consider whether or not the risk in any particular research, as far as it is possible to gauge that risk, is reasonable. To do this, a committee must assess independently any evidence of risks, from the proposed research to the human participants, and the nature and degree of that risk, as far as it is possible to judge. Some indication of the risk is needed so as to (1) consider whether any risk to subjects is reasonable having regard to the potential for the research to benefit others; (2) minimize the risks in whatever way is possible; and (3) reject those proposals which appear to entail an unacceptably high degree of risk to the participants.

INDUCEMENT AND EQUITY

It is clearly not possible to remove all risks. An experiment would not be an experiment if it was known in advance that the experimental procedure was safe. For this reason, those who volunteer for research should be those who clearly understand the extent and the nature of that risk. Comprehension of the risk is important. Furthermore, I claim that subjects should not be induced to disregard or downplay an appreciation of that risk by the offer of a financial reward.

Inducement needs to be considered in relation to the effect it has on a voluntary and free acceptance of the risks inherent in any research program. In the 1960s and 1970s various commentators suggested that the ideal research subjects would either be researchers themselves or people well educated who were capable of understanding all of the implications of the research program. The reason that inducement is particularly of concern is that those most susceptible to inducement may be the least able to assess the aims and technical information relating to the research and to decide on whether or not the risk is worth taking. It is already the poor and socially disadvantaged who volunteer for most research yet it is typically the better off members of society who benefit from research. The offering of financial inducement simply exacerbates this inequity and adds further to the risks for those disadvantaged people.

Wilkinson and Moore are concerned that inducement might lead to harm but only in the special case where an inducement would encourage people to withhold information about a medical condition so as to take part in research. For example, a person may be excluded from participation in drug research because of a heart condition.

The authors acknowledge that there might be an inducement for that person to deny a heart problem. In their view, however, this is not an argument against inducement. They consider that a committee should simply require adequate methods for establishing subject eligibility independent of self-reports.

This is far too narrow a concession in my view. It is already apparent that subjects are encouraged to volunteer for research by the offer of payments. These are often described as "payments for inconvenience, time spent and out-of-pocket expenses" as is noted in a footnote to Wilkinson and Moore's paper. Yet these payments are sufficiently attractive to act as inducements to volunteer. Advertising for subjects within a teaching hospital of my own University makes it obvious that researchers use "out-of-pocket" payments to attract students to volunteer. I agree with the authors that it is "hard to reconcile rejection of inducement" with the offer of these payments. In my view such payments cannot be justified when they act as an inducement to volunteer. Whilst it may be hard to draw the line between a genuine out-of-pocket expense and financial inducement, this is not an argument against drawing the line.

The basis of my argument against inducement is that it encourages people to expose themselves to risk of harm. This encouragement is greater for the impecunious. The difficulty is acute when the experiment has a clear potential for harm such as experimenting with chemical compounds (drug research) and other medical research. This is not simply a matter of individual autonomy. Society has an obligation, prior to the protection of individual freedom and autonomy, to establish basic safeguards that are equitable in their operation. It is not equitable that the poor are encouraged to expose themselves to risks of harm, by the offer of a financial inducement, especially when the potential benefit is to others.

For my part I concede that Wilkinson and Moore do have a case with research that has very little risk of physical, mental, emotional or social harm. For example a psychologist requiring subjects to perform a battery of repeated tests involving a task, where the biggest risk is that of boredom (and there is no other apparent risk), may be justified in paying people to participate in that research. In other words, financial inducement to take part in research can be justified when there is no known, and very little likelihood of, harm. The case against inducement is much more persuasive where there is a risk of harm to the subjects. There is something repugnant about offering money to relatively poor people, impecunious students, travelers and others, to take part in research which, by its nature, exposes them to risks of harm. The poor in our societies already have higher risks of poor health and other adverse life events. Inducement to take part in experimentation should not be allowed when it adds to those risks. Wilkinson and

Moore have argued that researchers should be allowed to pay subjects so as to get enough subjects for their research on the basis that subjects are happy to accept a financial reward with the result that both are better off and no-one is worse off. The inducement of money for participating in research is a factor which adds to their difficulty in adequately assessing the risks of participating. The acceptance of inducement to participate in research is likely to further increase the inequity of research conducted on the impecunious for the benefit of the well-off.

Part V

Informed Consent in Research

As we saw in Part I, the early history of contemporary research ethics often focused on the issue of informed consent. On one side, clinical researchers tended to affirm the scientific imperative, claiming that society must continue to give physician-investigators wide latitude regarding whether and how much to tell their research participants. They claimed that a rigid insistence on informing patient-participants would only serve to disconcert patients and impede the march of scientific progress. On the other side, lawyers, philosophers, and some physicians argued that such deference was incompatible with the autonomy and inviolability of potential research participants, who were first and foremost *human beings*. These critics also noted that the utilitarian ethical principle animating the researchers' resistance to a requirement of informed consent had provided philosophical support for some of the worst abuses of modern medicine, such as those of the Nazi doctors and the researchers at Tuskegee. The partisans of autonomy clearly prevailed in that great debate.

Important questions remain, however, about the precise nature, requirements, and scope of the duty to elicit informed consent. First, does the requirement of informed consent extend to each and every instance of clinical research—even, for example, to a comparison of two brands of disinfectant hand soap—no matter how small the risks or how indifferent patients would likely be to the prospect of being included in such studies? Second, exactly *how much* must patients be told about the risks and benefits inherent in the very format of the randomized clinical trial itself, such as random assignment of treatment, blinding, and control groups, *in addition to* whatever risks might be posed by the various interventions involved? This second question raises the issue of whether there might

exist serious psychological barriers to valid informed consent, many of which might be traced to a confusion in the minds of both researchers and participants between the goals of clinical medicine and those of biomedical research. The contributors in this part of the book explore these more sophisticated and difficult problems.

Our first contributor, Robert J. Levine, offers a comprehensive overview of the nature, functions, requirements, and limits of the duty to elicit informed consent in biomedical research. Levine begins with the observation that the consent requirement draws foundational support from a variety of important sources in philosophy, religion, and law. He then discusses the various functions of the consent requirement, taking care to distinguish genuine informed consent as a process of communication from its bureaucratic trappings in consent forms. Whereas the former is supposed to serve the rights and welfare of potential participants in research, the latter largely serves the legal and financial interests of researchers and their institutions. In this connection Levine raises the interesting question of whether the standards of informed consent in research should be the same as those governing medical practice. The bioethics literature and the vast bureaucracy built on the code of U.S. federal research regulations would appear to attest that higher, more demanding requirements should be imposed in the context of research, but Levine proposes that both patients and clinical research participants should be afforded the same rigorous degree of protection in this regard.

Levine next canvasses the crucially important elements or conditions of genuinely informed consent. First, consent must be freely given or truly voluntary. If the consent of a participant is obtained by means of fraud, deception, or coercion, it is not genuine consent and therefore cannot legitimize *using* this person in research. It is doubtful, however, whether any particular offer to participate in research is coercive in the requisite sense. Does this mean that any and all moral suasion or financial inducements are to be ruled out of bounds? Does it mean that the consent of desperately ill cancer patients must be considered invalid *simply* in virtue of the constraints imposed by their disease on free choice? Does it mean that the consent of medical students and prisoners must be considered suspect because of the power relations between teacher and student, warden and prisoner? And what about the consent of desperately poor patients infected with the human immunodeficiency virus (HIV), from developed and developing countries alike, who sometimes join studies as much for the free medical care provided as for the experimental intervention? Questions such as these underscore the need for more philosophically rigorous and context-sensitive inquiries into the various kinds of constraints on choice and their respective implications for the validity of informed consent.

Another related threat to the voluntariness of consent is the lack of mental or decisional capacity, or, as the law puts it, the "incompetence," of many persons to give genuine consent. In contrast to those who are coerced and constrained by the force of external circumstance, many potential research participants lack the requisite psychological capacities to give legitimate consent. This category includes children, those who are mentally challenged, and those suffering from cognitive and affective deficits such as schizophrenia and depression. The main focus of debate here centers on the most favorable interpretation of the criteria for the "capacity" to make decisions regarding one's participation in research. We shall revisit this broad category of research participants in Part VI.

The third major element of genuine consent is that it be sufficiently *informed*. As Franz J. Ingelfinger noted 30 years ago, the "trouble with informed consent is that it is not educated consent."[1] Ingelfinger's point—one that still has force today—was that, try as researchers might, the *provision* of information to prospective research participants is one thing; their *understanding* of that information is quite another. To ensure genuine consent, potential research participants must have sufficient information about a proposed trial in order to make a reasonable decision on the basis of their own values and preferences. As Levine notes, current U.S. federal regulations require that researchers disclose specific information bearing on (1) the purpose of a study, (2) its foreseeable risks and benefits, (3) the various alternatives to participation in the research, (4) protections of confidentiality, (5) the availability (if any) of compensation for research-related injury, and (6) conditions of participation, including reassurances that participants can leave a study at any time without penalty or forfeiture of their medical entitlements. Although there is broad agreement regarding the informational elements that must be disclosed, the problem in practice continues to be how best to ensure that prospective research participants understand this information. There has thus been no shortage of techniques employed over the years intended to ensure that "informed consent" is also "educated consent," to use Ingelfinger's language. The empirical literature on informed consent is vast and shows no sign of abating as researchers try new informational delivery techniques in the service of gaining genuine consent to research participation.[2]

Beyond this cluster of required disclosures, controversy surrounds the status of other facts that might be of interest to potential research participants.[3] For example, should patients be informed of various financial arrangements that could potentially engender a conflict of interest for researchers? Evidence indicates that patients want to know more about this kind of financial information than physicians think they should be told.[4] Moreover, suppose that a pharmaceutical company has offered to pay researchers a "finder's fee" of $3,000 for each patient enrolled in a particular study. Should potential participants know about this financial incentive?[5] Another emerging issue concerns whether the inherent risk of participation in a randomized clinical trial circumscribed by a rigid and restrictive protocol ought to be shared with potential participants.

Apart from the issue of the *kinds of information* that should be shared with potential participants, there remains the vexing problem of choosing between competing underlying standards for the disclosure of information. Exactly *how much* information must researchers share with potential participants? Should they be governed by the norm of standard medical practice in the community of researchers? If so, Dr. Chester Southam of the infamous Jewish Chronic Disease Hospital case described in Part I would most likely have been thought to have done no wrong because he was merely following standard practice among researchers at that time. One alternative norm is the so-called reasonable person standard, which requires that researchers provide the amount of information a reasonable person would need to know. Another norm is the "specific person" standard geared to the idiosyncratic, but not unreasonable, preferences of particular individuals. The latter standard is obviously most respectful of the value of individual autonomy, but it is difficult if not impossible to implement in the context of a relationship between investigator and potential participant—a relationship that most often exists between strangers.

Levine concludes his survey with a comment on some possibly legitimate exceptions to the general consent requirement in the context of biomedical research. One false start in this inquiry would be to assert a research-oriented equivalent to the doctrine of "therapeutic privilege" acknowledged in the area of medical practice. According to this doctrine, physicians may withhold information from patients when they judge the disclosure of such information detrimental to the patient's best interests. While this doctrine may justify the occasional withholding of information within a doctor-patient relationship, Levine rightly finds it difficult to imagine withholding information for this reason within a clinical research setting. Paternalism may infrequently be justified for the patient's own good, but never (or hardly ever) for the good of a research project. That, we must recall, was exactly the rationale invoked by Dr. Southam at the Jewish Chronic Disease Hospital.

A more promising exception to the general rule of consent falls under the general rubric of medical emergencies. Just as physicians who treat unconscious accident victims may rightly presume the consent of the latter to treatment, so emergency room clinician-researchers may well claim a legitimate exception to the consent requirement in the design of research protocols bearing on the treatment of accident victims and those suffering from stroke or heart attack. Patients in the midst of such crises often cannot pause or rouse themselves for a dispassionate discussion of alternative medical management strategies, and the time required may compromise the intervention. We must, then, either insist on informed voluntary consent even here, and thereby forego important advances in critical care medicine, or waive the requirement for contemporaneous informed consent. The U.S. Food and Drug Administration

(FDA) and Department of Health and Human Services (DHHS) followed the latter course in 1996 in allowing a waiver of informed consent for research on emergency treatments.[6]

We delve more deeply into the nature and requirements of informed consent with an exchange between the distinguished medical educator and editor, Franz J. Ingelfinger, and philosopher Benjamin Freedman. Ingelfinger worries that the so-called informed consent of ordinary research participants is routinely compromised on two fronts. First, such consent may pass muster according to our formalized legal rituals, but the average person is, he asserts, woefully ill equipped to truly comprehend and accurately assess the stakes of participating in a clinical trial. Second, Ingelfinger notes that there will usually be some element of duress that undermines the voluntariness of participants' consent. Incapacitated, frightened, and often unduly hopeful, many patients are unable to exercise genuinely free choice when an authority figure in a white coat amiably requests their consent to research. Ingelfinger concludes, echoing Henry Beecher, that while efforts to promote more educated consent are definitely in order, the research subjects' only real protection remains the conscience and compassion of the investigator and his or her peers.

Benjamin Freedman takes aim at a related but much more skeptical claim about informed consent. According to many opponents of the very notion of such a requirement, participants, lacking as they do the knowledge of a medical student or physician, can never be "fully informed" about the purposes and risks of medical research. While some researchers conclude from this that informed consent will always fall short of the ideal, others conclude that such a requirement is entirely bogus. Freedman attributes such responses to a flawed understanding of the informational requirement of informed consent. Instead of viewing this requirement as a demand for abstract information detached from any specific context, a demand that would always fall short of the "ideal" of total disclosure, Freedman urges us to recall that this information is required in the service of a very specific and limited purpose, that is, the making of a responsible decision. The proper test, then, is what the potential participant in research needs to know in order to decide responsibly. With the emphasis squarely on the issue of *responsibility*, Freedman makes the surprising and controversial claim that *ignorant* consent may on occasion be valid for that class of participants who wish to lodge their trust in their physician to do the right thing by them.[7]

Finally, with regard to Ingelfinger's concerns about duress, Freedman counters that such worries may be due to our failure to distinguish between choices forced by human decisions and choices "forced" by nature or fate. For example, a patient facing the unsavory choice between open-heart surgery and death may feel as though she has "no choice," but we would hardly say that her option for surgery is "coerced" in any morally meaningful sense of that term. Additionally, Freedman draws a distinction between offers that improve our situation above a baseline of minimal human decency and those that make the awarding of minimal goods contingent upon our participation in research. The former are not coercive, but the latter may well be. Thus a well-paid Hollywood stunt actor might voluntarily agree to undertake serious risks, while uninsured patients in dire need of hospitalization are indeed coerced if their receipt of medical care is conditioned upon their participation in a clinical trial.

Robert D. Truog, Walter Robinson, Adrienne Randolph, and Alan Morris further pursue the question of exceptions to the consent requirement in their contribution to this volume. In contrast to the legions of physicians who opposed a rigorous consent requirement prior to the imposition of the U.S. federal rules, these authors wholeheartedly endorse the rationale for informed consent in medical practice and clinical research. However, they question the necessity of this requirement for any and all varieties of research in the clinical context. The authors begin with a paradox in contemporary medicine—namely, that while physicians and surgeons are free to follow their hunches regarding "clinical innovation" in the practice of medicine, often without having to get consent for specific procedures or drugs in common use, as soon as they attempt any kind of explicit research in the clinical setting they are immediately encumbered by a robust consent requirement and institutional review board (IRB) review. They argue that in some cases, such as a comparison of two brands of antacid or of two similar and approved antibiotics for preoperative prophylaxis, these ethical requirements are excessive and often act as a barrier to the conduct of potentially useful and important clinical research. As a result, they allege, new procedures or new uses for existing drugs are often haphazardly introduced into the practice of medicine without the critical scrutiny they

deserve. Their proposed solution is to drop the requirement of "specific" informed consent to participation in research that falls within a rigorously defined range of exceptional cases.

Truog and colleagues propose five criteria for the justifiable waiver of informed consent in clinical research: (1) all the treatments offered in the trial must already be available for use outside the trial, (2) participation in the trial would not expose participants to more than minimal risk, (3) genuine clinical equipoise must exist between the various treatment arms, (4) no reasonable person would have a preference for one treatment over another, and (5) these very standards should be disclosed to all patients at the institution or in the clinical setting where the research is being conducted. Criterion 4 is crucial here, because it allows the authors to reconcile the waiver of consent with a proper concern for the self-determination of the participants. If one can argue that no reasonable patient would have a preference for one arm of a study over another, then a waiver of consent to such a trial would not adversely affect participants' rightful claims to bodily autonomy.

These authors insist that the responsibility for applying these criteria should rest not with individual researchers, but rather with IRBs, which would be obligated to interpret them "narrowly" and apply them "conservatively." This is an important proviso, because there seems to be significant congruence between these suggested criteria and Dr. Chester Southam's dubious rationale for bypassing consent in the Jewish Chronic Disease Hospital case. In both cases a great deal of weight is placed on a favorable risk-benefit ratio and on assurances that no reasonable patient would need or want to know the full story. Obviously, if these criteria are to be applied in a manner that will not threaten participants' well-being and rights to self-determination, IRBs must exercise great care to place themselves in the shoes not of a "reasonable physician," but rather of a "reasonable person." How best to determine the contours of "reasonableness" is, of course, a deep and problematic issue. However, as Rebecca Dresser has pointed out, IRBs granting this kind of waiver should consider expanding their rosters to include more community members.[8]

In some ways, the initial battle over informed consent was the "easy" part. The progressive elaboration of increasingly sophisticated and controversial methodologies for conducting clinical trials—such as the randomized, double-blind, placebo-controlled trial—has required us to radically rethink the informational elements of informed consent. In the past, it may have been enough simply to inform the potential participant that he or she was being asked to participate in a research study and to enumerate the likely risks and benefits. The advent of the randomized controlled trial (RCT), however, has posed new questions about the ethics of this rigorous scientific methodology itself, questions that have placed great stress on the ethics of the participant-researcher encounter. As numerous commentators have pointed out (see Part III), the RCT harbors several methodological requirements that threaten to undermine the traditional medical ethic of undivided physician loyalty to the individual patient. Although patients enroll in such trials based largely on the possible therapeutic gains to be had, their treatment is nonetheless randomly allocated regardless of their more particular needs. Adherence to the research protocol may preclude giving individualized attention to the specific and evolving needs of individual patients because the sine qua non of the RCT is an insistence on uniformity of intervention within each arm of the trial. Thus patients who remain in the study may not be allowed to take additional, nonstudy drugs, even if they or their physicians think doing so would advance their best interests. This proscription of nonstudy drugs is not absolute. Control interventions, which some patients are assigned at random, offer standard therapy to test promising new approaches and, when placebos are used for controls, often offer patients no pharmacologically active treatment at all. Finally, the RCT is typically double blinded, so contrary to good clinical practice, neither the patient nor his or her physician knows what therapeutic intervention the patient is receiving. Although some researchers continue to insist that participation in a rigorous clinical trial constitutes the best medicine for patient-participants, others see the RCT as placing the needs of research over the individual needs of patients. The question arises, then, as to how, if at all, researchers ought to inform potential participants of this ethical tension embedded within the very structure of the RCT.

This problem is greatly exacerbated by the widespread confusion in the minds of many researchers and patients alike between the goals of research and those of therapy. Throughout his illustrious career Yale psychiatrist and law professor Jay Katz has underscored the differences between these often conflicting enterprises, arguing forcefully that the legacy of "professionalism" among researchers leads them to overestimate the benefits and underestimate the risks of research and to shield much of their uncertainty and understanding of risks from patients on traditional paternalistic grounds. In his contribution to this volume Katz contends that the conversation between investigators and potential participants requires critical reappraisal and reform. In order to disabuse potential participants of the misplaced belief that participation in a clinical trial is first and foremost for their own benefit, Katz encourages physician-investigators to see themselves "as scientists only and not as doctors." Only by adopting this univocal self-image, he suggests, will investigators be able to avoid unwittingly becoming "double agents" with conflicting loyalties. Skeptics have argued that such a shift in self-perception is neither possible nor desirable. Katz also argues that conversations between investigators and potential participants must be firmly grounded upon an unwavering respect for the autonomy of the latter. If informed consent is not to be a coercive sham, he claims, investigators must subordinate both their paternalistic inclinations and their ideology of scientific progress to the ultimate values of patient dignity and self-determination.

Katz's claims regarding the common confusion of research with therapy received confirmation from an empirical study of research participants conducted by President Clinton's Advisory Committee on Human Radiation Experiments (ACHRE), included here. This study revealed that for most veterans of research in the fields of medical and radiation oncology and cardiology, the ritual of informed consent played little, if any, role in their decision to volunteer. Although many patients cited altruism and their belief in the importance of biomedical research as motivations for enrolling, the vast majority reported the decisive influence of two factors: (1) their trust in their physicians to recommend the best course of action for them and (2) their perception that participation in a clinical trial was a way to receive optimal medical treatment. Although most of these patient-participants expressed an awareness of the scientific goals of clinical trials, they generally expected or hoped to benefit personally from participating in their particular project. Echoing Katz's concerns with the continuing legacy of physician professionalism in biomedical research, the ACHRE commissioners note that the consent process was colored in large measure by patients' trust in their physician-investigators. For some patients, they report, the "consent form was the means by which patients could authorize trusted health professionals to do what they think is best." Of concern, many patients reported that they felt they had "no choice" but to participate in clinical trials in order to maintain hope and gain access to possibly beneficial treatments.

This confusion on the part of potential participants between research and treatment receives further empirical confirmation and deeper psychological scrutiny from our next contributors, Paul S. Appelbaum and colleagues. On the basis of their study of consent in the context of psychiatric research, these authors conclude that most participants suffer from a "therapeutic misconception"—that is, they systematically downplay or ignore the risks posed to their own well-being by participation in clinical research. The reason for this misconception, the authors assert, is the participants' deeply held and nearly unshakeable conviction that every aspect of their participation in research has been designed for their own individual benefit. Perhaps these authors' most disconcerting finding was that the therapeutic misconception colors the thinking of even patients who exhibit a clear-headed cognitive understanding of the various methodological elements of the standard RCT. The deeply embedded nature of this misconception is perhaps best illustrated by the case of a 25-year-old college-educated woman who had exhibited an excellent grasp of the nature, purposes, and methods of her particular study, including a clear understanding of the presence of a placebo intervention that would be assigned to participants at random. When asked, however, how *her* medication would be selected, she responded, "I hope it isn't by chance"; when asked what drug most people in the study would get, she suggested that each would probably receive the medication he or she needed.

This misconception on the part of potential research participants is matched, and partially fueled, by a corresponding misconception and perhaps misrepresentation on the part of researchers and their sponsors. As Mark Hochhauser observes in his contribution to this volume, researchers and their institutional or pharmaceutical sponsors routinely engage in practices designed to foster the impression that research is equivalent to treatment, even though the FDA reports that overall only 20 percent of clinical trials yield a marketable product. Hochhauser points

out, first, that clinical research has recently become a big business crucially dependent upon success in recruiting sufficient numbers of participants. Toward this end, researchers and their industry sponsors increasingly affix to their clinical trials "brand names"—that is, acronyms that have different uses and serve many functions. As Berkwits has recently argued, such clinical-trial brand names can serve pragmatic, heuristic, symbolic, expressive, or provocative functions.[9] Like the naming and marketing of products by the advertising industry, Berkwits claims that "branding" a research project is intended in part to describe the "product" as well as to elicit a favorable reaction from the "consumer," the potential research participant. Hochhauser is interested in what Berkwits calls the "provocative" function of clinical trial names, that is, names that are designed to inspire confidence in potential participants. Examples Hochhauser cites include MAGIC—MAGnesium In Coronaries—and MIRACL—Myocardial Ischemia Reduction with Aggressive Cholesterol Lowering. Given that the names of clinical trials are included on the consent form, prospective participants may often be under the impression that research participation affords them access to the latest and the best in medical therapy. Hochhauser claims that whenever possible the drafters of informed consent forms eschew the words "experiment" and "experimental drug" in favor of more hopeful expressions, such as "clinical research study" and "new investigational drug." Hochhauser cites a newspaper advertisement for a study of an "Innovative Pharmacological Therapeutic Intervention." In addition to this, advertising for clinical trials has reached the Internet, where in one case university sponsors contended, "Cancer patients and health care providers have access to these clinical research trials as part of the latest in cancer care." Hochhauser concludes that all of these practices jointly constitute a kind of "doublespeak" designed to deceive or confuse people into participating in the business of clinical research.

The causes of the therapeutic misconception are manifold. Our contributors focus on just two of these: the psychology of participants and that of the researchers who recruit them. Yet as Rebecca Dresser argues, the causes extend beyond the participant-researcher dyad and include government policies regarding access to research, the influence of industry sponsors, and the influence of the media.[10] As she claims, "Hardly anyone acknowledges the scientific constraints that research imposes on the care of trial participants. Furthermore, hardly anyone acknowledges the relative scarcity of cases in which clinical-trial participants have their lives significantly extended or improved. In this environment, it would be shocking if patients were *not* affected by the therapeutic misconception."[11]

The therapeutic misconception described by the contributors poses a disturbing challenge to the adequacy of the informed consent process and thus to the ethics of most clinical trials conducted today, although its full extent is unknown. What might be done to address this problem? Both Katz and Appelbaum and colleagues contend that researchers need to be much more clear and forthcoming with patients about the overarching scientific rationale of their protocols and about the risks posed by the various elements of the standard RCT. They agree, moreover, that researchers need to underscore in their conversations with patients that research is not a form of individualized treatment and that participation in an RCT may preclude the patient's receiving the therapy that his or her doctor would prescribe in view of an exhaustive assessment of the patient's idiosyncratic medical and psychological needs. Finally, Appelbaum and colleagues suggest that the consent process might be strengthened by the addition of a "neutral explainer"—that is, someone not on the research team who could supplement the investigators' disclosures with frank discussions bearing on the most problematic aspects of the research design and its implications for patients' welfare. Whether a "neutral explainer" would help or hinder informed consent has not been tested and is unknown, and some commentators suggest that it may be undesirable.

1. Franz J. Ingelfinger, "Informed (But Uneducated) Consent," *New England Journal of Medicine* 287 (1972): 465–66.

2. Jeremy Sugarman, Douglas C. McCrory, Donald Powell, et al., "Empirical Research on Informed Consent: An Annotated Bibliography," *Hastings Center Report* 29, no. 1 (1999): S1–S42.

3. T. M. Wilkinson, "Research, Informed Consent, and the Limits of Disclosure," *Bioethics* 15 (2001): 341–63.

4. John La Puma, Carol B. Stocking, William D. Rhoades, and Cheryl M. Darling, "Financial Ties as Part of Informed Consent to Postmarketing Research: Attitudes of American Doctors and Patients," *British Medical Journal* 310 (1995): 1660–61.

5. Jammi N. Rao and L. J. Sant Cassia, "Ethics of Undisclosed Payments to Doctors Recruiting Patients in Clinical Trials," *British Medical Journal* 325 (2002): 36–37.

6. The U.S. Food and Drug Administration rules regarding the waiver of informed consent are codified at 21 CFR 50.24, "Exceptions from Informed Consent Requirements for Emergency Research," available online at www.access.gpo.gov/nara/cfr/waisidx_00/21cfr50_00.html.

7. Benjamin Freedman, "The Validity of Ignorant Consent to Medical Research," *IRB: A Review of Human Subjects Research* 4, no. 2 (1982): 1–5.

8. Rebecca Dresser, "Is Informed Consent Always Necessary for Randomized, Controlled Trials?" [correspondence] *New England Journal of Medicine* 341 (1999): 449.

9. Michael Berkwits, "CAPTURE! SHOCK! EXCITE! Clinical Trial Acronyms and the 'Branding' of Clinical Research," *Annals of Internal Medicine* 133 (2000): 755–59.

10. Rebecca Dresser, "The Ubiquity and Utility of the Therapeutic Misconception," *Social Philosophy & Policy* 19, no. 2 (2002): 271–94.

11. Ibid., 284–85.

30 Consent Issues in Human Research

ROBERT J. LEVINE

"The voluntary consent of the human subject is absolutely essential." This, the first sentence of the Nuremberg Code, signals the centrality of the consent requirement in research involving human subjects. Before the Nuremberg Code was written in 1947 as a response to the atrocities committed in the name of science by Nazi physician-researchers, statements of medical and other professional organizations apparently made no mention of the necessity of consent. Ironically, the only nations known to have promulgated regulations that established a requirement for consent to research were Prussia and Germany. Subsequently, the tendency to focus on informed consent has been reinforced by public outcry over the inadequacy of consent in certain U.S. judicial landmark cases, such as Willowbrook, [the] Jewish Chronic Disease Hospital, [sociologist Laud Humphreys'] Tea Room Trade, and Tuskegee. Indeed, the issue of informed consent has so dominated recent discussion of the ethics of research that one might be led to think erroneously that other ethical issues (e.g., research design, selection of subjects) are either less important or more satisfactorily resolved.

GROUNDING OF INFORMED CONSENT

Philosophical basis. The philosophical foundations of the requirement for informed consent may be found in several lines of reasoning. Based upon the Hippocratic admonition "to help, or at least, to do no harm," one can justify seeking consent for the benefit of the patient; to do so provides a mechanism for ascertaining what the patient would consider a benefit. Allowing the individual to decide what he or she considers beneficial is consistent with the perspective affirmed in U.S. public policy that competent persons are generally the best protectors of their own well-being. However, a focus solely on patient benefit would allow physicians and scientists not to seek consent when they judge that doing so might harm patients or subjects. Thus this justification alone does not suffice to establish a requirement to seek consent.

The requirement can also be justified on grounds of social benefit: The practice of seeking consent may contribute to producing the "greatest good for the greatest number" by forestalling suspicion about research, thus ensuring a subject population and increasing the efficiency of the research enterprise. Again, however, the justification fails to stand alone, since it can also be used to justify not seeking consent; the social good might be better served by avoiding the inefficient and frequently time-consuming consent process. Some commentators express that, carried to its extreme, the social-benefit argument might support the use of unwilling subjects, as in Nazi Germany; such a position would necessarily rest on a very limited vision of the relevant social consequences.

The firmest grounding for the requirement to seek consent is the ethical principle "respect for persons," which according to the U.S. National Commission for the Protection of Human Subjects of Biomedical and Behavioral Research (hereafter, U.S. National Commission) "incorporates at least two basic ethical convictions: First, that individuals should be treated as autonomous agents, and second, that persons with diminished autonomy and thus in need of protection are entitled to such protection." [...] In a legal context, Justice Benjamin Cardozo in 1914 stated that "every human being of adult years and sound mind has a right to determine what shall be done with his own body." To return to the Kantian terms that will be used often in this article, this principle ensures that the research subject will be treated as an end and not merely as a means to another's end. Thus the purpose of the consent requirement is not to minimize risk but to give persons the right to choose.

Religious basis. Several fundamental tenets of the Judaeo-Christian tradition also provide grounding for the requirement to seek consent. This tradition affirms that each human life is a gift from God and is of infinite and immeasurable worth (the "sanctity of life"). The infinite worth of the individual requires that persons treat each other with respect and not interfere in each other's lives without consent. The consent requirement can also be grounded explicitly in the notion of covenant. Seeking consent is an affirmation of the basic faithfulness or care required by the fundamental covenantal nature of human existence.

Legal basis. The legal grounding for the requirement for consent to research is based on the outcome of litigation of disputes arising almost exclusively in the context of medical practice. There is virtually no case law on the basis of which legal standards for consent to research, as distin-

Robert J. Levine, "Consent Issues in Human Research," in *Encyclopedia of Bioethics,* ed. Warren T. Reich, 2nd ed. (New York: Macmillan Reference, 1995), 1241–50.

guished from practice, might be defined (there is one Canadian case, *Halushka* v. *University of Saskatchewan*). The law defines, in general, the circumstances under which a patient, or by extension, a subject, may recover damages for having been wronged or harmed as a consequence of failure to negotiate adequate consent.

The legal bases for the consent requirement—which also shed light on the ethical dimensions of consent—are twofold. First, failure to obtain proper consent was traditionally treated as a battery action. Closely related to the principles of respect for persons and self-determination, the law of battery makes it wrong *a priori* to touch, treat, or do research upon a person without the person's consent. Whether or not harm befalls the patient/subject is irrelevant: It is the unconsented-to touching that is wrong.

The modern trend in malpractice litigation is to treat cases based upon failure to obtain proper consent as negligence rather than battery actions. The negligence doctrine combines elements of patient benefit and self-determination. To bring a negligence action, a patient/subject must prove that the physician had a duty toward the patient; that the duty was breached; that damage occurred to the patient; and that the damage was caused by the breach. In contrast to battery actions, negligence actions remove as a basis for the requirement for consent the simple notion that unconsented-to touching is a wrong. Rather, such touching is wrong (actionable) only if it is negligent and results in harm; otherwise, the patient/subject cannot recover damages. Under both battery and negligence doctrines, consent is invalid if any information is withheld that might be considered material to the decision to give consent.

FUNCTIONS OF INFORMED CONSENT

Jay Katz and Alexander Capron identified the following functions of informed consent: To promote individual autonomy; encourage rational decision making; avoid fraud and duress; involve the public; encourage self-scrutiny by the physician-investigator; and reduce the civil and/or criminal liability of the investigator and his or her institution.

In general, the negotiations for informed consent are designed to safeguard the rights and welfare of the subject, while documentation that the negotiations have been conducted properly safeguards the investigator and institution. The net effect of the documentation may, in fact, be harmful to the interests of the subject. Retaining a signed consent form tends to give the advantage to the investigator in any adversary proceeding. Moreover, the availability of such documents in institutional records may lead to violations of privacy and confidentiality. Consequently, federal regulations permit waivers of the requirements for consent forms when the principal threat to the subject would be a breach of confidentiality and "the only record

linking the subject and the research would be the consent document."

Those who are interested in making operational the requirement for consent have a tendency to focus nearly all of their attention on the consent form. Federal regulations prescribe what information must be included in and excluded from these forms. This seems to reflect an assumption that the consent form is an appropriate instrumentality through which researchers might fulfill their obligation not to treat persons merely as means. Most commentators on informed consent disagree, however, seeing consent as a continuing process rather than an event symbolized by the signing of a form; for example, Robert Levine characterizes informed consent as a discussion or negotiation, while Katz envisions consent as a searching conversation.

Whether or not negotiations for informed consent to research should be conducted according to different standards than consent to practice is controversial. Alvan Feinstein observes that it is the custom to adhere to a double standard: "An act that receives no special concern when performed as part of clinical practice may become a major ethical or legal issue if done as part of a formally designed investigation." In his view there is less need for formality in the negotiations for informed consent to a relationship where the interests of research and practice are conjoined—for example, as in research conducted by a physician-investigator who has the aim of demonstrating the safety and/or efficacy of a nonvalidated therapeutic maneuver—than when the only purpose of the investigator-subject relationship is to perform research. Capron, on the other hand, asserts: "Higher requirements for informed consent should be imposed in therapy than in investigation, particularly when an element of honest experimentation is joined with therapy." Levine concludes that patients are entitled to the same degree of thoroughness of negotiations for informed consent as are subjects of research. However, patients may be offered the opportunity to delegate some (but not all) decision-making authority to a physician, while subjects should rarely be offered this option. The most important distinction is that the prospective subject should be informed that in research, in contrast with practice, the subject will be at least in part a means and perhaps primarily a means to an end identified by someone else. [. . .]

INFORMED CONSENT:
CONDITIONS AND EXCEPTIONS

According to the Nuremberg Code, to consent to participate in research one must (1) be "so situated as to be able to exercise free power of choice"; (2) have the "legal capacity" to give consent; (3) have "sufficient . . . comprehension" to make an "enlightened" decision; and (4) have "sufficient knowledge" on which to decide. Recent discussion emphasizes the knowledge or information component of consent—hence the term "informed consent." Nuremberg's focus on freedom of choice rather than on the quantity or quality of information transmitted is represented by its use of the term "voluntary consent," not "informed consent." [...] Most commentators agree that compromise of any one of the four conditions specified by the Nuremberg Code jeopardizes the ethical acceptability of the consent.

Free power of choice. The Nuremberg Code proscribes "any element of force, fraud, deceit, duress, overreaching, or other ulterior forms of constraint or coercion" in obtaining consent. Any flagrant coercion—for instance, when competent, comprehending persons are forced to submit to research against their expressed will—clearly renders consent invalid. There may be more subtle or indirect "constraints" or "coercions" when prospective subjects are highly dependent, impoverished, or "junior or subordinate members of a hierarchical group." Some argue that consent obtained from such persons violates the intent of the Nuremberg Code. This argument has been posed most sharply with respect to prisoners and other institutionalized populations, since institutionalization often involves both dependency and impoverishment. (Biomedical research involving prisoners as subjects has become quite rare since 1976 when the U.S. National Commission recommended very stringent standards for its justification.) Some argue that consent to participate in research is not valid when it is given (1) to procure financial reward in situations offering few alternatives for remuneration; (2) to seek release from an institution either by evidencing "good behavior" or by ameliorating the condition for which one was confined; or (3) to please physicians or authorities on whom one's continued welfare depends.

Cornel West argues, however, that such indirect forms of constraint do not constitute coercion in a strict sense and thus do not render consent involuntary. Coercion, says West, consists in a threat to render one's circumstances worse if one does not do something. Hence, a threat to withdraw basic necessities of existence, or in some other way to render a prison inmate's situation worse if he or she declines to participate in research, would constitute coercion and render consent invalid. Similarly, to condition release from prison upon participation would constitute coercion, since it would make the inmate's situation worse by removing normal alternatives for seeking release. But the provision of better living conditions in exchange for participation in research does not constitute a threat to make conditions worse; rather, it is an enticement to make conditions better. While enticement and bribery can invalidate consent by undermining the rational grounds for choice,

they do not undermine the voluntariness of the choice. Similarly, a desire to "get well" or to favorably influence institutional authorities is not an "ulterior" constraint in the strict sense of the Nuremberg Code, though it may be a very real psychological constraint.

Other commentators, however, are less concerned with a sharp distinction between coercion and other forms of constraint or undue influence. Even outside such total institutions as prisons there are many situations in which junior or subordinate members of hierarchical groups may be exploited or manipulated. Such persons may assume that their willingness to consent to research may be rewarded by preferential treatment or that their refusals could provoke retaliation by those in positions of authority in the system. Whether or not such assumptions are justified, it is the assumptions themselves that make such persons susceptible to manipulation. Examples of such persons are medical or nursing students, subordinate hospital and laboratory personnel, employees of pharmaceutical firms, and members of the military services. Other persons whose dependency status can be exploited include residents of nursing homes, people receiving welfare benefits, patients in emergency rooms, and those with incurable diseases. [...]

While most regulations and ethical codes proscribe undue material inducements, there is no consensus on what this means. Some commentators argue that in most cases in which competent adults are recruited to serve as subjects in research that presents only slight increases above minimal risk, the role of the research subject is similar to that of an employee. Consequently, the amounts of cash payments or other material inducements can be determined by ordinary market factors. Others protest that because participation in research entails "selling one's body" as opposed to "selling one's labor" the role of the research subject might be considered more akin to prostitution than to any other type of employment. According to this view, research subjects should not be paid at all; rather they should be motivated by altruism.

Attempts to regulate the amounts of permissible material inducements are inevitably problematic. Setting the rates at a low level results in inequitable distribution of the burdens of participation among those who have no opportunities to earn more money for each unit of their time. Higher rates may overwhelm the capacity of the impoverished to decline participation.

Competence and comprehension. The Nuremberg Code requires both "legal capacity" to consent (often called "competence") and "sufficient understanding" to reach an "enlightened" decision. Definitions of competence often include elements of comprehension, for example, to evaluate relevant information, to understand the consequences of action, and to reach a decision for rational reasons. [...]

Assessments of incompetence. The various standards employed for assessing competence are variations of four basic themes.

1. Reasonable outcome of choice. This is a highly paternalistic standard in that the individual's right to self-determination is respected only if he or she makes the "right" choice—that is, one that accords with what the competency reviewer either considers reasonable or presumes a reasonable person might make.

2. Factual comprehension. The individual is required to understand, or at least be able to understand, the information divulged during the consent negotiation.

3. Choice based on rational reasons. Individuals must demonstrate a capacity for rational manipulation of information. They may, for example, be required to show that they not only understand the risks and benefits but also have weighed them in relation to their personal situations.

4. Appreciation of the nature of the situation. Individuals must demonstrate not only comprehension of the consent information but also the ability to use the information in a rational manner. Furthermore, they must appreciate the fact that they are being invited to become research subjects and what that implies.

While there is disagreement as to the grounds for assessing incompetence, most commentators agree that such assessments are limited in several ways. First, a judgment of incompetence may apply only to certain areas of decision making, for example, to one's legal but not to one's personal affairs. Second, confinement to a mental institution is not in itself equivalent to a determination of incompetence. Third, some who are legally competent are functionally incompetent, while some who are legally incompetent are functionally competent.

The Nuremberg Code does not permit the use of subjects lacking legal capacity or comprehension. Most subsequent codes and discussions allow their use with certain restrictions: for example, that mentally competent adults are not suitable subjects, that the veto of a legally incompetent but minimally comprehending subject is binding, and that consent or permission of the legal guardian must be obtained.

According to the U.S. President's Commission for the Study of Ethical Problems in Medicine and Biomedical and Behavioral Research (hereafter, U.S. President's Commission), "decisionmaking capacity requires, to a greater or lesser degree: (1) possession of a set of values and goals; (2) the ability to communicate and understand information; and (3) the ability to reason and deliberate about one's choices." Moreover, individuals may have sufficient capacity to make some decisions but not others. In the words of the U.S. President's Commission:

> Since the assessment [of capacity] must balance possibly competing considerations of well-being and self-determination, [one should] take into account the potential consequences of the patient's decision. When the consequences for well-being are substantial, there is a greater need to be certain that the patient possesses the necessary level of capacity. . . . Thus a particular patient may be capable of deciding about a relatively inconsequential medication, but not about the amputation of a gangrenous limb. [. . .]

Disclosure of information. The Nuremberg Code requires that the subject be told "the nature, duration, and purpose of the experiment; the method and means by which it is to be conducted; all inconveniences and hazards reasonably to be expected; and the effects upon his health or person which may possibly come." These requirements have been modified by subsequent codes and regulations. U.S. federal regulations require (1) a statement of the purpose of the research and a description of its procedures; (2) a description of foreseeable risks and discomforts; (3) a description of benefits; (4) disclosure of appropriate alternatives, if any; (5) a statement of the extent of confidentiality; (6) an explanation of the availability of medical treatment for injury and compensation for disability; (7) an explanation of whom to contact for answers to questions; and (8) a statement that participation is voluntary and that neither refusal to participate nor withdrawal at any time will result in a loss of benefits to which the subject is otherwise entitled. The regulations further specify six additional elements of information to be provided when appropriate: (1) additional risks to the subject or to the fetus if the subject becomes pregnant; (2) circumstances in which a subject's participation may be terminated without his or her consent; (3) additional costs to the subject that may result from participation; (4) the consequences of a subject's decision to withdraw and procedures for orderly termination of participation; (5) a commitment to divulge significant new findings developed during the research that may relate to the subject's continued willingness to participate; and (6) the approximate number of subjects in the study. Finally, the regulations forbid requirements that subjects waive any of their legal rights as well as releases of the investigator, sponsor, or institution from liability for negligence.

While these requirements have the force of law, they are by no means exhaustive of possible standards for disclosure. To them one might add the following: A clear invitation to participate in research, distinguishing maneuvers required for research purposes from those necessary for therapy; an explanation of why that particular person is invited (selected); a suggestion that the prospective subject might wish to discuss the research with another person; and an identification of the source of funding for the research. [...] In short, there is no universal agreement on standards for disclosure of information or on what it takes for a person to have "sufficient knowledge" to give "informed" consent.

Those who agree on the need for disclosure of information in a particular category—the risks, for example—often disagree on the nature of the information that must be made known. The Nuremberg Code requires explication of hazards "reasonably" to be expected. Does this include a very slight chance of a substantial harm, or a substantial chance of a very slight harm? Neither the quality nor the probability of the risks to be divulged has been clearly determined legally.

Disagreements over particulars arise in part from disagreements about underlying standards: Is disclosure to be determined by (1) general medical practice or opinion; (2) the requirements of a "reasonable person"; or (3) the idiosyncratic judgment of the individual? While the legal trend may be shifting from the first to the second, it may be argued that only the third, the "subjective standard," is truly compatible with the requirement of respect for the autonomy of the individual person.

Yet even those who adopt the subjective standard disagree as to its implications. Freedman holds that the idiosyncratic judgment of the individual is overriding, to the point that the prospective subject can choose to have less information than a "reasonable" person might require. Veatch, however, argues that anyone refusing to accept as much information as would be expected of a "reasonable person" should not be accepted as a subject.

In the context of medical practice, two exceptions to the requirement for informed consent are recognized— "emergency exception" and "therapeutic privilege." The former, which permits the doctor to proceed without delay to administer urgently required therapy in emergencies, is included in a limited form in the regulations of the U.S. Food and Drug Administration; in some "life-threatening" emergencies in which informed consent is "infeasible," physician-investigators are authorized to employ investigational drugs and devices. There is continuing controversy over whether the emergency exception can be invoked to justify "deferred consent," that is, postponement of soliciting the consent of the subject or permission of the next-of-kin for up to several days after the subject has been enrolled

in a research protocol in an emergency. The therapeutic-privilege exception to the informed-consent rule permits the doctor to withhold information when, in his or her judgment, disclosure would be detrimental to the patient's interests or well-being. Most commentators agree that invoking the doctrine of therapeutic privilege to assure a subject's cooperation in a research project is almost never appropriate; it gives the investigator entirely too much license to serve vested interests by withholding information that might be material to a prospective subject's decision. U.S. federal regulations do not explicitly endorse the use of the therapeutic-privilege exception in research, although some authors have suggested that they could be interpreted as an implicit endorsement.

The success of some research activities is contingent upon withholding from the subjects information about their purposes or procedures or, in some cases, by deliberate deception (providing false information). U.S. federal regulations permit "waivers and alterations" of consent requirements if there is no more than minimal risk; if the waiver or alteration will not adversely affect subjects' rights or welfare; if without the waiver or alteration the research "could not practically be carried out"; and if the subjects will be debriefed (given a full and accurate explanation afterward) when appropriate. [...] Various proposals have been made to minimize the need for and harmful effects of deceptive practices: Subjects might be invited to consent to incomplete disclosure with a promise of full disclosure at the termination of the research; subjects might be told as much as possible and asked to consent for specified limits of time and risk; or approval of the plans to withhold information from or to deceive subjects might be sought from "surrogate" populations that resemble the actual intended subject populations in relevant respects.

CONCLUSIONS

The use of a person as a research subject can be justified only if that person, or one authorized to speak on his or her behalf, consents to such use. The legal and ethical requirement for consent is grounded in fundamental tenets of the Judaeo-Christian religious tradition as well as in basic ethical principles that create the universal obligation to treat persons as ends and not merely as means to another's end. The consent requirement also reflects the perspective that competent persons are generally the best protectors of their own well-being. Most major disagreements over the form and substance of the consent requirements derive from conflicting interpretations of one or more of the basic principles. [...]

31   Informed (But Uneducated) Consent

The trouble with informed consent is that it is not educated consent. Let us assume that the experimental subject, whether a patient, a volunteer, or otherwise enlisted, is exposed to a completely honest array of factual detail. He is told of the medical uncertainty that exists and that must be resolved by research endeavors, of the time and discomfort involved, and of the tiny percentage risk of some serious consequences of the test procedure. He is also reassured of his rights and given a formal, quasi-legal statement to read. No exculpatory language is used. With his written signature, the subject then caps the transaction, and whether he sees himself as a heroic martyr for the sake of mankind, or as a reluctant guinea pig dragooned for the benefit of science, or whether, perhaps, he is merely bewildered, he obviously has given his "informed consent." Because established routines have been scrupulously observed, the doctor, the lawyer, and the ethicist are content.

But the chances are remote that the subject really understands what he has consented to—in the sense that the responsible medical investigator understands the goals, nature, and hazards of his study. How can the layman comprehend the importance of his perhaps not receiving, as determined by the luck of the draw, the highly touted new treatment that his roommate will get? How can he appreciate the sensation of living for days with a multi-lumen intestinal tube passing through his mouth and pharynx? How can he interpret the information that an intravascular catheter and radiopaque dye injection have an 0.01 per cent probability of leading to a dangerous thrombosis or cardiac arrhythmia? It is moreover quite unlikely that any patient-subject can see himself accurately within the broad context of the situation, to weigh the inconveniences and hazards that he will have to undergo against the improvements that the research project may bring to the management of his disease in general and to his own case in particular. [...]

Nor can the information given to the experimental subject be in any sense totally complete. It would be impractical and probably unethical for the investigator to present the nearly endless list of all possible contingencies; in fact, he may not himself be aware of every untoward thing that might happen. Extensive detail, moreover, usually enhances the subject's confusion. [...] The inconsiderate investigator, indeed, conceivably could exploit his authority and knowledge and extract "informed consent" by overwhelming the candidate-subject with information.

Ideally, the subject should give his consent freely, under no duress whatsoever. The facts are that some element of coercion is instrumental in any investigator-subject transaction. Volunteers for experiments will usually be influenced by hopes of obtaining better grades, earlier parole, more substantial egos, or just mundane cash. These pressures, however, are but fractional shadows of those enclosing the patient-subject. Incapacitated and hospitalized because of illness, frightened by strange and impersonal routines, and fearful for his health and perhaps life, he is far from exercising a free power of choice when the person to whom he anchors all his hopes asks, "Say, you wouldn't mind, would you, if you joined some of the other patients on this floor and helped us to carry out some very important research we are doing?" When "informed consent" is obtained, it is not the student, the destitute bum, or the prisoner to whom, by virtue of his condition, the thumb screws of coercion are most relentlessly applied; it is the most used and useful of all experimental subjects, the patient with disease.

When a man or woman agrees to act as an experimental subject, therefore, his or her consent is marked by neither adequate understanding nor total freedom of choice. The conditions of the agreement are a far cry from those visualized as ideal. Jonas would have the subject identify with the investigative endeavor so that he and the researcher would be seeking a common cause: "Ultimately, the appeal for volunteers should seek . . . free and generous endorsement, the appropriation of the research purpose into the person's [i.e., the subject's] own scheme of ends." For Ramsey, "informed consent" should represent a "covenantal bond between consenting man and consenting man [that] makes them . . . joint adventurers in medical care and progress." Clearly, to achieve motivations and attitudes of this lofty type, an educated and understanding, rather than merely informed, consent is necessary.

Although it is unlikely that the goals of Jonas and of Ramsey will ever be achieved, and that human research subjects will spontaneously volunteer rather than be "conscripted," efforts to promote educated consent are in order. In view of the current emphasis on involving "the community" in such activities as regional planning, operation of clinics, and assignment of priorities, the general public and its political leaders are showing an increased awareness and understanding of medical affairs. But the orientation of

Franz J. Ingelfinger, "Informed (But Uneducated) Consent," *New England Journal of Medicine* 287 (1972): 465–66.

202   INFORMED CONSENT IN RESEARCH

this public interest in medicine is chiefly socioeconomic. Little has been done to give the public a basic understanding of medical research and its requirements not only for the people's money but also for their participation. The public, to be sure, is being subjected to a bombardment of sensation-mongering news stories and books that feature "breakthroughs," or that reveal real or alleged exploitation —horror stories of Nazi-type experimentation on abused human minds and bodies. Muckraking is essential to expose malpractices, but unless accompanied by efforts to promote a broader appreciation of medical research and its methods, it merely compounds the difficulties for both the investigator and the subject when "informed consent" is solicited.

The procedure currently approved in the United States for enlisting human experimental subjects has one great virtue: patient-subjects are put on notice that their management is in part at least an experiment. The deceptions of the past are no longer tolerated. Beyond this accomplishment, however, the process of obtaining "informed consent," with all its regulations and conditions, is no more than an elaborate ritual, a device that, when the subject is uneducated and uncomprehending, confers no more than the semblance of propriety on human experimentation. The subject's only real protection, the public as well as the medical profession must recognize, depends on the conscience and compassion of the investigator and his peers.

32   A Moral Theory of Informed Consent

BENJAMIN FREEDMAN

Most medical codes of ethics, and most physicians, agree that the physician ought to obtain the "free and informed consent" of his subject or patient before attempting any serious medical procedure, experimental or therapeutic in nature. They agree, moreover, that a proxy consent ought to be obtained on behalf of the incompetent subject. And informed consent is seen as not merely a legal requirement, and not merely a formality: it is a substantial requirement of morality.

Acceptance of this doctrine, however, requires the solution of a number of problems. How much information need be imparted? At what age is a person mature enough to consent on his own behalf? Can prisoners give a "free and informed consent" to be experimented upon? Lurking behind these and similar questions there are more fundamental difficulties. What are the functions of consent for the competent and the incompetent? What is the sense in which the patient/subject must be "free," "informed," and "competent"? It is by way of an approach to these latter questions that I shall attempt to respond to the more specific questions. [...]

THE REQUIREMENT OF INFORMATION

The most common locution for the requirement which I am discussing is "informed consent"—we require "in-

Benjamin Freedman, "A Moral Theory of Informed Consent," *Hastings Center Report* 5, no. 4 (1975): 32–39.

formed consent" to protect a doctor from legal liability resultant from his therapeutic endeavors, or to ensure the "ethicacy" of an experiment. But I believe "informed consent" to be a serious misnomer for what we do, in fact, want medical practice to conform to.

No lengthy rehearsal of the absurdities consequent upon taking the term "informed consent" at face value is necessary. The claim has been made, and repeated with approval, that "fully informed consent" is a goal which we can never achieve, but toward which we must strive. In order to ensure that fully informed consent has been given, it has seriously been suggested that only medical students or graduate students in the life sciences ought to be accepted as subjects for experimentation. *Reductio ad absurdum* examples of "fully informed consent" have been elaborated, in forms which list all the minutiae of the proposed medical procedure, together with all of its conceivable sequelae. With such a view of "informed consent" and its requirements, it is not surprising to find doctors who claim that since they cannot fully inform patients, they will tell them nothing, but instead will personally assume the responsibility for assuring the subject's safety.

In truth, a *reductio ad absurdum* of this view of "informed consent" need not be constructed; it serves as its own *reductio ad absurdum*. For there is no end to "fully informing" patients. When the doctor wishes to insert a catheter, must he commend to the subject's attention a textbook of anatomy? Although this, of course, would not suffice: he must ensure that the patient understands the text as well. Must he tell the patient the story of Dr. X, that bogey of first-year medical students, who, in a state of inebriation, inserted ("by mistake") his pen-refill instead of the catheter? With, of course, the assurance that *this* physician never gets drunk. ("Well, rarely, anyway.") Must the patient be informed of the chemical formula of the catheter? Its melting point?

The basic mistake which is committed by those who harp upon the difficulties in obtaining informed consent (and by critics of the doctrine) is in believing that we can talk about information in the abstract, without reference to any human purpose. It is very likely impossible to talk about "information" in this way; but impossible or not, when we do in fact talk about, or request, information, we do not mean "information in the abstract." If I ask someone to "tell me about those clouds" he will, ordinarily, know what I mean; and he will answer me, in the spirit in which he was asked, by virtue of his professional expertise as an artist, meteorologist, astronomer, soothsayer, or what-have-you. The meteorologist will not object that he cannot tell you the optical refraction index of the clouds, and therefore that he cannot "fully answer" your question. He knows that you are asking him with a given end in mind, and that much information about the cloud is irrelevant *relative to that purpose.*

That this "abstract information" requirement is not in question in obtaining valid consent is hardly an original point, but it is worth repeating. One of the leading court opinions on human experimentation puts it like this: ". . . the patient's interest in information does not extend to a lengthy polysyllabic discourse on all possible complications. A mini-course in medical science is not required. . . ."

The proper question to ask, then, is not "What information must be given?" That would be premature: we must first know for what purpose information is needed. Why must the patient be informed? Put that way, the answer is immediately forthcoming. The patient must be informed so that he will know what he is getting into, what he may expect from the procedure, what his likely alternatives are—in short, what the procedure (and forbearance from it) will mean, so that a reasonable decision on the matter may be made. This is the legal stance, as well as, I think, a "common sensical" stance; as Alexander Capron writes, the information component in valid consent derives in law from the recognition that information is "necessary to make meaningful the power to decide." The proper test of whether a given piece of information needs to be given is, then, whether the physician, knowing what he does about the patient/subject, feels that the patient/subject would want to know this before making up his mind. Outré, improbable consequences would not ordinarily, therefore, be relevant information. Exceptionally, they will be: for example, when there is a small risk of impotence consequent upon the procedure which the physician proposes to perform upon a man with a great stake in his sexual prowess. This is only sensible.

Our main conclusion, then is that valid consent entails only the imparting of that information which the patient/subject requires in order to make a responsible decision. This entails, I think, the possibility of a valid yet ignorant consent.

Consider, first, the therapeutic context. It is, I believe, not unusual for a patient to give his doctor *carte blanche* to perform any medical procedure which the physician deems proper in order to effect a cure. He is telling the doctor to act as his agent in choosing which procedure to follow. This decision is neither unwise nor (in any serious sense) an abdication of responsibility and an unwarranted burden upon the physician. We each of us choose to delegate our power of choice in this way in dealing with our auto mechanic or stockbroker.

It may be harder to accept an ignorant consent as valid in the purely experimental context. I think, however, that much of this difficulty is due to our paucity of imagination, our failure to imagine circumstances in which a person might choose to proceed in this way. We might approach such a case, for example, by imagining a Quaker who chooses to serve society by acting as a research subject, but who has a morbid fear of knives and pointed instruments. The Quaker might say to the physician-investigator that he wants to serve science but is afraid that his phobia would overcome his better judgment. He might consequently request that any experiment which would involve use of scalpels, hypodermic needles, and such, be performed without informing him: while, say, he is asleep or unconscious. He might further ask the doctor not to proceed should the experiment involve considerable risk. In such a case, or one similar, we would find an instance of a valid yet ignorant consent to experimentation.

The ostensible differences between the therapeutic and experimental contexts may be resolved into two components: in the therapeutic context it is supposed that the physician knows what the sequelae to treatment will be, which information, by definition, is not available in the experimental situation; and in the therapeutic context the doctor may be said to be seeking his patient's good, in contrast to the experimental context where some other good is being sought. On the basis of these differences it may be claimed that a valid yet ignorant consent is enough permission for therapy, but not for experimentation.

Closer examination, however, reveals that these differences do not necessarily obtain. First, because I believe it would be granted that a valid yet ignorant consent can be given in the "therapeutic-experimental" situation, where a new drug or procedure is being attempted to aid the patient (in the absence of any traditional available therapy). In the therapeutic-experimental situation, as in the purely experimental situation, the sequelae are not known (although of course in both cases some definite result is expected or anticipated). If a valid yet ignorant consent is acceptable in the one, therefore, it must be acceptable in the other.

Secondly, because it is patently not the case that we can expect there to be no good accruing to the subject of an experiment by reason of his participation. There are, commonly, financial and other "tangible" benefits forthcoming (laboratory training, and so on). And it must once again be said that the pleasures of altruism are not negligible. The proposed differences between experimentation and therapy do not stand up, and so we must say that if a valid yet ignorant consent is acceptable in the one it must be acceptable in the other. It must be remembered that this statement only concerns itself with one part of the consent doctrine, which is, itself, only one of the requirements which the ethical experiment must satisfy.

To mention—without claiming totally to resolve—two problems which may be raised at this point: First, it is said that a doctor often does not know what will happen as a consequence of a recommended procedure, and so cannot tell the patient what the patient wants to know. The obvious response to this seems to be right: the physician should, in that case, tell the patient/subject that he does not know what will happen (which does not exclude an explanation of what the doctor expects to happen, and on what he bases this expectation).

Second, it will be objected that the adoption of a requirement such as I propose would forbid the use of placebos and blind experiments. I am not sure that this is so; sometimes it must be the case that the subjects in an experiment may be asked (without introducing artifacts into the results) to consent to an experiment knowing that some will, and some will not, be receiving placebos. Another alternative would be to inform the subjects that the experiment may or may not involve some subjects receiving placebos. I am aware, however, that these remarks are less than adequate responses to these problems.

Our conclusion, then, is that the informing of the patient/subject is not a fundamental requirement of valid consent. It is, rather, derivative from the requirement that the consent be the expression of a responsible choice. The two requirements which I do see as fundamental in this doctrine are that the choice be responsible and that it be voluntary.

THE REQUIREMENT OF RESPONSIBILITY

What is meant by saying that the choice must be "responsible"? Does this entail that the physician may at any time override a patient's judgment on the basis that, in the physician's view, the patient has not chosen responsibly? Surely not; to adopt such a criterion would defeat the purpose embodied in the doctrine of consent. It would mean that a person's exercise of autonomy is always subject to review.

Still, some such requirement would appear to be necessary. A small child can certainly make choices. Small children can also be intelligent enough to understand the necessary information. Yet surely we would not want to say that a small child can give valid consent to a serious medical procedure. The reason for this is that the child cannot choose *responsibly.*

We are faced with a dilemma. On the one hand, it appears that we must require that the choice be responsible. To require only that the choice be free would yield counterintuitive results. On the other hand, if we do require that the choice made be a responsible one, we seem to presuppose some body which shall judge the reasonableness of choices; this represents a paternalism which is antithetical to the doctrine of consent. An elderly patient chooses to forgo further life-saving measures. How are we to judge whether or not this choice is a responsible one?

The path between the horns of this dilemma involves saying that the "responsibility" which we require is to be predicated not on the nature of the particular choice, but on the nature of the patient/subject. What we need to know is whether he is a responsible man ("in general," so to speak), not whether the choice which has been made is responsible. In this way, we avoid the danger of upholding as "responsible" only those choices which we ourselves feel are good choices. We can and do admit into the community of responsible persons individuals who make choices with which we do not agree.

In this sense, responsibility is a dispositional characteristic. To say that someone is a responsible individual means that he makes choices, typically, on the basis of reasons, arguments, or beliefs—and that he remains open to the claims of reason, so that further rational argument might lead him to change his mind. It is to say that a person is capable of making and carrying through a life-plan—that he is prepared to act on the basis of his choices. It is to say that a person is capable of living with his life-plan; he can live with the consequences of his choices, he *takes responsibility* for his choices. Of course, none of these are absolutes: all responsible people are at times pigheaded, at times short-sighted, at times flighty. That is to say, all responsible men at times act irresponsibly. Should the lack of responsibility persist, of course, to an extreme degree, we may say that the person has left the community of responsible folk.

VOLUNTARISM AND REWARD

The other requirement of valid consent is that it be given voluntarily. The choice which the consent expresses must be freely made.

We all know some conditions which, if satisfied, make us say that a consent has been given involuntarily. The case which immediately springs to mind occurs when an individual succumbs under a threat: we call this duress or coercion. But the threat need not be overt; and perhaps there need not be a threat at all to render consent involuntary.

Hence, the major problem currently engendered by the requirement of voluntariness. It is typified by the prisoner who "volunteers" for an experiment in the hope or expectation of a reward: significantly higher wages, an opportunity for job training, better health care while involved in the experiment, a favorable report to his parole board. Is the consent which the prisoner offers a voluntary consent? The problem may be stated more generally thus: At what point does reward render consent involuntary?

The problem of reward is particularly difficult, since it involves questions of degree. Is a prisoner's consent involuntary if the reward for his participation in the experiment is a three-month reduction of sentence? Is it relevant here that the prisoner is serving a twenty-year sentence, rather than a one-to-five-year sentence? Does a possible increase in wages from twenty-five cents per hour to one dollar per hour constitute duress? Should we consider the percentage increase, or the increase in absolute value, or the increase in actual value which the seventy-five cent disparity represents in the prison environment?

To some, of course, questions like these have little meaning. They have little meaning to those who are indifferent to the demands of justice and autonomy which the consent doctrine represents, to those who are willing to buy guinea pigs, rather than to reward human beings. And they have little meaning for those who are convinced that prisoners are inherently unfree, and who thus would call for a total cessation of prison experimentation. Each of these positions denies, in an *a priori* fashion, freedom to prisoners; each must be rejected. A recognition of the fact that decisions about consent may be over- as well as under-protective forces us to deal with this sort of question, complex though it may be.

As is so often the case, posing the question in a different way may facilitate response. We have been considering the question of how much reward nullifies the validity of consent, how much reward renders the subject unfree. But is it in fact the case that *reward* is the disruptive factor here?

This problem may be clarified by the following examples. Imagine an upper-middle-class individual, who can provide for his family all of their needs and most of the amenities of civilized life. Let us say that this person is offered one hundred dollars to cross the street—if you like, make it one thousand or ten thousand dollars. He chooses to cross the street. Is his choice *involuntary*? Despite the substantial reward, I think most of us would agree that the consent was freely offered (and would that we should have such problems!).

Consider a person who deeply wants to be an astronaut. He is told that as part of the program he must participate in experiments to determine resistance to high-G conditions. Is his consent to this invalid, involuntary? I think not. We would say, this is part of his job; he should have expected it; and if he can't stand the heat, he should get out of the kitchen. In this vein, consider Evel Knievel, a financially prosperous man who is offered millions of dollars to perform daredevil stunts. His choice may be bizarre, even crazy: but has his reward rendered it unfree?

Finally, consider a man who is informed by his doctor that he will most likely die unless he has open-heart surgery. His "reward" for consenting is life; the penalty for not consenting is death. Does this mean this man cannot give the doctor valid consent—morally valid consent—to proceed?

There are two distinctions which, I think, go a long way towards dispelling these problems. First, I think it must be granted that natural contingencies ("acts of God," things which come to pass naturally, those contingencies which we cannot hold anyone responsible for) do not render a person unfree, nor do they render unfree the choices which a person makes in light of those contingencies.

That natural contingencies do not render a man unfree is a point which is apt to be forgotten in the present context. I am not—in the morally relevant sense—lacking in freedom because I cannot, unaided, fly through the air, or live on grass. Nor am I unfree because my heart is about to give out. Nor am I unfree when, recognizing that my heart may give out, I choose to undergo surgery. I may, of course, be so crazed by knowing that I am near death's door that I am in a state of general impotence, and hence must have the choice made for me; but general incompetence is not in question here. The distinction between choices forced by man, and choices forced by nature, is, then, of importance.

The second distinction is between those pressures which are, and those which are not, in Daube's words, "consonant with the dignity and responsibility of free life." I would explain this as follows: there are certain basic freedoms and rights which we possess which *entitle* us (morally) to certain things (or states of affairs). We would all, no doubt, draw up different lists of these rights and freedoms; but included in them would be safety of person, freedom of conscience and religion, a right to a certain level of education, and, for some of us, a right to some level of health care. When the "reward" is such as only to give us the necessary conditions of these rights and freedoms—when all that the reward does is to bring us up to a level of living to which we are entitled, and of which we have been deprived by man—then the "reward," I think, constitutes duress. A reward which accrues to one who has achieved this level, or who can easily achieve it (other than by taking the reward-option), and which hence serves only to grant us "luxury" items, does not constitute duress, and hence does not render choices unfree, no matter how great this reward may be.

The rewards above the moral subsistence level are true rewards. In contrast, we may say (with some touch of metaphor) that the "rewards" which only bring us up to the level to which we were in any event entitled are properly viewed as functioning as *threats:* "Do this, or stay where you are"—when you should not have been "where you are" in the first place.

The astronaut, Evel Knievel, and the upper-middle-class street-crosser are being granted "luxury" items, and hence are capable of giving free consent. But consider a man who will not be admitted to the hospital for treatment unless he agrees to be a subject in an experiment (unrelated to his treatment). Those who feel, as I do, that we are, here and now, morally entitled to medical treatment would agree, I trust, that this illegitimate option coerces the man into agreeing. Or consider a man who has religious scruples against donating blood, who takes his daughter to a hospital for treatment. He is told that the doctors will not treat her unless the family donates a certain amount of blood. His freedom has been nullified; his "consent" to donating blood is morally invalid. Similarly, the college stu-

dent whose grade is contingent upon his participation in the instructor's psychological experiments is not validly consenting to serve. He is entitled to have his grade based upon his classroom work.

It yet remains to apply this distinction to our original problem, prison experimentation. The application will not be attempted here, for we would first need to be clear in our minds what rights and freedoms a prisoner is entitled to. I would not hesitate to say, though, that when a situation is created whereby a prisoner can only receive decent health care by participating in an experiment, he is being coerced into that experiment. I would have little hesitation in claiming that if subjecting himself to experimentation is the only way in which a prisoner could learn a trade which may be used "outside," then that prisoner is being coerced, his consent is not free. When we take into account the condition of our society, these would seem to be reasonable entitlements for the prisoner. Other rewards—for example, higher pay—may or may not constitute rewards above the moral subsistence level; if they are, then consent in light of these rewards could be freely offered. Perhaps too much has been said already; judgments like these must be made in an individualized fashion, one which is sensitive to the realities of prison life. [...]

---

33 Is Informed Consent Always Necessary for Randomized, Controlled Trials?

Robert D. Truog, Walter Robinson,
Adrienne Randolph, and Alan Morris

Consider this paradox: If a physician reads a case report about a novel method of ventilation for critically ill patients and wants to try it in the next several patients with respiratory failure he or she treats, the physician may do so provided the patients have given general consent for treatment. On the other hand, if a physician is interested in performing a randomized, controlled trial to determine rigorously which of two widely used antibiotics is more effective at treating bronchitis, he or she must prepare a formal protocol, obtain approval from the institutional review board, and seek written informed consent from po-

tential participants. In each case, the physician is performing an experiment. In each case, there is uncertainty about the best way to treat the patient. Yet in the context of clinical care, the experiment can be done with virtually no external scrutiny, whereas in the context of a clinical trial, the experiment is prohibited unless substantial hurdles are overcome. This is true even when the experimental therapy (e.g., a promising but risky method of ventilation) involves risks that are unknown or substantially different from those of the alternatives.

To put it another way, physicians can do almost anything they want in the name of therapeutic innovation, but only if there is no attempt to gain systematic knowledge from the intervention. Or, to paraphrase Smithells, "I need permission to give a new drug to half my patients but not to give it to all of them." In this article we argue that the current approach to informed consent is at least partially off

———
Robert D. Truog, Walter Robinson, Adrienne Randolph, and Alan Morris, "Is Informed Consent Always Necessary for Randomized, Controlled Trials?" *New England Journal of Medicine* 340 (1999): 804–7.

target, in that patients are often "protected" from clinical trials under circumstances in which the risks associated with participation in the trial are virtually nil, but they receive no protection from physicians who want to experiment with new treatments in the name of therapeutic innovation.

The reasons for the current approach are not mysterious. In a simplistic sense, all medical interventions may be characterized as either therapy or research. Research differs from therapy in many important ways. The goal of research is to gain new knowledge, and any benefits from the research are reaped primarily by future patients. The aim of therapy is to benefit the patient at hand. These differences have predictably led to an elaborate process designed to protect patients involved in clinical trials, whereas minimal constraints are placed on physicians providing clinical care. [...]

An analysis of the goals of informed consent can provide insight into the paradox described above. Informed consent is either general or specific. A patient gives general informed consent for treatment as part of the process of establishing a fiduciary relationship with a physician. Specific informed consent is necessary whenever the proposed intervention involves a high risk-benefit ratio, either in an absolute sense or in comparison with the alternatives, or whenever the preferences or values of the patient are relevant to the decision at hand. The distinction between these two tiers of informed consent is illustrated by the fact that physicians typically order routine tests and prescribe standard medications under the general consent for treatment but obtain specific consent before undertaking a major diagnostic or therapeutic procedure, before prescribing a potentially toxic medication, or whenever a patient's values and preferences would be expected to have a substantial influence on the clinical course chosen.

We suggest that the obligation to seek specific consent for research should likewise depend on the risk-benefit ratios of the intervention and the alternatives as well as the degree to which the patient would be expected to have preferences about the various options for diagnosis or treatment that are under investigation. We believe that as with clinical care, in the case of many randomized, controlled trials, the patient's participation can and should be considered to be authorized by his or her general consent for treatment and that specific consent should not be required.

Consider, for example, a hypothetical trial comparing two similar cephalosporins for preoperative prophylaxis. Both are widely used, but they differ markedly in cost, and their comparative efficacy in preventing wound infections is unknown. If both drugs have been in use long enough that their side-effect profiles are known to be similar, patients are unlikely to prefer one medication over another; it is also unlikely that the process of obtaining specific consent would serve the patient in any meaningful way. Other examples of this type of study are a randomized trial to assess whether low-dose heparin increases the longevity of intraarterial catheters in the intensive care unit, a randomized trial of two brands of antacid to control gastric acidity, and a randomized comparison of two methods of mechanical ventilation to determine which method results in more rapid resumption of spontaneous, unassisted breathing. These hypothetical trials share several characteristics, which we have integrated into the following proposed criteria for determining whether the requirement of informed consent for a randomized, controlled trial can be waived.

First, informed consent should not be waived unless all the treatments offered in the trial could be offered outside the trial without the specific informed consent of the patient. This is often the case when a trial is comparing two therapies that are already in use or when an existing therapy or drug is being used for a new indication. In the hypothetical trials described above, the specific informed consent of the patient would thus not be required for any of the options being offered.

Second, the treatments should not involve more than minimal additional risk in comparison with any of the alternatives. When the risks associated with each of the options are assumed to be similar, the patient could be treated outside the trial with any one of the interventions under study. Again, the examples we cited could meet this requirement. Of course, physicians would exclude a patient for a justifiable medical reason—for example, if the patient were known to be allergic to one of the medications being studied.

Third, genuine clinical equipoise must exist among the treatments. This state of balance is, of course, a general ethical requirement before a randomized, controlled study can be undertaken. There should be honest uncertainty about which treatment is superior. If the informed consent of the patient is judged unnecessary, investigators have an even greater burden of proof to ensure clinical equipoise.

Fourth, no reasonable person should have a preference for one treatment over any other, regardless of the differences between the treatments being compared. This standard would cover not only the direct effects of the intervention being studied but also the indirect effects associated with research, such as whether the study would require extra visits to the clinic or other inconveniences.

Although the reasonable-person standard is widely used in the law, it is far from perfect. For example, there is always the possibility that a patient may be unusual in ways that cannot be anticipated and that would lead the patient to have an unanticipated preference for one treatment over another. This problem arises with both general and specific informed consent, however, and cannot be addressed solely by demanding more rigorous standards for research.

The validity of the reasonable-person standard depends in large part on how it is implemented. We propose that studies for which a waiver of informed consent is requested should, like all other studies, be submitted to an institutional review board for review and approval. The institutional review board would therefore assume responsibility for applying the standard. Because an important function of the institutional review board is to ensure the involvement of the community through the representation of people without medical backgrounds, the board would be in the best position to apply the reasonable-person standard and to determine whether the informed-consent requirement could be waived.

How should the reasonable-person standard be applied with reference to the community in which the research is being performed? Since the abuses of the Tuskegee syphilis study, members of racial minority groups have been particularly sensitive to the implications of being involved in research without their consent. Although we believe that exemptions to informed consent should be considered only when potential subjects would have no reason to decline participation, we recognize that for some the refusal to participate in research may not be related to the pertinent facts of a particular study but, rather, may be based on important historical and cultural issues of concern. Depending on the community and the context of the research, these issues may be grounds for insisting on specific informed consent for participation in the research.

Fifth, patients should be informed that the institution or clinical setting in which they are being treated uses the standards that we have described as guidelines for determining the need for specific instead of general informed consent. Thus, patients would have the opportunity to obtain additional information about the policy or seek care elsewhere.

These criteria for the waiver of informed consent should be interpreted narrowly and applied conservatively. For example, a trial comparing a beta-blocker with an angiotensin-converting-enzyme inhibitor for treatment of hypertension should not be approved for a waiver of informed consent because of the substantially different side effects of the two classes of drugs. Similarly, comparisons of medical treatments and surgical interventions should always require specific informed consent, even if the outcomes are presumed to be similar, because of the probable relevance of patients' preferences to the decision. Finally, specific informed consent should be required whenever a study compares therapies that involve a trade-off between efficacy and safety, as would be the case in a trial of the use of an anticoagulant to reduce the morbidity associated with strokes. This decision requires the balancing of benefits against qualitatively dissimilar risks, necessitating the involvement and specific consent of the patient.

Our arguments may also have important implications for studies that fall under the heading of quality improvement. Consider, for example, a study that seeks to identify the more effective disinfectant hand soap by using one brand for patients in one hospital and a different brand for patients in another, with nosocomial infection rates as the outcome measure. The patients are to be randomly assigned to the wards. Should specific informed consent be sought from the patients enrolled in the study? If so, then what should be done if a patient chooses not to participate? (Should he or she be transferred to another ward, or should data not be collected on that patient?) Our criteria may be useful in determining the need for specific informed consent in a context such as this one.

Our arguments pull in two different directions. Greater respect for the autonomy of patients means that many experiments that are currently undertaken in the context of clinical care under the guise of therapeutic innovation should be subject to much greater scrutiny. Such a shift in thinking would have far-reaching consequences, from changing the way that surgeons approach consent for the use of new techniques in the operating room to altering the way that physicians prescribe drugs for indications for which they have not been approved by the Food and Drug Administration (FDA).

Yet we have argued that specific informed consent should not be mandatory for all randomized, controlled trials. Although this idea has been proposed before, many will nevertheless find it objectionable. They may argue that it backtracks from crucial elements of human rights at a time when we need to be as vigilant as possible and that essential principles enunciated at Nuremberg and Helsinki must not be compromised under any circumstances. Furthermore, they may claim that informed consent is an essential protection against the exploitation of patients by research investigators. These are important objections.

In response, our proposal should serve as a reminder that the process of informed consent is not a goal or ideal in itself. Rather, informed consent is important because it is frequently essential for ensuring that the patient's right to self-determination is respected. Our proposal not only supports this important objective but also provides grounds for criticizing the inappropriate use of what are termed therapeutic innovations without the specific informed consent of the patient.

There is little evidence to support the claim that informed consent, as currently practiced, provides protection against the exploitation of patients in research. Studies have shown that patients rarely demonstrate an adequate understanding of consent forms and often do not even understand the meaning or implications of randomization. The most effective protection against exploitation comes not from the process of informed consent but, rather, from the careful oversight and scrutiny of conscientious institutional review boards. Boards that approve questionable studies on the assumption that the informed-consent process will protect research subjects against abuse abrogate their responsibility to defend patients against unethical research. Our proposal recognizes and emphasizes the essential role of institutional review boards in this regard.

In addition, there is a price that is paid when one insists on specific informed consent for all randomized, controlled trials. Many worthwhile studies will not be conducted if investigators are required to obtain specific informed consent. Many small but meaningful improvements in the quality of care will not occur if clinicians are forced to engage every patient in a dialogue about informed consent, especially when there is no reason to believe that the patient would have any preference regarding participation in the research. When unnecessary roadblocks prevent the easy evaluation of the comparative efficacy of new forms of technology and new interventions, these innovations tend to be adopted uncritically into practice. And this result is unfortunate, given that many of them would probably be found worthless or even harmful if subjected to formal evaluation in a clinical trial.

These clinical and practical realities were recently acknowledged in the United States with regard to research under emergency conditions. For many years, research on emergency treatments was virtually paralyzed by the impossibility of obtaining informed consent from the subjects. For new therapies, such as the administration of hemoglobin substitutes in severe trauma and of thrombolytic agents in acute myocardial infarction, or new methods of performing cardiopulmonary resuscitation, systematic clinical trials could not be undertaken. In 1996, the FDA and the Department of Health and Human Services endorsed a waiver of informed consent for this type of research under certain clearly defined conditions. Although they acknowledged the importance of informed consent to medical practice, these agencies endorsed the waiver on the grounds that it would allow desperately ill patients access to new therapies and would result in important benefits to future patients. The agencies recognized that without the waiver, this important work would never be done.

We believe that the same rationale supports our proposal against the anticipated objections of those who prefer to see no exceptions made to the doctrine of informed consent. When benefits to society and to future patients can be gained without meaningfully compromising respect for patients' autonomy and without any serious increase in risk to those involved, blind insistence on informed consent is not only unnecessary, but also harmful.

34   Human Experimentation
       and Human Rights

JAY KATZ

[...]

VI. THE NATURE OF THE INFORMED CONSENT PROCESS IN CLINICAL RESEARCH

If the tensions between the inviolability of research subjects and the advancement of knowledge are to be resolved in favor of respect for the human rights of the subjects, the mindset which investigators bring to the invitation of participation, the ethical principles which govern the invitation, and the conversations which physician-investigators and patient-subjects must engage in require re-examination. I shall take up each in turn.

A.   The Mindset of Physician-Investigators

Physician-investigators, *before* approaching a potential patient-subject, must first rid themselves of the customary attitudes which in the past shaped, if not determined, their invitation to patient-subjects. A morally valid consent in research settings requires a radically new personal and professional commitment to the patient-subjects and the informed consent process: Physician-investigators must see themselves as scientists only and not as doctors. In conflating clinical trials and therapy, as well as patients and subjects, as if both were one and the same, physician-investigators unwittingly become double agents with conflicting loyalties. Only if they first know who they truly are can they begin to make the subject understand the burdens he or she is assuming when an invitation to participate in clinical trials is extended. Moreover, since loyalty to the research protocol will take precedence over faithful-

Jay Katz, "Human Experimentation and Human Rights," *St. Louis University Law Journal* 38 (1993): 7–54.

ness to the therapeutic mission, and since physician-investigators will tend to view the person before them as a patient and not as a subject, the tragic fact that human beings are used for the ends of others can readily become obliterated. It is then not surprising that physician-investigators, without fully knowing it, become confused about the nature of their task, as well as about their perceptions of themselves and their patient-subjects.

The investigators who appear before patient-subjects as physicians in white coats create confusion. Patients come to hospitals with the trusting expectation that their doctors will care for them. They will view an invitation to participate in research as a professional recommendation that is intended to serve their individual treatment interests. It is that belief, that trust, which physician-investigators must vigorously challenge so that patient-subjects appreciate that in research, unlike therapy, the research question comes first. This takes time and is difficult to convey. It can be conveyed to patient-subjects only if physician-investigators are willing to challenge the misperceptions that many patients bring to the invitation.

B.   The Primacy of Autonomy

Physician-investigators must extend the invitation to participation in research with a thoroughgoing commitment to the principle of autonomy. [...]

Respect for autonomy imposes numerous burdens on the physician-investigator. First, he must not allow disclosures to be shaped by paternalistic or beneficent concerns that patient-subjects will make decisions which are not in their "best interests." Second, he or she must not allow disclosures to be shaped by concerns that patient-subjects will learn that the customary treatments which they may continue to take, should they decline the more promising experimental treatments, offer no hope for the alleviation of their suffering. Nor should disclosures be shaped by concerns that patient-subjects' trust in medicine will be undermined once they learn about the uncertainties inherent in all medical treatments, nor by concerns over upsetting hospitalized patients if they were to appreciate that they, too, are being asked to yield their individual interests to the interests of scientific investigations.

Moreover, physician-investigators must reflect on the fateful impact of their commitment to the ideology of medical science—its ethos to acquire knowledge for the sake of mankind—on the invitation to participation in research. Medical scientists share with their colleagues from the natural sciences a commitment to the pursuit of truth, objectivity, and the advancement of knowledge. The commitment to objectivity invites investigators' thought processes to become objectified and, in turn, to transform the human beings who are the subjects of research into data

points to be plotted on a chart that will prove or disprove a research hypothesis.

Margaret Radin's observations about objectification illuminate this problem. In an article on women and people of color she noted that

> [o]bjectification comes about through *subordination* when one culture conceives of certain characteristics of persons . . . as marks of lesser personhood. These marks license manipulation of those who bear the marks, and also license refusal to recognize in them rights and other indices of respect otherwise conceived of as universally applicable to persons.

This license was usurped or conferred on physicians in clinical practice, and since the age of medical science has been extended to clinical research. Objectification begins with patients and becomes intensified when subordination is also affected by attitudes toward gender, color, religion, social and economic status, and, of course, by the scientific imperative of clinical research.

Furthermore, human beings should not be used lightly and cheaply to serve as means for the ends of others, even though they are so readily available in large numbers. Prior to extending an invitation to subjects, physician-investigators must give thought to the minimal number of subjects required for obtaining satisfactory answers to a research question and must conduct a literature search of existing studies which will make a repetition of an experiment unnecessary. Science's commitment to truth and progress, particularly when human beings are needed for purposes of research, ought to disdain inquiries where the truth is already apparent and progress already a reality.

Finally, as I have already suggested, physician-investigators must go to considerable length in extending the invitation to participate in clinical research so that they can rest assured that patient-subjects understand the implications of their consent. Pellegrino, in his discussion of "valid consent," sensitively describes the difficulty patients experience in "[separating] the physician-scientist role from the physician-healer." He further notes that "[t]he physician can easily obtain consent to an experimental protocol simply by emphasizing the hope of cure and downplaying the risk and the experimental nature of the treatment." He cautions physicians that "[a] legally adequate consent form may not be morally valid, [for a] morally valid consent aims at true 'con-sent,' an agreeing together."

Only respect for persons' autonomy and self-determination can guarantee "true 'con-sent,' an agreeing together"; otherwise, the invitation subtly becomes a request or even a demand. Invocation of the principle of beneficence, in the service of shielding patient-subjects from painful disclosures, can only mislead physician-investigators into "downplaying the risk and the experimental nature of the treatment." Whenever beneficence suggests withholding of information, the better solution would be to exclude patient-subjects from participation in clinical research.

C. The Conversation

To obtain a "morally valid consent [which] aims at true consent" is an inordinately difficult task. The physician-investigators must disclose to their subjects at least the following information: (1) that the subjects are not only patients and, to the extent to which they are patients, that their therapeutic interests, even if not incidental, will be subordinated to scientific interests; (2) that it is problematic and indeterminate whether their welfare will be better served by placing their medical fate in the hands of a physician rather than an investigator; (3) that in opting for the care of a physician they may be better or worse off and for such and such reasons; (4) that clinical research will allow doctors to penetrate the mysteries of medicine's uncertainties about which treatments are best, dangerous, or ineffective; (5) that clinical research may possibly be in the patient's immediate best interest, perhaps promise benefits in the future, or provide no benefit, particularly if the patient is assigned to a control (placebo) arm of a study; (6) that research is governed by a research protocol and a research question and, therefore, his or her interests and needs will yield to the claims of science; and (7) that physician-investigators will respect whatever decision the subject ultimately makes.

Conversing with patient-subjects in such a manner which will give them a clearer appreciation of the difference between clinical research and therapy is a daunting assignment. I have on occasions been asked, "How will investigators know when to stop the conversation?" My response has been that they will know when to stop once they have learned to begin the conversation with a commitment to respect for personhood; for only then will they not shirk their responsibility to be utterly forthright in disclosing the research dimension of their work and the alternatives available to their patient-subjects. It is the spirit in which the conversation begins which is the problem. If that problem is better resolved, the end will take care of itself.

Levine once wrote that in the current climate of extending the invitation to participation in research, "[the informed consent] requirement [serves] as a *pledge* made by researchers that in the pursuit of their salutary mission they will not exploit people; [or that i]ndividual persons will not be involved as research subjects without their awareness or approval." If he meant by "pledge" a symbolic gesture "to secure and maintain public confidence in scientific research," rather than a true commitment, I would agree.

Guido Calabresi years ago expressed his doubts about informed consent serving as a "control system" for the value conflicts inherent in the conduct of research. He did not believe that it could in practice serve such a purpose. His argument was that "[c]onsent or its semblance keeps us from blatantly [destroying] the fabric of our commitment to human dignity." I am not convinced that informed consent need only serve such a limited symbolic function once the idea of shared decision making becomes a guiding commitment. Levine's and Calabresi's observations, however, identify the mutual deceptions in which scientists and the public engage in order not to unduly impede scientific research. The public, propelled by its longings to benefit from the advancement of science, has made common cause with scientists' demand for freedom of inquiry by acquiescing to the human costs which research entails. The symbolic bow to informed consent then allows the public and scientists to have it both ways. Forcing a public debate on the morality of human experimentation may put an end to the all too silent evasion of confronting any tragic choices that must be made. To be sure, "public confidence in scientific research" is justified on the ground that physician-investigators will take great care in not exposing patient-subjects to unnecessary *physical* harm. But this is a different matter.

The disclosure obligations I have set forth so far emphasize the need to pay particular attention to explaining to patient-subjects how participation in research differs from how they would ordinarily be treated or would expect to be treated. Thus, the first task in extending the invitation is to be absolutely clear about the research dimension of the invitation, its implications and possible consequences. Such disclosures do not require patient-subjects to understand the esoteric knowledge of medicine and science. Indeed, at present, subjects are overwhelmed with unnecessary scientific information that clarifies little and serves more the purpose of obscuring the crucial information that they need to know, such as the risks, benefits, alternatives, and uncertainties which patient-subjects face by their participation in clinical research, and the impact of participation, known and conjectured, on the quality of their future lives. Investigators have an obligation to translate scientific information into language which is relevant to patient-subjects' life and interests. Informed consent forms are so incomprehensible because they are written at a higher reading level than is appropriate for the intended population. In addition, they include too much distracting technical information of little consequence to the decisions which patient-subjects must make. Put another way, current informed consent forms often provide IRBs [institutional review boards—eds.] rather than the subjects with a better understanding of investigators' intentions.

Physician-scientists will be reluctant to converse with patient-subjects in the spirit of the recommendation that I have outlined. Such conversations take time, may have to extend over hours, perhaps even days, and must be continued until one is reasonably certain that the patient-subjects understand. Of course, subjects may still make decisions which they later on will regret because they then believe, perhaps correctly so, that they had not given their participation the thought it deserved. This is inevitable, and physician-investigators must not allow that possibility to tailor their disclosures in order to avoid burdening subjects with guilt feelings over having made the wrong decision (another variant of beneficence) or that they will agree to what investigators believe to be in subjects' better interests. Autonomous persons must be held responsible for their own mistakes and must not be protected from making them by subterfuge. As Justice Stevens once put it when he spoke about a pregnant woman's distress in deciding whether or not to undergo an abortion, "[I]t is far better to permit some persons to make incorrect decisions than to deny all individuals the right to make decisions that have a profound effect upon their destiny."

Thus, recruitment of subjects will prove to be more time consuming. Completion of research may also be de-layed and, if too many patients refuse, selection bias will make some research impossible to conduct. Not only may scientific progress be impeded but physician-investigators' self-interests in recognition and advancement of their careers may be jeopardized. Scientific discoveries do not occur in isolation and, more often than not, scientists in many centers are pursuing similar inquiries. The imperative to publish first is of crucial personal significance, because so much depends on it in terms of recognition, fame, future grants and prospects. A commitment to disclosure and consent entails paying a great personal price which can be moderated, however, if the collectivity of physician-investigators embrace these responsibilities or find new ways of conducting research which will make forthright disclosures less of a burden. It is also a great professional price to pay because physician-investigators come to research out of a deeply felt dissatisfaction with the current state of medical knowledge and out of a painful awareness of the suffering of their patients. [...]

35   Subject Interview Study

THE PRESIDENT'S ADVISORY COMMITTEE
ON HUMAN RADIATION EXPERIMENTS

[...]

RESULTS

[...]

Distinctions Between Research and Medical Care

While the Brief Survey [consisting of a 5- to 10-minute interview of 1,882 patients in medical oncology, radiation oncology, and cardiology clinics at 16 institutions across the United States—eds.] did not address distinctions between medical treatment and research, this issue arose during the In-Depth Interview [a more detailed, 45-minute interview of a 103-person subset of those who completed the Brief Survey—eds.]. Here, patients' descriptions of their research experiences often included de-

The President's Advisory Committee on Human Radiation Experiments, "Subject Interview Study," in Final Report of the Advisory Committee on Human Radiation Experiments (Washington, D.C.: U.S. Government Printing Office, 1995), available online at http://tis.eh.doe.gov/ohre/roadmap/achre/report.html.

scriptions of their physical conditions, their own health care providers, or the hospitals at which their research projects were conducted. Research experiences, particularly for those patients who reported being in research evaluating potential treatments, were inextricably interwoven with their medical care experiences. One respondent described her research experience "as a means of treating what I have." Another respondent, when asked what she disliked about the project in which she was a participant, replied: "Nothing other than the fact that nobody likes to be sick and nobody likes to go to doctors."

While patients, if asked, were quite able to identify which procedures, tests, and staff were associated with their research, they did not themselves readily make distinctions between research and medical treatment. Particularly for patients with serious medical diagnoses, research often was viewed as one of the treatment options for their medical conditions. Not surprisingly, then, some participants evaluated their research experience in terms of whether they believed it would provide them with clinical benefit. One respondent noted, "I see results that indicate that the chemotherapy that I'm taking is working, and therefore, that is adequate enough to satisfy me."

Despite the tendency for some patients to fuse discussions of research and treatment, some clearly differentiated the two. This was especially true for those who reported that they were in diagnostic, epidemiologic, or survey research.

Deciding to Participate

BRIEF SURVEY

When asked whether specific factors contributed a lot, contributed a little, or did not contribute to their decision to participate in particular research projects, patients typically identified multiple motivations. Most patients reported that they had joined a research project to get better treatment (contributed a lot, 67 percent; a little, 11 percent) and because being in research gave them hope (contributed a lot, 61 percent; a little, 18 percent). Patients who cited the desire for better treatment as a reason for agreeing to be in research were more likely than other patients to be in a study that they viewed as "therapeutic," that related to the patient's medical condition, and that involved radiation.

In addition to this emphasis on the possibility of better treatment and the bolstering of hope, 135 patients agreed with the statement that they "had little choice" but to participate and that this belief contributed a lot to their decision. While it is difficult to ascertain precisely what these patients understood this statement to mean, patients elaborated on this motivation in the In-Depth Interviews, often saying that because of the serious nature of their medical condition and/or because other interventions had not been successful, they believed they had "little choice" but to try research. Patients reporting that they had little choice tended to categorize the projects in which they were subjects as treatment projects (compared with diagnostic or epidemiological), tended to report that the projects involved radiation, that they did not feel they had enough information, and that the research was related to their medical condition.

Altruistic reasons also played a part in many patients' decisions to participate in research. Specifically, most patients reported that they looked at participation as a way to help others (contributed a lot, 76 percent; a little, 18 percent) and as a way to advance science (contributed a lot, 72 percent; a little, 21 percent). Patients also frequently said that they had joined research projects because it seemed like a good idea (contributed a lot, 48 percent; a little, 17 percent), the project sounded interesting (contributed a lot, 53 percent; a little, 24 percent), and they had no reason not to participate in medical research (contributed a lot, 56 percent; a little, 15 percent).

IN-DEPTH INTERVIEW

In reporting how they had decided to participate in research, In-Depth Interview patients described many differ-ent processes, ranging from the very deliberate weighing of risks and benefits to the quicker decision of just taking action. Doctors (e.g., "my doctor," "the doctor," a particular doctor, or referring physician) were frequently identified as the key agent in the respondent's decision to participate in research.

Patients expressed a broad range of *reasons* they decided to participate in biomedical research. As in the Brief Survey, for people in therapeutic research, the primary reason for participating in research was to obtain benefits either through an experimental treatment they hoped would be better than standard treatment or through the closer medical attention they believed they would receive through research. One woman reported that she was participating in a treatment trial specifically to obtain an experimental drug that she believed looked promising. Furthermore, she wanted to receive it in a controlled environment where she could receive good follow-up and where researchers would document the drug's effects. Another respondent commented that since doctors at the military hospital where he received his care were very busy, he could receive closer attention and obtain appointments more easily by enrolling in research. Some patients who reported being in therapeutic research hoped that the research would give them more "time": "[A]ll I wanted at that point was five years to get my boys through high school"; "I want longevity . . . I don't see myself wanting to just pass away." Some patients decided to be in research because they believed that newer therapies might inherently be better: "If there's something new on the market that might be better than the traditional program they've been using, why not try it?"

Mirroring the Brief Survey finding that 31 percent of patients felt they had little choice in joining a research project, many In-Depth Interview patients who participated in therapeutic research remarked that they had joined because they believed they had "no choice," meaning they had no medical alternatives: "My doctor told me if I do not take the drug, in a couple of months I . . . [will] . . . die. So, I had no choice. Who wants to die? Nobody." Another respondent said, "I had one more option as he [the doctor] put it." Hope and desperation pervaded the remarks of many terminally ill patients. Patients said they wanted to "try anything" or that this was their "last resort." One man explained, "Well, what was driving me to say 'yes' was the hope that this drug would work. . . . When you reach that stage . . . and somebody offered that something that could probably save you, you sort of make a grab of it, and that's what I did." This same patient noted that he had first declined what he had considered a very aggressive therapy, "because at that point everything was pretty okay and there was no need for me to do any wild things." Later, when his condition worsened, he decided to participate in the research.

One of the most influential forces in patients' decisions to enroll was doctors' recommendations. One patient described the process of her enrollment: "He [the doctor] asked me if I wanted to go on it, and I said, 'If it's what you think I should do, yes, because you know more about it than I do.' . . . [H]e said, 'I think it would be a good idea to try it.'"

Along these lines, a theme of trust overwhelmingly emerged. Patients trusted specific physicians, medical professionals more generally, or the overall research enterprise. Trust in specific physicians was straightforward: "Basically, y[ou] know, we trust Dr. [So-and-so]. . . . [There] was no reason to . . . get a second opinion from another doctor." Another respondent exclaimed, "Oh, I love that man. He has kept me alive and I obey him and I do what he tells me to do. . . ." Some patients also communicated trust in the medical profession more generally: "I have this attitude. They know what they're doing. They wouldn't have you to do this if they didn't know what they were doing and . . . that's my attitude. . . ." Finally, there were a few patients who expressed trust in the overall enterprise of medical research as well as its oversight. One respondent stated: "I do not feel like the drug would be on the market if it were going to harm me, and if it would help in any way . . . I'm very willing to participate in this and perhaps other studies." Related were patients who said they decided to participate because of their trust in the institution where the research was being conducted. "I think I've got the best treatment down there [named hospital]. I don't think I could get any better." Rare were the patients who had less "blind trust" and considered themselves to be more of a consumer: "I sort of take my own treatment in my [hands] and tell them that I'm his client. It's not the other way around. . . ."

Elaborating on responses to the Brief Survey, the majority of patients mentioned altruism as a reason to participate. This desire to help others took many forms, including helping others who had the same medical condition, advancing medical science more broadly, and contributing to society. Most frequently, those in therapeutic research seemed to voice a combined motivation of seeking benefit for themselves and hoping to achieve benefit for others. Very representative was the comment, "I was hoping, if not for me, at least for the next people coming along. . . ."

For some patients who faced a life-threatening illness, participating in research seemed to offer them a greater sense of personal worth, a chance to contribute something of value to society. One woman said, "[I]f I can help find a cure for what seems to be so common [that is, cancer] these days, I would love to think I was part of finding that cure." For a small number of patients, this notion of helping others went further, to be a duty or obligation: "[I thought], well, I don't have to do this, and then I thought, well, here I am benefiting from literally thousands and thousands of experiments that have gone before and that are helping to save my life and this one sounded [very] reasonable to me and I was happy to participate." Similarly, one respondent replied, "I feel like that [participating in research and giving blood] is a moral obligation as a citizen. You put back into your community. . . . [O]pportunities to not only help yourself but other people are real important to me. . . ."

Only three patients cited monetary reasons for participating in research. [. . .]

DISCUSSION

[. . .]

Implications

[. . .] We learned a great deal from this project about why patients choose to be in research. The overwhelming majority of the patients we interviewed who were participants in research were subjects in studies investigating medical treatments. Almost all of these patients said that they had enrolled in research because they thought it offered them their best chance of personal medical benefit. Moreover, for many of them, their doctors had recommended it. Often these patients had very serious illnesses and had tried many treatments unsuccessfully; the opportunity to be in research offered them hope that improvement might still be possible. Many of these patients specifically said that they had "no choice" but to participate. They had tried everything else to improve their condition, and nothing else had worked. These patients felt constrained to participate because of their medical situation, not by their providers or the research investigators.

Not surprisingly, then, when asked to describe the research project they were in, most of the patient-subjects we talked with described the project as part of their therapy. Although, when asked, these patients appeared to clearly understand which interventions were associated specifically with the research, they also conceived of the research as their medical treatment. And despite the recognition by most of these patients that the goal of the enterprise of medical research generally was to advance science, when asked about their own specific project, they often believed that the project would benefit them.

It is likely that in some, and perhaps in many, of these cases, it was indeed in the patient's medical best interest to be enrolled in a research project. As demonstrated by the recent push for access to investigational drugs on the part of people with HIV infection and other serious illnesses where there may seem to be no truly efficacious standard therapies, many patients believe that their best chance of extending life is to take treatments that are still experimental. In some cases, patient-subjects were participating in treatment studies involving agents available only through research because their illnesses may have had no known efficacious treatments. From the perspective that holds extending life to be the primary concern, it would be in the patients' best interests to be in the research.

It is a separate issue whether participation in research is in a patient's *overall* best interests. Investigational interventions for devastating, life-threatening illnesses may be a patient's best chance—however small—of extending life. However, this chance may be at the expense of the person's ability to function and enjoy life for the time affected by participation in the research. Furthermore, the history of experimentation demonstrates that such therapies might also shorten life rather than extend it. Unfortunately, we did not pursue whether these sorts of trade-offs were clearly understood by the patient-subjects we interviewed. [. . .]

That patients viewed their participation as being in their best interests is consistent with patients' profound trust in their physicians, on whom they depend as their lifelines, and who they could not imagine offering something not in their best interests. We heard from several patients the belief that their doctors are the experts and that they know best what would be helpful. If a doctor recommended or even offered research, patients were certainly more inclined to decide to participate. The trust that patients placed in their physicians often was generalized to the medical and research community as a whole. Patient-subjects frequently expressed the belief that an intervention would not even be offered if it did not carry some promise of benefit; many certainly assumed that the intervention would not be offered if it posed significant risks.

It was largely because of this trust that most patient-subjects considered the consent process somewhat incidental to their decision to participate in research. When asked, almost all patients reported that they had been pro- vided with information, their questions had been answered, and they had been satisfied with the consent process. Nevertheless, doctors' recommendations and patients' own beliefs that the research was their best chance or even their only hope made the research an obvious decision for many patients, and the consent process and consent form were viewed as somewhat of a formality.

This framing of research as therapy is consistent with the very language used to describe research projects. We learned that patients attach very different meanings to the different terms associated with medical research. *Experiments* are considered by patients to involve unproven treatments of greater risk, often invoking the image of human beings as "guinea pigs," while terms such as *clinical investigation* or *study* convey less uncertainty to patients and a greater chance of personal benefit. [. . .]

It is often the case in clinical research that the participation of ill people in research and the medical treatment they receive for their illnesses are identical. When this occurs, it is not surprising that some patients conflate their being in research with therapy to the point that they no longer understand or remember that they actually are in a research project. Ironically, it may be especially when patient-subjects feel well cared for that they are most likely to feel like a patient only, and not like a research subject. At the same time, many patient-subjects told us of being reminded by research staff that they could leave the project at any time for any reason. It seems doubtful that the patients we interviewed whose self-report of participation was not consistent with research records had such an experience. [. . .]

---

36   False Hopes and Best Data

Consent to Research and the Therapeutic Misconception

<small>PAUL S. APPELBAUM, LOREN H. ROTH, CHARLES W. LIDZ, PAUL BENSON, AND WILLIAM WINSLADE</small>

Following a suicide attempt, a young man with a long history of tumultuous relationships and difficulty controlling his impulses is admitted to a psychiatric hospital. After a

Paul S. Appelbaum, Loren H. Roth, Charles W. Lidz, Paul Benson, and William Winslade, "False Hopes and Best Data: Consent to Research and the Therapeutic Misconception," *Hastings Center Report* 17, no. 2 (1987): 20–24.

number of days, a psychiatrist approaches the patient, explaining that he is conducting a research project to determine if medications may help in the treatment of the patient's condition. Is the patient interested, the psychiatrist asks? The answer: "Yes, I'm willing to do anything that might help me."

The psychiatrist returns over the next several days to explain the project further. He tells the patient that two medications are being used, along with a placebo; medications and placebo are assigned randomly. The trial is double-blinded; that is, neither physician nor patient will know what the patient is receiving until after the trial has been completed. The patient listens to the explanation and reads and signs the consent form. Since the process of providing information and obtaining consent seems, on the surface, exemplary, there appears to be little reason to question the validity of the consent.

Yet when the patient is asked why he agreed to be in the study, he offers some disquieting information. The medication that he will receive, he believes, will be the one most likely to help him. He ruled out the possibility that he might receive a placebo, because that would not be likely to do him much good. In short, this man, now both a patient and a subject, has interpreted, even distorted, the information he received to maintain the view—obviously based on his wishes—that every aspect of the research project to which he had consented was designed to benefit him directly. This belief, which is far from uncommon, we call the "therapeutic misconception." To maintain a therapeutic misconception is to deny the possibility that there may be major disadvantages to participating in clinical research that stem from the nature of the research process itself.

RESEARCH RISKS AND
THE SCIENTIFIC METHOD

The unique aspects of clinical research include the goal of creating generalizable knowledge; the techniques of randomization; and the use of a study protocol, control groups, and double-blind procedures. Do these elements create a body of risks or disadvantages for research subjects? The answer lies in understanding how the scientific method is often incompatible with one of the first principles of clinical treatment—the value that the legal philosopher Charles Fried calls "personal care."

According to the principle of personal care, a physician's first obligation is solely to the patient's well-being. A corollary is that the physician will take whatever measures are available to maximize the chances of a successful outcome. A failure to adhere to this principle creates at least a potential disadvantage for the clinical research subject: there is always a chance that the subject's interests may become secondary to other demands on the physician-researcher's loyalties. And the methods of science inhibit the application of personal care.

Randomization, an important element of many clinical trials, demonstrates the problem. The argument is often made that comparisons of multiple treatment methods are legitimately undertaken only when the superiority of one over the other is unknown; thus the physician treating a patient in one of these trials does not abandon the patient's personal care, but merely allows chance to determine the

assignment of treatments, each of which is likely to meet the patient's needs.

But as Fried and others have noted, it is very unlikely that two treatments in a clinical trial will be identically desirable *for a particular patient.* The physician may have reason to suspect, for example, that a given treatment is more likely to be efficacious for a particular patient, even if overall evidence of greater efficacy is lacking. This suspicion may be based on the physician's previous experience with a subgroup of patients, the patient's own past treatment experience, the family history of responsiveness to treatment, or idiosyncratic elements in the patient's case. Subjects may have had previous unsatisfactory responses to one of the medications in a clinical trial, or may display clinical characteristics that suggest that one class of medications is more likely to benefit them than another.

Ordinarily, these factors would guide the therapeutic approach. But in a randomized study physicians cannot allow these factors to influence the treatment decision, and efforts to control for such factors in the selection of subjects, while theoretically possible, are cumbersome, expensive, and may bias the sample. Thus reliance on randomization represents an inevitable compromise of personal care in the service of attaining valid research results. There are at least two reports in the literature of physicians' reluctance to refer patients to randomized trials because of the possible decrement in the level of personal care.

The use of a study protocol to regulate the course of treatment—essential to careful clinical research—also impedes the delivery of personal care. Protocols often indicate the pattern and dosages of medication to be administered or the blood levels to be attained. Even if they allow some individualization of medication, changes in time or magnitude may be limited. Thus patients who do not respond initially to a low dose of medication may not receive a higher dose, as they would if they were being treated without a protocol; on the other hand, patients experiencing side effects, which could be controlled by lowering their dosage, yet which are not so severe as to require withdrawal from the study, cannot receive the relief they would get in a therapeutic setting.

Analogously, adjunctive medications or forms of therapy, which may interfere with measurement of the primary treatment effect, are often prohibited. The exclusion of adjunctive medications, such as sleeping medications or decongestants, may increase a patient's discomfort. The requirement for a "wash-out" period, during which subjects are kept drug-free, may place previously stable patients at risk of relapse even before the experimental part of the project begins. And alternating placebo and active treatment periods may mean that a patient who responds well to a medication must be taken off that drug for the purposes of the study; conversely, patients who improve on placebo must be subject to the risks of active medication.

In sum, the necessary rigidities of an experimental protocol often lead investigators to forgo individualized treatment decisions.

The need for control groups or placebos and double-blind procedures can produce similar effects. In the therapeutic setting patients will rarely receive medications that are deliberately designed to be pharmacologically ineffective; the ethics of those occasional situations when placebos are employed clinically are hotly disputed. Yet, placebos are routinely employed in clinical investigations, without the intent of benefiting the individual subject.

Similarly, clinicians in a nonresearch setting will never allow themselves to remain ignorant of the treatment patients are receiving. Double-blind procedures, however, are necessary to ensure the integrity of a research study, even if they delay recognition of side effects or drug interactions, or have other adverse consequences.

Are these disadvantages so important that they should routinely be called to the attention of research subjects? That issue raises an empirical question: how prevalent is the therapeutic misconception?

STUDIES ON CONSENT

Our findings suggest that research subjects systematically misinterpret the risk-benefit ratio of participating in research because they fail to understand the underlying scientific methodology.

This conclusion is based on our observations of consent transactions in four research studies on the treatment of psychiatric illness, and our interviews with the subjects immediately after consent was obtained. The studies varied in the extent of the information they provided to subjects. Two of the studies compared the effects of two medications on a psychiatric disorder (one used, in addition, a placebo control group). A third study examined the relative efficacy of two dosage ranges of the same medication. And a fourth examined two different social interventions in chronic psychiatric illness, compared with a control group.

The populations in these studies ranged from actively psychotic schizophrenic patients to nonpsychotic, and in some cases, minimally symptomatic, borderline, and depressed patients. Our questions were based on information included on the consent form with regard to the understanding of randomized or chance assignment; and the use of control groups, formal protocols, and double-blind techniques. Eighty-eight patients comprised the final data pool, but since all of the issues addressed here were not relevant to each project the sample size varied for each question.

We found that fifty-five of eighty subjects (69 percent) had no comprehension of the actual basis for their random assignment to treatment groups, while only twenty-two of eighty (28 percent) had a complete understanding of the randomization process. Thirty-two subjects stated their ex-plicit belief that assignment would be made on the basis of their therapeutic needs. Interestingly, many of these subjects constructed elaborate but entirely fictional means by which an assignment would be made that was in their best interests. This was particularly evident when information about group assignment was limited to the written consent forms and not covered in the oral disclosure; subjects filled vacuums of knowledge with assumptions that decisions would be made in their best interests.

Similar findings were evident concerning other aspects of scientific design. With regard to nontreatment control groups and placebos, fourteen of thirty-three (44 percent) subjects failed to recognize that some patients who desired treatment would not receive it. Concerning use of a double blind, twenty-six of sixty-seven subjects (39 percent) did not understand that their physician would not know which medication they would receive; an additional sixteen of sixty-seven subjects (24 percent) had only partially understood this. Most striking of all, only six of sixty-eight subjects (9 percent) were able to recognize a single way in which joining a protocol would restrict the treatment they could receive. In the two drug studies in which adjustment of medication dosage was tightly restricted, twenty-two of forty-four subjects (50 percent) said explicitly that they thought their dosage would be adjusted according to their individual needs.

Two cases illustrate how these flaws in understanding affect the patient's ability to assess the benefits of the research. The first demonstrates the effect of a complete failure to recognize that scientific methodology has other than a therapeutic purpose. The second demonstrates a more subtle influence of a therapeutic orientation on a subject who understands the overall methodology but has certain blindspots.

In the first case, a twenty-five-year-old married woman with a high-school education was a subject in a randomized, double-blind study that compared the use of two medications and a placebo in the treatment of a nonpsychotic psychiatric disorder. When interviewed, she was unsure how it would be decided which medication she would receive, but thought that the placebo would be given only to those subjects who "might not need medication." The subject understood that a double-blind procedure would be used, but did not see that the protocol placed any constraints on her treatment. She said that she considered this project not an "experiment," a term that implied using drugs whose effects were unknown. Rather, she considered this to be "research," a process whereby doctors "were trying to find out more about you in depth." She decided to participate because "I needed help and the doctor said that other people who had been in it had been helped." Her strong conviction that the project would benefit her carried through to the end of the study. Although the investigators rated her a nonresponder, she was convinced that she had improved on the medication. She attributed her improvement in large part to the double-blind procedures, which kept her in the dark as to which medication she was receiving, thereby preventing her from persuading herself that the medication was doing no good. She was quite pleased about having participated in the study.

In the same study, another subject was a twenty-five-year-old woman with three years of college. At the time of the interview, she had minimal psychiatric symptoms and her understanding of the research was generally excellent. She recognized that the purpose of the project was to find out which treatment worked best for her group of patients. She spontaneously described the three groups, including the placebo group, and indicated that assignment would be at random. She understood that dosages would be adjusted according to blood levels and that a double blind would be used. When asked directly, however, how *her* medicine would be selected, she said she had no idea. She then added, "I hope it isn't by chance," and suggested that each subject would probably receive the medication she needed. Given the discrepancy between her earlier use of the word "random" and her current explanation, she was then asked what her understanding was of "random." Her definition was entirely appropriate: "by lottery, by chance, one patient who comes in gets one thing and the next patient gets the next thing." She then began to wonder out loud if this procedure was being used in the current study. Ultimately, she concluded that it was not.

In this case, despite a cognitive understanding of randomization, and a momentary recognition that random assignment would be used, the subject's conviction that the investigators would be acting in her best interests led to a distortion of an important element of the experimental procedure and therefore of the risk-benefit analysis.

The comments of colleagues and reports by other researchers have persuaded us that this phenomenon extends to all clinical research. Bradford Gray, for example, found that a number of subjects in a project comparing two drugs for the induction of labor believed, incorrectly, that their needs would determine which drug they would receive. A survey of patients in research projects at four Veterans Administration hospitals showed that 75 percent decided to participate because they expected the research to benefit their health. Another survey of attitudes toward research in a combined sample of patients and the general public revealed the thinking behind this hope: when asked why people in general should participate in research, 69 percent cited benefit to society at large and only 5 percent cited benefit to the subjects; however, when asked why *they* might participate in a research project, 52 percent said they would do it to get the best medical care, while only 23 percent responded that they would want to contribute to scientific knowledge. Back in the psychiatric setting, Lee Park and Lino Covi found that a substantial percentage of patients

who were told they were being given a placebo would not believe that they received inactive medication, and Vincenta Leigh reported that the most common fantasy on a psychiatric research ward was that the research was actually designed to benefit the subjects.

RESPONDING TO THE PROBLEM

Should we do anything about the therapeutic misconception? It could be argued that as long as the research project has been peer-reviewed for scientific merit and approved for ethical acceptability by an IRB, the problem of the therapeutic misconception is not significant enough to warrant intervention. In this view, some minor distortion of the risk-benefit ratio has to be weighed against the costs of attempting to alter subjects' appreciation of the scientific methods. Such costs include time expended and the delay in completing research that will result when some subjects decide that they would rather not participate.

Whether we accept this view depends on the value that we place on the principle of autonomy that underlies the practice of informed consent. Autonomy can be overvalued when it limits necessary treatment, as it may, for example, in the controversy over the right to refuse psychotropic medications. There, we believe, patients' interests would best be served by giving claims to autonomy lesser weight. But when we enter the research setting, limiting subjects' autonomy becomes a tool not for promoting their own interests, but for promoting the interests of others, including the researcher and society as a whole. We are not willing to accept such limitations for the benefit of others, particularly when, as described below, there may exist an effective mechanism for mitigating the problem.

Assuming that one agrees that distortions of the type we have described in subjects' reasoning are troublesome and worthy of correction, is such an effort likely to be effective? One might point to the data just presented to argue that little can be done to ameliorate the problem. The investigator in one of the projects we studied offered his subjects detailed and extensive information in a process that often extended over several days and included one session in which the entire project was reviewed. Despite this, half the subjects failed to grasp that treatment would be assigned on a random basis, four of twenty misunderstood how placebos would be used, five of twenty were not aware of the use of a double blind, and eight of twenty believed that medications would be adjusted according to their individual needs. Is it not futile, then, to attempt to disabuse subjects of the belief that they will receive personal care?

Various theoretical explanations of our findings could support this view. Most people have been socialized to believe that physicians (at least ethical ones) always provide personal care. It may therefore be very difficult, perhaps nearly impossible, to persuade subjects that *this* encounter is different, particularly if the researcher is also the treating physician, who has previously satisfied the subject's expectations of personal care. Further, insofar as much clinical research involves persons who are acutely ill and in some distress, the well-known tendency of patients to regress and entrust their well-being to an authority figure would undercut any effort to dispel the therapeutic misconception.

In response, more of our data must be explored. In each of the studies we observed, one cell of subjects was the target of an augmented informational process, which supplemented the investigator's disclosures to subjects with a "preconsent discussion." This discussion was led by a member of our research team who was trained to teach potential subjects about such things as the key methodologic aspects of the research project, especially methods that might conflict with the principle of personal care.

By introducing a neutral discloser, distinct from the patient's treatment team, we shifted the emphasis of the disclosure to focus on the ways in which research differs from treatment. Of the subjects who received this special education, eight of sixteen (50 percent) recognized that randomization would be used, as opposed to thirteen of the fifty-one (25 percent) remaining subjects; five of five (100 percent) understood how placebos would be employed in the single study that used them, compared with eleven of the fifteen (73 percent) remaining subjects; nine of sixteen (56 percent) comprehended the use of a double blind, while only fifteen of fifty-one (31 percent) remaining subjects did so; and five of seventeen (29 percent) initially recognized other limits on their treatment as a result of constraints in the protocol, compared with one of the fifty-one (2 percent) other subjects.

Our data suggest that many subjects can be taught that research *is* markedly different from ordinary treatment. Other efforts to educate subjects about the use of scientific methodology offer comparably encouraging results. There is no reason to believe that subjects will refuse to hear clearcut efforts to dispel the therapeutic misconception.

Novel approaches such as we employed may be one thing, of course, while routine procedures are something else. Perhaps our data derive from an unusually gifted group of patient-subjects. Will the complexity of explaining the principle of the scientific method defy understanding by most research subjects?

Undercutting the therapeutic misconception, thereby laying out some of the major disadvantages of any clinical research project, is probably much simpler than it seems. About the goals of research, subjects could be told: "Because this is a research project, we will be doing some things differently than we would if we were simply treating you for your condition. Not all the things we do are designed to tell us the best way to treat *you*, but they should help us to understand how people with your condition *in general* can best be treated." About randomization: "The treatment you receive will be selected by chance, not because we believe that one or the other will be better for you." About placebos: "Some subjects will be selected at random to receive sugar pills that are not known to help the condition you have; this is so we can tell whether the medications that the other patients get are really effective, or if everyone with your condition would have gotten better anyway."

One can quibble about the wording of specific sections, and complexities can arise with particular projects, but the concepts underlying scientific methodology are in reality quite simple. And as long as subjects understand the key principles of how the study is being conducted, investigators can probably omit some of the detail that currently clogs consent forms and confuses subjects about the minor risks that accompany the experimental procedures, such as blood drawing. Overall, then, we may end up with a much simpler consent process when we focus on the issue of personal care.

Who should have the task of explaining the therapeutic misconception to subjects? Clearly, investigators should be encouraged to discuss such issues with subjects and to include them on consent forms, but several problems arise here. First, it is decidedly *not* in investigators' self-interest for them to disabuse potential subjects of the therapeutic misconception. Experienced investigators, as we have reported elsewhere, view the recruitment of research subjects as an intricate and extended effort to win the potential subject's trust. One of our subjects in this study described the process in these words: "It was almost as if they were courting me . . . everything was presented in the best possible light." One could argue that it is unrealistic to expect investigators to raise additional doubts about the benefits that subjects can expect; any effort in that regard will result in resistance by investigators, particularly those who have yet to internalize the justifications for informed consent in general.

Second, even investigators who recognize the desirability of subjects making informed decisions may have great trouble conveying this particular information. When a researcher tells subjects that he or she is not selecting the treatment that will be given or that the medications being used may be no more effective than a placebo, the researcher is confessing uncertainty over the best approach to treatment, as well as the likely outcome. Harold Bursztajn and colleagues have argued that the essential uncertainty of all medical practice is precisely what physicians need to convey in *both* research and treatment settings. Yet, as Jay Katz points out, physicians have been systematically socialized to underplay or ignore uncertainty in their discussions with patients. In a recent report of physicians' reluctance to enter patients in a multicenter breast cancer study, 22 percent of the principal investigators cited as a major obstacle to enrolling subjects difficulty in telling patients that they did not know which treatment was best.

Third, few researchers who are also clinicians feel comfortable acknowledging, even to themselves, that the course of treatment may not be optimally therapeutic for the patient. Thus, there appear such statements as the following, which recently was published in *The Lancet:* "A doctor who contributes to randomized treatment trials should not be thought of as a research worker, but simply as a clinician with an ethical duty to his patients not to go on giving them treatments without doing everything possible to assess their true worth." The author concludes that since randomized trials are not really research, there is no need to obtain *any* informed consent from research subjects. Although this conclusion may be extreme, the example emphasizes the difficulties of getting investigators to admit to themselves, much less to their patient-subjects, the limits they have accepted on the delivery of personal care.

If there is concern with particular protocols, IRBs might consider supplementing the investigators' disclosure and the "courtship" process with a session in which the potential subject reviews risks and benefits with someone who is not a member of the research team. [...] The neutral explainer would be responsible to the IRB and would be trained to emphasize those aspects of the research situation about which the IRB has the greatest concern. This approach might be especially appropriate when the investigator is also the subject's treating physician and the methodology used is likely to be interpreted as therapeutic in intent. The model we employed of using a trained educator (nurses are natural candidates for the job) worked well. It is certainly more manageable and less disruptive than the oft-heard suggestions that patient advocates or consent monitors sit in on every interaction between subject and investigator.

There may be advantages to using a trained, neutral educator, apart from aiding subjects' decisionmaking. Subjects' perceptions of the research team as willing to "level with them," even to the point of explaining why it might not be in subjects' interests to participate in the study, may increase their trust and cooperation. On the other hand, failure to deal with the therapeutic misconception during the consent process could increase distrust of researchers and the health care system in general, if subjects later come to feel they were "deceived," as a few did in the studies we observed. Enough experiences of this sort could further heighten public antipathy to medical research, particularly if they are publicized as some have been. The scientific method is a powerful tool for advancing knowledge, but like most potent clinical procedures it has side effects that must be attended to, lest the benefits sought be overwhelmed by the disadvantages that accrue. With careful planning, the therapeutic misconception can be dispelled, leaving the subjects with a much clearer picture of the relative risks and benefits of participation in research.

37   "Therapeutic Misconception" and "Recruiting Doublespeak" in the Informed Consent Process

MARK HOCHHAUSER

About 20 years ago, Paul Appelbaum and his colleagues identified "therapeutic misconception"—the mistaken belief held by many research subjects that research projects will directly benefit them. Despite what they're told by the researcher (and read in the consent form), subjects may see no conflict between the goals of research and treatment, especially when the researcher is also their treating physician. They expect the research to help them, not harm them. Some may even think that they're getting state-of-the-art treatment, a drug that's so new (and so effective) that other people don't yet have access to it.

Mark Hochhauser, "'Therapeutic Misconception' and 'Recruiting Doublespeak' in the Informed Consent Process," *IRB: Ethics and Human Research* 24, no. 1 (2002): 11–12.

Over the past 20 years, medical research has morphed into the clinical trial industry, and subject recruiting has become big business. Delays in recruiting subjects and completing clinical trials can cost drug and device companies millions of dollars. Subjects must be recruited in a timely manner, and success or failure depends on what the researcher/personal physician tells potential subjects verbally and in writing during the recruiting and consenting process. It all comes down to words and what they mean.

EXPECTANCY EFFECTS

Most clinical trials now have a "brand name," which may contribute to a subject's therapeutic misconception by biasing his or her assessment of the experimental drug that he or she is taking. The clinical trial's "brand" is not just a convenient but meaningless acronym, but often an acronym that may subliminally suggest a particular perspective on the trial. For example, what meaning will subjects take from clinical trials with brand names such as ALIVE (Adenosine Lidocaine Infarct zone Viability Enhancement trial), BEST (Beta-blocker Evaluation of Survival Trial), MAGIC (MAGnesium In Coronaries), MIRACL (Myocardial Ischemia Reduction with Aggressive Cholesterol Lowering), or PROVED (Prospective Randomized study of Ventricular failure and the Efficacy of Digoxin)? [See Table 37.1 for further examples.—eds.]

Such trial brands seem to suggest the outcome even before the trial is completed! How can we realistically expect a prospective subject to appreciate fully the experimental nature of a trial presented with that kind of positive imagery?

WHAT'S THE DIFFERENCE BETWEEN AN EXPERIMENT AND A CLINICAL TRIAL?

The word "experiment" or "experimental" is one that seldom shows up in a consent form, perhaps because sponsors realize that while people may be willing to be part of a "clinical trial," they may not want to be part of an "experiment." I am a member of the IRB at North Memorial Health Care in Robbinsdale, Minnesota, and recently reviewed 29 consent forms randomly selected from all that were submitted between August 1999 and January 2002. I found that experimental research projects were described in the following ways. As a:

Study

Research investigation

Trial

Medical research trial

Research trial

Clinical research study

Research study

Clinical research program (study)

Research project

Clinical trial, a type of research study

None of these terms or phrases accurately reflects the experimental nature of the activity. While the consent forms usually refer to "research," the word experiment may or may not show up anywhere in them. Indeed, experiment/experimental showed up in only two of the consent forms I examined. And the IRB has no way of knowing if investigators explain accurately the experimental nature of the re-

Table 37.1
Clinical Trial "Brand Names"

AFFIRM	COURAGE	PRESTO
ALIVE	DEFINITE	PREVENT
APLAUSE	EXCEL	PROTECT
ASSET	FASTER	PROVED
AVERT	GREAT	PROVE IT
BEST	GUSTO	REDUCE
BETTER	HERO	RESCUE
BRAVO	HOPE	RESTORE
BRILLIANT	MAGIC	SAVED
CHAMP	MIRACL	STOP
CONVINCE	PRAISE	WIZARD

search during the consent process. While subjects might expect risks if they sign up for an experiment, they may not expect any risks if they sign up for a research study. If they believe that they're part of a "study," they may not pay attention to the riskier parts of the project.

DO SUBJECTS TAKE EXPERIMENTAL DRUGS?

Those same consent forms used a variety of terms to avoid saying that subjects would take an experimental drug, instead saying that subjects would be taking a(n):

Study drug

New drug

Study medication

Research (investigational) product

Investigational drug

Investigational (experimental) agent

New investigational drug

Several years ago, a newspaper ad in Minneapolis recruited subjects by offering an "Innovative Pharmacological Therapeutic Intervention." An "experimental drug" sounds as though it comes with some risks; a "study medication" sounds fairly safe.

ADVERTISING CLAIMS VS. REALITY

Online clinical trial research programs often overstate the benefits of being in a clinical trial, making claims that border on advertising hype. For example:

• "Cancer patients and health care providers have access to these clinical research trials as part of the latest in cancer care" (University of Minnesota—Cancer

Clinical Trials, www.cancer.umn.edu/page/protocol/index.html).

But clinical trials are research, not therapy.

• "Chosen for their interdisciplinary nature and potential benefits to patients, these programs range from fundamental investigations of the origin of disease to advanced clinical trials in which patients have access to the latest and most promising treatments" (Press release, University of California, San Francisco, www.ucsf.edu/pressrel/2001/10/102501.html).

"Latest" and "most promising" are not the same as effective, however.

• "Participants are among the first to receive new treatments before they are widely available" (Cancer Research Center of Hawaii, www.hawaii.edu/crch/SerCTBenefits.htm).

Unless, of course, participants receive a placebo or control drug.

• "Clinical trials offer high quality cancer care" (Cleveland Clinic, www.clevelandclinic.org/cancer/trial/default.htm).

But if a participant's personal doctor is also the investigator, how high is the quality of care he or she receives?

The FDA drug approval rate belies the optimism of such statements. About 70 percent of drugs make it through phase I, which primarily addresses safety and drug administration issues. About 33 percent of experimental drugs will be successful in phase II trials (for effectiveness and some short-term safety issues), while about 25 percent –30 percent will be successful in phase III trials assessing safety, dosage, and effectiveness. The FDA reports that overall only about 20 percent of drugs tested in clinical trials will ultimately be brought to market. Most subjects will not benefit from most clinical trials.

The clinical trial brand name, the turning of potentially risky experiments into relatively safe "studies," the administration of "study medications" instead of experimental drugs, and overestimating the therapeutic benefits of participating in clinical trials, are all forms of doublespeak: as *Webster's College Dictionary* defines it, "evasive, ambiguous, or high-flown language intended to deceive or confuse." How can subjects make informed decisions about whether to participate in risky research when the terms they're given do not adequately explain—in words they can readily understand—the real risks involved?

Part VI

Clinical Research with Special Populations

Hans Jonas once argued that the ideal research participant from an ethical perspective is one who can identify with the purpose of the research, understand and appreciate the details, and make a free choice about participation. Such participants can give informed consent based on a determination that research participation is compatible with their own interests and values. However, scientific progress relevant to the needs of certain populations often requires the inclusion of "special" or "vulnerable" populations in clinical research. Such persons, less capable of protecting their own interests and of understanding or identifying with the research, are included in order to answer questions of importance to understanding health and managing illness in these groups.

Research with such special groups raises additional ethical concerns because of their "vulnerability" or their diminished capacity to protect their own interests. There is a need for protection of their interests through means other than traditional informed consent, and thus special considerations and additional safeguards are recommended for research involving members of vulnerable groups. But who is vulnerable? What is the basis of their vulnerability? What are appropriate safeguards that should be used to protect vulnerable research participants? And what is the appropriate balance between protecting vulnerable persons and conducting important research needed to improve their health?

The selections in Part VI address these questions by focusing on certain "special populations" or groups of people thought to be vulnerable for a variety of reasons, including those with cognitive impairments, children, prisoners, and students. Since the source of vulnerability varies from a decreased capacity to appreciate or understand research to a decreased ability

to make a voluntary choice, appropriate safeguards and mechanisms for protecting the interests of these research participants also vary.

SECTION ONE. PEOPLE WITH COGNITIVE IMPAIRMENTS

The first three papers address the issue of clinical research involving subjects with mental illness. Our first contribution is a selection from a 1998 report produced by the U.S. National Bioethics Advisory Commission (NBAC) that deals with research involving persons with mental disorders. Although the NBAC commissioners recognized that limitations on decisionmaking capacity are not unique to persons with mental disorders, they chose nonetheless to focus their recommendations on those with mental disorders because of the long-standing regulatory gap in research protections for such persons. The NBAC report delineates 21 recommendations, several of which reiterate considerations important for the ethical conduct of any study involving humans. Specific additional recommendations designed to increase safeguards for research involving those with mental illness include: the addition to institutional review boards (IRBs) of members familiar with the concerns of persons with mental disorders, the creation of a special panel at the Department of Health and Human Services (DHHS) to review studies that involve greater than minimal risk, the requirement of independent capacity assessments for those invited to participate in studies that pose greater than minimal risk, and the legitimization of prospective authorization by participants and of permission by legally authorized representatives for some research studies.

In his response to the NBAC report, Robert Michels argues against the NBAC recommendations because they are likely to hamper critically needed research and because they try to "fix a problem that may not exist." He warns that NBAC's recommendations imply that mental illness and psychiatric research are both different from and more dangerous than physical illness and general medical research and, moreover, that researchers are not to be trusted. He notes that progress in mental health treatment is a result of the successes of clinical research and that, if the NBAC recommendations are endorsed, the result is likely to be a diminished treatment arsenal for those with mental disorders. He finds at least two particular problems with the NBAC recommendations, namely, that they raise unnecessary hurdles for research that presents greater than minimal risk and that they require independent capacity assessments of potential research participants.

The next contributor in this section, Carl Elliott, notes that there is often less concern about the cognitive ability and competence of participants in research on depression than in other psychiatric research. Since depression is a mood disorder, it is thought to not necessarily affect one's ability to reason, deliberate, or make decisions, capabilities thought critical for competence. Elliott challenges this view by asserting that although a depressed person may be aware of risks, he or she may not care about them, and this lack of concern is an intellectual impairment. He argues that since a competent consent decision is one for which an individual can be considered accountable and morally responsible, both intellectual ability and emotional state are relevant to valid consent. He offers two reasons why a depressed person's competence to consent to research should be carefully scrutinized: authenticity and self-interest. Since a person's values, beliefs, desires, and dispositions are dramatically different when she is depressed than when she is healthy, can they be authentic? And since a depressed person does not necessarily act in accord with concern for his or her own well-being or interests, he may in fact welcome research risks or at least not care about them.

SECTION TWO. CHILDREN

Children constitute a special population of research participants, legally and often developmentally incapable of granting valid consent or of protecting their own interests. Consequently, regulations and guidelines have sought to protect children from exploitation and harm in research primarily by restricting the level of acceptable research risk and by requiring a child's assent to participation, whenever possible, in addition to requiring the permission of the parent(s) or guardian(s). Three papers in this section discuss research with children by addressing issues of acceptable risk levels in pediatric research, parents as decision-makers, and the assent of children in research.

Our first contributor, Carol A. Tauer, examines the controversial case of a large randomized placebo-controlled study of growth hormone in children who were not deficient in human growth hormone production. Although she recognizes the scientific need to understand the safety and efficacy of long-term growth hormone use, Tauer nonetheless questions whether such studies are ethical in healthy children. She reviews the conclusions of a National Institutes of Health (NIH) ad hoc committee that the study conformed to the federal regulations at 45 CFR §46.406, but questions whether the intent of the regulations was truly met. In crafting §46.406, as Tauer explains, the National Commission for the Protection of Human Subjects of Biomedical and Behavioral Research intended to allow sick children to be included in research that presents greater than minimal risk whenever such inclusion would be needed to answer a question about their disease. Yet she questions whether short stature should properly be conceived of as a disease. Tauer recommends that the regulations be revised—especially the definition of "minimal risk"—because the growth hormone studies could otherwise set a precedent for the approval of research on children that poses greater than minimal risk in order to test uses of genetic therapies to enhance desired characteristics such as height in otherwise normal children.

Benjamin Freedman, Abraham Fuks, and Charles Weijer next examine the notions of "minimal risk" and "minor increment over minimal risk" in research with children. The authors recognize, as do others, that informed consent is not a moral solution for research with children, and they also note that research with children is critical lest children be left "therapeutic orphans." Minimal risk, as defined in the U.S. federal regulations, uses the risks of everyday life as an anchor or benchmark for the assessment of permissible risk. Freedman and colleagues contend that, given the imprecision of this definition, a determination of what counts as minimal risk cannot be made out of context and so must be made relative to a child's actual situation. They suggest that the term "minor increment over minimal risk" used in the federal regulations is not quantitative but should rather be thought of as a categorical judgment that focuses on the comparison of the risks of new experiences to those in the child's everyday life. Thought of in this way, risk can be seen to be both relative and substitutive (i.e., the risks entailed in one risky activity, such as research, *substitute for* the risks of forgone activities, such as other therapies or daily activities); moreover, risk determination is flexible enough to accommodate some cultural variance. Using the threshold of minimal risk, an IRB acts *in loco parentis* and judges whether the risks of research are acceptable in comparison to the risks a similar group of children routinely encounters.

Our final contributor to this section, Sanford Leikin, examines the conditions under which it is appropriate to seek a child's assent to research participation. Assent involves a child's understanding what is being asked of her, realizing that her permission is being sought independent of that of her parents, and making a choice free from outside constraint. Leikin reviews data regarding children's understanding of and reasoning about research and argues that individual variations in a child's development and ability to reason about the consequences of participation may be more important than age in their giving assent (at least in children over 9 years of age). Furthermore, Leikin argues that both natural developmental variations in voluntariness and in the desire of a child to please adults should be taken into account in assessment of the child's dissent. IRBs should thus recommend assent based both on the developmental characteristics of the child and also on the complexity of the decision to be made. When there is uncertainty, however, Leikin recommends that evaluation by a psychologist independent of the parents and the investigators might be useful. Leikin cautions against using a child's developmental limitations as an excuse not to engage her in an assent process and emphasizes the importance of informing and involving both minors and their parents whenever possible. He argues that dissent should always be honored unless the research protocol provides access to potentially beneficial therapy otherwise unavailable to the child. Leikin

also suggests that middle or late adolescents should be allowed independent assent, especially for research that presents minimal risk and perhaps for that which presents a minor increment over minimal risk.

SECTION THREE. CAPTIVE POPULATIONS: SOLDIERS, PRISONERS, AND STUDENTS

Captive populations are those that are convenient and readily available, but usually constrained in such a way that their movements and choices may be less than voluntary. These constraints may thus compromise their ability to give voluntary informed consent to research. Populations can be physically captive, such as prisoners or those who are institutionalized, but may also be captive by virtue of their positions in power relationships with authority figures, such as students and military personnel.

Jonathan D. Moreno, our first contributor in this section, presents a historical account of research with captive populations, in particular, military personnel. His overarching claim is that understanding the history of how specific populations came to be regarded as vulnerable is essential if one is to understand the current ethical and regulatory research environment. Moreno notes that there is currently a very low threshold of risk tolerance in military research and development, and briefly discusses the recent controversy over the use of pyridostigmine bromide in the Gulf War. Moreno concludes by arguing that in the selection of captive or convenient populations considerations of justice require additional and specific protections through institutional and public scrutiny, but not a priori exclusion.

Carl Cohen next discusses the ethics of including prisoners as participants in research. Concerns about research with prisoners include the possibility of compromised consent because of the totalitarian nature of prisons, in which coercion is common. Prisoners are physically unfree and are subject to careful surveillance and control; most are poor; boredom pervades prison life; and prisoners will do almost anything they think will help them get released early. Cohen argues that for these reasons research in prisons must be closely scrutinized, but he contends that prisoners are in fact capable of free consent. He argues that the term "coercion" is used too loosely and that even desperate circumstances and great pressures do not necessarily coerce or obviate voluntary consent.

Cohen concludes that there are strong moral reasons for permitting prisoners to participate in research, especially possible long-term benefits to society and to prisoners themselves.

Harold F. Gamble addresses research with students. He recounts how data showing that students did not feel coerced, felt free to say no, and derived educational benefit from research participation convinced two IRBs to reverse their initial decision to restrict students from participation in classroom research. Discussing whether a teacher's giving extra credit for research participation should be thought of as a threat or an offer, he recognizes that gaining extra credit through research may be more appealing than gaining it through other alternatives because research may require less effort and possibly be more interesting. However, since educational benefit is not the only reason to include students in research and since pressure to participate is certainly possible, he argues instead for an offer of cash payments, which he considers more consistent with the ideas of free choice and similar treatment for all student participants.

Nancy R. Angoff argues not only that special protections for medical students as research participants are unnecessary but that they constitute "overprotective paternalism." She argues that medical students are not captive or less free than anybody else but are in fact highly autonomous and smart and have good judgment. She contrasts Harvard University's policy that restricts the inclusion of medical students in research with a policy of the Yale Human Investigations Committee that actually recommends the inclusion of medical students as they are the participants most capable of understanding a highly invasive study. She also argues that cash payments are appropriate for medical students.

Section One

People with Cognitive Impairments

---

38   Research Involving Persons with Mental Disorders
      That May Affect Decisionmaking Capacity

THE NATIONAL BIOETHICS ADVISORY COMMISSION

EXECUTIVE SUMMARY

In this report, the National Bioethics Advisory Commission (NBAC) considers how ethically acceptable research can be conducted with human subjects who suffer from mental disorders that may affect their decisionmaking capacity; whether, in this context, additional protections are needed; and, if so, what they should be and how they should be implemented. In addition, this report provides an opportunity for investigators, IRB members, persons with mental disorders and their families, and the general public to become better informed about the importance of such research and what we believe are the appropriate protections for the human subjects involved.

[. . .] Much has changed in the research environment since the National Commission for the Protection of Human Subjects of Biomedical and Behavioral Research completed its work 20 years ago, and yet one finding is as true today as it was then: all research involving human beings as subjects must satisfy appropriate ethical and scientific standards. This moral imperative is especially acute for potentially vulnerable populations such as children, pregnant women, prisoners, or, NBAC believes, individuals with mental disorders that may affect their decisionmaking capacity.

Mental disorders—which can be heartbreakingly burdensome for patients and their families and frustrating for the professionals who treat them—have in recent years been the focus of research studies that have produced important new methods of diagnosis and treatment. At the same time, some of these investigations have generated public controversy, government sanctions, and at times

The National Bioethics Advisory Commission, Research Involving Persons with Mental Disorders That May Affect Decisionmaking Capacity, Volume I (Rockville, Md.: NBAC, December 1998), available online at bioethics.georgetown.edu/nbac/pubs.html.

lawsuits. Although existing federal regulations for research involving human subjects provide special protections for certain populations that are regarded as particularly vulnerable, persons with mental disorders (who may have impaired capacity to make decisions about research participation) have not received any such special protections.

NBAC believes that a cogent case can be made for requiring additional special protections in research involving as subjects persons with impaired decisionmaking capacity [. . .].

In its consideration of these issues over 18 months, NBAC received input through public comments provided at every meeting, expert testimony, commissioned papers, interactions with professional and patient groups, and a 45-day comment period during which interested parties could submit written comments on the final draft report. In addition, NBAC reviewed a sampling of research protocols and consent forms relevant to research on individuals whose decisionmaking capacity might be affected by mental illness. Based on these varied inputs and careful deliberations, NBAC came to the following conclusions:

• During the nearly two decades in which the current federal regulations for the protection of human subjects have been in place, important scientific research on the cause and treatment of mental disorders has continued and expanded. Further, NBAC believes that important opportunities to develop new therapies will continue to emerge, and that the research community may be on the verge of some momentous breakthroughs. NBAC's challenge, therefore, was to develop recommendations that would sustain the continued acquisition of new knowledge and the development of new therapies, while ensuring the protection of those who participate as subjects in such research.

• Although IRBs have considerable authority and discretion to review, approve, and monitor research involving persons with mental disorders, they have received little practical guidance for reviewing such protocols. However, more than additional guidance is needed. Because of significant gaps in the current federal regulations additional regulations are necessary at this time. NBAC believes that enhanced protections will promote broad-based support for further research by engendering greater public trust and confidence that subjects' rights and interests are fully respected.

• More research is being conducted than ever before, and the research environment has become far more complex, involving both a larger societal investment and a greater role for the private sector. NBAC shares what it believes to be a broad base of support for continuing efforts to more fully understand and treat mental disorders. NBAC recommends additional new protections with the deepest respect for the many people involved in research on these disorders: those with a disorder that may affect decisionmaking capacity, whose autonomy must be protected and, when possible, enhanced; the clinical investigators who are dedicated to the alleviation of these disorders; and informal caregivers, whose own lives are often absorbed by the tragedy that has befallen their loved ones. NBAC does not believe, however, that the additional protections recommended in this report will excessively burden research or hamper the development of effective new treatments. Moreover, it is useful to note that many share in the responsibility to protect the interests of those without whom this research could not be done—especially those who may be unable to give full informed consent and who may not themselves directly benefit from the research.

OVERVIEW OF THE REPORT

[...] The several recommendations for changes in federal regulations and for other governmental, institutional, and organizational actions are interconnected. Even though only a few recommendations are explicitly cross-referenced, it is important to view each recommendation in the context of the others. Only then is it possible to see exactly how NBAC proposes to protect human subjects with mental disorders that may affect decisionmaking capacity and also allow important research to proceed.

RECOMMENDATIONS

[...] Taken together, these recommendations would both enhance existing protections and facilitate broad public support for continued research on mental disorders.

Although NBAC proposes a number of recommendations that would require changes in the Common Rule, it is

aware that the time frame for such reforms might be long and the process labor intensive. Many of the regulatory proposals made by NBAC could, therefore, be accomplished by the creation of a new subpart in 45 CFR 46. Regardless of which regulatory route is selected, NBAC encourages researchers and institutions to voluntarily adopt the spirit and substance of these recommendations immediately. The recommendations are clustered into six sections related to: review bodies; research design; informed consent and capacity; categories of research; surrogate decisionmaking; and education, research, and support.

I. Recommendations Regarding Review Bodies

INSTITUTIONAL REVIEW BOARD MEMBERSHIP

Recommendation 1. All IRBs that regularly consider proposals involving persons with mental disorders should include at least two members who are familiar with the nature of these disorders and with the concerns of the population being studied. At least one of these IRB members should be a member of the population being studied, a family member of such a person, or a representative of an advocacy organization for this population. These IRB members should be present and voting when such protocols are discussed. IRBs that only occasionally consider such protocols should involve in their discussion two ad hoc consultants who are familiar with the nature of these disorders and with the concerns of the population being studied; at least one of these consultants should be a member of the population being studied, a family member of such person, or a representative of an advocacy organization for this population.

CREATION OF A SPECIAL STANDING PANEL (SSP)

Recommendation 2. The Secretary of the Department of Health and Human Services (DHHS) should convene an SSP on research involving persons with mental disorders that may affect decisionmaking capacity. The panel's tasks should include:

(A) reviewing individual protocols that cannot otherwise be approved under the recommendations described in this report, that have been forwarded by IRBs to the SSP for its consideration. If the SSP finds that a protocol offers the possibility of substantial benefit to the population under study, that its risks to subjects are reasonable in relation to this possible benefit, and that it could not be conducted without the proposed population, then the SSP may approve the protocol if it is satisfied that all appropriate safeguards are incorporated. Under no circumstance, however, should the SSP approve a protocol that reasonable, competent persons would decline to enter;

(B) promulgating guidelines that would permit local IRBs to approve protocols that cannot otherwise be approved under the recommendations described in this report. Such guidelines could suggest that a particular class or category of research, using specified research interventions with certain identified populations, could be considered by local IRBs without the need to resort to the SSP for further approval. Under no circumstances, however, should the SSP promulgate guidelines permitting IRBs to approve research that would enroll subjects who lack decisionmaking capacity in protocols that reasonable, competent persons would decline to enter.

The SSP should have members who can represent the diverse interests of potential research subjects, the research community, and the public. The panel's protocol approvals and guidelines should all be published in an appropriate form that ensures reasonable notice to interested members of the public.

Those federal agencies that are signatories of the Common Rule should agree to use the SSP, and the SSP's effectiveness should be reviewed no later than 5 years after inception.

II. Recommendations Regarding Research Design

APPROPRIATE SUBJECT SELECTION

Recommendation 3. An IRB should not approve research protocols targeting persons with mental disorders as subjects when such research can be done with other subjects.

JUSTIFYING RESEARCH DESIGN AND MINIMIZING RISKS

Recommendation 4. Investigators should provide IRBs with a thorough justification of the research design they will use, including a description of procedures designed to minimize risks to subjects. In studies that are designed to provoke symptoms, to withdraw subjects rapidly from therapies, to use placebo controls, or otherwise to expose subjects to risks that may be inappropriate, IRBs should exercise heightened scrutiny.

EVALUATING RISKS AND BENEFITS

Recommendation 5. Investigators should provide IRBs with a thorough evaluation of the risks and potential benefits to the human subjects involved in the proposed pro-tocol. The evaluation of risks includes the nature, probability, and magnitude of any harms or discomforts to the subjects. The evaluation of benefits should distinguish possible direct medical benefits to the subject from other types of benefits.

III. Recommendations Regarding Informed Consent and Capacity

INFORMED CONSENT TO RESEARCH

Recommendation 6. No person who has the capacity for consent may be enrolled in a study without his or her informed consent. When potential subjects are capable of making informed decisions about participation, they may accept or decline participation without involvement of any third parties.

OBJECTION TO PARTICIPATION IN RESEARCH

Recommendation 7. Any potential or actual subject's objection to enrollment or to continued participation in a research protocol must be heeded in all circumstances. An investigator, acting with a level of care and sensitivity that will avoid the possibility or the appearance of coercion, may approach people who previously objected to ascertain whether they have changed their minds.

ASSESSING POTENTIAL SUBJECTS' CAPACITY TO DECIDE ABOUT PARTICIPATING IN A RESEARCH PROTOCOL

Recommendation 8. For research protocols that present greater than minimal risk, an IRB should require that an independent, qualified professional assess the potential subject's capacity to consent. The protocol should describe who will conduct the assessment and the nature of the assessment. An IRB should permit investigators to use less formal procedures to assess potential subjects' capacity if there are good reasons for doing so.

NOTIFYING SUBJECTS OF INCAPACITY DETERMINATION AND RESEARCH ENROLLMENT

Recommendation 9. A person who has been determined to lack capacity to consent to participate in a research study must be notified of that determination before permission may be sought from his or her legally authorized representative (LAR) to enroll that person in the study. If permission is given to enroll such a person in the study, the potential subject must then be notified. Should the person object to participating, this objection should be heeded.

IV. Recommendations Regarding Categories of Research

RESEARCH PROTOCOLS INVOLVING MINIMAL RISK

Recommendation 10. An IRB may approve a protocol that presents only minimal risk, provided that:

(A) consent has been waived by an IRB, pursuant to federal regulations; or

(B) the potential subject gives informed consent; or

(C) the potential subject has given Prospective Authorization, consistent with Recommendation 13, and the potential subject's LAR gives permission, consistent with Recommendation 14; or

(D) the potential subject's LAR gives permission, consistent with Recommendation 14.

RESEARCH PROTOCOLS INVOLVING GREATER THAN MINIMAL RISK THAT OFFER THE PROSPECT OF DIRECT MEDICAL BENEFIT TO SUBJECTS

Recommendation 11. An IRB may approve a protocol that presents greater than minimal risk but offers the prospect of direct medical benefit to the subject, provided that:

(A) the potential subject gives informed consent; or

(B) the potential subject has given Prospective Authorization, consistent with Recommendation 13, and the potential subject's LAR gives permission, consistent with Recommendation 14; or

(C) the potential subject's LAR gives permission, consistent with Recommendation 14.

The research must also comply with Recommendations 7, 8, and 9.

RESEARCH PROTOCOLS INVOLVING GREATER THAN MINIMAL RISK RESEARCH THAT DO NOT OFFER THE PROSPECT OF DIRECT MEDICAL BENEFIT TO SUBJECTS

Recommendation 12. An IRB may approve a protocol that presents greater than minimal risk but does not offer the prospect of direct medical benefit to the subject, provided that:

(A) the potential subject gives informed consent; or

(B) the potential subject has given Prospective Authorization, consistent with Recommendation 13, and the potential subject's LAR gives permission, consistent with Recommendation 14; or

(C) the protocol is approved on the condition of its approval by the panel described in Recommendation 2, or falls within the guidelines developed by the panel, and the potential subject's LAR gives permission, consistent with Recommendation 14.

The research must also comply with Recommendations 7, 8, and 9.

V. Recommendations Regarding Surrogate Decision Making

PROSPECTIVE AUTHORIZATION

Recommendation 13. A person who has the capacity to make decisions about participation in research may give Prospective Authorization to a particular class of research if its risks, potential direct and indirect benefits, and other pertinent conditions have been explained. Based on the Prospective Authorization, an LAR may enroll the subject after the subject has lost the capacity to make decisions, provided the LAR is available to monitor the subject's recruitment, participation, and withdrawal. The greater the risks posed by the research protocol under consideration, the more specific the subject's Prospective Authorization should be to entitle the LAR to permit enrollment.

LEGALLY AUTHORIZED REPRESENTATIVES (LARS)

Recommendation 14. An LAR may give permission (within the limits set by the other recommendations) to enroll in a research protocol a person who lacks the capacity to decide whether to participate, provided that:

(A) the LAR bases decisions about participation upon a best estimation of what the subject would have chosen if capable of making a decision; and

(B) the LAR is available to monitor the subject's recruitment, participation, and withdrawal from the study; and

(C) the LAR is a person chosen by the subject, or is a relative or friend of the subject.

EXPANSION OF THE CATEGORY OF LEGALLY AUTHORIZED REPRESENTATIVES AND OF THE POWERS GRANTED UNDER STATUTES FOR DURABLE POWERS OF ATTORNEY (DPA) FOR HEALTH CARE

Recommendation 15. In order to expand the category of LARs:

(A) an investigator should accept as an LAR, subject to the requirements in Recommendation 14, a relative or friend of the potential subject who is recognized as an LAR for purposes of clinical decision making under the law of the state where the research takes place.

(B) states should confirm, by statute or court decision, that:

(1) an LAR for purposes of clinical decision making may serve as an LAR for research; and

(2) friends as well as relatives may serve as both clinical and research LARs if they are actively involved in the care of a person who lacks decision-making capacity.

Recommendation 16. States should enact legislation, if necessary, to ensure that persons who choose to plan for future research participation are entitled to choose their LAR.

INVOLVING SUBJECTS' FAMILY AND FRIENDS

Recommendation 17. For research protocols involving subjects who have fluctuating or limited decisionmaking capacity or prospective incapacity, IRBs should ensure that investigators establish and maintain ongoing communication with involved caregivers, consistent with the subject's autonomy and with medical confidentiality.

VI. *Recommendations Regarding Education, Research, and Support*

REVIEWING AND DEVELOPING EDUCATIONAL MATERIALS REGARDING RESEARCH

Recommendation 18. Professional associations and organizations should develop (or review their existing) educational materials pertaining to research involving persons with mental disorders to ensure that they are adequate to inform the health care community and the public of ethical issues related to the involvement of such persons as research subjects, and to convey the importance of measures to ensure that their rights and welfare are adequately protected.

EXPANDING KNOWLEDGE ABOUT CAPACITY ASSESSMENT AND INFORMED CONSENT

Recommendation 19. The NIH should sponsor research to expand understanding about decisionmaking capacity, the best means for assessing decisionmaking capacity, and techniques for enhancing the process of informed consent, and the possible roles of surrogate decision makers in research. It should sponsor research to evaluate the risks of various research interventions, and the attitudes of potential subjects toward the prospect of participating in research. Particular attention should be paid to attitudes toward participating in research of greater than minimal risk that does not offer the prospect of direct medical benefit to subjects. These data may be of particular value to the panel described in Recommendation 2.

The NIH should ensure that proposals for training grants and center grants include appropriate provisions for training and technical assistance in the issues discussed in this report. Where appropriate, the NIH and the Office for Protection from Research Risks [OPRR, now the Office for Human Research Protection, OHRP—eds.] should consider using consensus development conferences or workshops to advance discussion of these issues.

INSTITUTE OF MEDICINE REVIEW OF RESEARCH STUDIES

Recommendation 20. The DHHS should contract with the Institute of Medicine to conduct a comprehensive review and evaluation of the nature and extent of challenge, washout, and placebo controlled studies with subjects with mental disorders that may affect decisionmaking capacity.

INCREASED FUNDING TO SUPPORT NECESSARY PROTECTIONS OF HUMAN SUBJECTS

Recommendation 21. Compliance with the recommendations set forth in this report will require additional resources. All research sponsors (government, private sector enterprises, and academic institutions) should work together to make these resources available.

39   Are Research Ethics Bad for Our Mental Health?

ROBERT MICHELS

Patients with mental illness are much better off now than they were only a few decades ago. Diagnostic methods are more reliable, and treatments are more effective. Only a minority of psychiatric patients require long-term hospitalization, and the practice of psychiatry is now more like the practice of other medical specialties. At the same time, the prevalence of psychiatric disease is more clearly recognized. Five of the world's 10 leading causes of disability are psychiatric: depression, alcohol abuse, bipolar mood disorder, schizophrenia, and obsessive-compulsive disorder. Each of these disorders has important genetic determinants and biologic correlates. In the past 40 years, specific effective treatments for each have replaced nonspecific concern and support. We have developed pharmacologic agents for depression, mania, psychosis, obsessions, and panic, as well as agents that block the cravings for drugs of abuse, calm hyperactive children, and slow the progress of Alzheimer's dementia. We have also developed psychological treatments for depression and methods of psychosocial management for patients with schizophrenia. This progress has been based on the immense growth of both basic and clinical psychiatric research. By 1995, academic departments of psychiatry were second only to departments of medicine in terms of funding for research.

However, there has been concern about the ethical aspects of psychiatric research. Are mentally ill subjects especially vulnerable to exploitation? Are they competent to give informed consent? Are psychiatric research methods particularly dangerous? Are special procedures or regulations needed for such research? There have been attacks and defenses of psychiatric research in the courts, in the media, and in statements made by groups that advocate for the rights of the mentally ill.

Perhaps the most vexing ethical problem has concerned mentally ill patients who have a diminished capacity to consent to participate in research. The Nuremberg Code [. . .] stated that "the voluntary consent of the human subject is absolutely essential." Henry Beecher, a pioneer of research ethics, wrote in 1959 that this principle would "effectively cripple if not eliminate most research in the field of mental disease." Society has struggled with this ethical dilemma ever since. There is agreement that research on

human subjects requires informed consent but that, at the same time, we must learn as much as possible in order to improve the care of those who suffer from diseases that impair their capacity to provide informed consent. How do we proceed when these goals are in conflict, when conducting research on those who cannot themselves consent to participate in it is the route to improving their care?

[T]he Declaration of Helsinki softened the absolute ban of the Nuremberg Code by allowing the legal guardians of incompetent persons to provide consent on their behalf, at least for "therapeutic" research. In 1974, the National Commission for the Protection of Human Subjects of Biomedical and Behavioral Research, which was created after the revelation of the exploitation of subjects in the Tuskegee study of syphilis, discussed the special problem of the use of vulnerable groups as research subjects. Its recommendations moved beyond both the Nuremberg Code and the Declaration of Helsinki. The commission argued that "prohibiting such research might harm the class of mentally infirm persons as a whole by depriving them of benefits they could have received if the research had proceeded."

The commission suggested special regulations to govern research on "persons institutionalized as mentally infirm," but these regulations were viewed as overly burdensome and were never adopted. However, the commission's general comments paved the way for the so-called common rule. This is an executive order, first proposed in 1986 and issued in 1991, that governs the basic structure of regulations for research on human subjects conducted by the federal government or in facilities receiving federal funds. The common rule recognizes the special problems of "vulnerable populations," including the mentally disabled. It requires that institutional review boards (IRBs) include additional safeguards to protect the rights of such groups but provides no specific guidelines as to how IRBs should do so.

The National Bioethics Advisory Commission (NBAC) is the latest federal panel to address the issue. [. . .] Its report was released in 1998. [It is included in this volume. —eds.]

The NBAC reviewed judicial and public concerns about research on the mentally ill, including a 1992 lawsuit against the University of California at Los Angeles alleging that a research protocol involving a drug "washout" aggravated a patient's schizophrenic illness and led to his suicide. [. . .] The NBAC also reviewed the series of judicial decisions in New York State that challenged regulations gov-

Robert Michels, "Are Research Ethics Bad for Our Mental Health?" *New England Journal of Medicine* 340 (1999): 1427–30.

erning participation in research by persons who lack the capacity to give informed consent, and it reviewed media exposés. [. . .] The commission concluded that there were three justifications for its work: first, the perceived regulatory gap since the rejection of the recommendations of the earlier commission [. . .]; second, the apparently inadequate protection of human subjects in some cases [. . .]; and finally, the need to ensure public confidence in the research enterprise.

The ethical problems of research on the mentally ill seem somewhat different today from the way they did in the 1970s. The proposals rejected at that time referred to "persons institutionalized as mentally infirm," but today, clinical psychiatric research is performed largely in the outpatient setting. In the past, mentally ill persons were often viewed as broadly incompetent. Because of that view, their civil liberties were curtailed, and involuntary treatment was common. Today, there are few patients who are hospitalized against their will. Even those who are retain their rights, including their right to refuse treatment. Empirical studies suggest that impaired decision-making capacity may be less common among psychiatric patients (it is estimated to be present in about 52 percent of hospitalized patients with schizophrenia) and more common among those with serious medical illnesses (about 12 percent) than previously believed. For example, a survey of patients with medical disorders found that 6 percent of those who believed they had never participated in medical research had actually done so, and 7 percent of those who had participated in research did not understand that they had the right to withdraw from it.

The NBAC considered some of these changes, but nevertheless made the fundamental and highly controversial decision to focus its report on persons with mental disorders that may affect the capacity to make decisions rather than on all potential research subjects with actual or probable impaired capacity. In my view, this focus reflects the persistence of outmoded stereotypes. Psychiatric patients and psychiatric research are fundamentally similar to medical patients and medical research, respectively, and psychiatric patients should have the same rights, governed by the same safeguards and regulations, as those of medical patients. Regulations should be based on functional characteristics such as decision-making capacity rather than on diagnostic categories, particularly categories, such as mental illness, that have been subject to stigma.

The traditional definition of the capacity to consent to research requires that the subject understand the difference between treatment and research, the nature of the research being conducted, its risks and benefits, available alternatives, and the fact that he or she is making a decision and that the decision can be changed. The subject must not be swayed by a pathologic affective state, a false belief, or a dependent relationship that might interfere with the decision

or with his or her autonomy and must be capable of making a stable, reasoned choice and communicating it. The NBAC agrees with this definition. Its most controversial recommendations concern the process of assessing the capacity to consent to research, the arrangements for surrogate decision making if this capacity is impaired, and the evaluation of the risks and benefits of research.

Currently, the capacity to consent to research is assessed in much the same way as the more familiar capacity to consent to treatment—that is, by the health care professionals and care givers who are closest to the patient. The NBAC would change this approach for all research involving more than minimal risk. The category of "more than minimal risk" is quite broad. It includes, for example, noninvasive magnetic resonance imaging (MRI) of the brain (because the noise, confinement, and apparatus could be distressing to a subject) or explicit questions about sexual preferences (which might upset a subject). Such research would require an assessment by an "independent qualified professional"; even the treating clinician would be disqualified from judging the capacity to consent to research if he or she were either participating in the research or employed by the institution conducting it. The NBAC considers the present system for evaluating a patient's capacity to consent to dangerous treatment inadequate even to assess the capacity to consent to MRI for research purposes. A similar proposal to use independent monitors of consent was a major factor in the rejection of the 1978 recommendations. Many psychiatric researchers consider these recommended procedures expensive, cumbersome, and clinically insensitive to the experience of impaired subjects, and some patient advocates fear that the implied mistrust of care givers may have a negative effect on the doctor-patient relationship.

For subjects found to have an impaired capacity to make decisions, the NBAC recommended acceptance of surrogate consent by legally authorized representatives, but with strict limits on their authority. Surrogate consent for research involving more than minimal risk (again, this includes brain imaging) would require approval of the protocol by a federal review panel, not just the IRB. This represents an extraordinary shift of authority from the community in which the research is being conducted to a central body distant from both the subjects and the researchers.

There are two problems with this suggestion. The first concerns what might seem to be a detail but turns out to be crucial. Similar regulations concerning children specify three levels of risk: "minimal risk," "minor increase over minimal risk," and "greater than minor increase over minimal risk." The middle category allows flexibility; there might not be the same concern about an MRI or probing questions about sexual behavior (examples of a minor increase over minimal risk) that there would be about a muscle biopsy (an example of a greater than minor increase). The requirement that a federal panel review research involving only a minor increase over minimal risk will be a serious barrier to research that has been free of ethical difficulties, such as studies of psychosocial interventions designed to reduce high-risk sexual behavior in psychotic patients or to determine the value of brain imaging in elucidating the mechanism of action of psychotropic drugs.

The second problem relates to the NBAC's view not only that mental patients and psychiatric researchers are different from medical patients and medical researchers, but also that psychiatric research methods themselves entail special risks. The commission cites three such methods: challenge studies (such as the administration of ketamine, which causes transient increases in psychotic symptoms, to patients with schizophrenia), drug washouts or holidays (periods when drugs are withdrawn), and studies in which some patients receive placebos. The NBAC ignored the extensive literature on the actual risks of these research strategies [. . .], but it nevertheless concluded that they "require special attention." Yet cardiac stress tests and glucose-tolerance tests are also challenge studies, drug-withdrawal strategies are commonly used in nonpsychiatric pharmacologic research, and placebo studies are often required by the Food and Drug Administration for drug approval. The risks of research may be small or large and it may be difficult to evaluate them, but there is nothing special about the evaluation of risk in psychiatric research as compared with other types of medical research.

The NBAC has made some excellent suggestions. One is that a federal panel collect data on the risks of various research interventions and the views of potential subjects. This will allow future guidelines to be based on facts rather than speculation and impressions. Another good suggestion is that funds be provided to cover the additional expenditures that the commission's recommendations would require. Oddly, the commission ignores the practical and ethical questions of who should provide these funds and what might have to be given up to make them available. Many psychiatrists and advocates for the mentally ill fear that the most likely result of adopting this recommendation will be a reduction in psychiatric research.

Finally, the NBAC suggests that IRBs that consider proposals involving persons with mental disorders should include members who represent the interests of the group being studied. This is a good principle. Unfortunately, it was not followed in the creation of the NBAC itself. Its 17 members include ethicists, scientists, physicians, patient advocates, and even an executive of a pharmaceutical company, but neither clinicians nor researchers in the fields of psychiatry or neurology. The New York and Maryland working groups that were studying the same issues at the same time made far less intrusive recommendations; each

working group included at least 4 psychiatrists among its 13 or 17 members. The participation of psychiatrists might have ensured that the NBAC had a fuller understanding of contemporary psychiatric practice and research. Herbert Pardes, the psychiatrist who was chairman of the New York working group, has stated that as they stand, the NBAC recommendations would "set us back twenty years."

The NBAC saw the absence of special guidelines for research involving mentally ill persons with impaired decision-making capacity as a "regulatory vacuum" and rushed to fill it. The absence of special regulations, however, does not necessarily define a vacuum, and providing additional regulations is not the best solution to all problems. The NBAC recognized that "unless individual investigators understand their ethical responsibilities no regulatory system will function properly" and quoted Henry Beecher, who observed that for human research subjects, "there is the more reliable safeguard provided by the presence of an intelligent, informed, conscientious, compassionate, responsible investigator." One danger of excessive regulations is that they can actually undermine researchers' sense of moral responsibility as their attention shifts from their obligation to research subjects to their compliance with the regulations.

The NBAC also justified its efforts by alluding to cases in which the protection of research subjects appeared to be inadequate. This is, of course, the most important justification; if protection has been inadequate in some cases, this problem should receive the highest priority. However, the commission did not determine whether research subjects have had inadequate protection. It would have been wise to find out how the current system is working and what problems exist before recommending new regulations to correct them—that is, to establish a diagnosis before prescribing a treatment.

Finally, the commission wanted to enhance public confidence in the psychiatric research enterprise. Singling out research on the mentally ill for special regulatory oversight, particularly in the context of media attention to unevaluated and unconfirmed allegations of abuse, is not likely to enhance public confidence.

Mentally ill persons with impaired decision-making capacity do not have one problem in regard to research ethics; they have two. The focus of the NBAC report is that the inability of such persons to provide full informed consent may leave them vulnerable to exploitation. The greater problem is that too little research is conducted on their behalf. Psychiatric research is burdened by a long history of public fear of mental illness, prejudice against the mentally ill, and distrust of those who treat or study them. The methodologic problems of studying the brain and behavior and the clinical burdens of working with psychiatric patients have contributed to this problem in the past but are abating at present. It would be unfortunate if the NBAC's attempts to address the problem of impaired capacity not only were incomplete and ineffective but also had the unintended effect of impeding research on mental illness.

If the mentally ill are different in a way that raises questions about their civil liberties and prevents them from participating in research, and if psychiatric research is dangerous and researchers are not to be trusted, the strategy recommended by the NBAC has merit. On the other hand, if persons with psychiatric disorders are as able and entitled as those without such disorders to take part in and benefit from research, if creative researchers can design valuable, yet safe studies, if clinicians and researchers regularly place their research subjects' interests first, and if the public, patients, ethicists, researchers, and clinicians all share a common goal, then it is time to expand the dialogue and collect data about the strengths and weaknesses of the current system. We should search for solutions that will protect all persons who have impaired decision-making capacity without further stigmatizing the mentally ill, undermining the research agenda for mental illness, or diluting the moral responsibility of researchers.

---

40   Caring about Risks

Are Severely Depressed Patients
Competent to Consent to Research?

CARL ELLIOTT

Depressed patients are often asked to take part in clinical research, and often this research carries risks. A depressed patient might be enrolled in a protocol to evaluate a new antidepressant drug, for example, or in one that requires a washout period, in which the patient's current medication will be discontinued. Some institutional review boards continue to approve protocols that test new antidepressants against placebo controls. Any of these situations entail risks, primarily the risk that the depressed patient's condition will worsen. The potential harm can be considerable, and at the extreme end of the spectrum includes the risk for suicide.

Although the concept of competence to consent to treatment and research has been widely and thoroughly discussed, only a few accounts give any attention to depression. Sometimes depression is not even considered a warning sign that a person's competence to consent needs to be evaluated, largely because it is not thought to be the type of disorder that would ordinarily interfere with competence. It is only the rare depressed patient who is psychotic, and while depression may often interfere with a person's memory and concentration, often this interference is not severe enough to raise any warning flags. Most accounts of competence focus on intellectual capacity and abilities to reason, and depression is primarily a disorder of mood.

According to conventional thinking, depression is primarily about despair, guilt, and a loss of motivation, while competence is about the ability to reason, to deliberate, to compare, and to evaluate. Often these latter abilities are ones that depression leaves intact.

I want to challenge this account of competence and argue that depression may well impair a patient's competence to consent to research. Most crucially, it can impair a person's ability to evaluate risks and benefits. To put the matter simply, if a person is depressed, he or she may be *aware* that a protocol carries risks, but simply not *care* about those risks. This sort of intellectual impairment can be as important a part of patient competence as the more detached, intellectual understanding that most accounts of competence emphasize. If my argument is correct, then institutional review boards need to take special precautions in allowing researchers to enroll depressed patients in research protocols.

COMPETENCE AND ACCOUNTABILITY

Competence is conventionally defined as the ability to perform a task—in this case, to consent to enroll in a research protocol. What counts as competence to consent will then depend on what one counts as the abilities relevant to the task in question. According to a widely accepted account of competence, the 1983 U.S. President's Commission Report, the relevant abilities are (1) the ability to reason and deliberate, (2) the ability to understand and communicate information, and (3) the possession of values and goals. As conceptualized within this framework, a potential research

Carl Elliott, "Caring about Risks: Are Severely Depressed Patients Competent to Consent to Research?" *Archives of General Psychiatry* 54 (1997): 113–16.

subject takes in the relevant information, weighs it according to his or her goals and values, and then reasons to an informed decision.

This account of competence, however, is incomplete. If competence to consent to research is defined simply as the ability to make a decision to enroll in a research protocol, we face the familiar problem of what *counts* as that ability —of trying to decide whether a person is incompetent by virtue of making an irrational decision, or by virtue of coming to that decision in an unsystematic, illogical, or erratic way. Since even competent people are sometimes stubborn, obtuse, or unreasonable, we need an account of competence that explains why we sometimes believe that a person can be both competent and make bad, irrational, or even unreasonable choices.

What we really want to know when we ask if a patient is competent is whether that individual is able to make a decision *for which he or she can be considered accountable.* What we want to know is whether the decisions that a person makes—whether they are good or bad, rational or irrational—are decisions for which that person can legitimately be considered responsible. This is why we define certain mental abilities as relevant: we realize that certain conditions or disorders impair a person's mental abilities such that he is not a morally responsible agent. He can make decisions, but we would not feel comfortable ascribing him with the credit or blame for that decision. If a person is making a decision that will affect his life in momentous ways, we will naturally be concerned that he makes a sound decision. But because we recognize that a person generally has the right to make even unsound decisions, a judgment about competence ensures that whatever decision a person makes, it is truly *his* decision: a decision for which he can finally be held accountable.

Once we conceptualize competence in this way, it becomes clear that it is not just intellectual ability that is relevant to competence. A person's emotional state can also affect her decisions in ways that might lead us to say that she cannot be judged fully accountable for them. The criminal law recognizes this, for example, and often grants leniency when a person acts under severe emotional distress. We often make decisions in the heat of anger or under the cold weight of despair that are uncharacteristic, that we would not have made otherwise, that we later regret, and for which we believe we should not be considered fully accountable. Likewise, we often recognize that it would be unfair to hold a person to a decision that he or she made in the face of overwhelming fear. In emotional extremes, we value, think, and behave differently—sometimes so differently that we might later believe that the decisions we have made are not decisions for which we can be held completely and unproblematically responsible.

The importance of emotion and mood for competence has not been lost on psychiatrists. Some accounts of competence stipulate that persons must "appreciate" the consequences of their choices, rather than simply understand them factually, the term "appreciate" implying a fuller, deeper comprehension of how the decision will affect the patient's life. A patient who can flatly recite the effects of treatment may still seem to fail to appreciate fully just how the treatment is going to affect his or her health. Nor can affect be completely divorced conceptually from cognition. Bursztajn and his colleagues have pointed out how a patient's affect can influence competence by altering his or her beliefs. For example, a depressed patient, convinced that his situation will never change, may refuse treatment based on the unrealistic belief that it will not help him.

However, while some patients may have affective disorders that disrupt their cognitive, rational decision-making abilities, a slightly different sort of depressed patient presents other problems. This is the depressed patient who is capable of understanding all the facts about his illness and the research protocol to which he is enrolling, and who appreciates the risks and the broader implications of the protocol on his life, but who, as a result of his illness, is not *motivated* to take those risks into account in the same way as the rest of us. For example, these patients might realize that a protocol involved risks, but simply not *care* about the risks. Some patients, as a result of their depression, may even *want* to take risks. Roth et al. wonder about the competence of one such patient, a 49-year-old woman capable of fully understanding the electroconvulsive therapy for which she was being asked to consent, but who, when told that electroconvulsive therapy carried a 1 in 3000 chance of death, replied, "I hope I am the one."

Several writers have speculated about whether depression might lead patients to overestimate the side effects of interventions and underestimate the likelihood of benefit. Although there are apparently no empirical studies examining the question of whether depressed patients are more likely than nondepressed patients to consent to risky or uncomfortable research, Lee and Ganzini have studied the effects of depression and its treatment on the preferences of elderly patients for life-sustaining medical therapies. In a study of 43 depressed patients, a subgroup of 11 severely depressed patients were more likely to choose life-sustaining therapies after their depression had been treated than they were while depressed. However, while this suggests that severe depression might affect the way some patients evaluate risks and benefits, it is not clear whether evaluation of life-sustaining therapy is similar enough to evaluation of research risks to bear much comparison.

Nonetheless, it seems unlikely that severely depressed patients are in the best position to make important decisions about their welfare. The Royal College of Psychiatrists in the United Kingdom is one of the few bodies to recognize this explicitly, offering the example of a patient with depressive delusions who consents to risky research because he thinks he is guilty and deserves to be punished. However, given the sense of hopelessness and worthlessness that characterizes some severely depressed patients, it seems reasonable to worry about their decision making. The novelist William Styron describes his own agonizing depressive episode as

> the diabolical discomfort of being imprisoned in a fiercely overheated room. And because no breeze stirs this cauldron, because there is no escape from this smothering confinement, it is entirely natural that the victim begins to think ceaselessly of oblivion.

DEPRESSION AND COMPETENCE

Although other writers have suggested that affective disorders may interfere with a patient's competence to consent to treatment, none has considered competence to consent to research, and only a few have attempted to say *why* depression impairs competence. That is, while there are not many writers who would dispute that mood is a part of ordinary decision making, it is also normal for a person's mood to change from one time to another, and it is not immediately obvious why a depressed mood should invalidate a patient's competence.

There are 2 good arguments for the conclusion that some depressed patients are incompetent to consent to research, each of which is persuasive for a slightly different type of patient. The first might be called the argument from *authenticity*. When a person is caught in the grip of depression, his values, beliefs, desires, and dispositions are dramatically different from when he is healthy. In some cases, they are so different that we might ask whether his decisions are truly his. A decision may not be truly his in the sense that it reflects dispositions and values that are transient and inconsistent with much more deeply ingrained traits of his character. One might say "I wasn't myself" when looking back on a time of despondency, and a caricature of the authenticity argument would hold that we should take this declaration literally: I was not myself, so that decision is not mine. Yet underneath that caricature is a grain of truth. If a person is so deeply depressed that his decisions are wildly inconsistent with his character, it seems problematic to abide by his decisions, particularly if the depression is dramatic and reversible.

Here is where the notion of competence as accountability is helpful. If a person were to behave badly while mentally ill—say, in a full-blown manic episode—we would very likely think it unfair to hold him fully responsible for what he has done. His behavior was uncharacteristic; he would never have acted this way unless he was manic; his mania is temporary and reversible with lithium treatment. His actions in the manic state were not truly *his*. Similarly for the depressed patient being asked to consent to research: his mental state is such that his behavior and choices do not seem to be truly his. If something untoward were to happen to him during the research, for instance, we could not in good conscience say that he bears the full responsibility for undergoing that risk.

The authenticity argument supposes a person with a stable character and entrenched dispositions, who, while depressed, makes decisions so uncharacteristic that we feel bound to question whether those decisions were truly hers. However, sometimes this break between the depressed and predepression personality is not so dramatic. Some patients are chronically depressed, and others are depressed periodically. It would not be plausible to argue that the decisions of these depressed patients do not reflect their underlying characters—characters that are closely tied to their depression. Yet there comes a point where, if a person appears largely insensitive to her own welfare, we might believe that she is incompetent to consent to research. Why should this be so?

One answer lies in what might be called the argument from *self-interest*. Our ordinary relationships with other people are based on certain assumptions about their thoughts and behavior. One of these assumptions is that other persons have some minimal concern for their own welfare. For example, the assumption that other people ordinarily both have some minimal degree of self-interest and are best positioned to judge their own interests lies at the heart of the institution of informed consent.

However, if we have reason to believe that severely depressed patients do not have this minimal degree of concern, then a fundamental assumption underlying informed consent is undermined. We justify exposing patients to the risks of research by the assumption that the patient is evaluating that risk with some degree of concern for her welfare. A competent evaluation of risks involves taking into account one's own well-being: not necessarily taking it as an overriding or supremely important concern, but at least taking it into account. If a person is so depressed that she fails to take her interests into account in deciding whether to take a risk, then we can hardly be comfortable saying that she is accountable for taking that risk.

CONCLUSIONS

Two broad types of conclusions can be drawn from these arguments, one empirical and the other conceptual. First, more empirical research needs to be carried out to determine the ways in which severe depression might affect psychological factors relevant to competence. For example, it would be important to know the extent to which severe depression affects how much a person cares about his or her own well-being, or how it might affect a person's willingness to expose himself or herself to potential harm.

Second, these arguments suggest that we may need to alter our conventional ways of assessing competence. As I have argued, many conventional accounts of how competence should be assessed downplay the importance of emotional factors. However, if my arguments are convincing, it may not be enough for psychiatrists or researchers to evaluate competence simply by testing a person's memory and reasoning ability, such as with a Mini-Mental State Examination. Rather, it may be that evaluations should also be concerned with a person's affective and motivational state: whether a person's mood has dramatically changed recently, how concerned a patient appears to be about her own well-being, how carefully she looks at risks and benefits, and so on. Of course, sound and uniform ways of assessing these affective and motivational factors will need to be developed.

On a practical level, these arguments have potential implications for the conduct of clinical research protocols testing new treatments for major depression. For example, if it is concluded that severe depression does impair competence to consent, clinical research protocols involving subjects with depression will need to require explicitly that the competence of subjects be evaluated before entering the study. This requirement might be similar to that of psychiatric research protocols testing new antipsychotic drugs, which generally state that subjects either be competent to consent or that consent be obtained from an appropriate surrogate.

Finally, this view of competence could have practical implications for studies involving relatively poor risk-benefit ratios. Sometimes severely depressed patients are enrolled in protocols in which their depression is likely to worsen (e.g., as a result of being assigned to a placebo treatment arm). Researchers argue that exposing competent adults to these sorts of risks is justified at least in part by the institution of informed consent, with the corresponding presumption that potential subjects understand the risks of the protocol, consent to them, and can be judged accountable for undertaking them. But if severely depressed patients are incompetent, exposing them to the risk of having their illness worsen is much more difficult to justify.

Section Two

Children

41 The NIH Trials of Growth Hormone for Short Stature

Carol A. Tauer

In May 1993 the National Institutes of Health (NIH) resumed recruiting extremely short children for two studies of biosynthetic growth hormone. These studies had been suspended a year earlier because of concerns about the ethics and the safety of the research. Two outside panels were convened to review the protocols; one panel concentrated on the study involving medically normal but very short children, and the other focused on the study of girls with Turner syndrome. [...]

Carol A. Tauer, "The NIH Trials of Growth Hormone for Short Stature," *IRB: A Review of Human Subjects Research* 16, no. 3 (1994): 1–9.

THE NIH SHORT STATURE PROTOCOL

The title of the NIH short stature protocol describes many of its aspects: "A Randomized, Double-Blind, Placebo-Controlled Trial of the Effects of Growth Hormone Therapy on the Adult Height of Non-Growth-Hormone-Deficient Children with Short Stature." The trial is planned to include 80 subjects, with half of the children receiving biosynthetic growth hormone and half a placebo. The growth hormone (or placebo) is given by means of three subcutaneous injections per week until bone age X-rays show that wrist and hand epiphyses have fused, that is, until bone structure has reached maturity and growth has ended. Girls ages 9 to 14 may be admitted into the study, boys ages 10 to 15. Given the long period of time during which subjects will participate in the study, the total number of shots given to each child will range from 600 to 1,100. Since the study is double-blind, a child in the placebo group will receive the same number of saline injections, as well as undergoing all medical and psychological testing required for the children receiving the drug.

The two criteria for admission to the study that are stated in its title are "non-growth-hormone-deficient" and "short stature." Identification that the subjects are non-growth-hormone-deficient depends on their reaction to provocative tests using arginine-insulin and levodopa. Since the pituitary gland secretes growth hormone sporadically, human growth hormone [hGH] cannot be measured randomly. Drugs like those mentioned stimulate release of growth hormone and are used in clinical evaluations of the level of hGH secretion.

The research protocol uses the level set by the National Pituitary Agency for normal hGH response to provocative tests, 7 ng/ml, as the lower limit for a child's acceptance under this protocol. [. . .] Pediatric endocrinologists constantly note, however, that because of the difficulty of measuring a child's production or secretion of hGH, the boundary between "growth-hormone-deficient" and "non-growth-hormone-deficient" children is by no means a bright and clear line.

The protocol's criterion for "short stature" has changed several times. When the study was first proposed in 1984, growth hormone was scarce; so the children admitted as subjects were to be extremely short, with current height or predicted adult height at least 3.00 standard deviations below the mean. In 1987, with biosynthetic growth hormone available, the inclusion criterion was changed to 2.5 standard deviations below the mean, and later amended to 2.25 standard deviations. These variations cover a range of approximately two inches with respect to adult height. [. . .] For North American males, an adult height 2.5 standard deviations below the mean is 5'3"; for females it is 4'10.5". So the standards for adult "short stature" vary by about two inches across the three proposed criteria, and all three differ by 4.5" for males versus females. Besides selection criteria, the study protocol describes in detail the tests and procedures each subject will undergo. The child will be admitted to the Clinical Center at NIH for a 3-day initial evaluation that includes the provocative tests of hGH response, standard blood and urine tests, tests of growth and bone maturity including X-ray and MRI scans, nude photographs, regularly repeated blood samples to measure the levels of hGH and other hormones, and behavioral and psychological assessments. If accepted, the child's next 6-month growth rate will be recorded as baseline, and then he or she will begin to receive injections of Humatrope or placebo.

Every six months the child will return to NIH for blood and urine tests, body measurements, assessment of possible immune response (antibody formation) to the study drug, and bone age X-rays. At the end of the first six months of injections the child will be readmitted to the clinic for three days for additional overnight measurements similar to those in the initial evaluation. Nude photographs and the MRI are to be repeated yearly, psychological assessment at six months and then every two years. [. . .]

PURPOSES OF THE STUDY

In the practice of pediatric endocrinology, short stature is one of the most common presenting problems. In its extreme manifestations, it is described as a major developmental abnormality and a permanent adult handicap. Even if not extreme, it may create psychological problems and be socially stigmatizing for both children and adults. A number of studies show that even relative short stature may be economically disadvantaging. Many parents, increasingly aware of the availability of synthetic growth hormone, may insist on trying it for a short child even though the child does not demonstrate growth-hormone deficiency.

Endocrinologists recognize that clinical tests to measure natural secretion of growth hormone are not entirely definitive. In a particular series of tests, a child may appear to be nondeficient although he or she really lacks adequate growth hormone. Since hGH therapy is recommended for children who show a deficiency in natural secretion, why should it be denied to equally short children just because they appear to produce their own growth hormone? Given that the consequences of short stature are the same for both classes of children and that diagnostic procedures cannot clearly distinguish between them, endocrinologists argue that both classes have an equal right to hGH treatment. [. . .]

The NIH review committee estimates that up to half of approximately 15,000 children now being treated with hGH in the United States are children who do not have classical hGH deficiency. Given the current state of knowledge, however, treating physicians do not know whether they are actually increasing the adult height of these children by prescribing hGH for them. Several short-term studies have shown an increased growth rate over a 6- to 12-month trial period. But it is possible that hGH therapy in those children simply speeds up growth velocity and accelerates advancement of bone age, while eventual adult height will be no greater than originally predicted, and might even turn out to be less.

In the short-term studies, no serious adverse effects of drug therapy have been noted. However, experts list many possible risks of long-term use. For example, Louis Underwood [. . .] writes:

> The risks of using [GH] therapeutically in patients who are not GH deficient are not fully known. Of concern is the hormone's

possible diabetogenic effects; hypertension and over-growth of soft and bony tissues . . . are also potential side effects. . . . It is possible that side effects similar to those seen in patients with acromegaly might occur. . . . The observation that leukemia has developed in some GH-deficient children after therapy has raised concern about a possible stimulatory effect of GH on tumor formation and growth.

The Physicians Committee for Responsible Medicine cites studies which suggest that administration of hGH to non-deficient children could increase the long-term risk of solid tumor formation, particularly the incidence of breast cancer.

Thus, questions about long-term use of hGH in non-deficient children involve issues of both efficacy and safety. Since these are the two issues a clinical trial is intended to resolve, it is not surprising that clinicians have been advocating studies to investigate the risks and benefits of extended use of hGH. Their questions underlie the NIH short stature protocol, and are reiterated in that document. [. . .]

THE REVIEW COMMITTEE'S
JUSTIFICATION OF THE STUDY

The NIH review committee offers several reasons to justify the study of hGH therapy in short, non-GH-deficient children.

The first is the fact that hGH is already being prescribed to thousands of such children even though safety and efficacy issues are unresolved. It is likely that these numbers will increase substantially in the future, particularly after Eli Lilly loses the last "orphan drug" permit for biosynthetic hGH in February 1994. (Genentech's permit expired in 1992.) Beginning in March 1994, biosynthetic hGH may be produced by other companies, possibly even under a generic label, so that the present cost of up to $20,000 per year should drop substantially. With lower cost and greater availability, usage is expected to increase regardless of Food and Drug Administration approval. [. . .] Before the prescription of hGH further expands in populations where its efficacy and safety are unknown, the review committee believes it is essential that clinical trials provide the data needed to inform clinical practice.

Second, the review committee believes that the data from the study "could illuminate the public debate on the use of growth hormone. . . ." Here the committee has in mind the widespread and possibly cosmetic uses of hGH, say for normal-height children who would simply like to be taller, thus touching on the debate about enhancement uses of genetic technologies. This is an important concern, but the committee seems to be taking the position that the sci-

entific questions should be resolved before the ethical and social issues. It could just as well (and perhaps more logically) have taken the reverse position: that we should decide whether this kind of medical treatment is ethically and socially desirable before we do government-sponsored clinical trials of the treatment. [. . .]

Third, the review committee states that "determining the efficacy of hGH therapy is an important issue in pediatric endocrinology." It certainly is true that endocrinologists want this question answered. However, that in itself does not make the question important enough to justify use of government resources for its study. The committee does raise the issue of whether hGH therapy is a good use of scarce medical resources, but that concern is not its focus.

From an ethical perspective, the strongest argument the review committee gives to support clinical trials is its fourth one, which is based on justice and equality. Since these [non-GH-deficient—eds.] short children suffer the same "functional impairment and psychosocial stigmatization" as GH-deficient children "it could be considered unjust to deny access to treatment for [these short] children . . . simply on the basis of an unacknowledged, currently imprecise definition of 'deficiency.'" The issue then is whether the nondeficient children could expect the same benefits from hGH therapy as GH-deficient children receive. And this is the issue the study is intended to resolve.

Most of the justifications for the NIH study [. . .] are not strong arguments from an ethical perspective. The first one may be related to a possible mandate to conduct research on unvalidated therapies in wide use, but ethical assessment of that mandate requires consideration of additional factors.

However, the argument based on justice, equality, and nondiscrimination in relation to two classes of short children does provide at least one sound ethical basis for *considering* the conduct of clinical trials of hGH for non-GH-deficient short children. But do such trials themselves meet ethical standards for research involving children?

THE NIH PROTOCOL AND
RESEARCH INVOLVING CHILDREN

The NIH review committee [. . .] gave by far the most attention to the question asking whether the short stature protocol complied with the federal regulations on research involving children. In concluding that the protocol did satisfy the regulations, the committee espoused an interpretation of these regulations that subtly implied a position on controversial philosophical questions: the meanings of health, disease, disorder, and therapy. Its conclusions entail a substantive position on the classification of "short stature" in relation to these theoretical concepts.

In reaching its conclusions, the review panel painstakingly applied 45 CFR 46, Subpart D, especially sections 46.404, 46.405, and 46.406, which state the specific conditions under which the Department of Health and Human Services (DHHS) may conduct or fund research involving children.

Minimal risk research. According to 46.404, DHHS may conduct or fund research with children provided that the risk to the subjects is no greater than minimal risk. The concept of "minimal risk" is of great importance as a basic standard in the research regulations, and it is defined consistently throughout the regulations:

> The probability and magnitude of harm or
> discomfort anticipated . . . are not greater . . .
> than those ordinarily encountered in daily life
> or during . . . routine physical or psychologi-
> cal examinations or tests.

Ambiguities in this definition did not cause problems for the review committee; no one on the committee thought the risk to subjects in the short stature study was limited to minimal risk.

Research offering direct benefit. Since the study could not be approved under 46.404, the committee moved in turn to 46.405. This section permits DHHS to conduct or fund research with children that involves greater than minimal risk provided the intervention or procedure offers the prospect of direct benefit to the individual subjects. Three provisions must be satisfied:

(a) the risk is justified by the anticipated benefit to the subject;

(b) the risk-benefit ratio is at least as favorable as in alternative treatments;

(c) the parents give consent and the child assents to participation.

Since this section does not apply unless each individual subject can anticipate some direct benefit from participation in the study, the committee devoted most of its attention to the children in the placebo arm. Various potential benefits to these children were suggested, for example, long-term medical care of high quality, increased self-esteem from contributing to research.

In balancing risk against benefit, as required by 46.405(a), the committee found "the judgments . . . difficult and the comparisons troublesome," both for the experimental and the control group. In the end, only a minority concluded that the risk was justified by the anticipated benefit to each individual subject.

The majority believed that the discomfort and the burden of 600 to 1,100 shots and the periodic trips to NIH for

testing were not balanced by a corresponding benefit for the placebo group. For the treatment group, the prospective benefit of increased height had to be weighed against the burden of all the same procedures, as well as the risk that short-term acceleration of growth could hasten puberty and bone aging, so that final adult height might actually be less than without treatment. Both groups could suffer psychological harm from focus on their shortness or from disappointment if years of medical procedures did not have the desired effect.

In its deliberations, the panel accepted without question the protocol's identification of increased adult height as the prospective benefit or goal of hGH treatment. [. . .]

Research likely to yield generalizable knowledge. After rejecting 46.404 and 46.405 as inapplicable to this protocol, the panel turned to 46.406 and concluded "almost unanimously" that the protocol satisfied its requirements. Four provisions must be satisfied:

(a) the risks are only a minor increase over minimal risk;

(b) the research interventions are "reasonably commensurate with those inherent in [the subjects'] actual or expected medical, dental, psychological, social, or emotional situations";

(c) the expected knowledge is "of vital importance for the understanding or amelioration of the subject's disorder or condition";

(d) the parents consent and the child assents to participation.

46.406(a). The committee believed that most risks involved in the study were minimal or only slightly greater than minimal, because any serious problem would be detected quickly so that harm could be avoided, or because the risk was too low or too speculative to carry weight. However, the panel report describes the pain, discomfort, and inconvenience of the large number of shots given to each child as a risk "*significantly greater* than minimal" (emphasis added), especially for the control group subjects who had little prospect of compensating benefit.

After giving this characterization, however, the committee speculated that they were imposing an adult perspective, and noted that they had no data to suggest that children receiving the injections experienced them as unduly burdensome. Members asked, therefore, that the reactions of children in the study be assessed in order to provide a more informed basis for judging conformity with 46.406(a).

Examination of the literature indicates that there is already some information about children's reactions to long-term administration of growth hormone, cited in studies of GH-deficient children. Diane Rotnem [. . .] found that some treated children "saw themselves as victims of painful and useless injections, and persistently or intermittently resisted shots and directed angry feelings toward their parents [the administrators]."

The NIH panel is tentative in its assessment because of limited information, but its description of the risk of harm as "significantly greater than minimal" does not support approval under (a), which allows "only a minor increase over minimal risk." In order to move to (b) and (c), the committee had to question its own perception of the risk and to ask for further data to check conformity with (a). Later, however, the committee concluded that all the requirements of 46.406 were satisfied. There is no explanation as to how they reached this conclusion without the data needed to disprove their belief that the level of risk was "significantly greater than minimal."

It is also puzzling that the review committee did not give more attention to other risks possibly associated with the long-term administration of growth hormone. Because the committee became focused on risks to the placebo group as the group that could anticipate little compensating benefit, the harms they worried about were almost exclusively those associated with receiving the lengthy series of injections.

But long-term physical and psychological risks to the children receiving the drug (the experimental group) are currently unknown. In fact, determining the safety of long-term use of GH in nondeficient children is one of the reasons given for conducting the study. The parents' consent form states: "The study will also help show if Humatrope is safe for [long-term] use. . . . If there are any important abnormal tests or adverse effects, you will be notified immediately." (Interestingly, the children's assent form does not mention any risks, but does say there are "things that will hurt.") [. . .]

While there is no evidence of serious harm so far, and the risk is considered to be small, in this study the research population consists entirely of healthy children. Jeremy Rifkin [. . .] claims that this "is the first time the NIH has exposed healthy children to risk in order to make a scientific point." Historically that may or may not be true. However, it is certainly ethically questionable to expose healthy children to iatrogenic risks in the interest of scientific research. The review committee downplayed the significance of these risks, describing them as small, of little significance, speculative, or uncalculable—at the same time that Arthur S. Levine at [. . .] the sponsoring agency advocates the trial precisely because GH "could be dangerous."

46.406(b). In judging conformity of the study with (b), the committee referred to the understanding of the National Commission for the Protection of Human Subjects [the National Commission—eds.], the body that framed and recommended the research regulations to DHHS (then the Department of Health, Education, and Welfare). In explaining the phrase, "experiences . . . commensurate with those in their actual or expected medical . . . situations," the National Commission said it meant experiences that children with this condition "ordinarily experience (by virtue of having or being treated for that disorder or condition)."

The growth hormone review committee found that participation in the research study was commensurate with undergoing hGH treatment in a practice setting, except that children in the study would have a more rigorous follow-up to detect any problems. Since these tests and procedures were relatively benign and intended to detect risk, most members of the committee saw no problem with meeting the standard of 46.406(b).

Now while the review committee properly consulted the comments of the National Commission in interpreting 46.406(b), it did not go far enough. In the paragraph immediately following the passage cited above, the National Commission explains that the reason for provision (b) is to

> assist children who can assent to make a
> knowledgeable decision about their partici-
> pation in research, based on some familiarity
> with the intervention or procedure and its
> effects. [. . .]

For the children entering the NIH study, however, it is specifically an *exclusion* criterion if the child has received prior treatment with growth hormone, and of course, other treatments involving regular injections such as insulin therapy for diabetes. Thus prospective subjects in the short stature protocol are by definition excluded from having had prior experiences similar to the procedures the review committee considered most worrisome: the thrice-weekly injections over a long period of time.

While a short child whose parents sought and obtained growth hormone therapy would have had experiences similar to those in the protocol, the specific subjects in the study will not have had these experiences. Thus it seems a misconstrual of the intent of the National Commission to interpret 46.406(b) as satisfied by the short stature protocol. [. . .]

A more serious problem in satisfying 46.406(b) is the question of whether growth hormone treatment, or other drug therapy, *ought* to be the "actual or expected" response to short stature. To conclude that provision (b) is satisfied by the NIH protocol, the review panel had to make the assumption that a burdensome and costly drug therapy is an appropriate and, in fact, expected clinical recommendation for treating the condition of short stature. Thus a value-laden assumption lurks behind the committee's interpretation of 46.406(b).

The deliberations of the National Commission show that in drafting 46.406, commissioners had in mind the disorders and conditions commonly regarded as diseases. They speak of 46.406 as applying to diseased children in contrast to healthy children, or to sick children rather than to normal children. For children who are diseased or sick, onerous and risky procedures would often be an "actual or expected" part of their treatment and their lives. But it begs the question to assume that such treatments are an "actual or expected" part of the lives of children who are short but healthy and medically normal.

46.406(c). The review committee notes that most of its discussion of 46.406 focused on part (c). The committee finally agreed that because of the care with which the short stature protocol was designed, the status of NIH, and the lack of other systematic studies, the study did promise to yield knowledge "vital to understanding or ameliorating the disorder or condition under study." (Note that this conclusion is phrased differently from 46.406 (c) itself, which requires that the information be "of vital importance for the understanding or amelioration of the disorder or condition . . . ," a small variance that may have significance.)

While only a minority of the review committee believed that the protocol satisfied 46.405, a majority agreed that it satisfied 46.406. Hence the committee recommended that the study continue with some modifications: that the selection criterion be moved back from 2.25 to 2.5 standard deviations below the mean, that the assent of the children be renewed annually, and that some very commendable changes be made in consent forms. They also strongly recommended that a standing data safety and monitoring board be appointed to oversee the future conduct of the study, especially to act as an "early warning" system if any problems were developing.

THE NATIONAL COMMISSION AND RESEARCH WITH CHILDREN

The review committee's approval of the short stature protocol under provisions of 46.406 raises troubling questions. While the committee expresses its commitment to respect "the intent of the authors of the regulations both in general and with regard to the meaning of particular terms," in its interpretation of 46.406 it seems to have gone far beyond the intent of the authors. To evaluate this interpretation it is necessary to review some points in the history of the research regulations.

The National Commission, which was mandated to draw up guidelines for a variety of subject populations, always felt that "research with children, to the extent that it involves any exposure to otherwise nonexistent risks, raises a serious ethical question and calls for particular ethical

justification." Originally the commission intended to ban entirely any research involving children that carried more than minimal risk and did not promise compensating benefit to each individual child.

The first proposal for an exception to such a ban came from special consultant Robert Levine, who raised the issue of "a national epidemic or emergency." He suggested that in a critical situation, a national ethical advisory board might be consulted to approve research involving greater than minimal risk. (This mechanism was later established through 46.407.)

However, commissioners were concerned about requiring national review and public comment for large numbers of potentially valuable studies. Kenneth Ryan, chairman of the commission, posed the problem:

> We have a child that is sick, an ill child, with a specific disease process . . . it could be cystic fibrosis, it could be diabetes, in which there is an intent . . . to get fundamental information on . . . the disease process which would benefit all children with that specific disease process.

Thus was born the notion that it might be permissible to allow a child with a specific disease process to participate in a study carrying somewhat greater than minimal risk, provided that the study promised to benefit other children with that same disease process.

As the discussion progressed, Donald Seldin, the strongest proponent for permitting such research, was asked [. . .] what sort of benefit he thought would justify it. [He answered]: "the relief of pain, the mitigation of disability and the postponement of death, in the class of patients suffering from these derangements."

The sorts of disorders cited by Ryan: cystic fibrosis and diabetes (with cancer also mentioned frequently); and the conditions noted by Seldin: pain, disability, and premature death—these are what the National Commission had in mind when drafting 46.406. They intended to allow some research with sick children that would not be allowed for healthy children because of the seriousness of the condition under study.

Two commissioners out of eleven dissented from 46.406. Robert Turtle argued that there is no moral justification for treating sick children differently from healthy children with respect to research risks. While Turtle disagreed with the ethical conclusion of the majority of the commissioners, he agreed with them that 46.406 was about children who were sick. In fact, in responding to Turtle's dissent, Chairman Ryan reiterated this understanding:

> The Commission's intention in [46.406 is] . . . to permit the conduct of research intended to develop *important knowledge of disease states*

from which certain children suffer and for which they are the only appropriate subjects (emphasis added).

SHORT STATURE AS A DISORDER

What was the rationale of the NIH panel in using 46.406 to approve the short stature protocol? There are several possibilities:

(1) Perhaps the panel believed that short stature qualified as one of the disorders the National Commission had in mind: that shortness is equivalent to a disease state and that its consequences are similar to those of a disease.

The record of the National Commission's deliberations explicitly belies such an interpretation of 46.406. The commission's examples all represent disorders that are commonly called diseases or illnesses, carrying serious consequences relative to pain, disability, and life span.

The NIH panel states its commitment to be guided by the intent of the National Commission, and worries that children in the study might get "the harmful and *misguided* view that they are 'abnormal' on medical rather than statistical criteria" (emphasis added). Thus it is unlikely that the panel thought that short stature was the type of disorder or condition the National Commission had in mind.

(2) Perhaps the NIH panel believed that the ethical conclusion in 46.406 should be broadened. If sick children can be entered into somewhat greater than minimal risk research that benefits the class of children to which they belong, why cannot healthy children? The panel might argue that every child is a member of *some* class, and if a utilitarian argument justifies risk to a sick child to benefit a class of sick children, why would it not justify risk to a healthy child to benefit a class of healthy children?

There is no evidence to suggest, however, that the review committee considered such a position, or that it intended to call into question the ethical conclusions of the National Commission.

(3) Perhaps the NIH panel believed that although the National Commission did not intend to include disorders like short stature under 46.406, it is reasonable to include them. While short stature may not be a disease *per se,* it is damaging and disadvantaging to many children. If medical treatment is being offered in an attempt to modify the physiological basis for this damage and disadvantage, then it is important to conduct research on the effectiveness of that treatment.

The panel's report suggests that this position is the one it takes. It argues that because a nonvalidated therapy is already in wide use, research on efficacy and safety is necessary. The panel works backward, concluding first that the research is needed, and then seeking a provision under which it can be approved. Apparently it can be approved only by expanding the National Commission's concept of "disorder or condition" to include the condition of short stature.

Although the NIH panel states specifically that very short stature in non-GH-deficient children is a statistical rather than a medical abnormality, the panel applies a regulation explicitly designed for approving research on the medical treatment of sick children. Such an application of 46.406 creates a precedent for approving greater than minimal risk research with healthy children in order to study any condition researchers or clinicians would like to be able to modify. If there are people who regard the condition as disadvantaging and who seek "treatment" for it, then that condition would seem to qualify for studies under 46.406. [. . .]

REVISE THE REGULATIONS?

While it is troubling that the NIH review panel extended 46.406 to cover research on a condition that is not a disease, the need for this particular research project deserves further consideration. Many pediatricians and endocrinologists who oppose (as well as those who favor) the use of growth hormone for short non-GH-deficient children, nevertheless support continuation of the NIH trials. Opponents as well as advocates of such therapy would like to have the scientific question settled. [. . .]

I have argued that this study cannot properly be conducted under the current federal regulations on research with children. Moreover, I believe it is dangerous to "bend" the regulations in order to approve research that seems important though not strictly in accord with the regulations. It would be far better to invoke such research to raise the question of whether the regulations themselves need to be revisited.

When the regulations on research with children were first promulgated, some members of the National Commission as well as knowledgeable commentators expressed discomfort with 46.406. Two commissioners dissented, and James McCartney's analysis said:

> Despite the amount of time and energy expended on it, [46.406] still remains the weakest section of the report, and will no doubt engender confusion when institutional review boards attempt to interpret it.

The concept of minimal risk, and exactly what constitutes a minor increase over minimal risk, has been debated in IRB meetings and in the literature. Studies show there is vast disagreement among clinicians and researchers on the application of these concepts. In using 46.406 to approve the short stature protocol, the review panel short-changed the discussion of risks. But if they had wished to do a more detailed analysis, they would have had little guidance in applying the concept of a "minor increase over minimal risk." [...]

The federal research regulations are an important mechanism for protecting children, a vulnerable population, from harm and exploitation. It is time for the current regulations to be reviewed, and perhaps revised. If they are to be revised, it must be done cautiously, through a process as careful as that of the original National Commission. It must also be done by a body with public accountability and with opportunity for public comment. The worst possible sort of revision is ad hoc reinterpretation by individual IRBs and review panels.

42 *In loco parentis*

Minimal Risk as an Ethical Threshold for Research upon Children

BENJAMIN FREEDMAN, ABRAHAM FUKS,
AND CHARLES WEIJER

[...] Is it ever ethical to expose children to risks associated with research? If it is, what are the ethical limits to such risk? How can a specific threshold to research risk be formulated, justified, and applied? These questions have preoccupied pediatric researchers and others for many years. [...]

The [...] definition provided in the "common rule" states, "'Minimal risk' means that the probability and magnitude of harm or discomfort anticipated in the research are not greater in and of themselves than those ordinarily encountered in daily life, or during the performance of routine physical or psychological examinations or tests." Finding that a research study poses only "minimal risk" has some important procedural consequences for review. In this paper, though, we will focus upon another role: "Minimal risk" is the concept used in American regulation to serve as an anchoring measure of allowable risk (or—the other side of the coin—relative safety) in clinical research. The critical threshold of risk that may not be surpassed (short of special federal approval) is in fact one level higher: "minor increment over minimal risk." However, since the rule offers no independent definition or specification of "minor increment," attention must first be focused upon its anchor, "minimal risk." [...]

"Minimal risk" seems to raise more questions than it solves. This paper deals with a number of those questions: Do all forms of research upon children require the use of a threshold like "minimal risk"? What is the meaning, use, and justification of "minimal risk"? To what criticisms is the concept vulnerable, and what problems arise in its application? We will deal with these questions with the conviction that even if final answers remain elusive, clarification must be attempted. The many thousands of members of research ethics committees internationally that employ "minimal risk" or a similar concept must develop some shared understanding of what it means.

THE UBIQUITY OF RESEARCH RISK

In any ethical consideration of research, the question of the allowable maximum of research risk must inevitably arise. Every activity poses some risks to its participants, and research is no exception to this rule. Risk, commonly expressed as the magnitude of some harm multiplied by the probability of its occurrence, can never be eliminated, because—to take one common philosophic interpretation of probability—the eradication of risk would require reducing the harms associated with an activity to zero in this world and in all other possible worlds. William Clark has drawn a suggestive analogy between the European witch hunts of the sixteenth and seventeenth centuries and modern-day efforts to guarantee safety. In each case, the accused is required to prove a negative—I am not a witch; I bear no risk—that no finite series of empirical observations can establish. Absolute safety can therefore never be guaranteed to participants in clinical research. [...]

Robert Levine, realistically reexamining the usual research interventions, has suggested that most often the

Benjamin Freedman, Abraham Fuks, and Charles Weijer, "*In loco parentis:* Minimal Risk as an Ethical Threshold for Research upon Children," *Hastings Center Report* 23, no. 2 (1993): 13–19.

concept of minimal risk could be replaced by a clearer threshold:

> It is of value to distinguish risk of physical or psychological injury from various phenomena for which more fitting terms are "inconvenience," "discomfort," "embarrassment," and so on; "mere inconvenience" is a general term that may be used.... Research presenting mere inconvenience is characterized as presenting no greater risk of consequential injury to the subject than that inherent in his or her particular life situation.... The vast majority of research proposals present a burden that is more correctly described as mere inconvenience than as risk of physical or psychological harm. In general, prospective subjects are asked to give their time (e.g., to reside in a clinical research center, to be observed in a physiology laboratory, or to complete a questionnaire); often there is a request to draw some blood or to collect urine or feces. Although the withdrawal of venous blood may be momentarily painful and be followed by a bruise, no lasting physical harm is done.

Is "mere inconvenience" a better choice as a threshold? It more accurately reflects the consequences of participation in the run-of-the-mill protocol. Research subjects experience inconvenience—discomfort, annoyance, nuisance, and boredom—far more commonly than damage. However, "inconvenience" shares some of the ambiguity of "minimal risk," in that both measures refer to the risks of everyday life (to be examined further below). More seriously, "inconvenience" is a concept dealing with only a single variable: magnitude, the seriousness of resulting harm. As such, it cannot replace the concept of "minimal risk," which subsumes two variables: magnitude and likelihood of harm. For what if there is a potential for danger of much greater magnitude but minuscule likelihood? The language of "inconvenience" makes it impossible for us to consider this prospect, which the ethics and law of clinical research must encompass.

Weiss v. *Solomon et al.,* the first North American case to find that a research ethics committee had negligently approved a protocol, furnishes one example. In that case, the court found that the subject of a trial had died as a consequence of an anaphylactic reaction to fluorescein angiography, an investigation done purely for research purposes. There had been no reports of fluorescein causing death by anaphylaxis at the time of Mr. Weiss's death; only a few such reports have emerged since. In the overwhelming majority of cases, that is, the pure research intervention of fluorescein angiography poses no more than inconvenience—but not always. The same may be said of other common demarcated research interventions. Spending two days on a clinical research unit is not more than inconvenient—*unless* it results in a nosocomial infection like methicillin-resistant *Staph. aureus.* An antecubital venipuncture is "merely inconvenient"—*unless* it results in an uncommon complication like cellulitis or venous thrombosis. The more compendious concept of risk is needed to cover any magnitude of damage (ranging from nuisance to real damage), and any likelihood of any given magnitude.

The doctrine of informed consent to research constitutes one major response to the ethical challenge of research risks. Competent subjects with the capacity of understanding research risks and benefits, by consenting to serve as research subjects, voluntarily assume these risks. As the legal maxim states, *Volenti non fit injuria* (One who has agreed to an activity is not wronged by it). Conceivably, the same justification applies to research upon persons who have while competent executed a valid advance directive permitting specified forms of research to be performed upon them when their competency should lapse. This stratagem, the research analogue to treatment's "living will," may in the future serve an important role in research upon Alzheimer's dementia.

But no such solution is available on behalf of incompetent subjects who were never competent—most importantly, infants and small children but also those suffering from congenital intellectual handicaps. Unless safety is understood in a relative sense, permitting some small risk that falls below a specified threshold, these incompetent persons could never be permitted to participate in clinical research—a situation that would in the long run leave them "therapeutic orphans," and for that reason at even greater risk.

THE MEANING AND USE OF "MINIMAL RISK"

[...] Which procedures are said in the medical literature to impose no more than minimal risk? Such highly invasive maneuvers as splenectomy, transthoracic enucleation of esophageal leiomyomas, and pancreatic biopsies are all described as "of minimal risk." This characterization, on the surface so surprising, is nonetheless justifiable given the necessity for the procedure in the patient populations in question and the risks associated with alternative interventions. Clearly, the term cannot be defined without specifying a context: Minimal risk to what end, from whose point of view, and under which situations? On a semantic level, "minimal risk" is relational, context-dependent. To understand its meaning in the research context, we must examine that specific usage.

Even if we restrict the context to research interventions upon children, though, and even if we restrict our inquiry to investigators, significant disagreement remains. Janofsky and Starfield surveyed chairpersons of pediatric departments and directors of pediatric clinical research units in the United States to elicit their understanding of "minimal risk," "minor increment over minimal risk," and "more than minor increment over minimal risk." (Recall that "minor increment over minimal risk" is the critical threshold, determining whether a study could be approved by a local committee or would require approval by a special federal panel.) Respondents were asked to classify common research procedures as administered to pediatric subjects of different ages.

The results demonstrated serious disagreement among respondents: 14 percent thought tympanocentesis (puncturing of the ear drum) posed minimal risk or less, 46 percent classified it as a minor increment over minimal risk, and 40 percent thought it more than a minor increase. Expressed in practical terms, 40 percent thought research requiring tympanocentesis was impermissible, despite the importance of the research, without the approval of a federally authorized panel of ethics experts in addition to the approval of the parents. (With regard to a population of research subjects aged one to four years, respondents came close to the three-way mathematical maximum of dissension: 34% thought it minimally risky, 31% a minor increment, 35% more than a minor increment.) While these are extreme examples, substantial scatter across the categories was the rule rather than the exception throughout the study.

It does not seem, therefore, that "minimal risk" or the other thresholds it anchors may be clarified by examination of sense or signification within the medical literature, nor by usage of the community of clinical investigators. There appears to be no natural or uniform understanding of "minimal risk" upon which we can draw. If that is the case, we are left with only the definition of "minimal risk" provided in the regulations: the risk of daily life or that encountered in routine physical or psychological examinations. Although other interpretations are possible, this definition seems to set the risks of daily life as the baseline and the risks of routine examinations as an example of the risks of everyday life most similar to the kinds of interventions found in research studies—routine immunizations, developmental testing, and the obtaining of urine and blood specimens. An intervention's satisfaction of the minimal risk standard can therefore be demonstrated in one of two ways: directly, by showing that it falls within the definition; or indirectly, by showing that it is relevantly similar to other interventions known to fall within the definition.

But how is the definition itself to be interpreted? What is meant by "the risks of everyday life"? As Kopelman notes, the risks of everyday life may be understood in several different ways; for example, it may refer to all the risks any person might encounter or to those that all of us encounter. She rightly rejects the first possibility. The fact that some people commonly face very high risks (parachuting, fire-

fighting) could not justify allowing a similar level of risk in research upon children. The second characterization is much more restrictive, constituting a lowest common denominator of risk. Kopelman criticizes this interpretation of the risks of everyday life as follows:

> This interpretation assumes that we know the kinds of risks we all encounter and their probability and magnitude. Neither is obvious. Most of us drive cars, walk across busy streets, and fly in airplanes. Are these the everyday risks the definition refers to? How do we determine what risks are encountered routinely by all of us and estimate the probability and magnitude of these risks?

In the passage two distinct claims are made, one concerning the difficulty in *identifying* the risks of everyday life, the other, the difficulty in *quantifying* them. The first difficulty, though, is clearly exaggerated. While there will always be exceptions, within any given society daily life will present the bulk of its citizens with ordinary hazards at home, at work, at play, and in transit, crossing the street or taking a bath. It is not hard to identify this set of common social risks. We are, by definition, each acquainted with them; and, almost by definition, if we are unsure whether they belong within the set of common risks then they don't.

On quantification Kopelman seems on firmer ground. While we all ride in cars, few of us know the likelihood of our being in a fatal accident. And it is certainly true that institutional review boards (IRBs) or other research ethics bodies typically consider whether a given proposal is acceptable without recourse to actuarial charts of the risks of daily living.

Indeed, Kopelman could have posed a far more fundamental challenge to the concept. As noted above, the critical threshold for allowable research risk in children is not "minimal risk" itself, but rather, "a minor increase over minimal risk." What meaning attaches to the qualification "minor increase" that is not defined, specified, or characterized in any way within the regulations? If, as Kopelman believes, these thresholds are quantitative measures, verbal surrogates for numbers expressing the probability and magnitude of potential harms of everyday life, the question is unanswerable. This strongly suggests that an alternative, nonquantititative understanding of "minimal risk" is intended. To understand that, we need to turn to the basic principles that underlie committee research review.

THE PURPOSE OF "MINIMAL RISK"

A number of parties must concur in the judgment that a clinical study is ethically appropriate before that study will proceed. The first and probably most important decision-maker is the investigator, who must consider before developing a protocol whether the task may be ethically achieved, how risks may be minimized, how the study's goals and risks may be explained, and so forth. If the study is done upon competent persons, their consent represents another ethical decision node. If the subjects are young children the agreement of parents is required, as well as the assent of the child herself to the extent that she is capable of giving it.

What role does a research ethics committee play? The institution within which research proceeds, both in itself and as society's agent, has its own obligation to treat subjects in a trustworthy capacity. Research review by the ethics committee is a concrete expression of this institutional fiduciary responsibility. In addition, as investigators are sometimes overly enthusiastic or bold, committee review of the ethics of research serves in part as a fail-safe mechanism to curb inappropriate zeal. For example, in assessing any protocol, the IRB must determine that its risk-to-knowledge ratio is reasonable and that the scientific importance of the undertaking is proportional to the risks subjects will be undergoing. These issues should have been considered by the investigators; and usually they do that. Nonetheless, the research committee is charged not to take that for granted, to serve as a backup in case the investigator has not competently discharged his or her personal and professional obligation. Again, it is the inalienable obligation of the investigators properly to inform subjects prior to their participation in a trial. The IRB, in reviewing the study's consent form, serves as a fail-safe mechanism to ensure that the investigator's plan for informing subjects will satisfy ethical norms and the institution's own moral obligation to protect subjects.

The IRB plays the same backup role *vis-à-vis* parental (or guardian) approval of participation of a child (or other incompetent person) in research. Parents may be ignorant, apathetic, or merely inattentive. Cognizant of these and other possibilities, and of its own moral obligation to protect incompetent research subjects, the institution charges a review committee to act as surrogate for the scrupulous parent by filtering out those studies that would impose an unacceptable level of risk upon child participants. It is in this light that the threshold concept, "minor increase over minimal risk," needs to be understood. In applying this standard, the IRB is attempting to track those decisions that would be made by informed and scrupulous parents whose children are being invited to participate in research. This fail-safe measure does not ensure that parents will scrupulously evaluate studies; rather, it ensures that they will only have the opportunity to enroll a child in a study that could have passed such an evaluation.

Asking a parent to agree to the child's participation in research is asking for a decision for participation in a new situation, with new attendant risks. These decisions are not arrived at quantitatively, by calculating risks, but rather on a categorical basis. Consider another such choice. A child has been asked out to an overnight camping trip for the first time. The risks of the trip are not the risks of everyday life—it is a new experience. If the threshold of allowable risk never permitted anything other than the risks of everyday life, no new experiences could ever be enjoyed (something which itself in the not-very-long run would not be in the child's best interests). Rather, a mother asks herself, "Is the child ready for this? Should the child approach this by stages? *Are the risks sufficiently similar to those in my child's everyday life that I should allow this experience at this time?*" In discussion about whether to permit this involvement—with the mother resisting, and the child pressing—a certain logic may be discerned. Appealing to consistency, the child will say that he has been permitted, and successfully undergone, situations relevantly and roughly similar, though not identical—while the parent will focus upon difference.

In other words, the parental decision to permit exposure to new risks is not itself governed by, but rather anchored to, the risks of everyday life. And this point is of course exactly mirrored in our understanding of the regulations, in which the upper threshold of research risk is not governed by, but anchored to, the concept of minimal risk. Almost by definition, exciting and important research ventures into the unknown. A prohibition on such research involvement would be to the long-term detriment of this child and other children, just as a prohibition on new experiences is harmful to children over the long term. Therefore, the limit is set as a "minor increase over minimal risk." This limit is not quantitative, but represents a categorical judgment that focuses upon the comparison of new experiences to those of everyday life. It is this form of discussion that needs to take place in research ethics committees considering the approval of research involving children.

JUSTIFYING AND APPLYING THE THRESHOLD

Because children and their situations differ, a judgment anchored to the risks of everyday life, whether arrived at by parent or IRB, must be made relative to the child's actual situation. A diabetic child's everyday life includes pin-prick blood tests, and additional such tests required by a study protocol represent much less of a variation in that child's daily life than in the life of a healthy child. This relativistic understanding of minimal risk, held by the National Commission for the Protection of Human Subjects [National Commission—eds.] (with the exception of Commissioner Turtle), is in fact the current interpretation of the regulations.

We should also point out that by choosing the risks of everyday life as an anchor to an acceptable level of research risk, less net added risk is imposed upon the child than might be thought. The risks of research are to a degree substitutive, rather than additive: research risks are undergone, but the risks of alternative activities are forgone. Normal, healthy subjects of research would otherwise be pursuing their normally risky daily lives; and ill subjects who are not enrolled in research studies may nonetheless receive treatments and diagnostic tests under the rubric of therapy that are similar to those they would have experienced in research. Furthermore, although in principle any given level of risk associated with an activity can be reduced, there is substantial empirical evidence that past a certain point individuals cease efforts at risk reduction, and the efforts of third parties to reduce risk yield severely diminishing returns. [...] Insurance companies have long since identified the problem under the phrase "moral hazard": property owners who are insured against damage or theft take fewer pains to avoid these contingencies. People do differ in their propensity to trade off safety for other goods, but by specifying a threshold at or near the risks of everyday life we approximate a lowest common denominator of risk, the level at which most reasonable people feel "safe enough" so that their choices can be made without considering the small risk repercussions.

The concept, "risks of everyday life," has normative as well as descriptive force, reflecting a level of risk that is not simply accepted but is deemed socially acceptable. Without defining the scope of parental authority and discretion within the law, therefore, we may be reasonably certain that the risks of everyday life fall within those bounds. There is, however, no precise legal analogue to this level. Questions of child abuse deal with risks and harms far above this threshold; so does the question of parental refusal of medical treatment for a child on religious grounds. In some ways, the closest analogy arises in disputes over child custody, which consider and weigh the risks of a child's transferring to a new school, being exposed to (or shielded from) church teachings, and so on. But these cases, inevitably, are resolved on the relative basis of which parent is the better custodian rather than on the basis of whether parentally imposed risks fall beneath a threshold of acceptability.

One last aspect of the "risks of everyday life" should be discussed: its flexibility, in conformity to time and circumstance. Kopelman sees this as a serious drawback: "[T]he risks to children living in Belfast and Edinburgh are different; but we would not want to have this automatically influence what sort of research we think would be 'not too risky' for them." In our understanding developed above, the example is inapt—parental concern in Belfast may not be less than in Edinburgh—but the point that standards diverge across cultures is true.

However, this flexibility of the threshold is to our minds an advantage. Any society's notion of what demands on children are allowable changes over time. The routine labor expectations of children fifty years ago are considered

exploitative now, and those made one hundred years ago would now be actionable child abuse. The same is true of exposure to risk. Given the huge historical and geographical differences among cultures as to the degree to which children should be protected from risk or engaged in life's risky activities, only the most parochial would maintain that the currently prevailing view in Western Europe and North America is necessarily the one right approach. The ethical evaluation of research can and must insist upon the rigorous protection of subjects, but cannot in so doing lose all reference to common social norms. An ethics of research must be sufficiently flexible as to incorporate and accommodate cultural variance, as is done when "the risks of everyday life" is used as a categorical anchor for research risk. [...]

The final question remaining is that of applying the standard. When is the aggregated risk of research interventions an increase above a minor increment over minimal risk? The status of many of the most common research interventions, for example, blood sampling, dietary restrictions, and other measures listed by the National Commission is easily settled: they are associated with routine physical examinations and so are of minimal risk. Some other interventions not on that list because not associated with the risks of everyday life of healthy persons are minor interventions common to the lives of all ill children within the relevant class. In accepting the principle of commensurate risks, it follows that the form, and perhaps also the sum, of research risk for ill children may exceed that imposed upon their healthy counterparts. The question, "Is this research risk sufficiently similar to their daily experience?" could not receive the same answer in two groups whose daily experience of risk is so different as the healthy and the ill. On the other hand, some interventions—for example, liver biopsies—are so risky and unfamiliar that no colorable case could be made on their behalf.

What are the hard cases the threshold needs to address? One kind of problem is posed by the reiteration of minimally risky procedures for research purposes. One or two venipunctures are minimally risky; four, arguably so, but still not more than a minor increase over minimal risk. But what of five, ten, forty, or any number in between? Similarly, when testing a new treatment for meningitis it is acceptable to perform one lumbar puncture on a sick child to satisfy the protocol's scientific needs, but not five. Where is the break point? Another set of problems is posed by those procedures (arterial punctures performed upon healthy children, for example) that are qualitatively different from common procedures, although of low risk.

It is not to be expected that the threshold definition of minimal risk as the risk of everyday life will settle each of these questions in an unambiguous and nonarbitrary fashion. Neither this nor any other threshold definition is self-interpreting; each will require the exercise of judgment. But we can require that the threshold define the terms of the argument, the kinds of questions that will need to be posed in the committee's deliberations. This the threshold can do. The arguments will parallel those familiar to any parent considering allowing a child to undergo a new experience. The committee, acting *in loco parentis,* will need to debate whether the demarcated research intervention is similar to a common experience of this child, and whether the incremental research risks are similar to the risks this child or others like him runs on a routine basis. The debate takes place within a context recognizing that the committee owes a fiduciary duty to these subjects, and that this duty entails imposing upon a child no risks substantially above a socially defined minimum for any scientific end, however worthy. [. . .]

43 Minors' Assent, Consent, or Dissent to Medical Research

SANFORD LEIKIN

Agreement to participate in medical research differs between adults and minors. The presumption of competence in adults allows them to agree to participate by consent that is legally free of the desire of others. Minors are presumed incompetent, so that their participation not only requires their assent, but also their parents' permission. Seeking assent from minors who have limited autonomy raises important ethical issues related to their psychological development. It is the purpose of this paper to examine this aspect of assent with particular attention to when it is appropriate to seek minors' assent, and what it means to them when it is sought.

Assent was advanced as an important feature of children's participation in research by the National Commission for the Protection of Human Subjects of Biomedical and Behavioral Research. In its 1977 report, the Commission recommended that research should be conducted on children. Recognizing that children cannot give legal consent, the Commission recommended that prior to the child's participation the parents' permission should be obtained, and that assent be obtained from those children whom the institutional review board (IRB) judges are capable of assenting.

Requiring parental permission (as distinguished from consent) presumes that parents will act in the best interest of their child. Requiring the child's assent accords with the ethical principle of respect for persons. That principle requires not only respecting the decisions of autonomous persons, but also honoring the choices of individuals with diminished autonomy to the extent that they have developed the capacity to make choices.

The recommendations for parental permission and children's assent were subsequently incorporated into the federal regulations on children's research. The regulations define assent as "a child's affirmative agreement to participate in research." But according to the regulations, if the IRB determines that "the intervention or procedure involved in the research holds out a prospect of direct benefit that is important to the health or well-being of the children and is available only in the context of the research, the assent of the children is not a necessary condition for proceeding with the research." This statement indicates that either not seeking assent or overriding the child's veto is allowable in the conduct of research on interventions intended to be beneficial. The National Commission specifically recommended that in the conduct of research involving no beneficial procedures, "a child's objection to participation should be binding," but the federal regulations make no comment on the question of dissent to nontherapeutic procedures.

The regulations further state that "the IRB shall determine that adequate provisions are made for soliciting the assent of the children when in the judgment of the IRB the children are capable of providing assent." This judgment may be made for all children to be involved in research under a particular protocol or for each child individually. In determining whether to seek assent, IRBs are expected to take into consideration the "age, psychologic state, and the maturity of the children involved."

While these criteria are general gauges of decisionmaking ability by young people, they fail to reflect certain important attributes of their decisionmaking. These include current knowledge about the development of chil-

Sanford Leikin, "Minors' Assent, Consent, or Dissent to Medical Research," *IRB: A Review of Human Subjects Research* 15, no. 2 (1993): 1–7.

dren's cognitive capacities and their understanding and reasoning about health care research. Other features of youths' thinking also need to be considered when determining whether to seek assent and in pursuing it. The young person from whom assent is requested must be able to recognize and express fulfillment of his or her rights concerning participation in or withdrawing from the research. Other questions of voluntariness also occur when seeking assent. For example, should minors' conformity or nonconformity to the influence of authority figures be relevant to assent? Another issue is that of altruism. If seeking assent is to be viewed as a way to provide moral training for young people, we should also consider how young people of various ages perceive their obligation to others. Integrating knowledge about these aspects of young people's decision-making may improve our understanding of what assent means to those from whom it is being sought, enhance our ability to determine whether to seek assent, and help us ascertain how best to help those from whom assent is sought.

THE COGNITIVE DEVELOPMENT OF THE YOUNG

When a young person is asked to assent he or she must be able to conduct certain cognitive functions: (1) to understand what is being asked immediately and generally; (2) to have a notion that permission is being sought independently; and (3) to make choices free from outside constraints. All of these functions, but particularly the first, depend greatly on the cognitive system operational in each child or adolescent. Child developmentalists formerly thought that children pass through certain cognitive stages and that at each stage they exhibit all of the characteristics identified with it. Although most experts still believe that the cognitive systems of early childhood, middle childhood, and adolescence are qualitatively different from one another, there is growing doubt that the differences between them are as radical as formerly thought. Instead, developmentalists now believe that children's cognition progresses via a variety of developmental trends rather than clearly defined stages.

These trends overlap but involve the following processes: (1) information-processing capacity; (2) acquisition of knowledge in specific areas; (3) concrete operations (basing judgment on perceived appearances) and formal operations (basing judgment on inferences that go beyond surface appearance to the underlying reality); (4) quantitative thinking; (5) development of a sense of how things are supposed to go in cognitive enterprises; (6) metacognition (monitoring and evaluating one's cognitive processes and strategies); and (7) improvement in cognitive strategies. What is most significant is that there is considerable difference in the rate of development of each of these trends in

each individual. These variations make it difficult to speak of a certain age, or stage, at which minors have or do not have the cognitive capacity for decisionmaking.

CHILDREN'S CAPACITIES TO UNDERSTAND AND REASON ABOUT RESEARCH

Although just what assent to research requires of young people has not been specifically agreed upon, it is generally acknowledged that there should be some correlation with the characteristics of adults' competency to give consent. To give consent, an adult must be aware of his or her situation, that is, must understand the nature of his or her condition; must understand the proposed treatment, including risks, benefits, and alternatives; must be able to work rationally with the relevant information to arrive at a reasonable choice; and must have the capacity to act voluntarily.

Several studies have been performed to learn how children and adolescents understand and reason about certain aspects of health care and biomedical and psychologic research. In these reports, it is sometimes difficult to distinguish between the mental processes of understanding and reasoning. That distinction, however, is an important one because possessing either capacity does not signify having the other. For purposes of this article, the two processes may be somewhat arbitrarily categorized as follows: understanding about research and reasoning about research.

Understanding Research

Reports of studies of young people's understanding of biomedical and behavioral research are limited in number. One study found that the majority of children of all ages and adolescents who were on protocols with therapeutic components were knowledgeable about concrete informational elements related to the research: the duration of their treatment, what was required of them during participation, the personal benefits of participation, and the facts that participation was voluntary and they were free to ask questions.

Published studies also indicate, however, that most children and younger adolescents fail to recall the nature of the research enterprise and what role they play in it. For example, even after giving assent, most young people were not aware or did not acknowledge that they were research subjects. Children, particularly those under nine years of age, had difficulty in understanding the scientific purposes of research. One study also reported that the majority of young people were not knowledgeable about the benefits of the research to others, and could not recall alternative treatment(s) or the risks of the research procedures. In addition, most children participating in research were unaware that they were free to withdraw from the research.

The adult's ability to understand information related to the consent process for research has also been reported to be poor. Many adults fail to acknowledge what they have heard or read, to apply it to their own circumstances, or to admit that the procedures serve any interests other than their personal care. [. . .] Whether quantitative or qualitative differences exist between juveniles and adults in their understanding of research participation is not known. Comparative studies of these two populations should be pursued to explore this question.

Reasoning about Research

In an investigation of youths' decisionmaking about research, Lewis and associates reported on the responses of 213 school children, ages six to nine, who were presented the opportunity to participate in an experimental trial of swine influenza vaccine. In nondirective inquiry sessions, all groups of children except one, composed of six-year-olds, asked all of the questions that the investigators deemed relevant to the trial and its associated risks and benefits. This study was conducted in an experimental school with an "adult free" health service that allowed the children direct access to a nurse, who encouraged them to formulate treatment options and honored their choices. The report does indicate that when children over six years of age are appropriately conditioned, they are able to identify risks and benefits when they are interviewed in a group setting. Since no attempt was made to determine how the children incorporated these factors into their decisionmaking, it is not possible to draw any further conclusions about their reasoning.

Several studies demonstrate how the reasoning of older children and adolescents might relate to assent. Kaser-Boyd and colleagues assessed the ability of youth 10 to 19 years of age to process information about the risks and benefits of psychological treatment. Seventy-five subjects with varying psychological treatment histories were asked to identify statements about a proposed therapy as either risks, benefits, or irrelevant to therapy. They were then presented with four treatment dilemmas and asked to decide whether a minor in such a situation should enter therapy and to explain their reasoning. No significant age difference was found for these children on the measures of the ability to identify and weigh risks and benefits of therapy. The wide variability among the minors at different ages, reading comprehension levels, and demographic characteristics led the authors to suggest that it may not be age *per se* that determines the ability to deliberate about treatment. They recommended that determinations of "competency to consent" be based on the capacities of the individual child.

Weithorn and Campbell used four hypothetical medical and psychological dilemmas to test healthy subjects nine, 14, 18, and 21 years of age. Two dilemmas concerned physical illness (epilepsy and diabetes) and two concerned psychological problems (depression and enuresis). Information provided concerning each dilemma included a description of the problem, alternative treatments, expected benefits, possible risks, and the consequences of failure to receive treatment. The dilemmas presented varied in complexity for various age levels. Responses were subjected to criteria (i.e., reasonable outcome, factual understanding, and actual understanding).

Although the nine-year-olds made decisions similar to those of the older individuals, they focused their thinking upon one or two of the more salient pieces of information, often to the exclusion of other data. In choosing a treatment, for example, they might concentrate on its benefits and ignore its risks, or vice versa. The 14-year-olds did not differ significantly from the 18- and 21-year-olds in their consideration of key elements in the dilemmas. In general, 14- and 18- and 21-year-olds were more skilled than nine-year-olds at considering multiple and ostensibly contradictory information simultaneously and at performing a rather abstract risk-benefit analysis.

The responses of minors to proposals to participate in research were explored by Keith-Spiegel and Maas. Thirty-six minors, ages nine to 15 years, and 36 adults, 18 to 28 years, were tested. Brief descriptions of low- to moderate-risk research procedures were presented to the subjects, who were then asked to state whether they would agree to be in such a study and to state the reason for their decision. Striking similarities were found between the responses of these two groups, both in terms of patterns of agreement and the reasons for their decision. Minors said "no" as often as adults. Minors were somewhat more interested in the money involved at the lower amount ranges than were adults. Minors gave fewer "maybe" responses than did adults. Minors gave essentially no "off-target" or irrelevant reasons for their decisions; flip or silly reasons, while few in number, came from the adult sample. These investigators conclude that the reasoning of minors above nine years of age about research participation is similar to that of adults.

Additional information about adolescents' reasoning ability for health care decisions and for research participation is provided by Lewis, who tape-recorded interviews with 8th-, 10th-, and 12th-grade male and female adolescents concerning the advice that those subjects would give to their "peers" about consenting to cosmetic surgery, the choice of the custodial parent after divorce, and consenting to paid experimentation with an acne medication. She found a significant increase with grade level in mention of the potential risks and future consequences of a decision, in recognition of and caution toward individuals with "vested interests," and in advice to solicit independent professional opinions. Even at the 12th-grade level, however, only a minority (42%) of the students mentioned future consequences as a factor to be considered in these dilemmas. [. . .]

As shown by these studies, older children and adolescents have developed considerable reasoning ability concerning health care and health care research. The studies are inconsistent as to whether during this period the capacity to recognize and weigh risks and benefits increases. Differences observed among the studies may be due to the prior experiences or opportunities to make decisions of the various populations studied, variations in the psychological methods used or, in fact, further development of cognitive function.

JUVENILES' EXPRESSION OF THE FULFILLMENT OF THEIR RIGHTS AND THEIR VOLITION

Children's expression of fulfillment of their rights. A basic element of consent to research in adults assures anyone being solicited that he or she is always allowed to refuse to participate or to withdraw from the research. As previously mentioned, the federal regulations concerning children state that for research that affords access to a beneficial intervention that is not otherwise available, parents' decisions can legally prevail. Despite the lack of a specific statement about dissent in the regulations, however, to respect minors as persons, they should not be forced to participate or be compelled to continue in research having no therapeutic components. But to exercise any right effectively, the holder of the right must understand it fully. Children's ability to conceptualize their rights develops as their moral judgment matures. Melton interviewed first-, third-, fifth-, and seventh-graders about their conception of their rights. In his analysis of the results of the study, he suggests children progress through three levels of moral judgment: (1) young children believe they have rights only if adults allow them (Level 1); (2) with further cognitive development, children perceive rights based on elementary fairness associated with being "good" or "nice" or obeying the rules (Level 2); (3) later on, children see rights based on abstract universal principles, e.g., right to privacy, freedom of speech (Level 3).

"In essence," Melton concludes, "children move toward more mature views about rights in which the existence of a right is not dependent on the whim of powerful people. Even seventh graders, however, tended to give Level 2 responses based on fairness and social order rather than Level 3 responses based on abstract ethical principles." [. . .]

Young people's volition. Closely associated with the conception of their rights is young people's volition, i.e., their power of making an authentic choice. As Grisso and Vier-

ling contend, "Registering one's consent or dissent in treatment situations is a social act. One is asked to announce to a person of some prestige and authority one's decision regarding a proposed treatment."

It is known that preadolescents, in order to avoid negative consequences, are prone to defer to authority figures. In early adolescence this deference is amplified by an increased concern for social expectations, causing a greater tendency toward conformity at this age than at any other period of childhood. By middle adolescence, nonetheless, the tendency toward conformity diminishes. The tendency toward deference can be modified by the nature of the consent process; for example, the manner in which the situation is presented may amplify or diminish the likelihood of deference. Similarly, as Grisso and Vierling suggest, "the presence of parents who have agreed to the proposed treatment might produce an increased likelihood of conformity on the part of the minor and further reduce the probability of truly voluntary dissent or veto by the minor."

On the other hand, as Melton argues, it may be that dissent from adults' recommendations by some youngsters is also "involuntary." For some adolescents, such actions may be developmentally appropriate anti-conformist judgments that are in their own way as conformist and unreasoned as unquestioned obedience in young children. Both the intrinsic hindrances to voluntariness and the acquiescence of young individuals to authority figures need to be considered in the issue of children's assent to research.

CHILDREN'S ALTRUISM

When an individual is faced with a decision concerning whether to become involved in research, the perception of one's moral obligation to others may arise. Some authors, in fact, view the process of seeking assent as a way to raise moral awareness and provide moral training. Nevertheless, if agreeing to participate doesn't make moral sense (i.e., cannot be conceptualized by a young person), it will not be morally constructive to insist that he or she assent. Forcing the juvenile to participate may cause him or her to be confused or resentful. Thus, if assent is to be used as a way of encouraging moral sensitivity, it is important to know when young people become capable of recognizing their moral obligation to others.

As with logical reasoning, there is a developmental aspect to young people's moral reasoning. Although egocentric during the first months of life, by two years of age children come to realize that others' feelings are distinct from their own. Later they become aware that others' thoughts and feelings may sometimes differ from their own. By about four years of age most children can interpret signs of happiness or distress in others in simple situations.

Older children are able to anticipate the perspective of others, and thus to be more empathic towards them. They can also understand that action within a relationship can be transcended by an external standard that enables them to take a "third person" perspective, and to understand such moral principles as the Golden Rule.

During late childhood or early adolescence, youth begin to perceive themselves and others as interrelated persons, each with his or her own narrative and identity. They become aware that others feel enjoyment or suffering, not only in special circumstances but also in relation to their overall life events. Although they may continue to react to a person's immediate suffering, their concern heightens upon learning that it reflects a lasting state. As their cognition develops further, they may be able to understand the adverse circumstances not only of an individual, but also of a group or class of individuals, e.g., those who are sick, deprived, or in a vulnerable state. This progression in moral reasoning enables older youth to consider the societal benefit of their participation in research.

THE DETERMINATION OF WHETHER TO SEEK ASSENT

Depending upon the nature of the research and its attendant risks and benefits, the demands placed on the decisionmaker vary greatly. Some children's research involves benign procedures, e.g., being weighed. Decisions of this nature can be readily considered, even by young juveniles. Other kinds of research, such as those involving an investigational drug, are more complex and carry greater risk. Decisions concerning these kinds of research require more advanced psychological capacities. Given these varying demands, it would seem ethically appropriate to try to base the determination of whether to seek assent on the youth's abilities to make the necessary decision.

The responsibility for determining whether children are capable of providing assent is now assigned to the IRB and is supposed to be based on chronology or a certain psychological state. As noted above, studies of young people's reasoning [. . .] indicate that older children and adolescents (i.e., individuals over nine years of age) generally have sufficient cognitive capacity to be involved in decisionmaking concerning participation in most research. Thus, individuals of this age should be considered as potential candidates for assent.

However, the cognitive skills of young individuals of a certain age vary. This variability makes it difficult to accurately identify those young people who possess or do not possess the requisite abilities for making a particular assent/dissent decision. Some children less than nine years of age may be capable of making some decisions, particularly those involving simple interventions with immediate and minimal risk outcomes. Alternatively, some older children and young adolescents may be capable of deciding about interventions of a very complex nature that have either delayed or serious consequences or both.

When uncertainty exists about the young person's decisionmaking capacity, IRBs should seek assistance in determining whether or not to seek assent. In these situations, the child's parents could be involved. They are most familiar with the youth's life experiences and how he or she has deliberated upon them. They also know their child's vulnerabilities and may be able to sense when it will be too stressful to seek assent from him or her. Nevertheless, parents may have an interest in having—or not having—their child participate in research that may affect their judgment. While it might be helpful to consult them, because of their possible conflict of interest they should not have a predominant role in making these determinations. Similarly, the conflict of interest that investigators have concerning the recruitment of subjects also makes them ill-suited for making this assessment. The enlistment of a developmental psychologist who is independent of the research is a better alternative for assisting in determining the young person's ability to assent. Such a professional not only can give an expert evaluation of the minor's decisionmaking capacity, but can be helpful in advising how to best inform the minor about the research.

THE PURPOSES OF ASSENT

Assent serves three fundamental purposes: (1) providing information to the young person; (2) offering shared decisionmaking with the parents; and (3) honoring his or her dissent. An understanding of these purposes is essential to discussions of research participation.

Information giving. Providing information is a very important function in the assent process. Simply talking to the young person concerning a research procedure and explaining what it will entail acknowledges the personhood of the individual. He or she learns about what is proposed to be done and about any associated proximate or future harm (e.g., pain, discomfort, inconvenience, or separation from loved ones). Informing the child properly requires that the presentation be geared to his or her cognitive level. The presentation of information to younger individuals must be very concrete; in older adolescents it may be more abstract, but still not be at an adult level. The informational content should primarily be on those matters which are of greatest interest to the young person, rather than those of relevance to the investigator or what adults might be interested in. Additionally, an intense educational effort appears to have a better likelihood for improving understanding and retention of the imparted information than the usual single encounter. [. . .]

Shared decisionmaking. The minor's assent is different from an adult's consent because of the former's incompetency or limited competency. This incompetency, however, goes beyond the cognitive functions of understanding and reasoning. As described above, children and young adolescents also tend to defer to authority figures. This is not surprising, given that the young are not socialized to think in terms of their own choices. Children and young adolescents are taught that they should obey their parents and just about anyone else bigger than they are. [...]

Consequently, children and even young adolescents are unlikely to perceive themselves as having any decisionmaking authority about research participation, regardless of the "objective reality" of their legal status. Even when they have a personal reservation, and the offer is made in the form of a request, they may still agree to participate in the research simply because they believe they should be compliant. This lack of assertiveness in voicing their authentic choices and their inability to conceptualize their rights and demand their fulfillment raise serious questions about whether one can justifiably speak of "assent" when children or young adolescents are concerned. At the same time, one might easily conceive of a situation in which an adult would likewise consent to participate or continue in a research study for social reasons (i.e., to please their doctor or a family member). How different is this adult's situation from that of a child who defers to authority? Are these developmental limitations reason enough for not pursuing or for rejecting his or her assent? On the other hand, is it not unfair to take advantage of young people's tendency toward conformity? The answer to this quandary is not readily forthcoming. Of help in answering it would be more information about how minors' deference to authority figures and their conceptualization and expression of fulfillment of their rights figures in their decisionmaking about research participation.

Lacking this information, however, does not prevent us from developing a framework for involving the young person's parents when assent is sought. At that time, parents should take a major role in conducting a joint decisionmaking process (shared autonomy) with their child. This process should consist of an open and honest discussion of all aspects of the research, particularly its risks and its personal and societal benefits. There should be discussions not only about whether the young person will participate in the research, but if he or she participates, under what circumstances participation will occur. [...]

Dissent. In these discussions, parents also need to be particularly sensitive to any reticence that the young person may have about participating. When such is suspected, the young person needs to be encouraged to express his or her concerns. Such an expression may represent a very strong conviction on the young person's part. When this is the case an authoritarian approach by the parents or the researcher, insisting that the young person participate, should not be applied. Any attempt to compel the minor to assent or to continue in the research when it offers no or only slight benefit, especially if it is coupled with significant risk, is disrespectful to him or her. Overriding the minor's dissent breaks his or her trust with those involved, thus compromising future relationships with health care personnel. Furthermore, since we would honor the refusal of a nonconformist adult, even if the dissent represents the nonconformity of adolescence it should be respected. [...]

INDEPENDENT DECISIONMAKING OF MIDDLE AND LATE ADOLESCENCE

By middle or late adolescence most youth have developed significant decisionmaking capacity. Moreover, the acquiescence to authority figures has lessened and they are more likely to express fulfillment of their rights. Because of their budding self-awareness they desire more personal autonomy. Nonetheless, economic, legal, and emotional ties still bind them to their parents. Hence, cognitively and emotionally, mid-to-late adolescents seem to be at a transitional point.

Society recognizes these changes and by legal means has attempted to grant mid-to-late adolescents some degree of autonomy for their health care, yet still protect them. Many states now have laws that permit adolescents to make medical decisions for themselves under some circumstances (e.g., treatment for venereal disease, mental illness and drug and alcohol abuse, or contraceptive counseling). These laws allow minors to seek help for these conditions without their parents being informed. The courts have also determined that when a medical intervention entails only a small risk, emancipated minors and mature minors (i.e., those over 14 years of age) can decide whether to accept it without parental consent.

Since we now allow mature minors to make these minimal risk decisions independently, should we not afford them the same right when research involves no more than minimal risk? Doing so is both consistent with what is presently known about this age group's psychological capacities and supports their desire for self-determination. Therefore, I would recommend that adolescents who are more than 14 years of age be allowed to assent to minimal risk research without parental permission: that is, I recommend that in essence, such adolescents be allowed to give consent.

These adolescents might also be allowed to consent for research involving more than minimal risk that offers no benefit to the subject. In this case, the conditions to be met would be: (1) that the research bears no more than a minor increase over minimal risk; (2) that it is likely to yield generalizable knowledge about the subject's disorder or condition; and (3) that an "appropriate mechanism" is in place. The mechanism could be the use of a nurse, psychologist, or social worker, not associated with the project, to assist the adolescent in decisionmaking. By allowing them to be sole decisionmaker in these situations we would thus respect their autonomy.

CONCLUSIONS

We can briefly summarize our main points as follows:

1. In deciding whether to seek assent, the minor's age is an important criterion, but other attributes also need to be considered. These are the young person's ability to identify the benefits and risks of the research, and to be able to reason about the consequences of participation.

2. When there is uncertainty as to whether assent should be sought from the child or adolescent, an independent psychological examiner should be employed to help evaluate the minor's decisionmaking capacities.

3. Two valuable functions of seeking assent from the minor are providing information and involving the minor and his or her parents in joint decisionmaking.

4. In seeking assent, undue advantage should not be taken of the child's developmental limitations related to his or her voluntariness (acquiescence to authority figures and the lack of expression of fulfillment of his or her rights).

5. Dissent from participation or withdrawal from research is always to be honored unless the protocol affords access to a therapeutic intervention that is not otherwise available.

6. Middle and late adolescents should be allowed independent assent (consent) for minimal-risk research, and under certain conditions for research bearing a slight increase over minimal risk.

Section Three

Captive Populations

Soldiers, Prisoners, Students

---

44   Convenient and Captive Populations

JONATHAN D. MORENO

Clinical research is a complex, expensive, and valued social activity. One of the conditions that makes clinical research possible is a subject population that is convenient, both in terms of availability for recruitment and for monitoring through the course of a study. [. . .]

Jonathan D. Moreno, "Convenient and Captive Populations," in *Beyond Consent: Seeking Justice in Research*, ed. Jeffrey P. Kahn, Anna C. Mastroianni, and Jeremy Sugarman (New York: Oxford University Press, 1998), 111–30.

Some [. . .] populations are convenient in the sense that they are readily available, such as students. Others are not only readily available but also captive, that is, constrained in their movements and choices by virtue of explicit conditions formally imposed on them by societal decision. The paradigm case of a captive population is those who are imprisoned. Other populations seem to occupy a middle ground between short-term hospitalized patients and long-term prisoners, including students, institutionalized persons, and military personnel. Among the ways that these populations differ from others are their degree of availability, the greater likelihood that those who are captive can be coerced or manipulated into participation by virtue of their dependent status, and that captive populations are more likely than others to be readily available for research activities for extended periods, enhancing their attractiveness to the research enterprise.

This [article] suggests that the growing sensitivity to the use of such populations in research cannot be understood without an appreciation of the historical background. The history of research on these subject populations is important because it provides the rationale for classifying them as "vulnerable." Therefore, this [article] reviews the historic roles of [...] military personnel [...] in research activities. The discussion of [this] population also includes an account of the way the regulatory system has evolved to take account of historic abuses. [Discussion of prisoners, institutionalized persons, and students omitted.—eds.]

Because these groups are not convenient or captive—or even vulnerable—in the same ways, crafting a just, efficacious, and reasonable public policy in the use of these populations in biomedical and behavioral research is not easy. For instance, a rough notion of justice may find it acceptable to impose greater burdens on prisoners because of their debt to society. Similarly, it might be argued that those who are institutionalized may need to be used to serve some important research goal, especially if no other population so readily presents itself for study. Nevertheless, historically, these attitudes have sometimes had baleful consequences. Further, our intuitions about justice in research may yield inconsistent results. For example, turning soldiers into "guinea pigs" may either be offensive to patriotic sensibilities or seem reasonable in light of soldierly duties; while students and laboratory workers could be viewed either as too easily coerced into research or as the most appropriate candidates due to their ability to understand an experiment's purposes. [...]

Discussions such as this tend to focus on ethical abuses or areas of potential moral concern. It should be remembered, however, that much human-subject research has contributed greatly to human well-being and has been conducted according to sound ethical standards. Such standards include efforts to prevent the burdens of research from falling unfairly on any particular person or group. This [article] will show how attitudes toward certain populations from which research subjects may be drawn have changed, and to indicate some of the issues that remain to be resolved. [...]

JUSTICE ACROSS TIME

[...]

Military Personnel

Military personnel are convenient subjects in the sense that they are typically healthy, "normal" persons who can be fol-lowed for data collection for a number of years. However, their disciplined environment raises questions about the extent to which any consent they give can be considered truly voluntary. Thus, they may be at risk for disproportionate representation in research, especially in studies relating to national security. Yet military officials have long considered voluntariness an important condition for participation in research by military personnel, as evidenced by the use of the term "volunteer" or "informed volunteer" from at least the 1940s. The precise significance to be given the term under the circumstances is, of course, a separate but vitally important matter.

The American record in the use of military personnel in research has been mixed—a history of pioneering policies inconsistently applied. Around 1900, U.S. Army scientist Walter Reed obtained consent and asked potential subjects to sign a written contract for his yellow fever experiment in Cuba. The contract specified some of the risks, and offered nonmilitary personnel monetary compensation for participating; reportedly, soldiers declined the compensation. The $100 in gold Reed offered the Spanish workers who participated in the experiment was a significant amount of money at the time, perhaps enough to be considered coercive today. There was little opportunity to withdraw from the study. Reed's colleagues (but not Reed himself) on the Yellow Fever Commission also subjected themselves to the mosquito's bite that was correctly suspected as the source of infection. One of his colleagues died of the infection.

Though Reed began his dangerous experiment without his superior's approval, he felt obliged to ask his commanding officer's permission when he thought it necessary to expand the study. Since at least the 1930s, it appears that approval for soldiers' and sailors' participation in medical experiments was to be obtained at the highest level of the relevant uniformed service, usually from the service's surgeon general and often the service secretary as well. The assignment of military personnel to research is, after all, a deployment decision that should theoretically be made by the responsible officer in the chain of command.

There are also significant potential risks to the armed forces if an experiment goes awry, especially in terms of public opinion and legal liability, constituting another reason for proper authorization of human research. During the Second World War the Committee on Medical Research declared that uniformed personnel were not to be used as "guinea pigs" in the war-related research it funded. Throughout this period there was significant concern that the public would not be sympathetic if their heroes were to be used in this manner. Nonetheless, during World War II naval personnel were forced to remain in mustard gas experiments against their will.

By the late 1940s there was a growing view in the national security establishment that some human experiments were going to be necessary in the postwar environment, especially in reference to unconventional weapons: atomic, biological, and chemical. The effects of these weapons could not be gauged in animal studies, nor could their combat implications be assessed with other healthy subjects. Early 1950s studies of flashblindness following atomic detonations, for example, were classified by the Pentagon as medical experiments, though most other exposures to the atomic battlefield were considered to be part of necessary training.

The Department of Defense attempted to anticipate the problem of using military personnel in research by adopting the Nuremberg Code as its policy in 1953. Subsequently, troops deployed near the site of atomic tests were systematically observed and they sometimes filed self-reports of panic reactions near the blast site. "Release" forms were even filled out in at least some cases by troops who had "volunteered" to operate closer to ground zero than others, thus exposing them to a higher level of radioactivity. Yet in other studies involving military personnel and radiation there was no documentation of volunteer status except the statements of superior officers. In still other cases, such as the Air Force's mushroom cloud–penetration experiments that measured the amount of fission released by an atomic blast and its effects on crew members, there is strong evidence that at least some air force personnel were eager to experience the challenge and adventure associated with the project, while others viewed the job as part of their routine.

The military context presents a unique puzzle about distinguishing training, which does not typically fall under the constraints of medical ethics, from medical research, which does. For instance, the vast majority of the "atomic soldiers" deployed for exercise at the training facility at Camp Desert Rock in Nevada from 1951 through 1962 were kept at what was thought to be a safe distance from the atomic blast site; though any acute ill effects might have been noted, the primary goal of the activity was to learn about human factors such as panic reactions on the atomic battlefield. Although the tension between national security needs and ethical considerations was rarely a topic of public discussion during the Cold War, it played an important role in shaping the defense establishment's ambivalent posture toward human subjects issues.

The implementation of the Nuremberg Code–based policy appears to have been sporadic at best, perhaps partly because there was confusion about its scope and application. The Army Inspector General found in 1975 that the Army had failed to comply with its own rules for the use of soldiers in research with psychoactive drugs, as thousands of men [. . .] were used in LSD experiments in the 1960s. Even in the courts the Code has not proven to be an effective standard. When one of the men brought suit against the United States government for injuries he incurred due to this research, the Supreme Court ruled in favor of the government by a five-to-four majority on the grounds that the judicial branch should not undermine discipline by inquiring into military matters. Only the minority argued that the Nuremberg Code must prevail.

Today, medical research in the armed forces has both reduced its dependence on healthy, "normal" subjects and, like other sectors of American society, has established a very low threshold of risk tolerance in the development of new armaments, equipment, and materials. In 1991, the Department of Defense regulations on the use of human subjects were brought under the same requirements as other federal agencies that sponsor studies with human subjects. The additional regulatory obstacles to recruitment of military personnel for research are such that today this is among the most difficult populations from which to obtain subjects. Today, all research in the Army's infectious disease institute at Fort Detrick, for example, is governed by several regulations and all proposals involving significant risk must be reviewed by a local institutional review board, the Human Use Review and Regulatory Affairs Division of the United States Army Medical Research and Material Command, the Human Subjects Research Review Board of the Office of the Surgeon General, and the Office of the Surgeon General itself. In response to the recommendations of the Advisory Committee on Human Radiation Experiments [ACHRE], in 1997 President Clinton ordered expanded training for senior officials on the nature of human subjects research, and instituted a new policy that precludes officers from involvement in the recruitment of research volunteers.

Other recent events illustrate the special ethical difficulties associated with regulating the use of innovative drugs with military personnel during a national emergency. In late 1990 and early 1991, during Operations Desert Shield and Desert Storm, the Defense Department was concerned about possible exposure to biological and chemical warfare agents. The department successfully sought an amendment to the Food and Drug Administration's (FDA) informed consent regulations that would enable medical professionals to determine that it was "not feasible" to obtain the informed consent of a person receiving an investigational drug or vaccine under combat conditions. The rule was published on December 21, 1990, and upheld by the courts.

Shortly after the rule was published the Department of Defense requested and received waivers of informed consent for two investigational products: pyridostigmine bromide (PB) and botulinum toxoid (BT). Even though the waiver was obtained for both agents, Central Command elected on ethical grounds to give service personnel a choice about receiving BT, but not for PB, which was in common use as an approved drug for other populations and for which informed consent was not deemed necessary.

The Pentagon estimates that about 8,000 troops took BT and about 250,000 received at least one dose of PB.

Months after the war some veterans began complaining about numerous symptoms that when grouped together are termed "Gulf War Syndrome." The vaccination program was shrouded in secrecy when it took place to deny information to the enemy about the Allies' defensive measures, but as the story emerged, the agents, especially PB, were theorized by some as a factor in the veterans' medical problems. A federal advisory committee was appointed to investigate the health problems of Gulf War veterans, including an analysis of the waiver process.

However skeptical one might be about such claims of voluntariness against an admitted record of pressuring uniformed personnel to "volunteer," matters surely become far more complicated in the case of potentially prophylactic agents used under combat conditions. In this case it can be argued that access to compounds that have not yet been approved for use under ordinary circumstances may be ethical. The lack of approval could be due to technical or bureaucratic factors and there may be sound scientific evidence that the agent can be of significant potential benefit to troops in battle.

Underlying much of the criticism of the Pentagon's conduct in the use of unapproved drugs is a suspicion that it was a deliberate effort to circumvent research requirements in order to assess the agents' efficacy under combat conditions. There is no evidence that this is the case. Indeed, one shortcoming of the Defense Department's handling of this episode is precisely the fact that no system was in place to document the response of service personnel to the medications, including a failure to establish appropriate baseline measures of subjects' metabolism. The use of these compounds "in theater" could theoretically have been justified on scientific as well as beneficent grounds if the operation has been treated as a research study according to established methodological standards.

Had a systematic research dimension been part of the agents' use in Desert Storm, there then would have been an opportunity to assess the fairness of conducting research with military personnel. The assessment would have turned on the manner in which the study was conducted, for while soldiers facing combat conditions may be required to accept all medical interventions that hold the prospect of ensuring their availability for service, the innovative use of these drugs may not entail a requirement to accept them. But if the decision to use the agents could have been left to the troops themselves, with appropriate information at their disposal about known risks and benefits, then their participation would have been acceptable. Apparently this information was not made available in Desert Storm, in spite of an agreement between the Defense Department and the FDA that it would be provided. [...]

FUTURE TRENDS

[...] Since the Gulf War, a primary public policy concern has revolved around waivers of informed consent provisions involving unapproved drugs for military personnel under combat conditions. The suitability of such waivers may be loosely characterized as a matter of justice in research, but only if the program for which a waiver is sought is intended mainly to yield information that can be used in later conflicts. Considering that the primary goal of the waiver is not research (and indeed medical data-gathering was not part of the Pentagon's mission in Desert Storm), the problem here does not seem to be one of discrimination against soldiers as disproportionately recruited to be experimental subjects. Rather, the dilemma stems from a wish to provide the troops with whatever medical benefit might theoretically be available without unacceptable risk.

More pertinent to the topic of justice in research for the military in the future is whether and under what conditions men and women in the armed forces may be utilized in new research activities during peacetime. In general, for both political and moral reasons there has been a reluctance to use military personnel in research when others are available. This reluctance has been compromised when some new threat seemed imminent and other appropriate subjects were not available. Therefore, a source of tension in the future about the acceptance of using military personnel in research could be a suspected new and deadly weapons system in the possession of a foreign power or terrorist group, combined with regulatory restrictions on the use of other healthy subjects. [...]

CONCLUSIONS

Generalized discussions about justice are sorely limited concerning specific groups. In crafting a just public policy for the use of human subjects, especially those who may be considered convenient or captive, the historical and practical factors that could enter into judgments about justice will vary depending on what population is being considered. The respective situations of prisoners, institutionalized persons, military personnel, and students are quite different and require analyses tailored to each of them. Underlying all these cases are complex issues of social status and power as well as medical ethics.

As experience in modern research with human subjects has accumulated, a "protectionist" attitude toward the participation of these groups has emerged. Prisoners are no longer a rich source of subjects, and specific federal regulations greatly restrict their involvement in studies. Institutionalized persons have long been considered to generate specific ethical issues in research, a trend that has lately accelerated. Research with military personnel, always a sensitive problem for defense officials, must navigate numerous obstacles for approval by command authorities. Participation in research by students, employees, and others in differential power positions is a simmering issue that may well be the next frontier for protectionist approaches.

Historical experience has been accompanied by an evolution in the sense of justice in research, one that has tended to qualify crude utilitarian attitudes toward the use of human subjects. The notion that long-term prisoners owe a special debt to society that may be expressed in research participation, for example, is an implication of a once-popular notion of justice that has resonance only to the degree that it is abstracted from actual abuses associated with imprisonment, including the familiar problem of voluntariness. Similarly, the view that prisoners or other institutionalized persons may have to be used in risky studies addressing important public health problems must be tempered by the condition (already in current regulations) that they must themselves be likely to benefit from such research, either as individuals or, at the very least, as members of the affected group.

Once a more refined conception of justice in research becomes available it may have implications for groups it was not even intended to address. The notion that military service does not include duties to be in research that is not intended to improve combat readiness is one that the armed forces were already coming to accept by the mid-1970s, but the Tuskegee Syphilis Study scandal and the work of the National Commission surely helped reinforce an awareness of research ethics in the military, as it did in all other areas. Under the auspices of a modern conception of justice in research, the proposition that the role of student or employee does not generate an obligation to serve in an experiment is now becoming more obvious.

A protectionist stance towards special populations does not rule out the possibility that strong arguments for research participation can be mounted. Surely there are circumstances in which justice may permit, or even require, access to research for populations that have historically been abused by some researchers. One of these circumstances is the prevalence of a disease that poses a particular threat to members of that population, and which cannot be studied as effectively with other subjects. Protected status implies institutional and public scrutiny of proposed research participation, not *a priori* exclusion. With this understanding, and in light of the historical factors that have made these groups' participation in medical research a matter of special concern, protectionism continues to be a morally sound presumption.

---

45   Medical Experimentation on Prisoners

CARL COHEN

PROLOGUE

Ought we to permit medical experimentation on prisoners? The issue is both practically important and morally complex. Some argue as follows: No human subject may be used in a medical experiment without his informed and freely given consent. But prisoners, by virtue of their total custody, cannot give free and uncoerced consent. Hence prisoners—no matter how valuable experimentation with their cooperation may prove—must be excluded from all populations of subjects in medical experimentation.

This argument, when expanded and reinforced, is very persuasive, as I shall show. I aim also to show that its key premise is simply mistaken, and the argument unsound. [...]

Carl Cohen, "Medical Experimentation on Prisoners," *Perspectives in Biology and Medicine* 21 (1978): 357–72.

CAN A PRISONER GIVE VOLUNTARY CONSENT?

[...] It may well seem that, by virtue of the complete custody of their persons, prisoners lack the capacity to act with the kind of uncoerced voluntariness required. If they do lack it, they ought not be subjects. So I want now to put, more carefully than I have found it put anywhere, what precisely it is about the prisoner's condition that might render him or her unfit to be a consenting subject in a medical experiment.

The argument goes like this. The prison environment [...] is such that consent without coercion is not possible there. This is not because of any defect in prisoners; it flows from the deeply intrusive, literally totalitarian character of prisons. One may take this as a condemnation of prisons, or simply as an unpleasant but unavoidable fact about them. Attitudes about prisons are not in contention here. Prisons being what they are, their inmates are in a state of constant coercion, from which there is no escape within the walls. No matter what the prisoner says, or we say to him, coercion is the essence of his condition. In that condition no consent to put oneself at risk should be accepted as full consent. Hence medical experimentation on prisoners should be forbidden, flatly.

This is the general thrust. Now, more concretely and specifically, see how this coercive spirit permeates the prison environment.

First. The body of the prisoner is simply not under his own control. Orders committing persons to prison are very blunt about this, generally containing the phrase: "[T]he body of the defendant shall be delivered" to the custodial institution appropriately identified. No system of criminal punishment that relies upon prisons, however humane its intent, can evade this fact. [...]

Second. Not only is the prisoner's person unfree, but the control of that person, and the secure incarceration of his body, are his keepers' chief and overriding concerns. Prisons are closed, tightly guarded places. Anyone who has not visited a medium or maximum security prison can hardly imagine the impact of omnipresent locks, bars, and armed guards. Supervision of hour-by-hour conduct is close; inspection is constant; privacy is nil; coercion is the flavor of every moment.

Third. Most prisoners are very poor, and have tightly limited opportunity to earn the most puny wages. Some states pay no wages for prison labor; most states pay less than one dollar per day; only six states pay more than that. And even where wages are paid, not all prisoners have the chance to earn them. From this poverty any decent payment for service is partial rescue.

Fourth. Boredom, killing monotony, is that feature which, next to control, most pervades prison life. The state tells every prisoner when to sleep, when to rise, when to eat and what, when to work and when to play, what to do and how to do it—all with maddening sameness. From this barrenness, any change is relief.

Fifth, and finally. The dominant concern in every prisoner's life is release and the eventual date of it. In this country prison sentences of indeterminate length are very common. That single most important date is therefore subject to the judgment, even to the whim, of administrators whom the prisoner can rarely reach or even address. His behavior in prison—in ways he cannot be sure of—must affect, perhaps determine, his date of release. Even for those with determinate sentences, that date remains indeterminate if there is, as usually, a parole board to be pleased. The felt need to please officials—doing what (at least in their own minds) prisoners think might please those who might be in a position to effect a somewhat earlier release—is an unavoidable pressure upon the behavior of prisoners.

It is in this environment that voluntariness of consent to subjection to medical experimentation must be assessed.

However freely it appears that he consents, the prisoner is coerced so fully by his circumstances that even asking him must be unfair. His service as subject must be seen by him as a precious opportunity to escape, if only for short or infrequent periods, from the drabness and routine of prison life. [...] And he is further coerced by the monetary rewards [...] promising opportunity for riches not possible otherwise. The risks are overshadowed by the partial escape from state-imposed penury. [...] And above all, what an opportunity to prove one's good will, one's eagerness to pay his debt to society, one's sincere intention to make up for past evils and be good! [...] Surely it will not work against the prisoner when parole or release is being considered—and it may, it just may do some good. How can the rational prisoner not be coerced by such a concatenation of pressures? He cannot. It is not right (this argument concludes) even to ask the prisoner whether he wishes to put himself at risk when doing so is encouraged by his circumstances so strongly and so perniciously. [...]

The argument has two addenda.

1. Everything above applies to prison experiments even when delicately and justly supervised. But the de facto circumstances in real prisons are such as to make delicacy rare, and justice less than universal. There is enormous potential for abuse in prisons; there is a great deal of abuse in prisons. Knowing that, we cannot in good conscience undertake medical experiments that may, in fact, be tainted by that abuse in various ways, but above all in the selection of subjects.

2. Those who support medical experimentation in prisons quickly point to the great benefits they have yielded for mankind—experiments on polio virus strains, for example, which led directly to the selection of strains now used worldwide in the preparation of polio virus vaccine administered by mouth. Then there is the work on malaria, and dengue fever, and so on. All that is very fine—but if such experiments rely upon the wrongful use of human subjects, they simply should not be done. The critical issues here concern what is right, what is just—not the balancing of benefits. Until the justice of such experimenting on prisoners has been shown, the calculation of benefits simply cannot be reached.

A CLOSER LOOK AT COERCION

There is the case, and it is a strong one. But it is not strong enough. The argument is rightly cautionary. Its several considerations show, I submit, that medical experiments using prisoners as subjects must go forward, if at all, under rules more constraining, and supervision more strict, than such experimentation in more ordinary contexts. It has not been shown, I contend, that a prisoner cannot give full consent in the sense that being a voluntary subject requires full consent.

I begin by granting much of the factual description of the prison environment presented above—although that account was deliberately put in rather purple language. But it is so; prison life is controlled, barren, poor, monotonous. Coercion is the spirit of the prison. Regrettably, however, those who accept the argument above, or some variant of it, are led by their detestation of prisons to equivocate upon the word "coercion." When careful with it we find, reasonably enough, that there are respects in which the prisoner is coerced and respects in which he is not [...]. We need to identify carefully that sense of coercion employed when we say that coercion vitiates an apparently free consent. Then we must decide whether when given an opportunity to volunteer as subject, the prisoner is coerced in that sense. [...]

By "coercion" our common meaning is compulsion by physical or moral pressures. Thus A coerces B when B is compelled or constrained to act as A wishes him to, as a result of measures taken by A to effect just that result. The bandit coerces me, with his revolver, into handing over my wallet. The threat of criminal prosecution if I do not file an income tax return is a coercive instrument designed to constrain my behavior. We are tempted—and too many yield—to leap from this to calling coercive whatever restrains or limits or influences behavior. I may be coerced into giving to the United Fund, say, by the threat of discharge or defamation; but I am not coerced into charitable giving by my strong desire to be admired as a public benefactor. Again, if my wealth were unlimited I should sail the seas in splendor; my means being what they are, I cast an admiring glance at every ocean racing yacht, and go on splashing about in my little sailing dinghy. It is an elastic use of English to say I am coerced into doing so. There are, too, desires of the utmost intensity which influence my conduct and with which I must come to terms. But these desires are not imposed (unless one holds a satanic view of the human condition) in order to bend my volition; they are the normal matrix of my life. It is facile or confused to suppose that I am coerced by my own wants. [...]

We sometimes think powerful inducements, as well as threats, to be coercive. Sometimes they may be, but only when the subject in question is caused, by an extraordinary and deliberate temptation, to do what should not ever be done. If a poor person is tempted by a huge sum to accept a risk we think it not proper to urge upon anyone, the offer is there coercive. But if the reward be for conduct that is itself reasonable, the fact that one's condition renders that reward exceptionally attractive does not show that coercion has been applied. Professional football players are not coerced by huge salaries into risking their necks, nor are workers coerced into work by their need for earnings.

A definite account of coercion I do not seek to provide here. No doubt any account, however refined, will leave some rough edges. But moderately thoughtful reflection will show, I believe, that the coercion that full consent precludes is the coercion flowing from the deliberate effort on the part of one who offers the choice (or his agent) to pressure the offeree into a particular decision. The pressure must be such that the offerer could have refrained from exerting it, but deliberately did not refrain.

If I seek admission to a research hospital specializing, say, in eye disease, desperate about my failing sight, and I am admitted upon the condition that I put myself at serious risk in an experiment having nothing to do with my condition, I have indeed been coerced improperly. Even in matters involving minor risks, if I am subjected to a moral barrage regarding the social value of medical research and the importance of the experiment at hand to all mankind, when asked for my consent to serve as subject, I am coerced, if mildly, by the deliberate pressures of the investigator. We do not permit such distortions of potential subjects' volitions, rightly. But if I suffer from a serious disease for which cure is unknown, it is quite reasonable that I should find serving as subject, in an experiment aimed at enlarging knowledge about that disease, attractive in a way that one who does not suffer from that disease does not find attractive. My diseased condition does not coerce me. [...]

Our lives are led, and our decisions made, within a network of needs and wants, some natural, some arising from the acts of others, some aggravated by the acts of the state. We are all bored, or threatened, or tantalized in differing degrees by a perilous world, some hostile people, and a not very sensitive government. Sometimes, within that framework, we are coerced by the design of persons or institutions into choosing X rather than Y. Such design, introduced in order to manipulate our choosing, is the coercion here chiefly of concern to us. [...]

Let us now apply this view of coercion to the case of the prisoner giving informed consent to serve as a medical subject. The opportunity is given him, let us suppose, to respond by letter to a notice on a bulletin board, after which, if he proves a suitable subject, he is given full information about procedures, risks, pay, and the rest by a research investigator. Is he coerced into giving consent by the fact of his imprisonment? On reflection I think we will see that he is not.

The question is not, "Are prisoners coerced?"—for we agree that, in general, theirs is a condition in which many more choices are foreclosed, and decisions compelled, than in conditions of ordinary life. But the pervasive presence of restraints in the prison leaves open the question of whether, with respect to a particular option put before him, he is coerced. He has a chance, say, to participate as subject in a set of drug tests, requiring intermittent hospital visits, small to moderate risks, occasional days of complete bed rest, and paying $20 per month for the 6 months of the tests. Most experiments using human subjects involve less time, less money, and less risk. Some involve more. Take this one as a realistic illustration.

It is true that his participation may promise occasional release from boredom. Boredom, however, is not a condition over which the investigator has any control, or in which he has any interest. It is simply the condition that the potential prisoner-subjects (as well as a good many nonprisoner-subjects) were in when the choice of participating or not was encountered by them. They are no more coerced into consenting by their boredom than I am coerced into seducing by my lust. The conditions in which we find ourselves powerfully affect our response to choices put before us. If the standard of noncoercion be that potential subjects be free of all conditions that may significantly influence their willingness to consent, we will have no subjects and no experiments.

"But," the critic may reply, "although we are, indeed, all in conditions that constrain us in some respects, there remain enormous differences of degree. The prisoner's conditions are unusually severe, and that severity is what we underscore. When, for example, he supposes that giving his consent may help him, somehow, achieve an earlier release, he is in the special condition of desperately wanting release, and blindly hoping that someone up there will be more moved to help him because he did consent. That is what is unusual about his condition."

This reply will not work; it does not serve to distinguish the prisoner's case from the case of others whom we do not regard as improperly coerced. It is not only prisoners who have desperate desires that they hope may come nearer to fulfillment because of participation in [an] experiment. Indeed, while the prisoner's hopes along that line may be tenuous and largely the result of his own wishful thinking, many nonprisoners are faced with the opportunity to participate in experiments involving considerable risk, which offer more serious hope of fulfilling desperate wants. Consider the person with psoriasis covering much of his body, given the opportunity to participate in an experiment using a new and very powerful ultraviolet light that may increase the likelihood of developing cancer and may injure his eyes. No pressure whatever is brought to bear on him by the researcher. But he or she must feel very great pressures from the intense longing to be rid of that disfiguring affliction. Is that potential subject coerced by virtue of the desperation of his desire? Not in any sense that precludes his consent, surely; and if we thought he and others like him were truly coerced, we should have to forbid the experiment. [...]

If the researcher [...] had portrayed the patient's condition more grimly than the facts warranted, in order to get him to consent, we would think the patient to have been coerced, not by the intensity of his desire [...] but by that deceptive account. If the researcher had refrained deliberately from telling the patient of some alternative therapy offering equal hopes, in order to woo his participation, the patient would have been coerced, not by his needs or their grip on him, but by the manipulation of the investigator. Analogously, it is not the degree of boredom, or the passion of the desire for release, or the level of any condition that the prisoner is in, that can coerce him. It is only deliberate conduct, conduct designed to deceive, to pressure, to constrain, that would coerce in the sense required. Therefore the boredom, the desire for early release, the being under constant guard—these cannot in themselves constitute coercion of a potential subject.

The critic may take another tack. "I see now [he may say] that it is not the intensity of desire that marks off the prisoner's case, or renders him coerced. Yet the precariousness of his condition is the key to the immorality I've been driving at. It is the deliberate choosing of prison populations to do experiments we would not do with others, taking advantage of their desperation, that is coercive. This, I now see, is the root of my complaint. By using prisoners the researcher gets away with an exploitation of subjects that would be impossible elsewhere—and that calculated exploitation must not be allowed."

Here the critic gives a caution that deserves to be taken seriously; but its scope must not be overblown. If we do on prisoners experiments we would not do on others, believing that for ordinary persons the risks clearly outweigh the potential benefits, the calculated choice of a precariously placed population enabling us to get away with that would, indeed, be wrongful. What troubles so about it, however, is that experiments would then be done which ought not be done at all. In the same way, where great risk far outweighs potential benefit we would not tolerate huge sums used to inveigle the participation of indigent welfare recipients. To do with some, because we can get away with it, what we ought to do with no one is surely unconscionable. Some experiments in prisons, in the past, have been like that.

But this argument does not have the general force its advocates may suppose. When, for example, subject populations are enlisted both in and out of prisons on the same terms—as is often done—this objection has no place. When the judgment of experimental justifiability is made independently of the special circumstances of possible subject pools, an improper reliance upon those special circumstances cannot be complained of.

Moreover, the special circumstances of subjects may rightly enter when the experiment is of a kind that requires just that kind of subject for scientific reasons. Persons suffering from a given disease are reasonably chosen for experiments dealing with that disease, obviously, and any inclination they have to serve as subjects arising from that circumstance is neither avoidable nor pernicious. Again, some experiments have special requirements for long-term regularity and control, calling for subjects in unusually restricted circumstances. Seeking out those who fit the requirements of the investigation—an investigation whose worthiness is independently established—is equally reasonable, and no less so if those subjects be prisoners. It is a fact that for some scientific purposes prisoners are irreplaceable as subjects. Prisoners constitute extraordinarily stable populations, under constant and detailed observation. Diet, activity, whereabouts, and other factors possibly critical to the experiment are thoroughly known and dependable. [. . .] The short of it is that, for reasons having nothing to do with manipulative intent but everything to do with scientific reliability, prison populations serve medicine as no other populations can. The critic rightly insists that prisoners should not be preyed upon, that we must not do in prisons what should not be done. This is a long way from showing that no experiments ought be conducted in prisons, or that prisoners ought not to be allowed to volunteer as subjects.

What shall we say of payment to prisoners? That, after all, clearly is a factor under the researcher's full control. Moderate remuneration, of course, is widely given to subjects, in and out of prison. Insofar as those sums are deliberately offered to allure and tempt they are, in every case, manipulative. And of course their manipulative force is the greater as the potential subject is the poorer. This argues against payment to subjects in any context, and I think that is an alternative worthy of serious consideration. On the other hand, the prospect of a small money reward (which does serve as a major motivating force in prisons) neither threatens nor pressures nor tempts to do what should not be done. The very moderate sums involved [. . .] are also viewed by many not so much as lures as compensation for inconvenience. Some who would be pleased to volunteer cannot otherwise afford the time. In that spirit the sums involved do not coerce anyone. [. . .] One principle we surely wish to maintain is that prisoners not be in any way special targets for exploitation, and their not being special targets entails their being treated, in the matter of payment, just as nonprisoners are treated. They should be paid no more, no less. [. . .]

I conclude that the argument against permitting prisoners to choose in this sphere, by virtue of their necessarily coerced condition, is simply mistaken. It confuses a wide sense of constraint (rightly characterizing the prison environment) with a different, narrow sense of constraint in the decision at hand—of which the prisoner can, with care, be entirely free. In the sense that one's condition coerces him, we are all coerced, and many of us as severely or more severely than prisoners. In the sense that choices before us, given our condition, may be made by us without ulterior manipulation in view of the merits of the case, the prisoner can, if fairly treated, be as free to choose as the rest of us.

[. . .] Mine has been a moral concern, about the rightness of the rule that would forbid all experimentation on prisoners. The common argument supporting that rule, I conclude, is grounded on mistake, on a misunderstanding of what is required for genuinely free consent. [. . .]

---

46   Students, Grades, and Informed Consent

HAROLD F. GAMBLE

Harold F. Gamble, "Students, Grades, and Informed Consent," *IRB: A Review of Human Subjects Research* 4, no. 3 (1982): 7–10.

Human subjects must give informed consent to participation in research. Federal regulations specify that a subject's informed consent be freely given; force, fraud, deceit, duress, or any form of constraint or coercion must not be used. With this in mind, an institutional review board (IRB) at a state university discussed recently whether students who participated in research as subjects in exchange for extra-credit grade points were able to consent freely to their participation. Some committee members thought that this was a potentially coercive situation.

The issue arose when an investigator, who had a long-standing project that used students recruited by extra-credit [. . .], requested reapproval of this research from the IRB. [T]he IRB, after much discussion, reapproved this project only if the investigator dropped the use of extra-credit. Presumably a majority of committee members thought that students could not make free choices in these circumstances.

[T]he investigator appealed this decision, pointing out that the department's rationale for having students participate as subjects was to provide a unique educational opportunity for them to understand research firsthand. Students see research from the subject's perspective and during the debriefing from the investigator's viewpoint. And for their extra effort in obtaining a special education benefit, they earn extra-credit.

Responding to whether students felt free to participate when presented with the option of research participation, the investigator stated that students did not view the procedure as coercive and pointed out that all 29 students in one experiment denied emphatically that they felt coerced. In addition, the investigator reported that neither the department chairperson nor ombudsman had received student complaints about these recruitment procedures; even though complaints had been received about other aspects of departmental policy or faculty behavior.

Referring to the department's written guidelines for the use of human subjects, the investigator noted that they required not only written consent from students, but also informed them of their right to refuse participation and withdraw any time during an experiment. In order not to coerce students subtly into selecting the option of earning extra-credit as subjects, the guidelines also required course instructors to provide options that were comparable to research participation in terms of time and effort, and also in educational benefit; for example, short papers, special projects, book reports, and brief quizzes on additional readings. The department estimated that one-third to two-thirds of students chose these alternatives. Finally, the investigator pointed out that extra-credit is allocated only after the grading curve for a course has been determined by test scores.

After the investigator's presentation and further discussion, the IRB reversed its earlier decision [. . .] and allowed research to continue with the use of extra-credit. However, the committee voted unanimously to have this issue reviewed by a campus-wide IRB (CW-IRB), the parent committee of this IRB.

In meeting with the CW-IRB, the investigator and three other department colleagues presented new data. Surveys of populations of 40 subjects who anonymously completed questionnaires at the request of graduate students and 906 students who anonymously completed teacher evaluation forms revealed that only 10 percent checked "No" in answer to the question "Did you feel free to choose whether or not to be a subject in an experiment?" The written comments of 6 percent of these indicated that they thought they were not free because there were not enough experiments offered. The remaining 4 percent made no comments.

In presenting evidence of educational benefit to the CW-IRB, it was noted that when populations of 98 and 906 students were asked how much they had learned from serving as subjects, the distribution of responses in both samples was skewed favorably—more than is the case with many educational practices—toward responses indicating educational benefit. Students' written comments on these surveys indicated positive feelings such as "helps to understand concepts we are studying" and "more in depth than class coverage."

After the presentation and further discussion, the CW-IRB likewise approved recruiting student subjects with extra-credit.

EXTRA-CREDIT: A THREAT OR AN OFFER?

A difficult question, which committee debate raised about this investigator's method of recruitment, was whether the use of extra-credit coerces or only appropriately rewards students for research participation. To investigators and instructors who feel the pinch of IRBs and Department of Health and Human Services (DHHS) regulations, the answer to whether a practice is coercive may seem to depend upon whimsy—or perhaps upon who is voting approval of the protocol. Is there some more rigorous characterization of coercion that allows it to be identified more precisely than everyday notions permit? Unfortunately, it seems not. Consider one problem.

One means of distinguishing coercion from appropriate reward is to ask whether instructors present students with a threat or an offer by using extra-credit. Assuming that threats are coercive and offers represent appropriate rewards, the problem is to identify threats. The philosopher Robert Nozick has suggested that whether a person threatens or makes offers depends upon how the consequences for others change from what they would have been in the normal or expected course of events. If instructors make the normal or expected course of events better for students than ordinarily would be the case, instructors make students an offer. If, however, instructors make the normal or expected course of events worse for students than ordinarily would be the case, instructors threaten students.

Although Nozick's account seems intuitively correct, whether instructors make offers or threats depends upon the background used to evaluate the option of extra-credit. If the background, the normal or expected course of events, is that students have lower grade averages and have learned less without extra-credit alternatives, and they have no objections to research participation for extra-credit, then instructors make them better off and so present offers. If, however, the background is that students should not engage in research participation for extra-credit—perhaps because they think their desires for grades are being unjustly manipulated or they are learning little from the experience—then instructors make students worse off by having them do something that they should not have to do. And so instructors threaten students.

Since the background used to evaluate whether extra-credit is a threat or an offer is crucial to the judgment we make, the background requires justification. But if we know what the background should be, i.e., what the relationship should be between instructors and students, then it is superfluous to use this to identify threats and offers because, presumably, we would already know whether there are ethical objections to recruiting students with extra-credit. Thus this attempt to specify more precisely when a subject is being coerced does not seem helpful to an IRB.

EXTRA-CREDIT, EDUCATIONAL BENEFIT, AND FREE CHOICE

Since the distributions in two surveys with medium and large samples were skewed favorably toward responses indicating educational benefit, and there were positive student comments from all three surveys, the investigator has good empirical evidence of educational benefit.

Although the rationale of the investigator's department for using students as subjects is educational benefit and students receive this benefit from research participation, it seems unlikely that educational benefit is the only motive for using students as subjects. [E]xtra-credit is a means of recruiting subjects where otherwise it may be unreasonably expensive to obtain them.

The investigator's arguments that students were making free choices when selecting research participation are less convincing than the arguments for educational benefit. The empirical evidence that all students in one experiment denied being coerced is derived from a small sample (29 students) and the surveys of populations of 40 subjects and 906 students who were asked whether they felt free to choose whether or not to be subjects are inconclusive. [...]

The investigator's testimony that the chairperson and ombudsman in the investigator's department received no student complaints about subject recruitment with extra-credit while students had complained about other departmental policies may indicate only that students were reluctant to complain about this policy. Citing a lack of complaints is not good evidence that there are no complaints unless a department conducts an active monitoring system to present students with the opportunity to complain.

The investigator's argument that the alternatives of earning extra-credit by short papers, quizzes, special projects, and book reports are comparable to research participation in terms of effort, and that therefore students are not being subtly coerced into the research alternative is fallacious. Research participation may be easier because students earn extra-credit based on the amount of time spent as subjects [...].

The argument that extra-credit appropriately rewards students for extra effort in obtaining a special educational benefit overlooks that every student who completes 30 minutes of research participation receives the same reward. If this is a strictly educational system—as in a classroom or a quiz on library reading assignments—then rewards should be proportional to the educational benefit. Serving as a research subject is unquestionably educational, but the reward system indicates that benefits depend only on time spent as a subject; no attempt is made to measure educational benefit as is done in a classroom.

Research participation may also not be comparable to alternatives for earning extra-credit because with the former, students may be motivated by curiosity, altruism, or novelty—motives that may not be associated with the latter. For example, reading articles and being quizzed on them to earn extra-credit may be perceived as only more of the "old" routine associated with regular classroom work. Research participation, however, may be seen as a welcome holiday from the usual chores associated with extra-credit, and therefore may be more attractive to students. Thus the possibility of subtly coercing students still remains.

Department figures showing that one-third to two-thirds of students chose alternatives to research participation do not necessarily show equality of effort between research participation and other alternatives to earning extra-credit; the figures may indicate only that many students feel the need to do something to improve grades. Once again, a valid survey of students' perceptions might help to explain the motivation for choosing alternatives to research participation.

Finally, the policies of the investigator's department of allocating extra-credit only after establishing a grade curve for a course by test scores and not allowing extra-credit to exceed 5 percent of the maximum that can be earned by all course requirements demonstrate the attractiveness of any extra-credit option—including research participation. The investigator's department uses a seven-step grading system—A, AB, B, BC, C, D, F—with steps not necessarily of equal size. The investigator reports that the possible change in grade by a 5 percent increase in points is probably a one-half of a grade step or less; and while it is possible for a student who falls between two steps to achieve the higher through extra-credit, it is not possible to move from a B to an A.

Since students perceive that their future is largely determined by grades—and only A or B grades are acceptable—the chance of raising grades, which are close to an A or B, by an activity that does not involve risk must be considered attractive to them. Allocating extra-credit only after establishing a grade curve for a course prevents extra-credit from raising the minimum necessary for any grade, but this does not make extra-credit options less attractive.

In summary, the investigator has good evidence that research participation provides educational benefit to subjects although it seems unlikely that this is the only motive of the investigator's department for providing students with the option of research participation. The claim that students do not feel coerced is inconclusively supported as is the claim—in the absence of an active monitoring system—that students have no complaints about research participation. The argument that the alternatives to research participation are equal in terms of effort are fallacious since research participation and quizzes on library readings use different standards to award extra-credit. Finally, department policies designed to limit the effect that extra-credit may have on students' grades do not prevent research participation—or any of the alternatives—from being attractive to students close to A or B grades.

CASH PAYMENTS AND FREE CHOICE

A recruitment alternative more consistent with free choice than extra-credit is the use of cash payments to recruit students, since cash payments may not be as imposing as extra-credit. Extra-credit recognizes the position and desires of students. Students may participate in experiments, which otherwise would not interest them, only to secure this unique benefit. And while paid subjects may participate in experiments only for the money, this benefit is not necessarily related to career goals. Paid subjects might seek better pay at any other activity that offered it.

Cash payments treat students like other persons who volunteer as paid subjects. Paid subjects have to balance their immediate wishes about participation with the immediate advantages of payment; it seems fair to have students make the judgment other paid students make. This also makes is easier for students to make an informed decision about the benefits of being a subject since they have to consider only tangible benefits—cash payments—and not the intangible ones of career advantage or educational benefit. It is always difficult to measure the benefit to oneself in any consent transaction, but wherever possible we should have subjects balancing the same considerations before consenting to participate.

Using cash payments to recruit research subjects avoids some of the problems associated with extra-credit, but others remain. What, for example, is an appropriate level of reward?

Since research participation is a service that students perform—much like pumping gasoline or stocking grocery shelves—there should be a similar reward. A useful guideline is the minimum wage with consideration for possible pain, discomfort, or risk. Inconvenience, which may not be adequately measured by the time spent in an experiment, should also be considered. For example, it may be more in-convenient for students to be in several brief experiments than to spend an equivalent amount of time in one longer experiment. Accordingly, then, brief experiments may appropriately pay more per hour than longer ones. If research participation involves more than a service (venipuncture, urine, or blood collection) a customary payment schedule—which treats subjects equally—is appropriate.

Should a bonus be used to secure subjects' participation in a series of observations? For example, subjects may be paid $10 for each of six weekly sessions with a bonus of $30 for completing the protocol. The value of subjects' participation to an investigator may be enhanced considerably if subjects participate in an entire experiment rather than a part of it. But it is a condition of any research participation that subjects be free to withdraw from an experiment at any time. Is using a bonus to secure complete participation inconsistent with [a] subject's freedom to withdraw?

Presumably, a bonus encourages subjects not to withdraw from a protocol for trivial reasons—inconvenience or boredom, and motivates them not to forget research appointments. But a bonus should not function to restrain subjects from withdrawing from a protocol because of physical or psychological harms stemming from the experiment. Consequently, when using a bonus, the informed consent should contain a statement of the conditions under which subjects may withdraw from a protocol and still receive a prorated amount of a bonus. There should also be an understanding of general grounds on which participation may be terminated without subjects' consent and without payment of the bonus. With no risk or minimal risk research, legitimate excuses to withdraw from protocols should be rare, and subjects should be so informed.

In calculating the amount of a bonus, an investigator should consider what is an appropriate and necessary inducement to recruit subjects, and make the bonus a percentage of this total amount. Thus, the amount of the bonus is not an undue inducement.

Other arguments justifying the use of a bonus are derivative from arguments suggesting the appropriateness of restricting a subject's freedom to withdraw from an experiment. Since a bonus encourages complete participation in a protocol, it helps to conserve scarce resources, which may be wasted by subjects' withdrawal; a bonus also encourages subjects to honor agreements to participate in research.

If a standard level of cash rewards yields too few subjects, then an investigator needs to examine the design of "unpopular" experiments and the cash rewards. Alternative design may solve the problem of too few subjects by decreasing the time, trouble, inconvenience, or risk and should be an investigator's first recourse. While no level of cash payment distinguishes due from undue inducement, and the minimum level of payment necessary to recruit an adequate number of subjects does not guarantee subjects are being duly induced, the context of minimal risk or no risk research makes it unlikely that additional increments of payment needed to obtain a sufficient subject pool constitute undue inducement. This does not, however, resolve the general problem of the appropriate level of cash payment to recruit sufficient numbers of subjects where more than minimal risk research is involved.

CONCLUSION

While it is difficult to show that an investigator's use of extra-credit is coercive, there are good arguments that in-dicate that students may not be consenting freely under these conditions. Using cash payments removes a benefit unique to students and allows them to judge the advantages of research participation in the same manner as paid subjects.

I have not considered the objection that the exchange of extra-credit for student participation as subjects is an improper use of an academic grading system. While such an objection is important, it is not properly raised by IRBs, which are charged to protect human subjects, not to consider broader social effects of human experimentation.

---

47   Against Special Protections for Medical Students

NANCY R. ANGOFF

[. . .] Nicholas Christakis concludes that institutional review board (IRB) review of research involving medical students as subjects is sufficient to safeguard the students' rights and well-being. He feels that special guidelines like the "Rules Governing the Participation of Medical Students as Experimental Subjects" in effect at Harvard since 1956 are excessively paternalistic and restrictive. I agree with Mr. Christakis's viewpoint; furthermore, I believe that this sort of protection is really overprotection and serves to foster a distorted image of medical students having diminished autonomy.

Harvard's rules were formulated originally in response to an apparent escalation in the use of medical students as research subjects in "risky" experiments in the 1950s. The appropriateness of the rules at that time is not an issue since there were few review committees resembling present-day IRBs. However, given IRBs and other institutional safeguards for protecting the rights of all research subjects and encouraging ethical and professional behavior on the part of investigators, the rules seem extraneous in 1985. Their existence contributes to an incorrect view of medical students as a special population more in need of protection than the general population. In fact, the rules specify protection even greater than those afforded groups such as children and the mentally infirm, groups recognized as needing special consideration owing to their decreased capacity to evaluate fully the research experience. [...]

Nancy R. Angoff, "Against Special Protections for Medical Students," *IRB: A Review of Human Subjects Research* 7, no. 5 (1985): 9–10.

The need for special protections for medical student research subjects is based on a perception that ". . . while medical students may be more able to give informed consent, they are less able to give free consent." The proponents of these rules seem to believe that this decreased autonomy is the result of an interplay of selfish motivations on the part of students and faculty inherent in the highly competitive medical school environment. Students might try to insinuate themselves into the good graces of their professors by selling themselves as research subjects, and faculty investigators may take advantage of their students by applying undue pressure to get them to participate in "risky research" against the students' better judgment. All of this unchecked behavior could pose threats to a student's health and ability to manage his or her time carefully.

The basic question to be decided is whether medical students as a group are, in fact, "less free" than the general population by virtue of being "a captive population." Since I do not believe that they are, I shall argue that they ought to be left to evaluate freely any demands on their health or time and make decisions about participating in research accordingly. Of course, the IRB must assess the risks of particular research protocols as acceptable.

THE AUTONOMY OF MEDICAL STUDENTS

There are several telling reasons to consider medical students highly autonomous. These are people who have maneuvered successfully through a system that includes many hurdles to their present status. [...] Such strong candidates do not just lose their good judgment upon entering the hallowed halls. [. . .] Certainly, people who will be entrusted with making judgments about the health and well-being of others should be allowed to make choices about managing their own time and health.

How real a threat does research pose to a medical student's health? Probably not so great a threat as exposure to formaldehyde in gross anatomy lab or to infections incubating in a pediatric ward. In fact, Robert J. Levine writes, "On the basis of all of the empirical evidence of which I am aware, it seems proper to conclude that the role of research subject is not particularly hazardous in general. It follows that attempts to portray it as such and arguments for policies designed to restrict research generally because it is hazardous are without warrant."

How real is the problem of overly aggressive faculty pressuring students to participate in research against their wishes? Faculty who behave this way become known very quickly to medical students and those who are reluctant to be pressured will steer clear of them. In any case, behavior of this sort should not be tolerated by the institution whether it occurs with students, employees, or patients. But a policy to prevent it should be aimed at curbing the behavior, not limiting the choices available to students.

THE IRB'S ROLE

If it is agreed that IRB review of research involving medical students is sufficient to protect their welfare, the question then arises whether IRBs should impose more rigid criteria for participation of students than for the general public. The IRB at the University of Massachusetts adopted a policy that students may participate as subjects when "(1) the experiment has minimal risks; (2) there is no major physical or surgical intervention; (3) there is a minimal interruption of one's daily routine." In the case that gave impetus to the adoption of this policy, several students who had participated in research complained to the IRB that since they had experienced side effects they were not "in the best shape for classes and examinations."

If representatives of any other group complained to an IRB that side effects of a study treatment were more disabling than they had been led to believe, the most likely action of the IRB would be to insist that the investigator modify the consent form to reflect more accurately the apparent side effects. The information that the study may result in stomach irritation that could prevent one from performing as usual for a few days is material to anyone's decision about whether to participate, not just students. It is unlikely that any other adult group's complaints would result in an exclusionary policy. Do special considerations of this type lead to what Harvard calls "the development of highly qualified physicians capable of providing leadership in their chosen fields"?

A CASE IN POINT

One IRB decided differently. A research protocol involving multiple catheterizations, infusions of drugs, and radiation exposure equivalent to an amount received from two chest x-rays and an upper gastrointestinal series was approved by the Human Investigation Committee (HIC) at the Yale University School of Medicine. Given the complexities of the procedures and the attendant risks, the HIC decided that participation should be limited to those subjects who could comprehend and evaluate the information shared with them by the investigators. The HIC informed the investigators that, in its view, any component of this study could be explained satisfactorily to most normal volunteers. However, in the aggregate, the sheer volume of risk information seemed likely to overwhelm the average prospective subject.

The research clearly would not fit the criteria allowing medical student participation set by the University of Massachusetts IRB. Students would not be allowed to participate under the Harvard rules either. The HIC, however, directed the investigators to describe a proposed subject population that would assure their familiarity with the procedures, assure their capacity to assess the risks and discomforts of the procedures, and afford confidence that they could appreciate the importance of the knowledge being sought. The HIC suggested that one category of subjects would be third- and fourth-year medical students. One of the co-investigators on this protocol was a fourth-year medical student. It seems ironic to protect students from participating fully and under the same conditions in an experience such as one which they may one day request others to accept.

The HIC approved payment to subjects on this protocol of $100 for approximately seven hours of their time, not an unreasonable amount for a day's work involving so much discomfort. One concern of proponents of Harvard's rules, which also exclude payment to student research subjects, is that students ". . . might participate in studies in an attempt to garner better recommendations, better grades, or other favors (such as summer employment)." It seems logical that direct payment to students for a job well done would somewhat dispel any expectations by students that any other form of reward would follow. Earning money from participation in research is at least as reputable a way as a variety of others available to students such as selling their blood, tending bar, or babysitting for a faculty member's children.

Finally, treating medical students differently by applying different standards to their participation in research than to the participation of the general public has the flavor of elitism. One may wonder why it is acceptable to ask the masses to accept risk in the name of science but not the very people whose futures are linked to the successful perpetuation of biomedical research. Medical schools that create this impression are acting somewhat like parents who profess a belief in public education but send their children to private school.

If medical schools really are interested in training competent and sensitive future investigators, exposure to the total research experience should be available to students. How better to know what information truly is relevant to informed consent; how better to understand the difference between words on a consent form and a consent process; how better to appreciate what it feels like to be made a "thing" whose "being is reduced to that of a mere token or 'sample'"; how better to know what it is like to be a subject than to be one! We should not be making it more difficult for medical students to participate in research; rather, we should be making it easier.

Part VII

Special Topics in Research Ethics

When the oversight structure for research with humans was being established in the United States in the 1970s, most of the focus was on traditional physiological and therapeutic research. Over time, an awareness of ethical issues related to other types of research has increased. Several trends have contributed to this expanded focus. Among these trends are greater emphases on genetics in clinical research, the combination of methodologies (especially epidemiology) with tissue storage interventions, and the ethical examination of long-accepted but hitherto unexamined or underexamined research practices. Part VII of this volume focuses on the ethical considerations arising in clinical research that extend beyond the bounds of the traditional testing of drugs and interventions that served as the paradigm for the development of the federal regulations.

These areas of focus raise many overlapping ethical concerns. First, they tend to deal with humans who cannot provide consent or with situations in which securing consent can be logistically difficult, if not impossible. Consequently, questions are raised about consent: When can consent be waived? Are there ethically acceptable substitutes for consent? Second, several of the topics raise questions about confidentiality and disclosure of sensitive information about participants. Under what circumstances should research data be disclosed to participants? How will the confidentiality of research data be secured? Third, some of these topics raise concerns about risks. What constitutes minimal risk? What are the risks associated with research when there is no physical intervention, but rather only the retention of information about participants?

SECTION ONE. GENETICS RESEARCH

The first section of this part deals with the difficult issues raised by genetics protocols. With the rapid advances in understanding of the genetic basis of disease and the sequencing of the human genome, clinical genetics research has exploded. From pedigree studies to the use of genetic tests in traditional clinical research studies and the assessment of genetically determined variations in disease etiology, it can sometimes seem that all clinical research has a genetic component. The integration of genetics into research with humans has highlighted certain ethical dilemmas, especially because in many but not all cases, genetic information can have implications for individuals beyond the presenting patient.

In a series of three papers, Kathleen Cranley Glass and colleagues make helpful suggestions for institutional review boards (IRBs) that review different types of genetics research protocols: (1) gene localization and identification studies, (2) genetic diagnostic and screening studies, and (3) gene therapy studies. They specify seven core areas that need to be scrutinized by IRBs that correspond to the seven ethical requirements that are arguably applicable to all clinical research:[1] (1) background and justification of the research (value), (2) research design (validity), (3) procedures (validity), (4) subject (or participant) selection, (5) risks and benefits, (6) provision of information to participants (informed consent), and (7) commercial interests. Within each of these core areas, Glass and colleagues delineate specific questions that should guide an IRB's deliberations. One general point the authors repeatedly emphasize is that the evaluation of some genetic studies may require special expertise, such as expertise in biostatistics or in the use of viral vectors as gene delivery vehicles, and that "IRBs lacking such expertise must call on outside consultants to assist in the review."

With respect to gene localization and identification studies, Glass and colleagues focus on several issues of special concern. One important issue relates to family pressure. Integral to gene localization and identification are pedigree studies that require participation by many if not all family members. This creates a situation in which family members who desire the genetic information may place pressure on other family members who may not desire such information. As Lisa S. Parker and Charles W. Lidz note, the ethical concern in such situations is that if participation is not voluntary, informed consent is nullified.[2] As they point out, however, it is important to distinguish pressure from coercion; coercion—an irresistible threat—is inherently antithetical to the voluntariness required for a valid provision of informed consent. But families are often rife with (conscious or unconscious) pressures. To complicate matters considerably, familial pressure need not be thought of as problematic; it may indeed be part and parcel of healthy family life. It is important, however, to distinguish sharply between such internal familial pressure and external pressure exerted by investigators. As Glass and colleagues note: "Discussions family members might have with one another may be completely appropriate, whereas the same conversations would not be appropriate if they involved an investigator and prospective subjects."

With respect to the issue of pressure, the key question to focus on is this: When does pressure shade into coercion and thus become unethical? Such a determination is context dependent and depends upon the intention(s) of the person(s) applying the pressure, the perceptions of the person being pressured, and the norms of their interactions. Data on family pressure in other medical contexts suggest that most people do not experience pressure by their family members as coercive.[3] Indeed, Parker and Lidz note that "patients often perceived the pressure to which they have been subjected as being less coercive than did the clinicians or family members involved."[4] Drawing on empirical data and the current research regulations, Glass and colleagues argue that although IRBs should make efforts to ensure that investigators do not pressure people to participate in genetic studies, they "should not be concerned with eliminating family interactions, including those that are characterized as persuasion, manipulation, or even pressure."

Another important issue endemic to genetics protocols is that of privacy.[5] In certain types of genetics research, unpleasant family secrets such as adoption, incest, or nonpaternity might be revealed. This is no idle worry, since nonpaternity rates may be as high as 10 percent. Moreover, the disclosure of a familial disease about which some may prefer *not* to know may even occur in the recruitment process before a person has the opportunity to refuse participation in a study. These issues are particularly pressing in pedigree and gene localization studies because, as Glass and colleagues write, "for the most part participation offers subjects no benefit beyond the opportunity for altruism."

A different facet of the privacy issue is analyzed by another contributor to this section, Jeffrey R. Botkin. Botkin takes as his starting point a survey study conducted at Virginia Commonwealth University (VCU). The father of one of the research participants raised concerns about whether informed consent *from the participant's family members* should have been required by the VCU IRB given that the survey asked for sensitive and arguably private information regarding the participant's parents. The question that the VCU case raises for Botkin is whether family members of participants in survey and pedigree research should themselves be considered research participants and, if so, whether and when informed consent should be sought from them for the collection and retention of their personal information. The VCU survey study thus resembles pedigree studies in the issues they raise vis-à-vis privacy and the threats thereto.

Although Botkin is sensitive to the harms that may follow a breach in privacy, his analysis suggests that many pedigree studies may proceed without the explicit consent of family members. Current U.S. regulations apply only to those who are, as a matter of regulatory definition, human subjects. Botkin believes that family members of pedigree research participants will only rarely be readily identifiable by the investigators and in such circumstances are not to be considered participants in the research. If, however, family members are determined to be participants, the issue becomes whether the consent of family members can be waived. Waiver of consent arises as an issue because obtaining consent, not only from primary participants but also from their family members, is time-consuming and expensive for investigators and may halt or delay many research protocols. According to Botkin, much will hinge on the nature and extent of the research risk. If the research poses greater than minimal risk, investigators may have to obtain consent from family members if either (1) the private information retained about them is highly sensitive or (2) sufficient data security measures have not been put in place. On the other hand, if the research cannot be practically carried out without a waiver of consent, it may be permissible to waive the consent requirement provided that the research involves no more than minimal risk.

Yet another issue raised by genetics studies concerns giving patients access to the results of genetic tests before the meaning and utility of such results are proven. An autonomy-centered view is that patients should always be given test results and that they can then do whatever they wish with the information. A beneficence-centered view, on the other hand, is that patients should be given results of research related to gene identification or genetic diagnostics *only* when the data are validated and their clinical utility is established. Some commentators believe that a policy of blanket disclosure is not justifiable.[6] Disclosure of results to participants, according to Glass and colleagues, should be based on three considerations: (1) the magnitude of the threat posed to a participant by the putative genetic condition, (2) the accuracy with which the data can predict the threat, and (3) the potential that there can be an intervention to treat the threat. On this basis, they argue that disclosure should not occur if the genetic test results are uninformative, that is, if the results cannot affect an individual's risk assessment, as in the case of preliminary linkage studies.

SECTION TWO. STORED HUMAN BIOLOGICAL SPECIMENS

The National Bioethics Advisory Commission (NBAC) estimates that there are hundreds of millions of stored biological samples in the United States alone.[7] Over the past few years serious controversy has arisen over the proper ethical requirements for using such material: When is informed consent required? What constitutes an anonymous sample? Although almost all commentators see the use of biological samples for genetic studies as the paradigm, these biological samples have been used in many different clinical research studies, from studies evaluating new antibodies to those determining levels of proteins. Thus the issue transcends the use of such samples for genetic analyses.

Discussions concerning research using stored biological samples have been somewhat confused because of vague terms. The first contribution to this section of Part VII, a statement on informed consent for genetic research promulgated by the American Society of Human Genetics (ASHG), goes some way toward clearing matters up. The ASHG distinguishes

between four types of biological samples considered under two broad classes of such samples. The ASHG first makes a distinction between prospective and retrospective samples. Prospective samples are those that are collected from an individual explicitly for the purposes of research, while retrospective samples are those that have been collected in the past and are then used, at a later date, for research purposes. The ASHG then makes a further distinction that is applicable to both prospective and retrospective samples—between anonymous or anonymized samples on the one hand and identified or identifiable samples on the other. Thus prospective (or retrospective) samples may be anonymous in two senses: either they are collected anonymously (that is, without identifiers) or they are collected with identifiers but are later anonymized; similarly, prospective (or retrospective) samples may be identifiable in two senses: either they are collected with identifiers and retain such identifiers or the identifiers have been removed—but it is possible, usually through a code, to relink the samples and the person, thus making the samples identifiable.

A general consensus seems to exist on the consent procedures surrounding the use of identified or identifiable samples. For prospective samples, most commentators endorse seeking consent at the time of collection.[8] However, there is disagreement about the details of this consent, namely, to what patients and participants should consent. Some urge the use of extensive and lengthy consent forms. For instance, the National Action Plan on Breast Cancer (NAPBC) has devised a model consent form that asks permission for three courses of action: (1) use of the sample for research related to the same disease for which it was collected, (2) use of the sample for research on diseases unrelated to the disease for which it was collected, and (3) recontact to give the patient the option to participate in additional research.[9] (This consent form is included in the appendix to this volume.) Others urge the use of a more general consent form, arguing that patients and participants do not make the types of distinctions specified on the NAPBC form and that multiple questions may be too complex and confusing, thus undermining the consent process.

Commentators are similarly in broad agreement that for the use of retrospective biological samples—such as those used in pathology departments or stored from past research projects—informed consent is necessary if the samples retain personal identifiers. That is, if there is sufficient information, such as the patient's name or social security number, to link the sample with a specific person, then, barring unusual circumstances, the person should be contacted to provide informed consent for research using the sample. If the patient does not consent or provide permission for use of the specimen, it should be excluded from the research.

The real controversy centers on the requirements for research using retrospective samples when researchers plan to anonymize these samples and, in particular, what must be done to securely anonymize the samples. In 1995 a joint workshop of the National Institutes of Health (NIH) and the Centers for Disease Control and Prevention (CDC) examined the issue; in the second paper in this section, Ellen Wright Clayton and colleagues summarize the workshop's conclusions. They acknowledge that, according to existing regulations, research using existing samples that are anonymous—that is, samples with no patient identifiers and no way to link them to patients—are exempt from the Common Rule requirements for both IRB review and informed consent. However, they argue that IRBs should review research using anonymous samples for the social value and scientific validity of the proposed research and should determine whether it would be possible to obtain consent.

In addition, Clayton and colleagues argue that, for biological samples that will be anonymized for the purposes of research, consent can be waived only if four regulatory requirements are met: (1) the research involves no more than minimal risk, (2) the rights of participants will not be affected by forgoing consent, (3) it is impractical to carry out the research with informed consent, and (4) after participation the participants will be given information about the research. Clayton and colleagues seem to suggest that consent is still required for research in which a sample is linked to patient records but all specific patient identifiers, such as name, birth date, and social security number, are removed. Others disagree about the need for consent in such circumstances.

Our final contributors in this section, Jon F. Merz and colleagues, agree that research using samples from which personal identifiers have been removed "can proceed with little or no prior informed consent (typical of stored tissues)" provided that "procedural safeguards are in place to prevent inferential identifi-

cation or statistical matching." If researchers are going to use biological specimens and want updated clinical information to link their results with disease outcomes, there should be a "one-way link between patient records and research data sets," such as a computer system that encodes clinical data. The one-way link Merz and colleagues prefer is that of a "tissue bank trustee" who would merge tissue samples and clinical information, de-identify them, and then provide this information to researchers. The trustee would be independent of the researchers and clinicians, and any information generated in the process of the research would be prohibited from flowing back to the trustee in a way that could be relinked to the patient.

SECTION THREE. HUMAN EMBRYOS AND STEM CELLS

The ethical issue surrounding research using embryos arises from the conflict between two sets of values: those related to the potential good that might come from the research and those related to the moral status of the embryo. The potential good that might come from embryo and stem cell research is similar to that of all other clinical research, namely, the relief of suffering and the improvement of health. This goal is in tension with the fact that in the research process or in the creation of stem cells the embryo must invariably be destroyed.

Even among those who believe that some cases of embryo research are morally permissible, considerations about the moral status of the embryo may well restrict these permissible cases of research to instances where the embryos are already in existence, thus morally foreclosing the option of bringing embryos into existence merely for research purposes. Moreover, even some who hold strong antiabortion positions nonetheless claim that research on embryos already in existence is morally permissible. The morality of abortion and that of research using human embryos do not therefore stand or fall together.

For some commentators, such as John Robertson[10] and Ruth Macklin,[11] the destruction of embryos is not worrisome because the embryo has no special moral status, certainly not the status of personhood with an entitlement to a right to life. The embryo is just a collection of cells without the key qualities—such as sentience, rationality, or cognition—

that would give it any moral entitlements associated with being a person.[12] To say that the embryo commands respect because of its potentiality is a form of symbolic or expressive reasoning, but not, some say, an ethical argument. As Macklin observes: "Appeals to respect for embryos and reference to the dignity of embryos are linguistic attempts to invest this form of life with a moral status that would allow some actions but not others. However, neither linguistic maneuvers nor moral intuition can substitute for ethical arguments."[13]

However, there are those who believe that human embryos are not merely collections of cells. Even lacking the qualities indicative of personhood, human embryos would develop into human beings with these qualities and therefore have potentialities of personhood in a way that acorns or mouse embryos or even nonhuman adult mammals do not. There are many permutations of this view. The theological view, most closely associated with the Catholic Church, argues for the special status of embryos because each is endowed by God with a human soul. A genetic view might argue that the embryo has the full complement of human genes and thus that it should have special moral status. Others place emphasis on the developmental process and argue that as the embryo obtains more qualities of personhood, it should correspondingly receive enhanced moral consideration.

In 1994 the NIH Human Embryo Research Panel (HERP) met to engage in deliberations about whether the moral status of the ex utero embryo was compatible with the federal financing of research using embryos. Excerpts from their report lead off this section of Part VII. The HERP recommends that the federal government fund embryo research that is important, promising, and impossible to carry out through other means. A key recommendation of the panel is that a determination of the personhood of the embryo be based not on a single criterion, but rather on a "pluralistic approach." Such a pluralistic approach involves the consideration of a number of different qualities, including the following: genetic uniqueness, potentiality for development, sentience, brain activity, and degree of cognitive development. Other qualities often mentioned are human form, capacity for survival outside the mother's womb, and degree of relational presence (whether to the mother herself or to others). And, they continue, "Although none of these qualities is by itself sufficient to establish personhood,

their developing presence in an entity increases its moral status, until at some point, full and equal protectability is required."

Out of respect for the embryo, the HERP recommends the limited use of embryos up to 14 days of development and says that embryos should be obtained primarily through free and informed donation by couples who have undergone in vitro fertilization and no longer plan to use their embryos to initiate a pregnancy. Although the panel leaves open the possibility of other sources of embryos, President Clinton announced in December 1994 that NIH funding would not be used to support the creation of human embryos for research purposes.

In their response to the HERP report, the next contributors to this section, the Ramsey Colloquium, criticize as "morally repugnant and a grave injustice to innocent human beings" the panel's conclusion that government money could be used to conceive human embryos for research. Creating embryos for research is the epitome of using human beings solely as means, they argue. The authors criticize the panel's focus on protecting persons (a moral category) as distinct from human beings (a biological category) and argue that every human being is inviolable and thus deserves respect and protection. They also accuse the panel of circular reasoning, criticize the panel's focus on social utility as the justification for embryo research, and denounce the one-sidedness of the panel's membership. They conclude that the production of human beings solely for the purpose of research that will destroy them should be prohibited by law.

The next contribution to this section is an excerpt from the 1999 NBAC report Ethical Issues In Human Stem Cell Research. Like the earlier HERP report, the NBAC report is framed by recognition of a deep tension: that between the laudable aim of using the fruits of research for the betterment of humanity and the equally laudable aim of protecting human life. Both the HERP and NBAC reports thus raise similar, but not identical, issues.

The NBAC commissioners focus their attention on the ethical acceptability of federal funding of research using embryonic stem (ES) and embryonic germ (EG) cells. It is NBAC's view that both (1) research involving the derivation and use of EG cells from cadaveric fetal tissue and (2) research involving the derivation and use of ES cells from human embryos that remain after infertility treatments may ethically be carried out with the support of federal research funds. However, NBAC concludes that research using ES cells from embryos (1) created solely for the purpose of research and (2) created from somatic cell nuclear transfer into oocytes (i.e., cloning) should be banned from the receipt of federal research funding support.

The distinction between these two classes of research turns on the source of the ES and EG cells—embryos. In particular, it is NBAC's view that embryos cannot ethically be brought into existence merely for the purpose of research on such cells. In support of this conclusion, the NBAC commissioners argue for a number of important preconditions that must be satisfied if such research is to be ethically carried out. They thus articulate and defend requirements related to the donor's consent to donate embryos and argue for the necessity of a robust research oversight and review mechanism. The NBAC commissioners buttress these recommendations through helpful analyses of (1) the (causal and symbolic) association of cadaveric fetal tissue research with abortion, (2) the moral status of the embryo (where NBAC adopts an intermediate view according to which the embryo merits respect as a form of human life, but rather less respect than a fully human person), and (3) the distinction between discarded and specially created embryos and the implications of this distinction for current and future debates.

The final author in this section, Maura A. Ryan, raises other concerns. She first notes that those who perform cost-benefit calculations based on a comparison of special treatment for embryos versus the good of scientific progress never seem to think an enumeration of the *actual* (or at least the highly likely) products of science is needed. That such research will yield great returns, she claims, is assumed as a matter of fact. This suggests that such comparative calculations may be disingenuous. More important, she contends that the arguments that focus on the moral status of the embryo are "disembodied" because they ignore the social context in which embryos are created, namely, the context of assisted reproduction for the purpose of the "union of sexual intimacy, procreation, and parenthood." Ryan contends that only the relational goods of procreation and parenthood can justify the creation of an embryo; creating embryos for research violates the goods of intimacy, generativity, and nurturing and should thus be prohibited, while the use of "spare embryos," in contrast, is permissible.

SECTION FOUR. DRUG CHALLENGE AND DRUG WASHOUT STUDIES

In recent years psychiatric research has been embroiled in controversy. Part of the controversy surrounds the issue of informed consent by participants in psychiatric research. (See Part VI, Section One, of this volume.) Another aspect of the controversy surrounds the use of placebos in psychiatric research (see Part III, Section Three, of this volume).[14] Yet another feature of the controversy, which is the focus of this fourth section of Part VII, is related to unique issues of study design, especially the use of drug washout and challenge studies.

Such studies are arguably justifiable for several reasons.[15] First, since there are fluctuations in psychiatric symptoms it is necessary to have control groups as well as periods off medications. Second, to minimize confounding caused by medications and drug-drug interactions, periods off medications before initiation of new medications are necessary. Third, to understand the pathophysiology of psychiatric diseases and the mechanisms of action of drugs designed to treat them, it is necessary to evaluate patients experiencing symptoms or being provoked to have symptoms. Finally, because of the substantial side effects of many psychiatric drugs, research needs to be done to examine the discontinuation of treatment.

Much of the controversy over methodological issues in psychiatric research derives from the University of California, Los Angeles (UCLA) schizophrenia study that stopped drug treatment for patients. As Paul S. Appelbaum comments in the first contribution to this section, the primary objective of the UCLA study was to identify factors that predict which schizophrenic patients could successfully be managed without antipsychotic medications. This is important to know because the medications themselves have significant, and sometimes quite debilitating and irreversible, side effects. Indeed each year about 5 percent of patients taking phenothiazine-type neuroleptics develop tardive dyskinesia—involuntary muscle movements affecting the face, limbs, and other parts of the body that are often, but not always, irreversible. The UCLA study involved schizophrenic patients who received biweekly injections of Prolixin, a standard phenothiazine antipsychotic treatment, for a year. Participants who wished to continue were then enrolled in a three-month randomized, double-blind, placebo-controlled study to evaluate the discontinuation of the Prolixin. After three months patients were crossed over: those who had previously received the placebo injections were given Prolixin and those given Prolixin were then given placebo. Participants who had not relapsed were then taken off all antipsychotic medications and followed for at least one year or until they had an exacerbation or psychotic relapse. The UCLA study caused controversy because one participant committed suicide and another had a psychotic relapse shortly after the Prolixin was stopped, and it was alleged that the research team was slow in restarting medications.

Commentators have delineated the rationale for drug washout studies as well as various ways in which the design of the research might affect the risks and what mechanisms might be used to reduce the risks of the research. The design safeguards might include (1) excluding patients at greatest risk of adverse events and those who are responding well to current treatments, (2) slowly tapering off administration of antipsychotic medications rather than abruptly withdrawing them, (3) enhancing the monitoring and provision of social treatments for patients off medications, (4) limiting the drug-free periods to the minimum consistent with scientific objectives (specifically, limiting the drug-free periods to two to four weeks rather than the more commonly used four to ten weeks), and (5) providing all participants optimal treatment at the end of the study.

Even more contentious than drug washout studies are challenge studies or symptom-provoking studies. The rationale for these studies is to learn more about brain function and symptom expression en route to developing new drug therapies. Such challenge studies are well known in other areas of medicine. For instance, in infectious disease research, especially studies of vaccines and pathogenesis, challenge designs are used to generate preliminary data about protection and individual history.[16] Indeed challenge tests, such as stress tests for cardiac patients and glucose tolerance tests for diabetic patients, have become standard parts of clinical practice. Contributors Franklin G. Miller and Donald L. Rosenstein report that "for most symptom-provoking studies the level of risk is relatively low, since the psychic distress that they produce is typically brief and of mild to moderate intensity." They do note that the reactions reported in some published research have been significant. Such

risks can be balanced by important scientific benefits and, in some cases, better understanding by participants of their own illness. These authors make seven practical suggestions for ensuring that such symptom-provoking studies are conducted in an ethical manner, and these suggestions closely match the recommendations to enhance the safety of drug washout studies.

SECTION FIVE. RESEARCH WITH COMMUNITIES

The genetic studies on BRCA1 and BRCA2 (genes associated with breast cancer) among Ashkenazi Jews raised the issue of conducting research among identifiable communities. This is not the first research endeavor that targeted a community, nor is it the most risky or potentially stigmatizing, but it has focused discussion on whether communities targeted for research should be provided protections and, if so, what these protections might be.

The first contributors to this section, Morris W. Foster, Deborah Bernsten, and Thomas H. Carter, take seriously the idea that communities involved in research should be dealt with in a very different manner than should individuals. These authors, who have worked extensively with Native American populations, propose a model agreement for such research based on their experience with the Apache Tribe of Oklahoma. These authors invoke as a reason for community protections the fact that genetics has often been a basis for discrimination and racism. They argue that research could entail harms for communities over and above the harms faced by individuals and therefore that "new protections against collective risks to identifiable populations" are necessary. Central to the new protections Foster and colleagues suggest is a process for community consultation and involvement. They describe the process of community consultation they used with the Apache people and the resulting contract covering topics from intellectual property rights to use and disposal of biological specimens.

Others disagree. In particular, our next contributor, Eric T. Juengst, acknowledges that "groups face significant risks from population-genomics research," yet argues against the provision of special group protections—or, as he puts it, a "gatekeeping role" for groups—for three principal reasons. First, there is a mismatch between groups that are likely to be targeted for genomics research, those in which genetics is determinative of membership, and social and political groups that would be approached for consent, those in which self-identification is determinative of membership. As Juengst writes, "The human groups that are picked out, described, and compared in the course of population-genomics research are not the named social groups in which we all claim membership." Put differently, social and political groups are not genetically determined. Recognition of this fact prompts Juengst's second concern: Lurking under this kind of reasoning is a form of genetic determinism, and he thinks that this is almost always a key step on the path to discrimination and racism. Juengst is thus at odds with Foster and colleagues on the relationship between genetics and discrimination and on the need for community protections. Finally, given the facts of intercultural migration and the frequent presence of the same "genetic group" within different "social groups," seeking the consent of local social groups would be ineffective in protecting the genetic groups from the (possibly) negative harms of population-genomics research.

This section rounds out with two companion pieces by Charles Weijer and colleagues. Like Foster and his colleagues, Weijer and his endorse community protections and articulate criteria for the determination of the types of communities to which their proposed protections should apply. They do so out of an appreciation of the fact that, given the different kinds of human groupings to which the term "community" can refer, a one-size-fits-all approach to community protection is bound to fail. They contend that the morally salient factor in these debates is not the nature of the research per se, but rather the fact that certain human groupings are targeted for research as distinct, identifiable communities.

After a review of some existing guidelines for the protection of communities, they note that protections can be divided into five broad categories with 23 specific requirements. They then argue that communities must be distinguished according to ten characteristics, and that the protections apply only to communities that have certain specific characteristics. They identify and support three basic regimes of protections: (1) community consultation and consent, which applies to aboriginal and political communities; (2) community consultation without consent, which applies to religious, disease-based, and ethnic communities; and (3) no specific community protec-

tions, which applies to occupational and virtual communities.

SECTION SIX. INTERNATIONAL RESEARCH

The final section of Part VII attends to some of the issues that arise in the context of international research. This has been a particularly controversial area of medical research and academic inquiry of late, and controversy seems to be intensifying. Many questions have been asked: Should the standard of care against which research interventions are compared be tied to what is available in the host country or to that of the sponsor?[17] Are all instances of cross-cultural research exploitative if the researchers come from developed nations to conduct research on participants of poorer, developing nations? What, as a matter of justice, are prospective research participants in developing countries entitled to, both during and after a study?

The first three papers in this section focus upon a group of contentious placebo-controlled trials that were carried out in several African countries, in Thailand, and in the Dominican Republic by researchers from the developed world. Much of the recent literature has been written in response to the first contributors to this section, Peter Lurie and Sidney M. Wolfe, who review what they consider the problematic cases of international placebo-controlled trials for the reduction of maternal-fetal transmission of the human immunodeficiency virus (HIV). The central issue for Lurie and Wolfe is this: Given that there is a standard therapy in the United States and Europe (namely, AZT, or zidovudine), what is an ethically acceptable control arm to use in research in countries within which AZT (or any other intervention) is not made readily available to the citizenry? Lurie and Wolfe argue that a placebo control arm in such research is ethically unjustifiable. First, they believe that a shorter course of AZT for HIV-positive pregnant women, one that is both more affordable and more easily administered, should be the intervention that is compared to the longer, more expensive, and more complicated AZT regimen that is standardly administered to such women in the United States and Europe. This is so because, based upon available data, physicians have reason to believe that a shorter regimen of AZT will be more effective than placebo. This fact, they argue, disturbs clinical equipoise and makes the use of a placebo control unethical.

Second, Lurie and Wolfe claim that the standard of care available in developing countries—no treatment—is a product not of sound public health policy, but rather of the sheer poverty endemic to such countries. Therefore, those who carry out research in developing countries have a duty to ensure that all arms of the protocol conform to the standard of care in the sponsoring country, namely, some form of AZT therapy. Otherwise, they say, the precedent for a dangerous double standard of research ethics will be set. Finally, Lurie and Wolfe claim that an equivalency study[18] wherein all participants would receive some AZT would be a better alternative to the placebo-controlled design and would only moderately increase the length of time required to complete the study.

The next contributors, George J. Annas and Michael A. Grodin, raise slightly different concerns. They are also opposed to the use of placebo controls, but their objection revolves around the claim that studies using placebos exploit the women and children in the developing world. As Annas and Grodin argue, absent a specific plan designed to ensure that those in the developing world receive the AZT that they require after completion of a trial, researchers from developed countries are exploiting the people in impoverished countries for the developed countries' own good. Moreover, in ways not unlike those seen in the Tuskegee syphilis study, researchers are avoiding ethical principles and instead are using professional consensus to justify such research. Finally, Annas and Grodin contend that, securing free and informed consent from the impoverished populations in which such research is carried out is likely to be impossible.

Robert A. Crouch and John D. Arras disagree both with Lurie and Wolfe and with Annas and Grodin. They offer a qualified defense of the placebo-controlled AZT trials based upon three lines of argument. First, a proper understanding of clinical equipoise entails that the entire context of a study must be taken into account when determining what may or may not be offered in research. Thus, all of the following facts must be considered: that there are real safety concerns regarding the use of anemia-inducing AZT in women who are already anemic; that the administration of the long-course AZT regimen can be difficult or impossible in a population that does not routinely present for prenatal care; and, most important, that the governments of developing countries could never afford to provide their citizens with the long-course AZT therapy. Given such facts, they argue

that while clinical equipoise has been disturbed in more developed countries, it has not been disturbed in many developing countries; a placebo control is therefore justifiable.

Second, Crouch and Arras argue that it is by no means clear that the citizens of developing countries have a moral entitlement to receive the expensive antiretrovirals that are required to reduce the vertical transmission of HIV. And this is so, they argue, even if the current baseline level of holdings in such developing countries is unjust, as they believe it to be. The problem here, they argue, is that even against a background of unjust holdings, it is unclear *what in particular* is owed to citizens of developing countries, whether antiretroviral therapy or basic public health measures. Further, it is unclear *upon whom* the duty to discharge this entitlement falls, whether researchers from developed countries or governments of developed countries. Moreover, the plausibility of an entitlement to expensive antiretrovirals depends upon the successful completion of the placebo-controlled trials. Only with a placebo control, they argue, will the governments of developing countries be provided with the information they need in order to make sound public health decisions.

Finally, Crouch and Arras raise objections to the charge that the proposed placebo-controlled studies exploit the women in the countries in question. They make a distinction between exploitative intentions and exploitative execution, and argue that the intentions of the researchers were clearly nonexploitative. Then, although they agree that sponsors must give some form of prior assurances that the study interventions will be made reasonably available to local populations, they raise a number of empirical and normative issues to which people must attend in determining whether a trial has been exploitative in execution or in the final analysis.

Next the participants in the 2001 Conference on Ethical Aspects of Research in Developing Countries focus on the idea of "reasonable availability" in their contribution to this volume. The authors advance several claims. First they argue that prior discussions have focused too narrowly on reasonable post-trial availability of study medications. This, they argue, is just one of many benefits that may accrue to the local population. Moreover, assurances that study medications will be made reasonably available to local populations after the study is completed are themselves insufficient as a protection against the exploitation of research participants. The authors thus articulate and defend the "Fair Benefits framework," which speaks directly to the issue of exploitation. The Fair Benefits framework, itself a moral prerequisite for research in developing countries, requires that (1) benefits, broadly construed to include more than the study medication, be distributed fairly; (2) all elements of the research be a product of a collaborative partnership between outside researchers and local populations; and (3) all discussion and collaboration be transparent and subject to public scrutiny.

The second theme discussed in this section centers on the manner in which informed consent is elicited from prospective research participants in developing countries, particularly when the researchers do not share their cultural background. Some have claimed that the informed consent requirements present in developed nations should not be applied when researchers from the developed world conduct research in developing nations. The informed consent requirement, based as it is on the Western value of autonomy, may be foreign in locales where autonomy and individual decisionmaking are valued to a lesser degree. Thus, some argue, international research can proceed without the individual informed consent requirement; rather, informed consent may be obtained from a trusted community leader, or similar surrogate, on behalf of the community members and prospective research participants.

The first author in this thematic subsection, Marcia Angell, frames her discussion with the following question: "Should ethical standards be substantially the same everywhere, or is it inevitable that they differ from region to region, reflecting local beliefs and custom?" It is Angell's view that investigators must always elicit first-person informed consent from research participants, no matter where they may reside. Failure to do so, she argues, implies that ethical standards are "matters of custom" rather than universal and substantive, much as human rights are often said to be. And while Angell is clear that local beliefs and values should be respected during the process of informed consent elicitation, she nonetheless believes that there is no ethically justifiable substitute for individual informed consent.

Nicholas A. Christakis takes a broader approach to this issue, attending to the manner in which informed consent should be elicited (and much else besides) by first asking a fundamental question: "Which ethics should govern transcultural clinical research?"

Christakis proposes, and ultimately rejects, four answers to this question: (1) there should be no transcultural research, (2) such research should satisfy both ethical systems, (3) a universal system of ethics should be abstracted from cross-cultural analysis, and (4) Western research ethics should apply universally. A problematic feature of all of these answers is that they fail to acknowledge that ethical systems are themselves cultural systems of thought. The solution that Christakis offers is one that engages the transcultural ethical differences such that both participant and researcher understand the other's ethical expectations in the research context. Therefore, Christakis rejects both ethical relativism and universalism (as he understands these positions) and opts instead for a form of ethical pluralism. Through negotiation and mutual understanding researcher and participant will, Christakis hopes, achieve the best possible solution to the practical problems raised by transcultural research, including informed consent elicitation.

This section closes with an in-depth case study and analysis by Richard R. Love and Norman C. Fost. The authors outline a novel approach to the problem of informed consent for a breast cancer study they conducted through the University of Wisconsin in Vietnam, where, the authors argue, patients rarely take an active medical decisionmaking role for themselves and choose instead to defer to their physician's judgment regarding treatment options. Love, the principal investigator of the study, felt that certain elements of the research design—namely, alternative treatment choices and randomization—would have to be omitted if informed consent were realistically to be elicited in this population. In other words, he proposed that women be randomized to a particular intervention; then their physician would inform them of the treatment they would receive without mention of alternatives or the fact that their treatment was chosen at random. He therefore met with two surrogate consent groups: Vietnamese immigrants living in the United States and "moral leaders" living in Vietnam, such as directors of the Vietnamese Women's Union. As Love and Fost point out, the approval of both surrogate groups—which was eventually granted—was an ethical prerequisite for the study to go forward. The University of Wisconsin IRB, however, called both for changes to the consent process to bring it more in line with U.S. regulations and for a consent-monitoring process to be initiated after the participants had been enrolled. As Love and Fost conclude, through the use of surrogate consent groups a slightly less rigorous consent process was successfully used in this study, with participants demonstrating an acceptable level of understanding regarding most features of their participation.

1. Ezekiel J. Emanuel, David Wendler, and Christine Grady, "What Makes Clinical Research Ethical?" *JAMA* 283 (2000): 2701–11.

2. Lisa S. Parker and Charles W. Lidz, "Familial Coercion to Participate in Genetic Family Studies: Is There Cause for IRB Intervention?" *IRB: A Review of Human Subjects Research* 16, nos. 1 and 2 (1994): 6–12.

3. Roberta G. Simmons, Susan K. Marine, and Richard L. Simmons, *The Gift of Life* (New Brunswick, N.J.: Transaction Books, 1987).

4. Parker and Lidz, 8.

5. Barbara P. Fuller, Mary Jo Ellis Kahn, Patricia A. Barr, et al., "Privacy in Genetics Research," *Science* 285 (1999): 1359–61; and Charles L. Earley and Louise C. Strong, "Certificates of Confidentiality: A Valuable Tool for Protecting Genetic Data," *American Journal of Human Genetics* 57 (1995): 727–31.

6. Eric Kodish, Thomas H. Murray, and Susan Shurin, "Cancer Risk Research: What Should We Tell Subjects?" *Clinical Research* 42, no. 3 (1994): 396–402.

7. National Bioethics Advisory Commission (NBAC), Research Involving Human Biological Materials: Ethical Issues and Policy Guidance (Rockville, Md.: NBAC, August 1999).

8. American College of Medical Genetics (ACMG) Storage of Genetics Materials Committee, "Statement on Storage and Use of Genetic Materials," *American Journal of Human Genetics* 57 (1995): 1499–1500; American Society of Human Genetics (ASHG), "Statement on Informed Consent for Genetic Research," *American Journal of Human Genetics* 59 (1996): 471–74; and William Grizzle, Wayne W. Grody, Walter W. Noll, et al., Ad Hoc Committee on Stored Tissues, College of American Pathologists, "Recommended Policies for Uses of Human Tissue in Research, Education, and Quality Control," *Archives of Pathology and Laboratory Medicine* 123 (1999): 296–300.

9. National Action Plan on Breast Cancer, "Consent Form for Use of Tissue for Research," May 1997. This consent form is included in the appendix of this volume and is available at the (U.S. DHHS) National Women's Health Information Center Web site at www.4woman.gov/napbc/catalog.wci/napbc/consent.htm.

10. John A. Robertson, "Symbolic Issues in Embryo Research," *Hastings Center Report* 25, no. 1 (1995): 37–38.

11. Ruth Macklin, "Ethics, Politics, and Human Embryo Stem Cell Research," *Women's Health Issues* 10 (2000): 111–15.

12. John A. Robertson, "Ethics and Policy in Embryonic Stem Cell Research," *Kennedy Institute Ethics Journal* 9 (1999): 109–36.

13. Macklin, 114.

14. Charles Weijer, "Placebo Controlled Trials in Schizophrenia: Are They Ethical? Are They Necessary?" *Schizophrenia Research* 35 (1999): 211–18.

15. William T. Carpenter, Nina R. Schooler, and John M. Kane, "The Rationale and Ethics of Medication-Free Research in Schizophrenia," *Archives of General Psychiatry* 54 (1997): 401–7.

16. Franklin G. Miller and Christine Grady, "The Ethical Challenge of Infection-Inducing Challenge Experiments," *Clinical Infectious Diseases* 33 (2001): 1028–33.

17. Alex J. London, "The Ambiguity and the Exigency: Clarifying 'Standard of Care' Arguments in International Research," *Journal of Medicine and Philosophy* 25 (2000): 379–97.

18. Marc Lallemant, Gonzague Jourdain, Sophie Le Coeur, et al. for the Perinatal HIV Prevention Trial (Thailand) Investigators, "A Trial of Shortened Zidovudine Regimens to Prevent Mother-to-Child Transmission of Human Immunodeficiency Virus Type 1," *New England Journal of Medicine* 343 (2000): 982–91.

Section One

Genetics Research

48 Structuring the Review of Human Genetics Protocols

Gene Localization and Identification Studies

KATHLEEN CRANLEY GLASS, CHARLES WEIJER,
ROBERTA M. PALMOUR, STANLEY H. SHAPIRO,
TRUDO LEMMENS, AND KAREN LEBACQZ

[...] Institutional review board (IRB) members have begun to ask whether or how genetics protocols fit into the ordinary review structure. [...] The challenge in their review of genetics research is to recognize when a particular protocol raises new issues, and if so, whether they are addressed appropriately by the investigators. [...]

GENE LOCALIZATION AND IDENTIFICATION PROTOCOLS

All gene localization and identification studies share the common goal of placing information about human genes in a systematic linear order according to their relative positions along each chromosome. The intent of these studies is to identify genes that cause or contribute to a disease or trait. This is typically done first by finding the approximate chromosomal position of the gene ("mapping"), and then by determining the identity of the gene.

There is no single, ready review model that will be appropriate for every protocol or every IRB. In the schema provided in Table [48.1], we have suggested a number of questions that will be relevant for many gene localization and identification studies. [...]

Kathleen Cranley Glass, Charles Weijer, Roberta M. Palmour, Stanley H. Shapiro, Trudo Lemmens, and Karen Lebacqz, "Structuring the Review of Human Genetics Protocols: Gene Localization and Identification Studies," *IRB: A Review of Human Subjects Research* 18, no. 4 (1996): 1–9.

DISCUSSION

Evaluating a protocol's validity and value. [...] Gene localization and identification studies pose some special questions for the evaluation of validity and value.

[...] IRBs must evaluate the concordance between the hypothesis and methodology used. A research design that leads to false conclusions may be unethical because actions based upon those conclusions may have adverse consequences. Invalid research also raises ethical issues of justice if scarce resources are wasted. [...]

[I]nclusion criteria for a pedigree study create an extremely narrow group of potential subjects who are not interchangeable in the same way subjects in other protocols may be. IRBs need to ask how valid the results will be if investigators do not succeed in recruiting everyone they have identified. Another factor affecting subject selection relates to how carefully cases and controls must be matched for ethnicity in a "gene-hunting" study using this design. Expertise in research design and statistics as well as background knowledge in genetics will be required to evaluate a protocol's validity. IRBs lacking such expertise must call on outside consultants to assist their review. [...]

Is it within the IRB's mandate to evaluate the wider social impact, positive or negative, of a protocol? Should it ask whether the proposed research has sufficient value to offset any risks, not just to the subjects, but to wider populations? United States regulations appear to answer these questions in the negative, stating that the IRB should not consider as "research risks over which it has responsibility" the possible long-range effects of applying the knowledge gained in the research. The effects of the research on public policy are cited as an example (45 CFR 46.111(a)). While there are indications that this requirement was established specifi-

Table 48.1
Schema for IRB Review of "Gene-Hunting" Protocols

[Questions marked with an asterisk refer to issues of particular relevance in genetics protocols.—eds.]

BACKGROUND AND JUSTIFICATION

What questions does the research address? Has the investigator demonstrated that the research has scientific or medical value? How does the proposed study relate to previous work? Does it provide a rational continuation of this work?

> *If not,* have the innovative aspects been adequately justified?

RESEARCH DESIGN

Is the scientific method to be employed valid? Has it been used previously, and if so, how has it been assessed? What quality controls are built into the method?

Is the planned statistical analysis appropriate (i.e., is it likely to provide valid and unbiased answers to the study question)?

> * If a full genome scan is planned,
> Does the sample size provide sufficient power to identify one or more loci with a reasonable degree of certainty?
> Are population-specific allele frequencies already known? If not, how will they be determined?
> * If the trait to be mapped is complex, will robust nonparametric methods of analysis (which do not necessarily require a Mendelian model) be used first?
>> *If not,* is there good justification for this?
> * If the study is a case-control study, are the cases and controls carefully matched for ethnicity?
> * Is there adequate consideration and/or statistical correction for multiple comparisons (which may number in the hundreds for genome scans), and is the procedure to be used described clearly?

PROCEDURES

What procedures are involved in the study (e.g., medical examinations, blood draws, tissue/tumor donation, questionnaires, interviews, etc.)? How many? How often? How much time will they take?

Are all of the procedures in this study required to answer the research question? Can any be eliminated?

Will procedures for obtaining or maintaining information involve a data/DNA bank? Is stored tissue involved? Will the data/DNA be destroyed at any point? Will identifiers be maintained with the stored data/DNA?

> * Will subjects be asked to allow investigators to contact them in the future for more information or to participate in further research?
> * Who will have access to information about those studied (including information about "nonparticipating" family members)? Will informed consent be sought to use the data/DNA in other studies? Under what conditions, if any, will data or DNA be released to other investigators?
> * Are the procedures for maintaining confidentiality of data/records/database information specified clearly (e.g., encryption, use of unique identifiers, sequestering of records, security measures)? Are they adequate?

SUBJECT SELECTION

How is the study population defined? Does it include affected and/or unaffected individuals, related or unrelated? Are healthy controls included?

Table 48.1. Continued

Have the eligibility criteria been justified? Do they strike a defensible balance between scientific validity and generalizability (i.e., is the study population sufficiently restricted to yield interpretable results without being unduly restrictive)?

How are subjects to be recruited? Will they be remunerated?
   If so, is the amount or nature of the remuneration appropriate?

   * If the study involves families, how will family members be recruited? By the proband [affected person—eds.]? By the family physician? Through support groups or lay organizations? By investigators directly?
   * Will the proposed recruitment process place undue pressure on other family members to participate?
   * Might recruitment itself "inflict" unwanted information about risk status on family members?
Are adequate procedures in place to protect the interests of these people?
   * Does the protocol involve "nonparticipating" family members about whom subjects will provide personal/medical information?
   * Does the protocol include incompetent subjects (young children or incompetent adults)? Is there a valid alternative to their participation in this protocol?
   If not, have provisions been made for assent and/or proxy consent?
   * Does the protocol involve other vulnerable populations (e.g., patients with Alzheimer disease or psychosis who have periods of fluctuating competence)? Have their special needs been taken into account?

RISKS AND BENEFITS

Is the importance of the research question sufficient to justify risks associated with the procedures specific to the research (i.e., the dedicated research procedures)?

Have risks been minimized to the extent possible?

   * Will participation in the protocol result in any benefit to subjects? Will the results have any predictive value for subjects in terms of life or health choices (e.g., marriage, reproductive choices, choice of employment, medical treatment, disease prevention)?
   * Are instances of nonpaternity or incest likely to be uncovered by the research? How will these be handled (e.g., disclosure of the possibility in consent materials, withdrawal of the samples from the research)?
   * Will the knowledge gained by the subjects about their current or future health or their carrier status pose additional risks to them, such as risks to insurability, employability, immigration, paternity suits, or social stigma? Have adequate provisions been made for privacy and confidentiality of subject information, including for "nonparticipating subjects"?
   * Could the research result in stereotyping or stigmatizing a particular community or cultural group? Have investigators taken steps to approach the group involved and solicit comments where appropriate?
   * Will a family pedigree be published? Will the method or occasions of publication or presentation of findings contain the potential for identifying family members?
   If so, have the affected individuals given consent to the publication or presentation of private information about them?

INFORMATION TO SUBJECTS

Does the information provided to prospective subjects adequately inform them of what is being studied and why, details about study procedures, known risks and benefits as well as uncertainties about risks and benefits, and alternatives to participation?

   * If there is no individual benefit to subjects, has this been disclosed?

(continued on next page)

Table 48.1. Continued

* Have subjects been told of their right to withdraw from the research without penalty or loss of benefits to which they are otherwise entitled? Have they been advised of any consequences of withdrawal? Are there any limitations on the ability of subjects to withdraw their data or DNA samples?

> *If so,* has this been adequately disclosed?

* Is it clear to subjects what information will be revealed to whom and under what circumstances (e.g., participants may learn about other family members' risk status)?

* Will subjects be informed of any special risks associated with the study (e.g., changes in family relationships, risks to privacy, confidentiality, insurability, employability, immigration status, paternity suits, educational opportunities)?

* Will the general study results be made available to subjects?

* If no immediately useful or interpretable information of relevance to subjects is likely to result from the study, has this been adequately explained?

* If information that is clinically relevant to subjects is likely to result, will counseling by genetic counselors be made available?

* Have subjects been given the option of individually choosing not to receive their study results?

* Could other clinically relevant information be uncovered during the study? If so, how will it be disclosed to subjects? Who will disclose it (e.g., investigators, genetic counselors, the family physician)?

Will there be any costs associated with participating (including the cost of genetic counseling or psycho/social counseling) that are not covered by the investigator or the institution? If so, has this been disclosed?

COMMERCIAL INTERESTS

* Does anyone have a commercial interest in the research?

> *If so,* who (e.g., third parties, the investigator)? Have the subjects been informed of these commercial interests?

* Where commercial products may eventually be developed from biological materials removed from the subjects in the course of the research, will subjects be asked to waive any rights or control over the tissue?

> *If they refuse,* will they be allowed to participate?

cally to deal with social science research, [...] the regulations as written reflect a model from clinical treatment—that of the physician and patient in a private relationship of two autonomous individuals. While such a model may be appropriate for protocols in which the risks are borne entirely by the individual subject, it may not serve well in the context of some genetics protocols, where the adverse impact may be felt by other individuals or an entire community. Ethics guidelines for social science research that require attention to the welfare and integrity not only of the individual subject, but of the particular collective, may be helpful. Risks to subjects and families and to wider communities can be reduced (though not eliminated) with stringent requirements for confidentiality of information or, where appropriate, collaboration with community groups in trial design and procedures for disseminating results to minimize any adverse impact.

[...] Judgments of value must include a view about the significance of the hypothesis itself for reasons of its nov-elty, clinical and/or scientific interests, and also for any other social implications. This requires the participation of an inter-disciplinary group, going beyond clinical and scientific expertise to include those with experience in law and ethics as well as representatives of the community in general. [...]

Genetics and the family. The existing paradigm of research ethics is the autonomous individual who makes an informed choice about participation. This paradigm emphasizes the importance of full disclosure of material information to prospective subjects, who should be free to make their choices without undue influence, coercion, or pressure. [...]

Many genetics protocols challenge this paradigm in at least two ways. First, genetic information is by its nature about families. [...] Second, cooperation of family members may be relevant to obtaining information that is key to the success of the research. [...] For a successful study, not only must family members be willing to participate, in some research they must also agree to share information about their genetic constitutions with other family members as well as with investigators. [...]

[...] As part of a family, we may be morally required to make decisions on the basis of thinking about what is best for all concerned, not simply what is best for ourselves. The Danish Council of Ethics goes so far as to suggest that since genetic information can be of crucial importance for allowing others to make appropriate health care decisions, genes are, in a way, a part of the "public domain."

While genetic research certainly challenges our traditional notions of the autonomous individual as research subject, we are not convinced that any moral obligation family members may have toward each other is enforceable, particularly by investigators or IRBs. [...]

In the absence of a paradigm that could protect subjects as well as "voluntary informed choice" while at the same time incorporating notions of interactive relationships and family solidarity, we can highlight several elements that IRBs should consider in their review of protocols requiring the participation of families.

Pressure on family members to participate in protocols.

[...] Genetic research involves close personal relationships entailing a range of actions and emotions—love, affection, obligation, gratitude, jealousy, advice, support, criticism, fear of disapproval, argument, security, or insecurity. No one can control how families will deal with genetic issues, nor can they predict individual coping strategies. [...]

Appelbaum and Lidz distinguish between pressures that affect human behavior so extremely as to deprive it of legal consequences, and those pressures that form a necessary component of socialization and education. "Human interaction can never be free of pressures that one person consciously or unconsciously places on another. Many pressures are inherent in such interaction and constitute a normal and often desirable part of relationships." These pressures exist naturally within families and are often intended to influence another's behavior. An IRB should not be concerned with eliminating family interactions, including those that are characterized as persuasion, manipulation, or even pressure, but with minimizing opportunities for going beyond this natural boundary by using undue influence or coercion that inhibits a voluntary consent to participate.

Making judgments concerning the nature of pressures is difficult because of individual family dynamics and the impact of context on a particular action. Actions that might be coercive in one family or circumstance might not be in another. Discussions family members might have with one another may be completely appropriate, whereas the same conversations would not be appropriate if they involved an investigator and prospective subjects. IRBs would therefore have difficulty establishing policies that define in advance what any particular family member might perceive as coercive. They can, however, impress upon investigators their obligation to inform prospective subjects in a nonthreatening, noncoercive manner. Where a protocol calls for family members to inform relatives about the study, the information they present should emphasize that each individual has the right to choose whether to participate. Where there are obvious reasons to suspect coercion or undue influence, investigators could explore with potential subjects their motivation for participation. Obviously the desire to help a relative is not an automatic indication of coercion. Such a motive may be purely altruistic.

Unwanted information and the right "not to know."

[W]hat if the recruitment process itself has the potential to harm a prospective subject, before that subject has the opportunity of choosing whether to participate? Such may be the case where family members are recruited into gene localization or identification studies. Persons who are unaware of the incidence of a disease in their family, who have not sought information concerning their own risk of developing the disease based on family patterns, or who may resolve their anxiety or emotional conflict by denying that the disease is an issue for them, may have a right "not to know" they and their families are at risk. [...] "Inflicting" unwanted information about risk status on family members could conceivably pose risks for privacy, confidentiality, employability, insurability, immigration status, paternity suits, as well as create the potential for a duty to warn relatives of at-risk status.

Protocol implementation may also disturb family secrets, either contemporary or from past generations, that could affect a genetic analysis. Facts such as adoption, incest, artificial insemination, nonpaternity, pregnancies, or permanent institutionalization because of mental illness are frequently hidden from at least some family members. Participation in research should not jeopardize family relationships by imposing information on those who have not sought to have it; nor should it "extract" secrets from those unwilling to share them.

The issue of harm is particularly sensitive in gene localization and identification studies since for the most part participation offers subjects no benefit beyond the opportunity for altruism. [...] While investigators should use the most sensitive recruiting techniques possible, the potential for this harm cannot be eliminated completely. This fact should alert IRBs to the necessity for careful review of the protocol's value [...].

Research subject access to test tesults.

[T]he principle of respect for persons is tempered by the principle of beneficence: the decision to disclose test results must involve a consideration of the risks and benefits of disclosure. Geneticists have exhibited a strong commitment to both principles and to the sharing of genetic information with research participants. Some geneticists—perhaps taking the principle of respect for persons to its extreme—believe that test results must always be disclosed at the subject's request, even when the meaning of a test result is uncertain. [...]

Reilly, among others, argues convincingly that the decision to disclose the results of a genetic test in the context of research must involve some consideration of the harms and benefits of disclosure as well as the accuracy of the test information. He argues that the IRB policy on disclosure in an individual study should be based on consideration of at least three factors:

> (1) the magnitude of the threat posed to the subject, (2) the accuracy with which the data predict that the threat will be realized, and (3) the possibility that action can be taken to avoid or ameliorate the potential injury.

Based on this analysis, test results can be grouped into results that must be disclosed, those that may be disclosed, and those that ought not to be disclosed. [...]

While this sort of calculus can be applied to any individual study, can we define a set of cases in which *in principle* test results ought not be disclosed? One conceivable approach is that the results of tests that are not clinically validated should not be revealed. [...] This approach is untenable [...]. [T]he criterion fails to take into account the fact that some experimental genetic tests may reveal information that calls for action. For example, while not enough is known about the efficacy of prevention strategies for women carrying the BRCA1 gene, a woman with the gene certainly requires close medical follow-up and the option of unproven prevention strategies (mammography, mastectomy, tamoxifen) ought to be discussed with her.

Might we, then, take the position that experimental test results that do not entail clinical action—i.e., useless test results—should be withheld from subjects? Kodish, Murray, and Shurin argue for just such a standard. Acknowledging a general obligation to disclose test results, they point out that:

> There exists . . . a threshold below which the meaning of scientific data does not attain clinical relevance, and for which there is no corresponding obligation to disclose results. We suggest that this threshold be defined as data that are sufficiently clear in clinical implications to affect the medical care of the subject.

Upon examination, this stance, as a blanket criterion, seems untenable. Even if a test result has no direct clinical implications (i.e., there are no known prevention strate-

gies), subjects may nonetheless benefit from information that reduces uncertainty regarding the condition for which they are at risk. [...]

[W]e are left with a restricted set of cases in which disclosure would be inappropriate: test results that are uninformative. If respect for persons implies a right to medical information, this cannot include a right to test results that are not "information." When a test is so preliminary that results are unlikely to affect the individual's risk assessment, the subject's autonomy is not furthered by knowing these results. Such circumstances are, of course, not uncommon in "gene-hunting" studies. Obvious cases in which test results are unlikely to be informative include: preliminary linkage or association studies, studies involving a population in which the association between genotype and disease is not established, and those where the subjects' genotypes at the many marker loci are not found to be linked to the disease gene.

One study [...] provides a useful illustration of how such a case might be handled by an IRB. The study in question proposed to examine the association between apolipoprotein-E [APO-E4] and Alzheimer disease (AD) in a cohort of Jewish and French-Canadian individuals. Although the association between APO-E4 and AD is fairly well established, the association had not been documented in this patient population. Indeed, a pilot project by the study investigators (with 40 patients) failed to reveal any association between APO-E4 and AD in this population. The study planned to enroll 100 persons with Alzheimer disease, 100 with cognitive impairment not yet diagnosed, and 288 age-matched healthy controls. All subjects would be tested for the APO-E genotype.

Believing that research participants have a right to know their own test results, the investigators planned to inform subjects of their APO-E status. The IRB questioned the propriety of disclosing results to subjects if indeed it was not known what those results meant. The committee's letter to the investigator stated:

> Why are subjects being offered the test result when the pilot showed no relationship between the allele and AD? If it means nothing, or at least, is not currently known to mean anything, subject autonomy is not served by informing them. We recommend that you include an information waiver—"I understand that the results of this test will not be made available to me. . . ." [...]

When test results are so preliminary as to be uninformative, patient autonomy is not served by sharing this information with subjects. In the context of gene-hunting studies, we suspect that this will often be the case. If subjects will not be informed of test results, they must be made aware of this fact up-front, at the time when they are approached for consent. This does not imply that test results must be disclosed in all other cases. Rather, the decision to disclose "informative" test results should be based on considerations of respect for persons and beneficence as outlined by Reilly.

[Glossary omitted—eds.]

49 Structuring the Review of Human Genetics Protocols, Part II

Diagnostic and Screening Studies

KATHLEEN CRANLEY GLASS, CHARLES WEIJER, TRUDO LEMMENS, ROBERTA M. PALMOUR, AND STANLEY H. SHAPIRO

[...]

GENETIC DIAGNOSTIC AND SCREENING PROTOCOLS

Distinguishing diagnostic and screening tests. Genetic tests are used in two distinct sets of circumstances: diagnosis and screening. Clinicians use diagnostic tests either to confirm or to exclude certain diagnoses in their patients. [. . .] Screening has been defined as the identification, among apparently healthy individuals, of those who are sufficiently at risk of a specific disorder to justify a subsequent diagnostic test or procedure. [...] *Genetic screening* differs from a diagnostic test in that a screening test may be insufficiently sensitive [. . .] to allow definitive diagnosis, and therefore calls for further testing, rather than immediate therapeutic intervention. [...]

Levels of genetic testing. There are five operational levels of genetic testing based on different screening techniques:

Clinical phenotype: structural or functional changes associated with the genotype may be obvious or easily identifiable. [...]

Chromosomes: the number and structure of chromosomes may be surveyed in appropriately cultured and stained cells using a light microscope. This is done with amniocytes when women of advanced maternal age are screened to detect a fetus affected by chromosomal aberrations, or in infants suspected of having Down syndrome or other chromosomal abnormalities.

Metabolite level: blood, urine, and other bodily fluids may be tested for evidence of metabolic disorder secondary to genetic disorder. Measurement of phenylalanine in neonatal blood as a screen for PKU is an example. Diagnosis of Lesch-Nyhan disease may be suspected on the basis of elevated levels of urinary uric acid.

Polypeptide or protein level: the mutant protein, that is, the gene product itself, may be identifiable. In Tay-Sachs, carriers may be identified by electrophoresis or measurement of serum hexosaminidase A activity. Enzyme assay is the most generalizable way of diagnosing Lesch-Nyhan disease.

DNA level: the DNA itself may be analyzed for genetic mutations known to occur in specific populations or families. Molecular testing is used in a variety of circumstances, including general population screening, screening groups at risk, or diagnostic tests for individuals at risk. Techniques such as polymerase chain reaction (PCR), single strand gel electrophoresis, single strand conformational polymorphism (SSCP), multiplexing, and direct sequencing of DNA are used.

Developing a genetic test: There are a number of stages in developing diagnostic and screening tests. Institutional review boards (IRBs) will encounter protocols in all of these stages before they are incorporated into clinical practice. Initially, an indication may emerge from a basic study that a test might reveal, in a cost-effective manner, a condi-

Kathleen Cranley Glass, Charles Weijer, Trudo Lemmens, Roberta M. Palmour, and Stanley H. Shapiro, "Structuring the Review of Human Genetics Protocols, Part II: Diagnostic and Screening Studies," *IRB: A Review of Human Subjects Research* 19, nos. 3 and 4 (1997): 1–11, 13.

tion that would benefit from medical attention or that might be useful to members of the general public. The test would operate at one of the levels discussed above [...] and could then be used to assist diagnosis. To move such a test into screening, the condition should be relatively common in the population selected for screening. Pilot projects would then be required to assess the test's performance (sensitivity and specificity, discussed below). Until this is established, test results are meaningless to the individuals. For this reason, many of these pilot studies are done with anonymous samples. Once performance has been demonstrated, additional studies may be done to determine the cost effectiveness of applying the test to larger populations. Psychosocial or other issues that may emerge from having the test available may also be studied. [...]

SCHEMA FOR REVIEW

Table [49.1] contains a series of questions IRBs may want to ask when reviewing testing and screening protocols. [...]

DISCUSSION

[...] The discussion below is limited to three issues that we believe are of central importance for appropriate review of these protocols: uncertainty of clinical prediction, research with communities [omitted—eds.], and confidentiality of test results.

Genetic testing and screening and the uncertainty of clinical prediction. [...] Receiving accurate information on the anticipated predictive value of a testing or screening protocol is important to an IRB for a number of reasons. First, the accuracy of the results and their consequent usefulness to research subjects will be a determining factor in the investigator's and the IRB's consideration of whether individual research test results should be disclosed to subjects. Second, in undertaking its risk-benefit analysis, the IRB must weigh the scientific, clinical, and in some cases, social usefulness of the test or screen. The predictive value will likely affect all of these. [...]

Quality of the technology, equipment or laboratory facilities, and personnel. How good is the technology or equipment being used for the test? How difficult are the results to interpret and how skilled are those charged with the interpretation? What quality control procedures are in place for dealing with ambiguous results? [...] Test results are [...] only as good as the equipment and personnel involved. [...] Subjects who receive test results must know whether those results are in any way limited or compromised.

In the United States, the Clinical Laboratories Improvement Act (CLIA) requires the accreditation of virtually all laboratories providing genetic test results.

Sensitivity or specificity of the test. [...] First, if the disease (or genetic mutation or gene product) is present, what is the likelihood that the test result will be positive? In other words, how *sensitive* is the proposed test? Second, if the disease (or genetic mutation or gene product) is absent, what is the probability that the test result will be negative? That is, what is the *specificity* of the proposed test?

IRB members should ask how frequently a result is expected to be falsely negative or falsely positive, and what impact this will have on the person receiving the results. For example, there should be a very low false negative rate for screening tests, such as the maternal alpha-fetoprotein exam, and a low false positive rate for the follow-up diagnostic test (chromosome analysis or ultrasound visualization of abnormalities) because of the potential for erroneously aborting an unaffected fetus.

The role of false positives and false negatives should be thoroughly explored in the context of the importance of the results and the existence of confirmatory testing. The prenatal alpha-fetoprotein test, for example, gives many false positive results, and it becomes relevant, therefore, how these results are handled. What steps will be taken with a positive test result? Will the test be repeated? [...] Is there an additional diagnostic tool that can be employed (e.g., ultrasound, amniocentesis) to confirm the accuracy of the testing process?

Penetrance, age of onset, and clinical expression. Genetic information concerning many disorders remains probabilistic in nature. [...] Even in monogenic conditions, there may be variability in the expression of the disease. The degree of severity cannot usually be predicted by a genetic test, even a test for a particular mutation. [...] Both the protocol and the information provided to subjects should accurately reflect how these variables apply to the condition being tested.

Reliability of the results. When is a genetic test ready for clinical use? [...] Investigators should provide IRBs with information concerning the stage of development of the test.

Availability of therapy or prevention or implications for life choices. Diagnostic tests are generally used when patient clinical care or life choices can be influenced. Where safe and effective therapy or prevention strategies exist that have been accepted as standard practice, providing the information necessary for patients to make appropriate choices is clearly in their best interests. [...] Where there is no therapy, and prevention strategies are unproven, as with BRCA1, the question of testing is ethically more questionable. [...]

IRBs should distinguish between diagnostic testing of individuals and screening programs aimed at groups by

Table 49.1
Schema for IRB Review of Genetic Diagnostic/Screening Protocols

Questions marked with an asterisk refer to issues of particular relevance in genetics protocols.

BACKGROUND AND JUSTIFICATION

What questions does the research address? Has the investigator demonstrated that the research has scientific or medical value?

How does the proposed study relate to previous work? Have any innovative aspects been adequately justified?

   * If the study concerns a diagnostic test, in what (clinical or other) situations will this test be helpful?

RESEARCH DESIGN

Is the scientific method to be employed valid? Has it been used previously, and if so, how has it been assessed? What quality controls are built into the method?

Is the planned statistical analysis appropriate (i.e., is it likely to provide valid answers to the study questions)?

   * For diagnostic studies, how is the condition (or risk thereof) currently diagnosed? Will the new diagnostic strategy be compared with the best available standard test?
   * What is known about the nature and frequency of genetic polymorphisms related to the study condition?
      If the study is a diagnostic protocol: How does the existence of polymorphisms affect the ability to define risk thresholds (cutoffs)?
      If the study is a screening protocol: How does the frequency of polymorphisms affect the feasibility of population screening?
   * Is it likely that other genes are required for full trait expression?
   * If subjects will be informed of the test results, does the study design provide for an adequate assessment of the psychosocial impact of genetic testing?

PROCEDURES

What research-specific procedures are involved in the study (e.g., physical examinations, blood tests, tissue/tumor donation, questionnaires, interviews, etc.)? How many? How often? How much time will they take? Are they all required to answer the research question?

   * If long-term follow-up is required, over what period of time will this take place?
   * What are the procedures for obtaining or maintaining information in a data/DNA bank (e.g., use of identifiers, limitation on access, need for a second consent, sharing with other investigators, duration of storage, future subject contact)?
   * Are adequate procedures in place for maintaining security and confidentiality of data/records/database information specified clearly (e.g., encryption, use of unique identifiers, sequestering of records)?

SUBJECT SELECTION

(for questions related to recruitment of families at risk, see our earlier paper [included in this volume—eds.])

   * How is the study population defined?
      If the study is a diagnostic protocol: Does it include affected and/or unaffected individuals, related or unrelated? Are healthy controls included?
      If the study is a screening protocol: How is the population at risk defined and why was it chosen? (General population? Targeted population—prenatal, newborns, young children, adolescents, adults, at-risk population?)

Have the eligibility criteria been justified? Do they strike a defensible balance between scientific validity and generalizability (i.e., is the study population sufficiently, but not unduly, restricted so as to yield interpretable results)?

(continued on next page)

Table 49.1. Continued

How are subjects to be recruited? If remuneration is provided, is the amount or nature appropriate?

* Does the protocol target members of an indigenous or other identifiable community? Have appropriate measures been included to take account of this fact (e.g., approaching community leaders, soliciting collaboration where appropriate)?

* Does the protocol include or target newborns or other young children? If so, is the study condition one that manifests or requires initiation of preventive measures in childhood? Have provisions been made for children's assent, where appropriate, and consent of the parents/guardians?

* Does the protocol include or target adolescent subjects? If so, is the study condition one which has implications for health at this age? For reproductive planning? Have provisions been made for counseling, taking account of any special needs of subjects in this age group?

* Does the protocol include incompetent adults? Is there a valid alternative to their participation? If not, have provisions been made for assent, where appropriate, and/or proxy consent?

If children or incompetent adults are included in the protocol, is there any conflict of interest between the research subjects and the parent/guardian giving consent? If so, how will the subjects' interests be protected?

* Does the protocol involve other vulnerable populations (e.g., patients with Alzheimer disease or psychosis who have periods of fluctuating competence)? Have their special needs been taken into account?

RISKS AND BENEFITS

(for questions related to nonpaternity, publication of pedigrees, and risks resulting in discrimination, see our earlier paper [included in this volume—eds.])

Is the importance of the research question sufficient to justify the research-specific risks? Have risks to subjects been minimized?

* Will participation in the study result in any benefit to subjects? Will the results be informative for participants in terms of life or health choices?

* Will knowledge gained by the subjects about their current or future health or their carrier status pose additional risks to them, such as risks to insurability, employability, immigration, paternity suits, educational opportunities, or social stigma? Have adequate provisions been made for privacy and confidentiality of subject information?

* Could the research result in stereotyping or stigmatizing a particular community or cultural group?

Have investigators taken steps to approach the group involved and solicit comments where appropriate?

* Is psychological support required for those determined to be at risk? How will it be provided?

INFORMATION TO SUBJECTS

(for questions pertaining to the participation of families, see our earlier paper [included in this volume—eds.])

Does the information to be provided to prospective subjects adequately inform them of what is being studied and why; details about study procedures, known risks, discomforts, and benefits; and alternatives to participation?

* Will subjects be adequately informed if the study objective is to assess unknown risks?

* Will subjects be adequately informed of any limitations of the test/screen results as a predictor of clinical risk?

* Will subjects be informed of any special risks associated with the study (e.g., risks to privacy, confidentiality, insurability, employability, immigration status, paternity suits, educational opportunities, or social stigma)?

Table 49.1. Continued

 * If no immediately useful or interpretable information of relevance to subjects is likely to result from the study, will this be disclosed adequately to subjects in advance of their participation?
 * Will subjects be told of their right to withdraw from the research without penalty or loss of benefits? Will they be advised of any consequences of, or limitations on, withdrawal, including withdrawal of data or DNA samples?

Will the general study results be made available to subjects?

 * Could other clinically relevant information be uncovered during the study? Who will disclose it (investigator, genetic counselor, family physician)?
 * Will genetic counselors be available to transmit relevant information to subjects?
 * Will subjects be given the opportunity *not* to receive their test results?
 * Will there be any monetary costs to the subject associated with participation (including the cost of counseling)? Will this be disclosed to subjects?

COMMERCIAL INTERESTS

 * Will subjects be informed of anyone having a commercial interest in the research (e.g., investigator, pharmaceutical or biotechnology company sponsor, university or hospital, government agency)?
 * When commercial products may eventually be developed from biological materials removed from subjects, will subjects be asked to waive any rights or control over the tissue? If they refuse, will they be allowed to participate?

asking what role the test results will play in the lives of the recipients. An individual patient for whom diagnostic testing is recommended should be in a position to understand his or her risk status and discuss the advantages, disadvantages, and implications of a genetic test with a knowledgeable physician or genetic counselor before making a choice as to whether to undergo a genetic diagnostic test. This would include any health or life choices that might be affected by the knowledge the test would bring, as well as the psychosocial impact of receiving test results. This is not the case with genetic screening programs, which are generally undertaken with groups of apparently healthy or asymptomatic individuals to determine who is predisposed to a disease or risks passing it on to descendants. In general, there is no professional-patient relationship, no opportunity to assess the psychosocial impact of testing on any single individual. It is therefore important when undertaking screening programs of the general population or certain at-risk groups to have specific objectives in mind, including therapy or preventive strategies. The programs should then be designed to best achieve those objectives. [...]

[...] Knowledge of one's genetic profile may have little value for its own sake. It may have advantages and disadvantages for specific reasons, many of them personal. As a consequence, in undertaking their assessment of projected risk and anticipated benefit, IRB members must ask what purpose will be served by giving subjects their test results. [...]

Genetics, risk assessment, and confidentiality. Genetic information, perhaps more than any other health information, could have harmful social consequences for individuals when used in contexts such as employment, insurance, and immigration. Cases have been reported of people with asymptomatic genetic predisposition who were excluded from employment or insurance. [T]his has raised the question of how researchers can best protect the confidentiality of genetic data in their studies. [...]

Confidentiality: promises and waivers. Research consent forms normally contain clauses of confidentiality. Moreover, codes of professional ethics impose a duty of confidentiality on physicians, geneticists, and other health care workers. They can be held liable for the consequences of illegitimate release of confidential information. Personal information contained in medical files belongs to those to whom this information pertains. These individuals can thus decide who should, and who should not have access to these intimate data, and thus can waive their right to confidentiality. Insurance contracts normally contain a clause permitting insurers to access medical files. While physicians and other health care workers are obliged to respect the confidentiality of medical information, they must also respect a patient's or subject's explicit authorization to give access. Codes of professional ethics provide that health care workers can divulge medical information when the patient permits them to do so.

Furthermore, the same codes contain another exception: physicians must divulge medical information if the law obliges them to do so. Not only does the law provide that health care workers have to respect the contractual stipulations of those toward whom they have a duty of confidentiality, but courts can also oblige physicians to give access without explicit waiver of confidentiality. This will be the case in court procedures where the issue is the state of health of a person and where parties obtain access to medical files in order to prepare a full and fair defense. Legal disputes related to life and health insurance frequently focus on the pre-existing medical condition of applicants. In these cases, insurers may obtain access to medical files, even when there is no explicit waiver of confidentiality.

Confidentiality and research files. [. . .] When access to medical files is requested, either by courts or on the basis of a waiver of confidentiality, can researchers adequately protect research subjects by refusing access?

There appears to be no standard for how or where research results should be maintained. Research subjects are recruited into genetics trials in a variety of ways: by their physicians who are also investigators; by probands who in turn recruit family members; by investigators—both physicians and nonphysicians—who advertise publicly or recruit through support groups or other lay organizations; by trial groups such as those associated with the National Cancer Institute who seek DNA samples from symptomatic subjects enrolled in trials of nongenetic therapies. There is also variety in how and where research data are kept. [. . .]

As a consequence of the variety of circumstances for both investigators and subjects, and also because of a lack of any clear policy direction or standard of practice, research results of an individual's genetic tests may be kept in patient medical files, or within a health care institution but intentionally separate from medical files, or within files in a research establishment unconnected with patient care.

[. . .] The first question researchers and research ethics boards have to ask is whether it is appropriate to keep all such data out of medical files. This might not be appropriate if these data have clear clinical relevance for the treatment of patients, and integration in medical files is important for future treatment decisions or prevention strategies.

But even if genetic test results are maintained entirely separate from medical records, will researchers always be able to maintain confidentiality against access by courts or insurers? When subjects have been informed about test results indicating an increased risk for health, can, or should, researchers promise that this information will remain confidential and will never be accessible to insurers? [. . .] To avoid adverse selection, insurance laws provide that contracts can be declared null and void if applicants withhold information that a reasonable insurer would have taken into consideration for determining insurability. This normally implies that applicants have to declare to insurers all relevant health information of which they are aware. They have to declare the results of genetic tests if these are relevant for assessing their health risks. [. . .]

It might be argued that if subjects have not been informed about genetic test results, they do not know more than insurers. Applicants cannot use information that they do not possess. In these circumstances, the argument goes, they are not in a position that undermines the consensual basis of the contractual agreement. However, if people have been informed, they clearly have an obligation to declare the results of the tests. Courts might oblige researchers to give access to the results of these tests because they were relevant to assess the insurability of applicants. [. . .]

[. . .] Investigators and IRBs who want information about the relevance of such legislation to research files, or under what circumstances research files could be accessed by the courts, should seek local legal advice.

Investigator and institutional responsibilities. What should IRBs expect from investigators concerning protection of confidentiality and what should investigators legitimately offer? Researchers and IRBs need to be clear whether and why research results will or will not be disclosed to subjects. Prospective subjects should *always* be informed that genetic information carries with it social risks, both from personal knowledge and from third-party knowledge. For protocols where it is reasonable to provide test results to subjects, they should always have the option of *not* receiving them. And the clinical relevance of the genetic knowledge to be gained from the particular trial *for the individual research subject* should not be exaggerated by investigators. As for the measures necessary to protect confidentiality of patient data or DNA samples, protocols must describe an explicit plan for doing so. IRBs should ensure that adequate measures have been taken, whether by encryption, use of unique identifiers, mandatory stripping of identifiers after a stated time period, encoding requiring IRB approval to re-link data with subject or patient files, sequestering of records, or, where appropriate, physical security measures. [. . .] This is a larger policy question for institutions, which should have in place mandatory procedures that protect research results to the maximum allowed by law.

CONCLUSION

IRBs need to assure that genetics protocols undergo the same rigorous review as nongenetics protocols. The schema provided integrates some of the new issues involving genetic research into the existing IRB review structure, accommodating the "critical path" we have suggested for an IRB to follow in reviewing genetic diagnostic and screening protocols. IRBs should use the issues addressed by the schema not only to review individual protocols, but also to determine whether they or their institutions ought to develop local policies relevant to such issues as DNA banking, commercial interests, disclosure, or consent.

Our discussion of issues suggests that IRBs must recognize any uncertainties involved in clinical prediction and assure that they are clearly disclosed to prospective subjects. [. . .] And individuals entering genetics protocols should be able to expect confidentiality for their data or samples to the greatest possible extent. Current limits on the ability to protect confidentiality may require changes in law or social policy. Where there are limits to what is feasible, those limits must be adequately disclosed to prospective subjects.

[Glossary omitted—eds.]

---

50   Structuring the Review of Human Genetics Protocols, Part III

Gene Therapy Studies

KATHLEEN CRANLEY GLASS, CHARLES WEIJER,
DENIS COURNOYER, TRUDO LEMMENS, ROBERTA M. PALMOUR,
STANLEY H. SHAPIRO, AND BENJAMIN FREEDMAN

[. . .]

GENE THERAPY PROTOCOLS

Gene marking, gene supplementation, and gene surgery. Gene therapy could be defined as the introduction of genetic material into patients to treat a genetically inherited or an acquired disorder. Gene therapy is often contrasted with "gene marking," in which new genetic information is transferred into cells in order to be able to detect these cells and study what happens to them once they are given back to the patient. Existing technologies do not yet permit the direct repair of specific gene mutations. Instead, a normal copy of the gene of interest (or its smaller "coding sequence") is introduced into an appropriate target cell type. This sequence can then express a function that was defective or normally absent in those cells. This approach is termed gene "supplementation," in contrast to gene "surgery," which would constitute the direct repair of mutations. Although gene surgery is technically feasible (by a procedure termed "gene targeting"), its minimal efficiency precludes utilization in the treatment of human disorders at this time.

Gene supplementation may also be used to counter the effects of an acquired disease, such as cancer. This is intended to augment normal immune function, to introduce drug-susceptibility genes, to inhibit oncogene expression, or to protect against the toxic effects of cancer chemotherapy. [. . .]

Gene delivery strategies. At this state of development, there are three principal strategies for delivering genes to cells: *ex vivo, in vivo,* and micro-encapsulation. In the *ex vivo* approach, somatic cells that are to be genetically modified are removed, cultured, and exposed to viral or nonviral vectors or "free" nucleic acids containing the gene of interest. After transduction or insertion of the gene of interest into these cells, they are readministered to the patient. The human cells that are genetically manipulated may come from the patient (autologous cells) or from another individual (allogenic cells).

With *in vivo* gene therapy, the genetically altered viral or nonviral vectors or "free" nucleic acids are administered directly to the patient, locally or systemically depending on the purpose of the genetic intervention. Local delivery is appropriate where tissue is accessible. For example, bronchoscopy or aerosol has been used for delivery to the lungs, insertion into the portal circulation for liver uptake, local delivery to the epithelial surfaces of the colorectum, or the use of sophisticated catheter systems to gain access to spe-

Kathleen Cranley Glass, Charles Weijer, Denis Cournoyer, Trudo Lemmens, Roberta M. Palmour, Stanley H. Shapiro, and Benjamin Freedman, "Structuring the Review of Human Genetics Protocols, Part III: Gene Therapy Studies," *IRB: A Review of Human Subjects Research* 21, no. 2 (1999): 1–9.

cific components of the vascular endothelium, such as the coronary vasculature. Local delivery into tumors by direct injection is used to enhance immune recognition in malignant disease. Some protocols require systemic delivery with some forms of targeting of particular cells or organs. The exact site of introduction may be irrelevant, provided gene expression takes place and the therapeutic molecule is released and can reach the intended site of action. [...]

Gene delivery vehicles. [...] In contrast to the retroviruses, adenoviruses can be used to introduce genes into both dividing and nondividing cells. In this vehicle, the virus/gene construct does not integrate into the host cell genome and is eventually lost from proliferating cell populations, requiring repeated administration to be effective. Adeno-associated virus vectors have also been investigated for gene therapy applications. These have the advantage of being nonpathogenic and capable of stable integration into the host cell genome. Vectors based on herpes virus, which do not integrate into the host chromosomes but are stably maintained extra-chromosomally, are particularly attractive for gene transfer into the nervous system because of their neural tropism. Herpes viruses have very large genomes and thus offer a very high potential for incorporating large foreign coding sequences.

Liposome complexes have been employed in a number of gene therapy protocols, in most cases using in vivo delivery to a local anatomical site. Liposome sacs can be filled with DNA, which is then delivered into human cells by fusing the liposomes with the recipient cells. Two major advantages of this vector system are that there is no possibility for replication or recombination to form an infectious agent and that the absence of proteins reduces the risk of unwanted immune or inflammatory reactions. [...]

Another approach under study involves a combination of *in vitro* and *in vivo* gene delivery procedures known as cell grafting. In this method, genes are transferred into cells that have been removed and that can, upon their return to the body, metabolically cooperate with cells that cannot be removed. The removable cells are harvested, cultured, and subjected to gene transfer using one of the in vitro methods described above. When the corrected cells are replaced in a living organism, they produce the desired gene products and should transmit them to the cells where they are needed.

Researchers have generally agreed that currently there is no single vector ideal for all situations. Each of the available vectors has some advantages and disadvantages. New vectors are under development in many laboratories. Research into genomic DNA-based strategies independent of the viral vector approaches, such as gene targeting and human artificial chromosome technology, is also being pursued. If successful, these strategies would have the major advantage of maintaining the integrity of the endogenous gene.

SCHEMA FOR REVIEW

Table [50.1] contains a series of questions institutional review boards (IRBs) may want to ask when reviewing gene therapy protocols. [...]

DISCUSSION

[...]

Forum for review. [...] Local review boards will be more familiar with both the investigators and the patient populations within their own institutions. On the other hand, gene therapy often generates scientifically difficult and ethically demanding questions. Because it is extremely specialized, of great public interest, and raises a number of new issues, national review has a number of advantages. It permits greater access to experts from across the country, allowing for a broader perspective and additional analytic resources. A national review committee could maintain consistency, providing standardization of requirements across the country for what may be controversial projects. It may help avoid the conflicts of interest local reviewers might face with protocols from their home institutions. Unlike the local review process, national review allows for collecting results from around the country, monitoring the progress of protocols, and rapidly disseminating the results. It should assist in avoiding overlap or duplication in protocols. [...]

Under a national review structure, local IRB approval may be a prerequisite for national review. A two-step process was originally established in the United States for federally funded gene therapy research, with review first by the IRB of the local institution, and then, if this review was positive, by the Recombinant DNA Advisory Committee (RAC) of the National Institutes of Health. The role of the RAC has recently been modified to include review only of vector systems that are entirely new in addition to its social policy role. [...]

Where national review does not exist, regional or intra-university committees might be helpful. They could offer some of the advantages of national review, especially if they provided greater access to specialized analytical resources. Regional review is required in some jurisdictions. In Denmark and France, for example, all human subjects research must be reviewed by regional committees; there are no local review mechanisms.

Where the relevant expertise in either genetics or research ethics is not available within a single institution, such as a university hospital or research institute, there may be advantages to establishing a university-wide IRB to review genetics protocols involving human subjects. The mandate of such a board does not necessarily have to pre-empt approval by a local IRB. It could offer an alternative review that, if positive, the local boards could accept or reject.

Table 50.1
Schema for IRB Review of Gene Therapy/Gene Transfer Protocols

BACKGROUND AND JUSTIFICATION

- Why is this disease a good candidate for gene transfer or gene therapy?
- What previous work has been done, including studies of animals and cultured cell models? Does the work demonstrate effective gene delivery? How does the proposed study relate to previous work?
- Is the disease course sufficiently predictable to allow for meaningful assessment of the results of the treatment proposed?
- What level of gene expression is presumed to be required to achieve the desired effect?
- *Given responses to the above questions, is there a sufficient justification for the investigator to proceed at this point to a clinical trial?*

RESEARCH DESIGN

- What are the objectives of the proposed study (e.g., establishing feasibility or relative safety of the gene transfer, determining therapeutic effectiveness, establishing a safe dose range, demonstrating proof of principle, etc.)?
- Is the goal of the study to ameliorate or cure disease or to enhance healthy individuals?
- What is the target tissue for gene transfer (e.g., bone marrow cells, skeletal muscle cells, respiratory epithelial cells, central nervous system tissue, etc.)?
- What method(s) (e.g., direct injection, inhalation, *ex vivo* genetic modification with injection of modified cells) and reagent(s) (e.g., vectors based on retroviruses, adenoviruses, adeno-associated viruses, herpes viruses) will be employed for gene delivery? What is the rationale for their use? Are other methods or reagents known that are more appropriate with regard to efficacy, safety, and stability?
- How will the investigator determine the proportion of cells that acquires and expresses the added DNA?
- How will the investigator determine if the product is biologically active?
- Is the planned statistical treatment appropriate (i.e., is it likely to provide valid answers to the study question)?
- *Is it reasonable to expect that the research design proposed will meet the investigator's objectives?*

PROCEDURES

- What research-specific procedures and research-specific investigations are required by the study over and above those that would be required for patients receiving standard clinical care (e.g., physical examinations, venous or arterial blood tests, collection of target cells, imaging procedures, irradiation, chemotherapy, direct injection of vector, reinjection of genetically modified cells, organ or tissue transplantation, surgery, tissue/tumor donation, questionnaires, interviews)?
- Is long term follow-up appropriate or essential for this protocol? If long term follow-up is proposed, is there justification for the number of visits and the length of time required? Is such follow-up feasible in the case of this protocol (e.g., have provisions been made for subjects who move, is adequate funding available for such follow-up)?
- What are the procedures for obtaining or maintaining information in a data/DNA bank (e.g., use of identifiers, limitation on access, need for consent, sharing with other investigators, duration of storage, future subject contact)?
- *Are all of the research-specific procedures necessary? In combination with data collected in the course of clinical care, is it reasonable to expect that the information produced by this study will be sufficient to answer the research question?*

CONFIDENTIALITY

- *Are the practical steps for maintaining confidentiality of data/records/database information clearly specified and adequate (e.g., encryption, use of unique identifiers, sequestering of records, security measures)?*

(continued on next page)

Table 50.1. Continued

SUBJECT SELECTION

- How has the study population been defined?
- Has an adequate rationale been provided for each eligibility criterion (e.g., safety considerations, definition of disease, avoidance of additional concurrent therapies, administrative considerations)? Do they strike a defensible balance between scientific validity and generalizability (i.e., is the study population sufficiently, but not unduly, restricted so as to yield interpretable results)?
- How will the subjects be recruited? If a cohort of eligible patients exists, how will selection be made amongst them? If several trials exist for which the same patients are eligible, how will this be presented to prospective subjects?
- *Does the definition of the research population reflect appropriate scientific, clinical, and ethical norms? In recruiting and negotiating with potential subjects, have the norms of nondiscrimination been respected?*

RISKS, DISCOMFORTS, AND BENEFITS

- What risks and discomforts are associated with the research-specific procedures and investigations (e.g., surgery, chemotherapy, radiation, bone marrow transplantation)? Have they been minimized?
- If a virus-mediated gene transfer is proposed, what is the potential for the presence of a replication-competent or pathological virus or other form of contaminants? How sensitive are the tests to detect such viruses or contaminants? What level of viral presence or other form of contamination would be tolerable in this protocol?
- Has the possibility of vertical transmission (i.e., gene insertion into germ cells or a fetus) or horizontal transmission (e.g., to family members or health care staff) been considered? What measures have been taken to minimize the risks of transmission? Are other measures possible? If transmission were to occur, what would be the consequences?
- What are the risks for the vector to activate an oncogene or inactivate a tumor suppressor gene leading to vector-related malignancy?
- *Are the risks and discomforts of the study justified given the potential benefit to subjects and the scientific importance of the research?*

INFORMATION TO SUBJECTS

- Have prospective participants been adequately informed of the following:
  1. What is being studied and why, given details about study procedures, known or potential risks, discomforts and benefits, and alternatives to participation;
  2. Their rights: (a) to information on an ongoing basis, confidentiality with regard to their participation and handling of their data, and the right to consult with others before making a decision whether to participate; and (b) to withdraw from the study without penalty or loss of benefits, as well as of any health consequences of withdrawal for themselves or their immediate contacts, or limitations on withdrawal, if any;
  3. Any special issues related to this gene therapy trial, such as uncertainty associated with short and long term risks and benefits or the possibility of media attention; and
  4. Any commercial or financial interests in the research.
- Have prospective participants been provided this information in simple language, using translation where necessary, with answers to their questions, referral to other sources of information, and adequate time to make up their minds whether to participate?
- If there is no individual benefit from participation in the research, has this been appropriately disclosed?
- Will the general study results be made available to subjects?
- Do all of the elements of the consent process combine to allow subjects a full opportunity to make an informed choice?

Safety: risks to subjects, risks to society. Risks associated with gene therapy studies can be classified as risks to individuals and risks to society. As with other clinical research, the IRB has an obligation to ensure that "risks to subjects are minimized." [...] After almost a decade of experience with gene therapy, many risks are more completely characterized.

[...] No single roster of risks is applicable to all gene therapy studies. The risks posed to participants vary with the technique used to transfer the genetic material into the subject's body. [...]

Contamination during vector preparation. [G]ene therapy carries risks that stem from inadequate control of the biological source, the production process, and the bulk and final product. These risks include transfer of an unwanted gene or genes to the subject, administration of replication competent virus, or bacterial contamination of the vector preparation. The IRB has an obligation to ensure that the technical and animal data are reviewed and that every precaution has been taken to minimize risk to subjects.

Immune response. Certain delivery systems may trigger a significant immune response and in some cases this may interfere with treatment efficacy. For example, an attempt to transfer a "therapeutic dose" of CFTR genes in patients with cystic fibrosis seems to have been thwarted by an immune response to the adenovirus vector. [...]

Malignancy. Some viral vectors, including retrovirus and adeno-associated virus, permanently incorporate into the research subject's genetic material. Since this occurs in a relatively random manner (less so for adeno-associated viruses), the vector integration may disrupt important host genes, such as tumor-suppressor genes, or may activate oncogenes, in either case promoting the occurrence of a malignancy. [...] A reliable assessment of the risk of cancer will require long-term follow-up of large numbers of patients.

Viral recombination, replication, and shedding. Great care is usually taken in the preparation of viral vectors to ensure that they are incapable of virus reproduction. Nonetheless, there remains a theoretical possibility, perhaps particularly with adenoviruses, that the vector might combine with a virus in the environment and regain the capacity to reproduce. Therefore, both persons who receive gene therapy and those with whom they are in contact (e.g., friends, family, and health care workers) might be at risk of infection with virus-carrying genes with powerful biological functions. Experience to date indicates that the risk of a virus regaining its reproductive potential is less than was previously feared.

Risks to society. A number of risks to society have been suggested in the literature. Concerns regarding the effect of gene therapy on the "gene pool" may be dispensed with immediately. While it is true that any therapy directed against genetic disease may increase the frequency of disease-causing genes, gene therapy is most often directed against recessive conditions in which affected individuals are rare relative to carriers. As a result, gene therapy will have a very small effect on allele frequencies. [...]

Other concerns are less easy to dismiss. While the use of gene therapy is currently restricted to the insertion of new genes into somatic cells, gene therapy could be used in other ways. It could be used to treat a disease once and for all by replacing the defective gene in germinal cells, thereby eliminating the transmission of disease to subsequent generations. [...]

Genetic enhancement. [...] Using genetic technology to promote socially desirable personal characteristics rather than to cure disease may become feasible.

The debate on enhancement is not new and not limited to gene therapy. In our society, effective treatments tend to undergo progressive expansion in use. Prozac, which has been enormously successful in the treatment of clinical depression, now is used by some to treat a wide variety of symptoms, including low self-esteem. [...]

The line between treating disease and changing characteristics not associated with disease can be easily blurred, making it difficult to agree on what exactly qualifies as enhancement. [...] Clear demarcations between appropriate and inappropriate uses of therapy—for example, between medical treatment and nonmedical enhancement—are often lacking. [...]

Despite the weightiness of these concerns, it would be unjust—and contrary to U.S. regulations—for IRBs to saddle individual protocols with these slippery slope arguments. But whether the pursuit of genetic enhancement runs counter to important values should be the subject of further debate. Where then is the proper forum for these issues? In the U.S., the RAC is the natural locus for these matters to be addressed. [...]

INTERVENTIONS AFFECTING THE GERM LINE: INTENTIONAL AND UNINTENTIONAL

Permanent effects on the germ line may occur both accidentally and intentionally. The accidental transmission of genetic material to the germ cells could happen if the vector unintentionally transferred genetic information into the genome of germ cells. This could occur in the recipients of the gene therapy or in persons who come in contact with them. It is one of the risks that the IRB must weigh against the potential benefits of a gene therapy study.

Intentional genetic modification of the germ cells is more controversial. While significant technical problems would have to be overcome to achieve germ-line genetic intervention, work with animals has demonstrated success using a limited number of techniques.

Advantages and disadvantages of germ-line therapy. [...] Many geneticists, ethicists, policy analysts, and legislators have expressed hesitancy about—and in many cases opposition to—deliberate manipulation of germ cells. [...]

Principle-based argumentation focuses on the effect that germ-line manipulation will have on future generations, who will have no opportunity to consent to the changes. The use of human embryos in the development of the technologies raises further consent issues. The issue of consent is not only theoretical. There are practical questions concerning moral and legal responsibilities to those future generations who may be harmed by an intervention.

An argument based on the right to be born with one's genome, or genetic patrimony, intact has been particularly strong in Europe. Making heritable changes denies that right. [...]

While arguments in favor of germ-line interventions stress society's obligations to relieve and to prevent human suffering and premature death from genetic diseases, agreement on any natural demarcation between "healthy" and "unhealthy" genes may be impossible. Experiences cited above with pharmacotherapy such as Prozac [...] indicate that we have not yet succeeded in making these distinctions. [...]

IRBs are unlikely to review protocols involving intentional germ-line manipulation for some time to come. Nonetheless, members should be aware that the techniques now being developed for somatic cell therapy will also facilitate germ-line research. [...]

[Glossary omitted—eds.]

51   Protecting the Privacy of Family Members in Survey and Pedigree Research

JEFFREY R. BOTKIN

[A]bsent from much of the discussion in research ethics is a consideration of rights and responsibilities that arise through family and social relationships. Since each of us lives within a complex web of biological and social ties, decisions by and information about one person have implications for others. [T]he obligations of investigators to protect the privacy and welfare of family members and social contacts of research subjects have not been determined.

A recent controversy at Virginia Commonwealth University (VCU) highlights this complex set of ethical issues in biomedical research with families. [...]

The VCU case involved an adult woman who was being recruited to participate in a twin study. Her father read a mailed survey instrument that included questions about the health of her parents and other family members. The questionnaire reportedly asked, among other items, whether the subject's father suffered from depression and whether he had abnormal genitalia. The father was concerned that providing this information constituted a threat to personal and family privacy and that informed consent should have been sought from family members. The father contacted the National Institutes of Health's Office for Protection from Research Risks [OPRR, now the Office for Human Research Protections, or OHRP—eds.], which ruled that the VCU institutional review board (IRB) should have considered whether family members were human subjects of this research by virtue of their relationship to the respondent and the nature of the family information obtained from the respondent. After review of the IRB procedures, the OPRR and the Food and Drug Administration suspended human subject research at VCU stating that the IRB had inadequately documented its monitoring of research protocols. The VCU case forces consideration of the broader question of whether family members of the primary subject become research subjects themselves (secondary subjects) and if informed consent is necessary from secondary subjects to retain their information. [...]

The IRB review of research protocols in this regard involves 2 levels of analysis. First, determine whether family members should be deemed human subjects of the research. Second, if family members are deemed human subjects, when must informed consent be sought for the retention of private information? [...]

Jeffrey R. Botkin, "Protecting the Privacy of Family Members in Survey and Pedigree Research," *JAMA* 285 (2001): 207–11.

HUMAN SUBJECTS

[...] The following is the definition of human subjects in the Common Rule:

> *Human subject* means a living individual about whom an investigator (whether professional or student) conducting research obtains (1) data through intervention or interaction with the individual, or (2) identifiable private information.... Private information must be individually identifiable (i.e., the identity of the subject is or may readily be ascertained by the investigator or associated with the information) in order for obtaining the information to constitute research involving human subjects. [45 CFR §46.102(f), included in this volume—eds.]

[T]he standards do not recognize a right of individuals to control all personal information. Not all individuals about whom information is obtained are considered human subjects [...]. The standards focus on protecting individuals from harm during research, and ensuring that consent is obtained if modest risks are posed, rather than ensuring that individuals are afforded absolute privacy and control over all personal information. A breach in privacy is not considered a harm per se, rather it is the risk of harm that may result from a breach that is the relevant consideration. Therefore, the standards represent an attempt to balance risk conferred by potential breaches in privacy with the social benefits of health research. [...]

READILY IDENTIFIABLE INDIVIDUALS

If unique individual identifiers are being obtained on family members from the primary subject, then family members are readily identifiable. In contrast, family members would not be readily identifiable in at least 2 circumstances. First, if the primary subject is anonymous and if no unique identifiers are obtained for family members. Second, the family data are rendered anonymous by unlinking them from an identifiable source. If the investigators primarily are seeking epidemiologic information, then rendering the primary subject or family data anonymous may be feasible without limiting the productivity of the research. [...]

[...] The question is whether family members can be readily identified from simply knowing the identity of the primary subject and the family relationship involved. In most circumstances, a family relationship alone is a poor lead for identifying relatives. Surnames are often widely shared in the population, names of women typically change through marriage, and family members often are geographically dispersed. [...] Unless the investigators were provided specific identifiers such as names, addresses, a unique job description, or Social Security numbers, family members would be virtually impossible to identify with any degree of certainty. [...]

In general, family members of adult individuals are not readily identifiable to third parties based on family relationship alone. [T]he regulations clearly state that individuals must be readily identifiable to the investigator, so that it is not relevant that specific family members are readily identifiable to other family members based on family relationship alone, or to individuals who have a social relationship with the family. [...]

PRIVATE INFORMATION

The regulations require that information on an identifiable individual obtained in research be private for the individual to be considered a research subject. The Common Rule does not provide a relevant definition of private information. [...] One consistent aspect of informational privacy is the idea that people want substantial personal control over information they consider private. [P]ersonal information that is generated or shared in intimate relationships between individuals typically would be considered private. A relationship with a physician, a counselor, an attorney, an employer, or a teacher involves personal information over which most individuals want and can exert control. [P]rivate information is personal information over which individuals typically want and can exert control.

[...] There are different spheres of privacy and a decision to share information with close friends and relatives does not imply a willingness to share information more broadly. [M]ost information about the health status of relatives of the primary subject should be considered private information.

WAIVER OF CONSENT

[...] If family members are subjects, then a determination must be made whether informed consent can be waived. There are 4 requirements for the waiver of consent listed in the regulations. All of the following criteria must be satisfied: (1) the research involves no more than minimal risk to the subjects; (2) the waiver or alteration will not adversely affect the rights and welfare of the subjects; (3) the research could not practically be carried out without the waiver or alteration; and (4) whenever appropriate, the subjects will be provided with additional pertinent information after participation. Of particular concern for this discussion are points 1 and 3.

Minimal Risk

With respect to the concept of minimal risk, the regulations stipulate:

Minimal risk means that the probability and magnitude of harm or discomfort anticipated in the research are not greater in and of themselves than those ordinarily encountered in daily life or during the performance of routine physical or psychological examinations or tests. [45 CFR §46.102(i), included in this volume—eds.]

[...] Many IRBs may consider virtually all survey research to be of minimal risk. [R]esearch projects that generate new health information are much more likely to confer risk than projects that simply document existing health information. In the context of survey research, health information on secondary subjects obtained from the primary subject is by definition existing information. Therefore the question for the IRB is whether the documentation of existing health or personal information through a research project poses greater than minimal risk to secondary subjects.

Judgments concerning minimal risk require an assessment of both the likelihood of harm and the magnitude of harm involved. Likelihood in this context is the probability that a breach of privacy will occur combined with the probability that the breach will lead to adverse events. [...]

The magnitude of the harm resulting from a breach in privacy for secondary subjects will depend on the nature of the information and on the relationship of the subject to the person who inappropriately receives private information. Fortunately, access to research data on secondary subjects by insurers or employers is highly unlikely. [I]nvestigators and IRBs must be particularly alert to protocol features that might allow histories obtained from one family member to be shared with other family members.

An IRB must make a determination about minimal risk based on the security of the data and on the general sensitivity of the information being obtained in the research protocol. [...] It may be appropriate for an IRB to consider protocols to be greater than minimal risk for secondary subjects when the family history pursued includes [...] highly sensitive information [such as alcoholism, schizophrenia, or sexual orientation]. In contrast, IRBs may consider protocols to be of less than minimal risk when the family history includes only information about existing health conditions of low or moderate sensitivity, such as heart disease, cancer, or diabetes, and when strong data security measures are in place. [...]

CONCLUSIONS AND RECOMMENDATIONS

Table [51.1] lists recommendations that investigators and IRBs should consider in the conduct of research in which primary subjects are asked for information on family members or social contacts. [...]

There can be no question that the issues raised by the VCU case are legitimate and complex. The interests of secondary subjects warrant careful attention and protection by investigators, IRBs, and funding agencies. The burden and expense of these protections are not justifications for forgoing these efforts. However, this analysis suggests that it is justifiable to proceed with research without the explicit consent of family members for many research protocols that meet the outlined criteria.

Table 51.1

Recommendations for Investigators and IRBs Regarding Privacy of Family Members in Research

I. Are the family members human subjects?
  A. Are family members readily identifiable by the investigators?
  - Yes, if unique identifiers are associated with individual data of primary subjects and their family members.
  - No, if the primary subject and family members are anonymous.
  - No, if data on family members are unlinked from the unique individual identifiers of the primary subject.
  - No, in most circumstances, if family members are linked by family relationship alone to an identifiable primary subject.

  B. Does the information obtained from the primary subject about family members constitute private information?
  - Yes, if the information consists of health status, health history, reproductive history, behavior history, etc.
  - No, if the information consists only of the family relationship and commonly available personal data such as age, race, or occupation.

  Responding yes for item IA and for IB means the individual is a human subject. Responding no for either item IA or IB means the individual is not a human subject.

Table 51.1. Continued

II. If family members are human subjects, can informed consent be waived?
   A. Does the research involve more than minimal risk?
      • Yes, if the information obtained is highly sensitive such as psychiatric history, sexual orientation, criminal history, etc.
      • Yes, if strong data security measures have not been prepared and the information is considered sensitive or highly sensitive.
      • No, if the information obtained on family members is not highly sensitive and strong data security measures are detailed in the proposal.
   B. Does the waiver adversely affect the rights and welfare of the subjects?
   C. Can the research be practically carried out without the waiver?
   D. When appropriate, can the secondary subjects be provided pertinent information after the completion of the research?

Responding no for items IIA, IIB, and IIC and yes for section IID means that informed consent can be waived for secondary subjects.

Section Two

Stored Human Biological Specimens

52   Statement on Informed Consent for Genetic Research

THE AMERICAN SOCIETY OF HUMAN GENETICS

This is the final and official statement of the Board of Directors of the American Society of Human Genetics. [...]

GENERAL CONSIDERATIONS

[...] Because of a variety of important and complex issues surrounding the use of previously collected biological samples, investigators are encouraged to develop procedures for obtaining informed consent when prospectively collecting specimens for genetic research purposes. [...]

[I]t is strongly recommended that research results only be transmitted to subjects by persons able to provide genetic counseling. Because of the sensitive nature of genetic

The American Society of Human Genetics, "Statement on Informed Consent for Genetic Research," *American Journal of Human Genetics* 59 (1996): 471–74.

information, even those institutions not covered by federal regulations should develop a process for human subjects review. [...]

RESEARCH USING PROSPECTIVELY COLLECTED SAMPLES

In genetic studies that are designed to collect new biological samples from individuals, the investigators generally have the opportunity to communicate with potential subjects in advance and involve them in the research by obtaining their informed consent (Figure [52.1], Table [52.1]). This should be encouraged, except for the prospective studies in which samples are collected anonymously, or have been "anonymized."

Studies that maintain identified or identifiable specimens must maintain subjects' confidentiality. Information

Table 52.1

Suggested Guidelines on the Need to Obtain Informed Consent in Genetic Research, by Type of Study Design and Level of Anonymity

	Study Design	
Level of Anonymity	*Retrospective*	*Prospective*
Anonymous	Not applicable	No
Anonymized	No	No
Identifiable	Usually yes (except if a waiver is granted)	Yes
Identified	Yes	Yes

Study Design

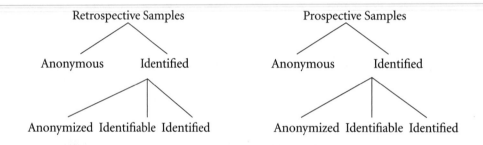

Figure 52.1

Flow diagram of types of biological samples used in genetic research, by type of study design and level of anonymity. Prospective research studies are those in which the collection of the new samples is part of the study design. Retrospective research studies utilize previously obtained samples collected for a purpose that is different from that of the project under study. Anonymous biological materials were originally collected without identifiers and are impossible to link to their sources. Anonymized biological materials were initially identified but have been irreversibly stripped of all identifiers and are impossible to link to their sources. This process does not preclude linkage with clinical, pathological, and demographic information before the subject identifiers are removed. Caution must be exercised so that the amount and type of linked information does not invalidate anonymity. Identifiable biological materials are unidentified for research purposes, but can be linked to their sources though the use of a code. Decoding can be done only by the investigator or another member of the research team. Identified biological materials are those to which identifiers, such as a name, patient number, or clear pedigree location, are attached and made available to researchers.

from these samples should not be provided to anyone other than the subjects and persons designated by the subjects in writing. [. . .] Investigators should indicate to the subject that they cannot guarantee absolute confidentiality.

Research results or samples should not be given to any of the subject's family members by the investigator without the explicit, written permission of the subject, except under extraordinary circumstances. [. . .]

CONSENT DISCLOSURES

Subjects providing consent to prospective studies should be told about the types of information that could result from genetic research. [. . .]

During the course of molecular genetic diagnosis, the results may indicate that the child is not the offspring of one or both of the presumed parents. The investigator therefore should consider including in the consent form a statement that misidentified parentage will not be disclosed. [. . .]

Additional risks that should be disclosed to subjects of certain genetic research studies include the possibility of adverse psychological sequelae, disruption of family dynamics, and social stigmatization and discrimination. All genetic research studies involving identified or identifiable samples in which disclosure of results is planned should have medical geneticists and/or genetic counselors involved to ensure that the results are communicated to the subjects accurately and appropriately. [. . .]

DISPOSITION OF SAMPLES
AND RESULTS

Depending on the study, subjects may be given the opportunity to determine if they want to be informed of the results of their testing. Subjects should be informed if the sample will be stored for later study, but they also need to be told that there is always the possibility of storage failure. [. . .]

In some studies researchers may wish to disclose results to subjects. If so, it is the obligation of the subjects to keep the investigator informed of how they may be con-

tacted. Investigators should indicate to study subjects that certain results may not allow definite answers until an analysis of the entire study has been completed (and, sometimes, not even then). [. . .]

Subjects involved in studies where the samples are identified or identifiable should indicate if their sample should be used exclusively in the study under consideration. If the sample is to be used more generally, subjects should be given options regarding the scope of the subsequent investigations, such as whether the sample can be used only for a specific disease under investigation, or for other unrelated conditions. It is inappropriate to ask a subject to grant blanket consent for all future unspecified genetic research projects on any disease or in any area if the samples are identifiable in those subsequent studies.

Subjects involved in studies in which the samples are identified or identifiable should indicate if unused portions of the samples may be shared with other researchers. If the subject is willing to have the sample shared with other researchers, it is the responsibility of the principal investigator to distribute the sample, so as to ensure that the agreement embodied in the informed consent is upheld. [. . .]

RETROSPECTIVE STUDIES
OF EXISTING SAMPLES

We endorse the use of anonymous samples for genetic research. Importantly, in retrospective research proposing to use samples collected anonymously or anonymized, there is no possibility, or need, to obtain consent.

For many studies, there may be benefits to making identifiable samples anonymous, because this effectively protects subjects from some of the risks of genetic research. Importantly, making samples anonymous will eliminate the need for recontact to obtain informed consent. This will also reduce the chance of introducing bias due to inability to recontact some, or the possible refusal of others to participate. [. . .]

For research involving identifiable samples, the investigator should be required to recontact the subjects to obtain consent for new studies. [. . .]

53   Informed Consent for Genetic Research on Stored Tissue Samples

ELLEN WRIGHT CLAYTON, KAREN K. STEINBERG, MUIN J. KHOURY,
ELIZABETH THOMSON, LORI ANDREWS, MARY JO ELLIS KAHN,
LORETTA M. KOPELMAN, AND JOAN O. WEISS

A workshop consisting of scientists, ethicists, lawyers, and consumers was convened jointly by the National Institutes of Health and the Centers for Disease Control and Prevention to develop recommendations for securing appropriate informed consent when collecting tissue samples for possible use in genetic research and for defining indications for additional consent if samples in hand are to be used for genetic studies. [. . .] The role of informed consent has been much less clear for research that can be performed using tissue samples. At present, much genetic research requires only DNA, which can be isolated from any nucleated cell.

People may not understand, however, that tissue samples they provide may be used for genetic research. They may have had any of a variety of reasons for providing the tissue—for medical screening and diagnostic testing, for tests following surgical procedures, and for clinical and epidemiologic research focusing on individuals, families, or populations—some of which are unrelated to the research in which the samples are used. Patients may expect that tissue samples will be used only for tests to provide information for their medical care. They may believe that samples will be discarded after testing, although the law often requires that samples be retained. When samples are obtained as part of medical care, patients may not be told about the possibility that these samples will be stored and used for research. In some relatively rare situations, such as state-mandated newborn screening, patients or those who make health care decisions for them may be unaware that tissue samples have been obtained.

THE NEED TO OBTAIN INFORMED CONSENT FOR RESEARCH

Increasing the fund of knowledge generally is a good both for society and for the individuals whose care is improved by more complete understanding. Society rightly values research and the contributions of those who participate as subjects in research. But despite the desirability of increased knowledge, research can risk harming the individuals who are being studied.

Yet obtaining consent entails costs. Federal law has long defined conditions under which research can be undertaken without obtaining consent. Some states have enacted laws that specifically allow investigators within an institution to obtain medical records for research without seeking patient consent.

ANONYMOUS SAMPLES FOR RESEARCH

According to federal regulations, the following is exempt from the requirements for protection of human subjects:

> Research involving the collection or study of existing data, documents, records, pathological specimens, or diagnostic specimens, if these sources are publicly available or if the information is recorded by the investigator in such a manner that subjects cannot be identified, directly or through identifiers linked to the subjects. [45 CFR §46.101(b)(4), included in this volume—eds.]

Thus, use of anonymous samples for research is exempt as long as two stringent criteria are met. First, the samples must already be existing at the time the research begins. Second, as interpreted by workshop participants, identifiers must be irretrievably removed from the information or samples that will be studied. Samples are anonymous if and only if it is impossible under any circumstances to identify the individual source. Samples are not anonymous if it is possible for any person to link the sample with its source. Even if the researcher cannot identify the source of tissue, the samples are not anonymous if some other individual or institution has this ability.

REMOVING IDENTIFIERS FROM EXISTING SAMPLES

There was much discussion about the appropriate use of already-existing samples that still retain identifiers at the

Ellen Wright Clayton, Karen K. Steinberg, Muin J. Khoury, Elizabeth Thomson, Lori Andrews, Mary Jo Ellis Kahn, Loretta M. Kopelman, and Joan O. Weiss, "Informed Consent for Genetic Research on Stored Tissue Samples," *JAMA* 274 (1995): 1786–92.

time the research is designed. Federal regulations currently permit investigators to take such samples without seeking consent, make them anonymous by removing identifiers, and then use them in research [45 CFR §46.102(f), included in this volume—eds.]. Such an unidentified data set might fit within the strict language of the exemption or cease to qualify as a "human subject" under the regulations and so be exempt from review or might fit within the provisions for waiver. Some of the workshop's participants argued that "anonymizing" samples without the sources' consent is ethically acceptable and that there is no possibility for stigmatization of the individual once identifiers are removed. Others argued, however, that anonymizing samples without consent is problematic because researchers had an opportunity to seek consent but did not exercise it.

There was consensus that, where use of anonymous tissue samples for specific research projects is anticipated at the time that the samples are obtained, sources' informed consent should be procured unless it can be waived in accordance with other provisions of the regulations. Given the frequency with which genetic researchers use stored tissue samples, one could argue that consent for use for research should be obtained whenever a tissue sample is collected in the future. However, one could argue that obtaining consent at the time samples are collected in the course of clinical care may pose formidable logistical and practical problems, particularly when there is little chance that any one sample will be used for research.

These and other problems led the workshop participants to agree that institutional review boards (IRBs) could usefully review research proposals to use currently anonymous samples and to make currently identifiable tissue samples anonymous without the sources' consent. [...]

USE OF LINKABLE OR IDENTIFIED SAMPLES FOR RESEARCH

[...]

Potential Consequences for the Individual of Genetic Research on Identifiable Samples

[...] Undertaking genetic research using identifiable samples without the consent of the sources can wrong them even if no direct harms that give rise to legally enforceable claims actually occur. Capron argues that, just as individuals are wronged if others enter their houses without consent, so too are they wronged if others obtain access to private information about them. In addition, undertaking research without consent fails to respect the preferences of some people who might have chosen not to provide the tissue samples at all or to put explicit limitations on their use. For example, some people may wish to limit the use

of their samples to noncommercial entities. Others may wish to forbid the use of their samples to investigate certain disorders. [...] In addition, retaining tissue samples or immortalizing cell lines may violate cultural or religious beliefs. [...]

Is Use of Identified or Linkable Samples Permissible with Less than Full Informed Consent?

Federal regulations allow IRBs to approve research protocols in which subjects' consent is limited or not obtained only if all the following requirements are met:

> (1) the research involves no more than minimal risk to the subjects; (2) the waiver or alteration will not adversely affect the rights and welfare of the subjects; (3) the research could not practicably be carried out without the waiver or alteration; (4) whenever appropriate, the subjects will be provided with additional pertinent information after participation. [45 CFR §46.116(d), included in this volume—eds.]

In deciding whether research on stored tissue samples involves more than minimal risk and whether limited consent will adversely affect the rights and welfare of the subjects, it is necessary to consider the magnitude of the psychosocial risks posed (which may be minimal in studies to detect genetic polymorphisms that are suspected to contribute to multifactorial disease) and the likelihood that research results will be revealed to the source and to third parties. [...]

Protocols that propose conveying genetic information to the source or to a third party generally pose more than minimal risk and so would require informed consent.

Even when disclosure is not planned, there may be some, albeit often small, risk that genetic information may be made available to the sources or third parties. Adopting strict procedures to minimize the release of information to anyone other than the investigators, including obtaining a certificate of confidentiality [...] may make it permissible to designate a protocol as presenting no more than minimal risk.

Another issue is whether informed consent for use of stored tissue samples can be limited because obtaining it would be impracticable. [...]

[...] Given that talking with people always entails some costs, consent cannot be waived on the simple assertion that seeking it would be tedious, burdensome, or costly. Rather, there must be proof that requiring consent would be so burdensome or expensive, as might be true were it necessary to contact the entire population, that the research could not go forward. [...]

What Information Should Be Given to Sources to Enable Them to Decide Whether to Permit Their Samples to Be Used for Research?

The sources' consents will generally be required for research using linkable and identified samples. The investigator who proposes the research is responsible for ensuring that consent has been obtained from subjects. Obtaining permission from the institution or individual having custody of the samples without review of the initial consent will not suffice. [...]

Regardless of who actually makes contact with the person who provided the tissue, federal regulations require extensive disclosure about a wide array of topics [45 CFR §46.116(a), included in this volume—eds.]. [T]he IRBs should require that copies of previous informed consent forms be examined to evaluate whether the new research conforms with or goes beyond the provisions of the original informed consent. [...]

In addition to receiving the federally mandated disclosures, sources might want to hear about the possibility that research using their samples could lead to the development of commercially valuable products. [...]

Under What Conditions Should Research Results Be Shared with Tissue Sources?

[...] When research involves the use of anonymous samples, recontact is impossible, a point that should be made clear to people who agree to the use of their samples for anonymous research. [...]

To avoid uncertainty about sharing research results and to limit possible liability, the best course is to inform people whose linkable or identified samples are going to be used in research about what types of information they can expect to have provided by the investigators. If the investigator wishes to recontact subjects, the circumstances under which this will and will not occur should be carefully delineated at the time consent for the use of the samples is obtained. These subjects must also be offered the opportunity to refuse recontact.

USE OF SAMPLES OBTAINED FROM PEOPLE WHO HAVE SINCE DIED FOR GENETIC RESEARCH

Under the federal regulations governing the protection of human subjects, people are subjects only during their lifetime [45 CFR §46.102(f), included in this volume—eds.]. [...]

PUBLIC HEALTH INVESTIGATIONS

Investigations of disease clusters may present different considerations from those involved in research. Specifically, timely determination of the cause of disease in a community may not be viewed as research but rather is needed to determine what, if any, intervention is warranted to avert the occurrence of new cases. To this end, investigators may wish to examine an array of potential causes, from infectious, environmental, nutritional, and occupational factors to genetic susceptibility, and they may search for gene-environment interactions as the cause of disease. The interventions performed in the name of public health can vary depending on the cause of the disorder. Detecting a primarily infectious cause may lead to a dramatically different response compared with finding that the incidence of disease depends heavily on genetic susceptibility. The extent to which the public through its agents can undertake these investigations and act to limit the incidence of disease or disability without seeking the consent from patients or subjects traditionally sought in medical care or research raises questions beyond the scope of this discussion. At a minimum, however, the state's power to act is clearest in cases of medical or public health emergency and wanes as the health problems pose less immediate threat to individuals and the community.

SPECIFIC RECOMMENDATIONS

The major observation of this workshop is that current federal regulations require IRB review and often the sources' consent for many proposals to use stored tissue samples for genetic research. The specific implications of the federal regulations for genetic research are described herein.

Use of Biologic Samples That Have Already Been Collected

DETERMINING HOW TO PROCEED WHEN SAMPLES ARE NOT ANONYMOUS AT THE TIME THAT THE RESEARCH IS PROPOSED

Informed consent that complies with the requirements defined in the "Collection of Samples in the Future" section is required if the investigator wishes to use identifiable or linked samples. Before requiring that a source be recontacted to obtain consent, the investigator and the IRB should determine whether the person who provided the sample previously agreed to the use of the sample for genetic research. Even in the absence of specific language about DNA testing, it may be appropriate to infer consent if the source wished for the sample to be used to determine why his or her family had a particular inherited disorder. By contrast, rarely does the language in typical operative and hospital admission consent forms provide an adequate basis for inferring consent to genetic research. If the IRB determines that the proposed research was agreed to by the source at the time the sample was obtained, then there is no need for further consent. [...]

Limitation or waiver of consent may be appropriate in some circumstances under the regulations or in emergency public health situations. The burden is on the investigator to justify seeking an exemption from obtaining full consent by meeting all the [applicable] regulatory requirements [45 CFR §46.116(d), included in this volume—eds.]. [...]

IS THERE ANY ROLE FOR IRB REVIEW OF PROTOCOLS THAT WOULD USE SAMPLES THAT HAVE ALREADY BEEN STRIPPED OF IDENTIFIERS?

Such protocols are exempt from review under current regulations. The workshop attendees agreed that IRBs nonetheless could usefully review such protocols to determine whether they are scientifically sound (particularly for protocols that have not already been subjected to peer review), whether they propose to address a significant problem, and whether the desired information could be obtained in a protocol that allows individuals to consent.

Collection of Samples in the Future

People should have the opportunity to decide whether their samples will be used for research. This option should be presented when samples are collected for whatever reason if it is likely that the samples will also be used for research. In addition, the possibility of future research should generally be discussed whenever tissue samples are collected for any research project. [...]

54   Use of Human Tissues in Research

Clarifying Clinician and Researcher Roles and Information Flows

JON F. MERZ, PAMELA SANKAR, SHEILA E. TAUBE, AND VIRGINIA LIVOLSI

[...] We propose that identifiability is directly related to the risks involved in tissue research and that the scope of informed consent must be directly correlated with it. Further, we posit that subject identifiability reflects a co-mingling of research and clinical roles, which we believe is particularly problematic and incompatible with the use of stored tissues in research. [...]

TISSUE BANKING AND RESEARCH

[...]

De-linking and De-identifying Research Data

[Figure 1 omitted—eds.]
[...] We assert that the more identifiable the subjects are, the more important it is to secure prior informed consent. There are two reasons for this. First, the identifiability of individuals whose tissues are used in research is directly related to the risks arising from possible misuse or improper disclosure of research data. The more tissues or data are identifiable the more likely it is that research data may find its way into files and databases where confidentiality cannot be assured. Second, subject identifiability raises the potential for use of research information in the clinical management of patients. Such use requires that prior consent be secured to ensure adequate counseling before developing information about the patients and to permit them to exercise a right not to know about genetic risks or pre-disposition to disease. [...]

[R]esearch with de-linked tissues may proceed with little or no prior informed consent (typical of stored tissues) if procedural safeguards are in place to prevent inferential identification or statistical matching. [...] In preparing consent documents, investigators and institutional review boards should anticipate what information will likely be generated in the research and what will be done with that information.

Separation of Research from Clinical Roles

[W]hen information of potential clinical relevance is a possible result of research activities, then a decision must be made prior to performing the research about whether to de-link the tissues for study or to secure detailed informed consent from subjects, specifically addressing the disclosure and use of such information. [...]

Jon F. Merz, Pamela Sankar, Sheila E. Taube, and Virginia LiVolsi, "Use of Human Tissues in Research: Clarifying Clinician and Researcher Roles and Information Flows," *Journal of Investigative Medicine* 45 (1997): 252–57.

A PROPOSED SOLUTION: THE TRUSTEE MODEL OF TISSUE BANKING

A link between tissues used in research and patient records is often useful for research purposes. Tissues without a link are of limited use because of the inability to update outcomes data, to link with related clinical, outcomes, or utilization data, or to solicit subjects for more information or for participation in follow-up studies. However, we agree with Clayton et al. [included in this volume—eds.] that law and ethics require strict protection of subject identity in tissue banks, absent consent to specific disclosures. [. . .] This suggests that we should consider methods to create a one-way link between patient records and research data sets, rather than the potentially burdensome expansion of consent requirements for all research with stored tissues. A one-way link can satisfy a researcher's needs for updating research data, as well as to ensure adequate de-identification justifying modification of informed consent requirements commensurate with planned research uses.

A one-way link could be technological, perhaps using a computer system that permits the creation and periodic updating of a de-identified research database in parallel to the medical record but which would not permit an inverse link to be made for any purpose. [. . .]

[T]he mechanism could be institutional, such as by interposing a banking repository between those who collect or store identified tissues (such as surgeons and pathologists) and researchers. [. . .] The repository trustee [. . .] would effectively de-identify tissues that it then provides to researchers. [. . .] This model precludes a researcher from filling the trustee role for projects in which he or she is involved because the researcher is barred from having access

to a subject's identities. Pathologists in particular will encounter problems when they try to work on their own collections. [. . .] [Figure 2 omitted—eds.]

[R]esearchers who desire access to relatively current outcomes data will want the trustee to link research samples with medical records, cancer registries, or other updatable records. There also will be value in enabling researchers to share research results, such as by developing a banked research database for use in future research projects. Whatever form the linked database takes, the key challenge will be to maintain isolation of it to protect subject identity and control the flow of research information.

[. . .] Because not all outcomes can be anticipated, the clearest ethical guideline is that a firm demarcation between clinical and research data must be maintained. Unless prior informed consent to the feedback of information and further contact for research purposes is secured from those persons whose tissues are being used in research, such feedback and contact must be prohibited.

CONCLUSION

[. . .] We have presented a model that should protect patient privacy and minimize research risks to human subjects in most research situations. These ends can be achieved by clarifying the proper uses of research and clinical data, by managing the risks of disclosure and breach of confidentiality, and by devoting appropriate efforts to securing informed consent. Toward this end, significant efforts are ongoing nationwide to develop informed consent processes and documents that will help individuals decide whether and under what constraints to allow their tissue to be used for research.

Section Three

Human Embryos and Stem Cells

55   Report of the Human Embryo Research Panel, Volume 1

AD HOC GROUP OF CONSULTANTS TO THE ADVISORY COMMITTEE TO THE DIRECTOR, NIH

EXECUTIVE SUMMARY

CHARGE TO THE PANEL

The mandate of the National Institutes of Health (NIH) Human Embryo Research Panel (the Panel) was to consider various areas of research involving the *ex utero* preimplantation human embryo and to provide advice as to those areas that (1) are acceptable for Federal funding, (2) warrant additional review, and (3) are unacceptable for Federal support. [. . .]

The Panel's charge encompasses only research that involves extracorporeal human embryos produced by *in vitro* fertilization or from other sources, or parthenogenetically activated oocytes. Research involving *in utero* human embryos, or fetuses, is not part of the charge. [. . .]

PRINCIPLES AND GUIDELINES FOR PREIMPLANTATION EMBRYO RESEARCH

[. . .] Any research conducted on the *ex utero* preimplantation human embryo or on gametes intended for fertilization should adhere to the following general principles as well as the more specific guidelines relevant to the nature of the particular research.

• The research must be conducted by scientifically qualified individuals in an appropriate research setting.

• The research must consist of a valid research design and promise significant scientific or clinical benefit.

Ad Hoc Group of Consultants to the Advisory Committee to the Director, NIH, Report of the Human Embryo Research Panel, Volume 1 (Bethesda, Md.: NIH, September 1994), available online at www1.od.nih.gov/osp/ospp/ pdf/volume1_revised.pdf.

• The research goals cannot be otherwise accomplished by using animals or unfertilized gametes. In addition, where applicable, adequate prior animal studies must have been conducted.

• The number of embryos required for the research must be kept to the minimum consistent with scientific criteria for validity.

• Donors of gametes or embryos must have given informed consent with regard to the nature and purpose of the specific research being undertaken.

• There must be no purchase or sale of gametes or embryos used in research. Reasonable compensation in clinical studies should be permissible to defray a subject's expenses, over and above the costs of drugs and procedures required for standard treatment, provided that no compensation or financial inducements of any sort are offered in exchange for the donation of gametes or embryos, and so long as the level of compensation is in accordance with Federal regulations governing human subjects research and that it is consistent with general compensation practice for other federally funded experimental protocols.

• Research protocols and consent forms must be reviewed and approved by an appropriate institutional review board and, for the immediate future, an ad hoc review process that extends beyond the existing review process to be established by NIH and operated for at least 3 years.

• There must be equitable selection of donors of gametes and embryos, and efforts must be made to ensure that benefits and risks are fairly distributed among subgroups of the population.

• Out of respect for the special character of the preimplantation human embryo, research involving preimplantation embryos should be limited to the shortest time period consistent with the goals of each research proposal and, for the present, research involving human embryos should not be permitted beyond the time of the usual appearance of the primitive streak *in vivo* (14 days). An exception to this is made for research protocols with the goal of reliably identifying in the laboratory the appearance of the primitive streak. [. . .]

CHAPTER 3. ETHICAL CONSIDERATIONS IN PREIMPLANTATION EMBRYO RESEARCH

INTRODUCTION

Current federal regulations [. . .] apply to "the product of conception from the time of implantation," and, without making any determination of the moral status of the postimplantation embryo *in utero,* they apply to it the same protection given fetuses. Thus, postimplantation embryos and fetuses may not be the subject of any research that carries more than minimal risk, unless such research is intended to be directly therapeutic to the individual embryo or fetus. These regulations apply equally to fetuses intended to be aborted, as well as to fetuses who are expected to develop to full term.

The regulations do not, however, address the status of *ex utero* preimplantation embryos, when research was made possible only through the development of human in vitro fertilization [IVF] techniques in the 1970s. [. . .]

APPROACHES TO ANALYZING THE MORAL STATUS OF THE HUMAN EMBRYO

Two broad approaches have been taken in debates over the moral status of the human embryo. One approach begins by proposing some single criterion of moral personhood. Beings that meet this criterion are believed to merit full and equal moral respect; those that do not are either denied respect or accorded a lesser status. The second approach is pluralistic. It sees moral respect and personhood as deriving not from one or even two criteria but from a variety of different and interacting considerations. [. . .]

Single Criterion Views

[. . .] One view holds that the embryo is a person, a being meriting full and equal moral respect, from the moment of conception or fertilization because at this moment a unique diploid genotype comes into being. For those who hold this view, humanness, in a moral sense, is the possession of a distinctive human genetic identity.

Others arrive at this same conclusion by emphasizing the significant increase in potential for development that accompanies the transition from gametes to embryo. [They] are agreed that the moment of fertilization/conception, however defined, is the crucial beginning of personhood.

For all who believe that moral personhood begins at conception the embryo ought to have the same moral rights as any other human research subject. No experimentation on the human embryo is permissible that would not also be allowed on the fetus *in utero* or on a newborn child.

Moral positions emphasizing genetic identity or developmental potential [. . .] create paradoxes in logic and run counter to many widely accepted practices, including the use of the intrauterine device and other contraceptive methods that work by preventing implantation. The equation of genetic diploidy with personhood leads to a logical paradox because twinning and the aggregation of two or more morula-stage embryos (sometimes inaccurately called "recombination") can occur well after fertilization. The emphasis on potential for development raises, but does not answer, the question of just *how much* potential is needed for moral respect. It also ignores the facts that even though developmental potential increases at conception, it remains relatively low at least until implantation. [. . .] As the British Royal College of Obstetricians observes, "[I]t is morally unconvincing to claim absolute inviolability for an organism with which nature itself is so prodigal."

[. . .] One position bases full moral personhood on sentience—the ability to feel or to experience pain. A second view emphasizes the beginning of brain activity or brain function. This view derives from the belief that the brain is the essential organ underlying our specifically human capacities. It is also an effort to render an account of the beginning of life that is consistent with the criterion of whole-brain death as the end of life. A third position takes as the marker for the beginning of personhood certain well developed cognitive abilities such as consciousness, reasoning ability, or the possession of self-concept.

While these views can lead to different conclusions as to when personhood begins, all support the conclusion that the preimplantation embryo does not merit the same degree of moral protection given to children or adult human beings. The absence of a nervous system until after gastrulation or neurulation makes it certain that the preimplantation embryo cannot experience pain, has no brain activity, and is not conscious or self-aware.

[. . .] Insistence on sentience as the criterion of personhood, for example, might require extending equal moral respect to animals. [. . .] Equating personhood with an earlier stage such as the commencement of brain activity raises the same parallel with animal rights and a further question of what is meant by brain activity in this context.

[. . .] Finally, a view based on consciousness, reasoning, or the possession of self-concept might lead to the exclusion of newborns from the class of protected subjects.

A Pluralistic Approach

[A pluralistic approach] does not focus on a single criterion of personhood [. . .] but emphasizes a variety of distinct, intersecting, and mutually supporting considerations. According to this view, the commencement of protectability is not an all-or-nothing matter but results from a being's increasing possession of qualities that make respecting it (and hence limiting others' liberty in relation to it) more compelling.

Among the qualities considered under a pluralistic approach are those mentioned in single-criterion views: genetic uniqueness, potentiality for full development, sentience, brain activity, and degree of cognitive development. Other qualities often mentioned are human form, capacity for survival outside the mother's womb, and degree of relational presence (whether to the mother herself or to others). Although none of these qualities is by itself sufficient to establish personhood, their developing presence in an entity increases its moral status until, at some point, full and equal protectability is required.

According to this view, the increased potentiality for development that marks the transition from gametes to zygote—and the establishment at this stage of at least the beginnings of biological uniqueness—counsel giving the preimplantation embryo a measure of respect that is not due the sperm or egg. However, the absence at this stage of almost all other qualities evoking respect makes it unreasonable to think of personhood as beginning here and places limits on the degree of respect accorded. [. . .] Formation of the primitive streak at 14 days of development and the beginning of cellular differentiation and organization of a single body axis marks yet another stage of development that merits an enhanced degree of protectability. As gestation continues, the further development of human form, the onset of a heartbeat, the development of the nervous system leading to brain activity and with this at least some of the physical basis for future sentience, relational presence to the mother, and capacity for independent existence all counsel toward according an increasing degree of protectability. This line of thinking culminates at birth, where substantial development and independent existence outside the mother's womb provide the moral basis for full and equal personhood. [. . .]

Implications for Public Policy

[. . .] From the perspective of public policy, the weight of arguments appears to support the permissibility of embryo research within a framework of stringent guidelines. Each of the single criterion views considered by the Panel poses unresolved conceptual and practical difficulties, but, in any case, only one of these positions attributes personhood and full moral protectability to the preimplantation embryo. The remaining positions accord it either limited or no moral status. The pluralistic approach, with its emphasis on a variety of intersecting and mutually reinforcing criteria, is less subject to the specific criticisms aimed at each of the single criterion views. This approach also corresponds with the steady increase in moral respect many people give to prenatal life in its various stages from conception to birth. In contrast to many of the single criterion positions, the pluralistic approach accords some moral weight to the preimplantation embryo but it does not rule out well-justified research. The absence of developmental individuation, the lack of even the possibility of sentience and most other qualities considered relevant to personhood, the very high natural mortality at this stage, and the important human benefits research might achieve all support the conclusion that embryo research may be conducted under strict guidelines. In terms of public policy, this conclusion appears to be the most compelling one available.

This conclusion regarding the permissibility of research involving the preimplantation embryo is based on an assessment of its moral status and not solely on its location *ex utero*. [. . .] One implication of the Panel's conclusion that research on the *ex utero* human embryo is permissible is that such research may sometimes occur at a slightly later stage than would be permitted with an embryo that has implanted in the uterus. [. . .]

DISTINCTIONS BETWEEN EMBRYOS INTENDED FOR AND NOT INTENDED FOR TRANSFER

It is important to recognize that when transfer to a uterus is intended, the preimplantation embryo is a research subject whose treatment raises distinct ethical issues. These issues are raised because research on the preimplantation embryo could result in harm to the child who will be born. Both in law and ethics, it is clear that fetuses who are brought to term are considered persons with full moral status and protectability. It would therefore be unacceptable to transfer an embryo or embryos if it is reasonable to believe that children who could be born from these procedures will suffer harm as a result of the research. Even when research involves a diagnostic procedure, an embryo or embryos may not be transferred unless there is reasonable confidence that any child born as a result of the procedures has not been harmed by them. This distinction in treatment between embryos that will not be transferred and those that will is warranted by the need to avoid harms to the child who will be born. [. . .]

FERTILIZATION OF OOCYTES
FOR RESEARCH

[...] Invoking deeply held and widely shared beliefs about the significance of fertilization as the first step in bringing a potential human being into existence, those opposed to fertilization of oocytes for research argue that this step ought not be taken solely for research purposes, no matter how important these purposes might be. They maintain that development of embryos expressly for research is inherently disrespectful of human life, as well as being open to significant abuses. They also fear that this practice will lead to the instrumentalization of the preimplantation embryo and, by extension, of other human research subjects. They are particularly concerned that the development of embryos for research may result in the commodification of embryos and even their commercialization.

Many of those who hold this view believe that research on embryos remaining from infertility treatments (or preimplantation diagnosis) may be justified as a byproduct of the otherwise well-intentioned act of trying to conceive a healthy child, whereas the express fertilization of oocytes for research purposes lacks even this minimal justification.

Those who would permit the fertilization of oocytes expressly for research often argue that the resulting embryos have equivalent moral status to embryos remaining from infertility treatment, and thus they should be acceptable for research under similar guidelines. [...] However, those who would permit the fertilization of oocytes expressly for research also offer a number of arguments based on moral concerns such as the safety and health of women, children, and men. First, a ban on fertilizing donated oocytes for research would rule out much important research on oocyte maturation that may be of potentially great clinical benefit. In studying oocyte maturation, it is essential to find out whether the oocytes are fertilizable and whether they develop normally during cleavage stages. There is reason to believe that the low viability of some IVF embryos may be due to the rapid maturation of oocytes following hormonal stimulation. [...]

Research on oocyte maturation might also obviate the need for hyperstimulation in women undergoing *in vitro* fertilization or serving as egg donors. [...]

Second, a ban on the fertilization of oocytes for research purposes would preclude much research on the process of fertilization itself. Such a ban would hinder studies on the efficacy and safety of new contraceptives that work by interfering with the interaction of egg and sperm. Attempting fertilization is the only way to verify whether such contraceptives work.

Research on the freezing and thawing of unfertilized eggs would be seriously impeded, since the only way to determine the safety and efficiency of this process is to fertil-ize the eggs and study their resulting chromosomes and rates of cleavage in vitro. [...]

Third, a ban on the fertilization of oocytes for research purposes might preclude very important research on the effect on gametes and embryos of potentially harmful drugs or chemicals administered to women or to which women are exposed. [...]

Fourth, a ban on the fertilization of oocytes for research purposes could impede particular kinds of research of great scientific and therapeutic value and for which an adequate number of embryos is essential to ensure validity. An example is research on genetic abnormalities or chromosomal imbalances arising or manifest during early embryogenesis and associated with birth defects and childhood or reproductive cancers.

Fifth, in certain cases, permitting the fertilization of oocytes might be justified based on the limited number and suitability of embryos remaining from IVF treatments. [...]

A final reason for permitting the fertilization and study of oocytes is that a complete prohibition in this area is likely to be very difficult—if not impossible—to enforce and is even likely to result in practices that exploit or harm women in infertility programs. [...]

These arguments suggest that studies that require the fertilization of oocytes are needed to answer crucial questions in reproductive medicine. Reviewing all these considerations, the Panel concluded that it would not be wise to prohibit altogether the fertilization and study of oocytes for research purposes. The Panel had to balance important issues regarding the health and safety of women, children, and men against the moral respect due the preimplantation embryo. [...] Given the conclusions the Panel reached about the lesser moral status of the preimplantation embryo, it concluded that the health and safety needs of women, children, and men must be given priority.

The Panel recognizes, however, that the preimplantation embryo merits respect as a developing form of human life and should be used in research only for the most serious and compelling reasons. [...] In order to minimize this, the Panel believes that the use of oocytes fertilized expressly for research should be allowed only under the following two conditions:

• When the research by its very nature cannot otherwise be validly conducted. Examples of studies that might meet this condition include oocyte maturation or oocyte freezing followed by fertilization and examination for subsequent developmental viability and chromosomal normalcy and investigations into the process of fertilization itself (including the efficacy of new contraceptives).

• When the fertilization of oocytes is necessary for the validity of a study that is potentially of outstanding scientific and therapeutic value. [...]

56   The Inhuman Use of Human Beings

A Statement on Embryo Research

THE RAMSEY COLLOQUIUM

[...] After carefully studying the Report of the Human Embryo Research Panel, we conclude that this recommendation is morally repugnant, entails grave injustice to innocent human beings, and constitutes an assault upon the foundational ideas of human dignity and rights essential to a free and decent society. The arguments offered by the Panel are more ideological and self-interested than scientific; the actions recommended by the Panel cross the threshold into a world of apparently limitless technological manipulation and manufacture of human life. [...]

[...] We urge a comprehensive public debate and intense congressional scrutiny regarding the proposals emanating from the National Institutes of Health. The research recommended by the Panel should not be funded by the government. It should not be done at all.

We are confident that most people, to the extent that they are aware of the Panel's recommendation, experience an immediate and strong revulsion. This is not to be dismissed as an irrational reaction. It signals a deep, intuitive awareness of lines that must not be crossed if we are to maintain our sometimes fragile hold upon our own humanity. [...]

The ominously new thing in the Panel's Report is that embryonic human life should be treated simply as research material to be used and discarded—and should even be brought into being solely for that purpose. The Report readily acknowledges that the embryos to be used are instances of human life. It does not hesitate to answer the question of when a new human life begins. Indeed, indisputable scientific evidence leaves no choice: a new human life begins at conception (or, as the Report usually prefers, "fertilization"). The Report speaks of the embryo from the earliest moment as "developing human life." We are at various points told that the very early embryo deserves "serious moral consideration," "moral respect," "profound respect," and "some added measure of respect beyond that accorded animal subjects."

Honesty requires that we speak not simply of human life but of a human being. Skin and intestinal tissue, even eggs and sperm, are human life. But, unlike such instances of human life, the embryo from the earliest moment has the active capacity to articulate itself into what everyone acknowledges is a human being. The embryo is a being; that is to say, it is an integral whole with actual existence. The being is human; it will not articulate itself into some other kind of animal. Any being that is human is a human being. If it is objected that, at five days or fifteen days, the embryo does not look like a human being, it must be pointed out that this is precisely what a human being looks like—and what each of us looked like—at five or fifteen days of development. [...]

[...] It is one of the most treasured maxims of our civilization that human beings are always to be treated as ends and never merely as means. In a partial dissent from the Report, Professor Patricia A. King, member of the Panel, writes, "The fertilization of human oocytes [female eggs] for research purposes is unnerving because human life is being created solely for human *use* [...]." [...]

In order to decide which human embryos are usable and which are "protectable" from such use, the Report leans very heavily on the concept of "personhood." The question is switched from "When does the life of a human being begin?" to "When does a human being become a person?" Persons are protectable; nonpersons or those who are deemed to be something less than persons are not protectable. But the only reason they are not protectable is that they will not be protected. Although they are obviously protectable in the sense that we are capable of protecting them, they are designated "not protectable" because we have decided not to protect them. And we decide not to protect them because they are not persons. Whether they are persons, and therefore protectable, depends upon their possessing certain qualities that we associate with persons and think worth protecting. [...]

The question is not whether the embryo is protectable but whether it is in need of protection. [...] The principle espoused by the Report leads to the suggestion that our obligation to afford protection to a human being is in inverse proportion to his or her need for protection. Put differently, those who are fully and undoubtedly persons are protectable because they are, by and large, able to protect themselves.

[...] The classical conviction of our culture has been that, contrary to the Report, it is "an all or nothing matter."

The Ramsey Colloquium, "The Inhuman Use of Human Beings: A Statement on Embryo Research by the Ramsey Colloquium," *First Things* 49 (1995): 17–21. Please see the end of the paper for a list of signatories to this Ramsey Colloquium statement.

We are implicated in the fate of all; every human being is inviolable. [...]

[...] Personhood is certainly not a scientific concept. As used by the Panel, it is an ideological concept, an idea in the service of a program aimed at changing dramatically our civilization's understanding of human life and community. In this Report, personhood is a status that we bestow. [...] We are told that protectability increases with an "increasing possession of qualities" that we find compelling. It follows that protectability decreases with the decreasing possession of such qualities.

[...] In the current language of the academy, personhood is entirely a "social construct." Whether someone is too young or too old, too retarded or too sick, too troublesome or too useless to be entitled to personhood is determined by a "decision on our part." [...]

The Panel claims to have established clear lines and clear time limits regarding what it is permissible to do with human embryos. That claim is false, and it seems that the panelists know that it is false. The Report says that research with these living human beings "should not be permitted beyond the time of the usual appearance of the primitive streak in vivo (14 days)." (The primitive streak is a groove that develops along the midline of the embryonic disk, and its appearance is viewed as one of several milestones in the embryo's continued development.) But this time limit is clearly arbitrary and chosen as a pragmatic compromise [...].

The panelists all know that development is continuous and it offers no such bright natural line to those who would "ascribe personhood." Moreover, this "time limit" is by no means firm, as is evident in the Report's assertion that it should serve "at the present time," and "for the foreseeable future." [...]

"Throughout its deliberations," we are told, "the Panel relied on the principle that research involving preimplantation embryos is acceptable public policy only if the research promises significant scientific and therapeutic benefits." But a principle that says something should not be done unless there are strong motives for doing it is no principle at all. The claim to have set limits is vitiated by the repeated assertion that exceptions can be made for "serious and compelling reasons." [...] There is no reason, in principle, why such license would be confined to very small and very young human beings.

[...] As for therapeutic benefits, the Report holds out the promise of improved success with *in vitro* fertilization, new contraceptive techniques, new prospects for genetic screening, the production of cell lines for use in tissue transplantation, and, more vaguely, treatment of cancer and other diseases. [...]

Is this the future that we want? Who should decide? That brings us to the makeup and role of the Panel itself.

"Americans hold widely different views on the question of the moral value of prenatal life at its various stages," the Report notes. "It is not the role of those who help form public policy to decide which of these views is correct. Instead public policy represents an effort to arrive at a reasonable accommodation to diverse interests." [...] In fact, however, in order to legitimate morally what it recommends, the Panel does adopt a particular philosophy that it believes cuts through the complexities and controversies. That philosophy is ordinarily called utilitarianism. It is a primitive and unreflective version of utilitarianism, to be sure, but the message is unequivocal: the end justifies the means. If there are "serious and compelling reasons," it would seem that the end would justify any means. Certainly it justifies producing, using, and destroying human beings who are valued only for their utility as tools serving the purposes of scientific research. The Panel's is not a "multifactorial" judgment. There is ultimately only one factor: scientific utility. [...]

The production of human beings for the purpose of experiments that will destroy them should be prohibited by law. The use of human beings for experiments that will do them harm and to which they have not given their consent should be prohibited by law. It matters not how young or how small, how old or how powerless, such human beings may be. Some nations ban or severely restrict the research proposed by the Panel (e.g., Norway, Germany, Austria, Australia). [...]

The shamelessly partisan and conceptually confused Report of the Human Embryo Research Panel should be unambiguously rejected. Limits that are "for the present time" and "for the foreseeable future" limit nothing. They are but unconvincing reassurances that scientists are going carefully where they should not be permitted to go at all. If the course recommended by the Panel is approved, the foreseeable future is ominously clear: it is a return to the past when people contrived "conceptual frameworks" for excluding categories of human being, born and unborn, from our common humanity.

Hadley Arkes
Matthew Berke
Gerard V. Bradley
James T. Burtchaell
Francis Canavan
Rabbi David G. Dalin
Midge Decter
Thomas S. Derr
Fr. Ernest Fortin
Jorge Garcia
Marc Gellman
Robert P. George
Mary Ann Glendon

Stanley Hauerwas
John Hittinger
Russell Hittinger
Robert W. Jenson
Leon R. Kass
Ralph McInerny
Richard John Neuhaus
David Novak
Michael Novak
James Nuechterlein
David Singer
George Weigel
Robert L. Wilken

57 Ethical Issues in Human Stem Cell Research

NATIONAL BIOETHICS ADVISORY COMMISSION

EXECUTIVE SUMMARY

INTRODUCTION

In November 1998, President Clinton charged the National Bioethics Advisory Commission with the task of conducting a thorough review of the issues associated with human stem cell research, balancing all ethical and medical considerations. [...]

SCIENTIFIC AND MEDICAL CONSIDERATIONS

[...] Many kinds of stem cells are found in the body, with some more differentiated, or committed, to a particular function than others. [...] Although the term stem cell commonly is used to refer to the cells within the adult organism that renew tissue (e.g., hematopoietic stem cells, a type of cell found in the blood), the most fundamental and extraordinary of the stem cells are found in the early stage embryo. These embryonic stem (ES) cells, unlike the more differentiated adult stem cells or other cell types, retain the special ability to develop into nearly any cell type. [...]

[S]cientists have long recognized the possibility of using such cells to generate more specialized cells or tissue, which could allow the generation of new cells to be used to treat injuries or diseases, such as Alzheimer's disease, Parkinson's disease, heart disease, and kidney failure. Likewise, scientists regard these cells as an important—perhaps essential—means for understanding the earliest stages of human development and as an important tool in the development of life-saving drugs and cell-replacement therapies to treat disorders caused by early cell death or impairment. [...]

ETHICAL AND POLICY CONSIDERATIONS

[...] Although we believe most would agree that human embryos deserve respect as a form of human life, disagreements arise regarding both what form such respect should take and what level of protection is required at different stages of embryonic development. Therefore, embryo research that is not therapeutic to the embryo is bound to raise serious concerns and to heighten the tensions between

National Bioethics Advisory Commission, Ethical Issues in Human Stem Cell Research, Volume 1 (Rockville, Md.: NBAC, September 1999), available online at bioethics .georgetown.edu/nbac/pubs.html.

two important ethical commitments: to cure disease and to protect human life. For those who believe that the embryo has the moral status of a person from the moment of conception, research (or any other activity) that would destroy the embryo is considered wrong and should not take place. For those who believe otherwise, arriving at an ethically acceptable policy in this arena involves a complex balancing of a number of important ethical concerns. [...]

For most observers, the resolution of these ethical and scientific issues depends to some degree on the source of the stem cells. [...] With respect to embryos and the ES cells from which they can be derived, some draw an ethical distinction between two types of embryos. One is referred to as the research embryo, an embryo created through in vitro fertilization [IVF] with gametes provided solely for research purposes. Many people, including the President, have expressed the view that the federal government should not fund research that involves creating such embryos. The second type of embryo is that which was created for infertility treatment, but is now intended to be discarded because it is unsuitable or no longer needed for such treatment. The use of these embryos raises fewer ethical questions because it does not alter their final disposition. Finally, the recent demonstration of cloning techniques (somatic cell nuclear transfer) in nonhuman animals suggests that transfer of a human somatic cell nucleus into an oocyte might create an embryo that could be used as a source of ES cells. The creation of a human organism using this technique raises questions similar to those raised by the creation of research embryos through IVF. [...]

CONCLUSIONS AND RECOMMENDATIONS

This report presents the conclusions that the Commission has reached and the recommendations that the Commission has made in the following areas: the ethical acceptability of federal funding for research that either derives or uses ES or EG [embryonic germ] cells; the means of ensuring appropriate consent of women or couples who donate cadaveric fetal tissue or embryos remaining after infertility treatments; the need for restrictions on the sale of these materials and the designation of those who may benefit from their use; the need for ethical oversight and review of such research at the national and institutional level; and the appropriateness of voluntary compliance by the private sector with some of these recommendations. [All recommendations omitted.—eds.] [...]

ETHICAL ISSUES RELATING TO THE SOURCES OF HUMAN EMBRYONIC STEM OR EMBRYONIC GERM CELLS

Research involving human ES cells and EG cells raises several important ethical issues, principally related to the current sources and/or methods of deriving these cells. If, for example, ES and EG cells could be derived from sources other than human embryos or cadaveric fetal material, fewer ethical concerns would be involved in determining a policy for their use for scientific research or clinical therapies. At present, however, the only methods available to isolate and culture human ES and EG cells involve the use of human embryos or cadaveric fetal tissue. Therefore, careful consideration of the ethical issues involved in the use of these sources is an unavoidable component of the advancement of this type of research.

This chapter first considers the ethical issues arising from research involving the derivation and/or use of ES or EG cells from three potential sources: cadaveric fetal tissue, embryos resulting from and remaining after infertility treatments, and embryos created solely for research purposes either by IVF or somatic cell nuclear transfer (SCNT) techniques. [...]

RESEARCH WITH EG CELLS DERIVED FROM CADAVERIC FETAL TISSUE

Many of the ethical questions regarding research involving the use of cadaveric fetal tissue were analyzed in depth by the 1988 National Institutes of Health (NIH) Human Fetal Tissue Transplantation Research Panel. What is new in the present context is that, in the near term at least, the materials derived from this tissue would not be transplanted; rather, gonadal tissue (both male and female) would be used as a source for human EG cells. Initially, these cell lines would be used in basic research to determine their nature, to understand their relationship to human development, and to identify differentiation factors that enable such cells to develop into particular tissue types. Later, such cell lines also might be used for the development of transplantation for particular tissue types. The value of cadaveric fetal tissue already has been demonstrated; a broad variety of research materials and reagents derived from cadaveric fetal tissue currently are used in federally funded research.

The ethical acceptability of deriving EG cells from the tissue of aborted fetuses is, for some, closely connected to the ethical acceptability of abortion. Those who believe that elective abortions are morally acceptable are less likely to identify insurmountable ethical barriers to research that in-volves the derivation and use of EG cells derived from cadaveric fetal tissue. This group might agree that it is necessary to restrict such research by requiring that the decision to donate fetal tissue be separate from the decision to terminate the pregnancy. The purpose of such a requirement would be to protect the pregnant woman against coercion and exploitation rather than to protect the fetus. In addition, even those who find it acceptable to use cadaveric fetal tissue in research might hold that certain uses of such tissue—for example, uses that treat it as nothing more than any other bodily tissue—should be ruled out as disrespectful.

Those who view elective abortions as morally unjustified often—but not always—oppose the research use of tissue derived from aborted fetuses. They usually have no moral difficulty with the use of tissue from spontaneously aborted fetuses or—if they recognize exceptions to the moral prohibition on abortion—from fetuses in cases that they believe are morally justifiable abortions (e.g., to save the pregnant woman's life). However, in general they do not believe that it is possible to derive and use tissue from what they believe are unjustifiably aborted fetuses without inevitable and unacceptable association with those abortions. This association, they believe, usually taints the actions of all those involved in using these materials or in financing research protocols that rely on such tissue. Nevertheless, some opponents of elective abortions believe that it is still possible to support such research as long as effective safeguards are in place to separate abortion decisions from the procurement and use of fetal tissue in research. For them, when appropriate safeguards are in place, using cadaveric fetal tissue from elective abortions for research is relevantly similar to using nonfetal cadavers donated for scientific and medical purposes.

Association with Abortion

Opponents of the research use of fetal materials obtained from elective abortions dispute the claim that it is possible to separate the moral issues surrounding the abortion from those involved in obtaining and using fetal material. They argue that those who obtain and use fetal material from elective abortion inevitably become associated, in ethically unacceptable ways, with the abortions that are the source of the material. They identify two major types of unacceptable association or cooperation with abortion: (1) causal responsibility for abortions and (2) symbolic association with abortions.

1. CAUSAL RESPONSIBILITY

Some believe that those who provide cadaveric fetal tissue in research are indirectly, if not directly, responsible for the choice of some women to have an abortion. Direct causal responsibility exists where, in this case, someone's actions directly lead a pregnant woman to have an abortion—for example, the researcher offers financial compensation for cadaveric fetal tissue and this compensation leads the pregnant woman to have an abortion she would not otherwise have had. In part because of concerns about direct causal responsibility, the Human Fetal Tissue Transplantation Research Panel recommended the following safeguards to separate the pregnant woman's decision to abort from her decision to donate fetal tissue:

- The consent of women for abortions must be obtained prior to requesting or obtaining consent for the donation of fetal tissue.

- Those who seek a woman's consent to donate should not discuss fetal tissue donation prior to her decision to abort, unless she specifically requests such information.

- Women should not be paid for providing fetal tissue.

- A separation must be maintained between abortion clinic personnel and those involved in using fetal tissue.

- There should be a prohibition against any alteration of the timing of or procedures used in an abortion solely for the purpose of obtaining tissue.

- Donors of cadaveric fetal tissue should not be allowed to designate a specific recipient of transplanted tissue.

[S]everal of these safeguards were later adopted in federal legislation regarding the use of aborted fetal tissue in transplantation research, and they appear to be sufficient to avoid direct causal responsibility for abortions in human EG research as well as in transplantation research.

Those involved in research uses of EG cells derived from fetal tissue could be indirectly responsible for abortions if the perceived potential benefits of the research contributed to an increase in the number of abortions. Opponents of fetal tissue research argue that it is unrealistic to suppose that a woman's decision to abort can be kept separate from considerations of donating fetal tissue, as many women facing the abortion decision are likely to have gained knowledge about fetal tissue research through the media or other sources. The knowledge that having an elective abortion might have benefits for future patients through the donation of fetal tissue for research may tip the balance in favor of going through with an abortion for some women who are ambivalent about it. Some argue that the benefits achieved through the routine use of fetal tissue will further legitimize abortion and result in more permissive societal attitudes and policies concerning elective abortion.

It is impossible to eliminate the possibility completely, however slight it may be, that knowledge of the promise of research on EG cells derived from fetal tissue will play a role in some elective abortion decisions, even if only rarely. However, it is not clear how much moral weight ultimately attaches to this possibility. One might be justified in some instances in asserting that if it were not for the research use of fetal tissue following an abortion, a woman might not have chosen to terminate her pregnancy.

But one could assign this kind of causal responsibility to a number of factors that figure into abortion decisions without making ascriptions of indirect causal responsibility, or what is sometimes called moral complicity. For example, a woman might choose to have an abortion principally because she does not want to slow the advancement of her education and career. She might not have had an abortion in the absence of expectations that encourage women to develop their careers. Yet, we would not think it appropriate to charge those who promote such expectations and/or policies as complicit in her abortion. In both this case and that of research, the opportunity to choose abortion is a consequence of a legitimate social policy. The burden on those seeking to end such policies is to show that the risks of harm—both the probability and the magnitude of harm—resulting from the policies outweigh the expected benefits. This criterion minimally requires evidence of a high probability of a large number of elective abortions that would not have occurred in the absence of those policies. There is, however, no such evidence at present. [. . .]

2. SYMBOLIC ASSOCIATION

People can become inappropriately associated with what they believe are wrongful acts for which they are not causally responsible. Particularly problematic for many is an association that appears to symbolize approval of the wrongdoing. For example, James Burtchaell maintains that those involved in research on fetal tissue enter a symbolic alliance with the practice of abortion in producing or deriving benefits from it.

A common response is that persons can benefit from what they might consider immoral acts without tacitly approving of those acts. For example, transplant surgeons and transplant recipients may benefit (the latter more directly than the former) from donated organs from victims of murder or drunken driving but nevertheless condemn those wrongful acts. A researcher who uses cadaveric fetal material in studies to answer important research questions or to study its potential therapeutic effects or the patient who receives the donated tissue need not sanction the act of abortion any more than the transplant surgeon who uses the organs of a murder victim approves of the homicidal act.

Some opponents of fetal tissue research maintain that it implicates those involved in a kind of wrongdoing that cannot be attributed to the transplant surgeon in the example above. Unlike drunken driving and murder, abortion is an institutionalized practice in which certain categories of human life (the members of which are considered by some to have the same moral status as human adults) are allowed to be killed. In this respect, some opponents of abortion go so far as to suggest that fetal tissue research is more analogous to research that benefits from experiments conducted by Nazi doctors during World War II.

But whatever one thinks of comparisons between the victims of Nazi crimes and aborted fetuses—and many are outraged by these comparisons—it is possible to concede the comparisons without concluding that human stem cell research involving cadaveric fetal tissue is morally problematic. Of course, some believe that those who use data derived from Nazi experiments are morally complicit with those crimes. For example, William Seidelman writes:

> By giving value to (Nazi) research we are, by implication, supporting Himmler's philosophy that the subjects' lives were "useless." This is to argue that, by accepting data derived from their misery we are, post mortem, deriving utility from otherwise "useless" life. Science could thus stand accused of giving greater value to knowledge than to human life itself.

But one need not adopt this stance. Instead, one can reasonably believe that a scientist's actions must be understood and judged not by their consequences or uses but rather by several other factors, including the scientist's intentions, the social practices of which his or her actions are a part, and the social context in which those practices are embedded. As philosopher Benjamin Freedman wrote:

> A moral universe such as our own must, I think, rely on the authors of their own actions to be primarily responsible for attaching symbolic significance to those actions.... [I]n using the Nazi data, physicians and scientists are acting pursuant to their own moral commitment to aid patients and to advance science in the interest of humankind. The use of data is predicated upon that duty, and it is in seeking to fulfill that duty that the symbolic significance of the action must be found.

It is likewise reasonable to maintain that the symbolic significance of support for research using EG cells derived from aborted fetal tissue lies in the commitment and desire to gain knowledge, promote health, and save lives. This research is allied with a worthy cause, and any taint that might attach from the source of the cells appears to be outweighed by the potential good that the research may yield.

Consent and Donation

In previous debates about the use of fetal tissue in research, questions have been raised about who has the moral authority to donate the material. Some assert that, from an ethical standpoint, a woman who chooses abortion forfeits her rights to determine the disposition of the dead fetus. Burtchaell, for instance, argues that "the decision to abort, made by the mother, is an act of such violent abandonment of the maternal trusteeship that no further exercise of such responsibility is admissible." By contrast, John Robertson argues that this position mistakenly assumes that the persons disposing of cadaveric remains act only as the guardians or proxies of the deceased. Instead, "a more accurate account of their role is to guard their own feelings and interests in assuring that the remains of kin are treated respectfully."

In our view, obtaining consent to donate fetal tissue is an ethical prerequisite for using such material to derive EG cells, even though the woman or couple are not research subjects per se, and even though the cadaveric fetus is not a human subject. This view is consistent with the conclusion of the Human Fetal Tissue Transplantation Research Panel, which held that "[e]xpress donation by the pregnant woman after the abortion decision is the most appropriate mode of transfer of fetal tissues because it is the most congruent with our society's traditions, laws, policies, and practices, including the Uniform Anatomical Gift Act and current Federal research regulations." According to this panel, a woman's choice of a legal abortion does not disqualify her legally and should not disqualify her morally from serving "as the primary decisionmaker about the disposition of fetal remains, including the donation of fetal tissue for research." She "has a special connection with the fetus and she has a legitimate interest in its disposition and use." In addition, her decision to donate fetal tissue would not violate the dead fetus's interests. The panel concluded that "in the final analysis, any mode of transfer other than maternal donation appears to raise more serious ethical problems." Fetal tissue should not be used without the woman's consent. Not only should her consent be necessary, it should also be sufficient to donate the tissue, except where the father's objection is known.

We concur with the Human Fetal Tissue Transplantation Research Panel that a woman undergoing an elective abortion should be authorized to donate fetal tissue, unless the father is known to object. We further agree with the panel and with subsequent federal legislation that it is important to establish safeguards to separate the pregnant woman's decision to abort from the decision to donate cadaveric fetal tissue. The guidelines already in place for fetal tissue transplantation research generally are appropriate and appear to be sufficient if they also apply to research involving human EG cells. [...]

RESEARCH WITH ES CELLS DERIVED FROM EMBRYOS REMAINING AFTER INFERTILITY TREATMENTS

[...]

The Moral Status of Embryos

To say that an entity has "moral status" is to say something both about how one should act towards that thing or person and about whether that thing or person can expect certain treatment from others. The debate about the moral status of embryos traditionally has revolved around the question of whether the embryo has the same moral status as children and adult humans do—with a right to life that may not be sacrificed by others for the benefit of society. At one end of the spectrum of attitudes is the view that the embryo is a mere cluster of cells that has no more moral status than any other collection of human cells. From this perspective, one might conclude that there are few, if any, ethical limitations on the research uses of embryos.

At the other end of the spectrum is the view that embryos should be considered in the same moral category as children or adults. [...] In contrast, scholars representing other religious traditions testified that moral status varies according to the stage of development. [...] Other scholars from Protestant, Jewish, and Islamic traditions noted that major strands of those traditions support a view of fetal development that does not assign full moral status to the early embryo. [...]

On this issue, the Commission adopted what some have described as an intermediate position, one with which many likely would agree: that the embryo merits respect as a form of human life, but not the same level of respect accorded persons. A standard approach taken by those who deny that embryos are persons with the same moral status as children and adults is to identify one or more psychological or cognitive capacities that are considered essential to personhood (and a concomitant right to life) but that embryos lack. Most commonly cited are consciousness, self-consciousness, and the ability to reason. The problem with such accounts is that they appear to be either under- or over-inclusive, depending on which capacities are invoked. [...]

Those who deny that embryos have the same moral status as persons might maintain that the embryo is simply too nascent a form of human life to merit the kind of respect accorded more developed humans. However, some would argue that, in the absence of an event that decisively (i.e., to everyone's satisfaction) identifies the first stage of human development—a stage at which destroying human life is morally wrong—it is not permissible to destroy embryos.

The fundamental argument of those who oppose the destruction of human embryos is that these embryos are human beings and, as such, have a right to life. The very humanness of the embryo is thus thought to confer the moral status of a person. The problem is that, for some, the premise that all human lives at any stage of their development are persons in the moral sense is not self-evident. Indeed, some believe that the premise conflates two categories of human beings: namely, beings that belong to the species *Homo sapiens,* and beings that belong to a particular moral community. According to this view, the fact that an individual is a member of the species *Homo sapiens* is not sufficient to confer upon it membership in the moral community of persons. [...]

The Importance of Shared Views

In [Alta] Charo's view, once one recognizes that the substantive conflict among fundamental values surrounding embryo research cannot be resolved in a manner that will satisfy all sides, the most promising approach is to seek to balance all the relevant considerations in determining whether to proceed with the research. Thus, although it is clear that embryo research would offend some people deeply, she would argue that the potential health benefits for this and future generations outweigh the pain experienced by opponents of the research.

It is, however, questionable whether Charo's analysis successfully avoids the issue of moral status. It might be argued, for example, that placing the lives of embryos in this kind of utilitarian calculus will seem appropriate only to those who presuppose that embryos do not have the status of persons. Those who believe—or who genuinely allow for the possibility—that embryos have the status of persons will regard such consequentialist grounds for destroying embryos as extremely problematic. [...]

We believe that the following would seem to be a reasonable statement of the kind of agreement that could be possible on this issue:

> Research that involves the destruction of embryos remaining after infertility treatments is permissible when there is good reason to believe that this destruction is necessary to develop cures for life-threatening or severely debilitating diseases and when appropriate protections and oversight are in place in order to prevent abuse.

Given the great promise of ES cell research for saving lives and alleviating suffering, such a statement would appear to be sufficient to permit, at least in certain cases, not only the use of ES cells in research, but also the use of certain embryos to generate ES cells. Some might object, however, that the benefits of the research are too uncertain to justify a comparison with the conditions under which one might make an exception to permit abortion. But the lower probability of benefits from research uses of embryos is balanced by a much higher ratio of potential lives saved relative to embryonic lives lost and by two other characteristics of the embryos used to derive ES cells: first, that they are at a much earlier stage of development than is usually true of aborted fetuses, and second, that they are about to be discarded after infertility treatment and thus have no prospect for survival even if they are not used in deriving ES cells. In our view, the potential benefits of the research outweigh the harms to embryos that are destroyed in the research process. [...]

RESEARCH WITH ES CELLS DERIVED FROM EMBRYOS CREATED SOLELY FOR RESEARCH

Ever since the NIH Human Embryo Research Panel [whose report is included in this volume—eds.] recommended that under certain conditions embryos could be created solely for research purposes, there has been an ongoing discussion about the ethical and scientific merit of such a practice. [...]

Embryos Created Using IVF Procedures

There are two significant arguments in favor of creating human embryos using IVF technologies solely for stem cell research: The first is that there may be an inadequate supply of embryos remaining after infertility treatments. The second is that important research that could be of great medical benefit cannot be undertaken except with well-defined embryos that are created specifically for research and/or medical purposes. However, recommending federal funding for research using or deriving ES cells from embryos expressly created for research purposes presents two ethical problems. First, unlike in the case of embryos that remain following infertility treatments, there does not appear to be sufficient societal agreement on the moral acceptability of this practice at this time. Second, it is unclear whether an adequate supply of ES cells from embryos is available to meet scientific need or whether specialized cells are needed.

We do not, at this time, support the federal sponsorship of research involving the creation of embryos solely for research purposes. However, we recognize that, in the future, scientific evidence and public support for this type of stem cell research may be sufficient in order to proceed. Therefore, to promote ongoing dialogue on this topic, we offer the following discussion.

The "Discarded-Created" Distinction: On the Importance of Intentions

Various parties have discussed whether there is a moral difference between conducting research on embryos created with the intention of using them for reproduction and conducting research on embryos created with the intention of using them for research. Embryos created with the intention of using them for reproduction become available for research only when it is known that they are no longer intended to be used for infertility treatments; only then are they considered discarded, and only then do they become potentially available for research. The second group of embryos—research embryos—are those that are created without the intention that they will be used for procreative purposes. Rather, they are developed solely for research purposes or to generate research and medical materials such as stem cells or other cell lines, clones, DNA sequences, or proteins. [...]

An ethical intuition that seems to motivate the "discarded-created" distinction is that the act of creating an embryo for reproduction is respectful in a way that is commensurate with the moral status of embryos, while the act of creating an embryo for research is not. Embryos that are discarded following the completion of IVF treatments were presumably created by individuals who had the primary intention of implanting them for reproductive purposes. These individuals did not consider the destruction of these embryos until it was determined that they were no longer needed. By contrast, research embryos are created for use in research and, in the case of stem cell research, their destruction in the process of research. Hence, one motivation that encourages serious consideration of the "discarded-created" distinction is a concern about instrumentalization —treating the embryo as a mere object—a practice that may increasingly lead us to think of embryos generally as means to our ends rather than as ends in themselves. [...]

58　Creating Embryos for Research

On Weighing Symbolic Costs

Maura A. Ryan

[. . .] For those who object to the experimental use of human embryos under any circumstances, there is no point in asking whether it is ethical to create embryos solely for the purpose of experimentation. If it is wrong to use embryos as experimental subjects, it is wrong to create them so that you can use them. If experimentation on human embryos cannot be conducted without violating obligations of informed consent or violating a human life, as theologian Paul Ramsey argued almost 30 years ago, it makes little difference whether we are contemplating the use of "spare" embryos. [. . .]

Alternatively, what if we hold that at least some kinds of embryo research can be justified? [. . .] In that case, is there any reason to object to the production of embryos for research use? [. . .] Does the creation of research embryos weaken or insult our communal respect for the sanctity of human life or the integrity of human reproduction in some way that in vitro fertilization (IVF) or the experimental use of "spare embryos" does not?

[I] argue that it is possible to draw a valid distinction between research involving the deliberate creation of embryos and research involving byproducts of medically assisted reproduction. [. . .] My position does not rest on claims about the moral status of the preimplantation embryo or assertions concerning the "rights" of embryos. Rather, I show that the most persuasive argument offered in defense of the deliberate creation of embryos for experimental use neglects fundamental questions concerning the proper or just use of procreative technologies. [. . .] I argue that reproductive interventions are justified only insofar as they serve the goals of responsible and human reproduction: The bringing forth of new life in loving and nurturing relationship. Creating embryos for research is incompatible with the goals that legitimate and should direct reproductive interventions. [. . .]

Maura A. Ryan, "Creating Embryos for Research: On Weighing Symbolic Costs," in *Cloning and the Future of Human Embryo Research,* ed. Paul Lauritzen (New York: Oxford University Press, 2001), 50–66.

STEINBOCK AND THE INTEREST VIEW

According to Bonnie Steinbock, "We may choose to respect embryos and preconscious fetuses as powerful symbols of human life, but we cannot protect them for their own sake." It is the failure to acknowledge the distinction between choosing to protect embryos and preconscious fetuses because of what they represent to us and claiming to protect the interests of embryos and preconscious fetuses, argues Steinbock, that accounts for a persistent confusion and inconsistency in our approach to the treatment of the unborn. [. . .]

[T]here is an important and, in Steinbock's view, frequently neglected difference between acknowledging the moral and social value of human embryos and according embryos moral standing. To have moral standing is to count morally, to be the sort of being whose interests must be considered, whose interests exert a claim on the behavior of others. Following Joel Feinberg, Steinbock argues that a "being can have interests only if it can matter to the being what is being done to it . . ." and ". . . if nothing at all can possibly matter to a being, then that being has no interests." [. . .] Because a human embryo or a presentient fetus has no interests, its interests need not, indeed cannot, be taken into account; thus, human embryos and presentient fetuses lack moral status.

In the interest view, sentience is both a necessary and a sufficient condition for moral standing. Only a being that is conscious and aware of its own experience can have a stake in what is or is not done to it. [. . .] Sentience acts, therefore, as a threshold as well as a dividing line for the interest view: "mere things and nonconscious living things fall below the moral status line; animals and people lie above it."

[. . .] As potential persons, embryos and fetuses have a symbolic value that precludes, for example, using them in unnecessary experiments or for purely commercial gain. In the interest view, however, it does not make sense to talk about moral obligations to avoid harm to or to promote the welfare of preconscious or presentient embryos on the grounds that we are "experimenting on unconsenting human subjects." Embryos do not have moral status.

[T]he moral reasons we give for protecting a flowering tree or a Picasso or a national flag have to do not with obligating features of the thing in question but with the symbolic or material value we have conferred on it. In the same way, when Steinbock argues that embryos or presentient fetuses should not be used in frivolous research or for crassly commercial purposes, it is not because to do so violates the interests of the embryo or presentient fetus or causes harm to them but because of the potentially brutalizing effect of such use on society—the possibility of undermining "commonly held fundamental values" such as respect for human life.

[...] In determining the boundaries of permissible research, however, the moral reasons for pursuing certain kinds of research must be weighed against the moral reasons for deciding not to pursue them. [...] Whatever the social or symbolic value of the embryo or presentient fetus, it does not outweigh the interests of real persons in access to goods and services they need and desire. Moreover, respect for human life is hardly expressed when embryos or presentient fetuses are protected at the expense of the "vital human interests" of already existing persons. [...]

WEIGHING THE SYMBOLIC

[...] At least for those who agree that fertilized ova and early embryos are not fully persons in a moral sense, the controversy over experimentation on human embryos is about what it means to display respect for embryos not as persons but as potent symbols of human life.

As Gilbert Meilaender reminds us [...] it is a serious mistake to ignore such concerns as "merely symbolic." Human thought and language is inescapably symbolic. [...] To overlook or dismiss the symbolic is to "cut ourselves off from what is most important in the life of human beings who are, after all, symbol-making animals."

In the case of embryo research or human cloning, overlooking or dismissing the symbolic evades what is really at stake in conflicts over where to draw the line. It is only when we recognize our anxieties about what we are doing when we fertilize human eggs in vitro or reproduce asexually as acknowledgements that we are close to, and may be violating, some of the deepest and most basic of human matters—procreation, kinship, marital intimacy—and our unwillingness to pay disrespect to human embryos as a powerful statement of our societal commitment to the value of human life generally that we come to the important questions [...].

[Steinbock] merely assumes rather than argues for the importance of the information to be gained through embryo research: Possible goals of embryo research include "developing more adequate contraception, determining causes of infertility, investigating the development and potential transformation of moles into malignant tumors, evaluating the effects of teratogens on the early embryo and understanding normal and abnormal cell growth and differentiation." Embryo research "may be particularly valu-

able for understanding, preventing, and treating cancers, and for studying and treating genetic disease." [...]

[...] As Daniel Callahan points out, however, the Human Embryo Research Panel (HERP) report [included in this volume—eds.] gives us simply a list of research possibilities rather than a substantive argument for proceeding at this time. Although it contains an extensive discussion of the moral status of the preimplantation embryo, there is no discussion of what he calls "the moral status of the proposed research." [T]he report is "utterly silent on how research claims and possibilities should be evaluated for their moral weight and benefit" [...]. [T]he HERP report makes no mention of results achieved or benefits gained.

Sheldon Krimsky and Ruth Hubbard contend that the panel conflates "scientific interest" and "human benefit." There is no question that research into the processes of fertilization, early cell division, implantation, and embryonic development is of immediate scientific interest and that it holds some therapeutic promise [...]. Why assume, however, that advancing the state of procreative technology should be a research priority or that overcoming infertility should lay a serious claim on medical resources and public funds? [...]

[...] The claim to be seeking a balance between respect for the human embryo as a potential form of life and the imperatives of research, however, risks being disingenuous, where the importance of the research in question is merely taken for granted and where no serious attention is given to the existence of genuine conflicts between competing and qualitatively different interests. [...]

[Steinbock] takes it as obvious that we should find the creation of human embryos for crassly commercial purposes or for use in frivolous research distasteful. Equally distasteful is the prospect of human embryos generated merely to have an ample supply of research material.

It is not at all clear, however, why this should be obvious, particularly why we should find the latter so obviously distasteful. [...] If we do not recognize the human embryo as potential life, as laying some claim on us morally that distinguishes it from a tree, as having a significance independent of our bestowal, what prevents us from producing as many embryos as we need for research just as we grow trees for furniture or auction art for charity? [...] Yet is not the embryo or presentient fetus "a powerful symbol of human life" precisely when it is recognized as having a transcendent value, a moral standing that, even if not equivalent to full personhood, distinguishes it from things and non-human forms of life? [...]

THE DEEP CONTEXT: MEDICALLY ASSISTED REPRODUCTION

There is a more immediate and even more important "social context" that is obscured in arguments from moral status. It should seem obvious that we cannot separate the business of embryo research from its setting in the practice of medically assisted reproduction. It almost goes without saying, as Krimsky and Hubbard observe, that without the medicalization of infertility and the public acceptance of IVF as a proper scientific and medical response, there would be no way to justify the collection of eggs and their fertilization outside a woman's body.

In vitro fertilization is the "port of entry" for human embryo research in both a practical and a conceptual sense. [. . .] In the short term, women undergoing assisted reproduction are likely to be the major source of research ova. More important, the mainstreaming of IVF as a treatment for infertility signified a radical shift in personal, social, and scientific relationships to reproduction. [. . .] IVF undeniably opens up possibilities for reproductive and genetic manipulations far beyond assisted reproduction. [. . .]

Yet, the debate over the limits of embryo research prescinds unselfconsciously from judgments about goals and methods in reproductive technology. In this sense, the debate is "disembodied." It is as if eggs did not come from within particular women or embryos were not formed from the gametes of particular individuals. [. . .] Rather, the problem is that the question of how we ought to treat the preimplantation embryo is abstracted from the larger question of what we are doing when we intervene in the process of reproduction. [. . .] By "re-embodying" the debate, we raise up what the moral status or interest view neglects, the intrinsically physical, social, and relational character of procreation; the ambiguity attached to our expanding power to alter the conditions under which fertilization and gestation occur, and the relationship between the expansion of reproductive technologies and the social meanings of sexuality, procreation, and parenthood. [. . .]

[M]edically assisted reproduction is not without risks. Drug regimes used to provide multiple ova for therapies such as IVF, Gamete IntraFallopian Transfer [GIFT], and Zygote IntraFallopian Transfer [ZIFT] pose long-term and short-term threats to women's health. [L]ong-range effects of the drugs used to initiate and sustain assisted pregnancies on the reproductive capacities of offspring are still unknown. Women conceiving through IVF and IVF-related therapies experience higher rates of ectopic pregnancy, miscarriage, and multiple gestation.

Perhaps more important and more relevant for our purposes are the emotional, relational, and social costs. Specialized treatment for infertility can be invasive, intrusive, emotionally draining, and financially exhausting. [I]t can also draw patients deeper into the repeated cycles of hope and despair that characterize the experience of infertility. The appearance of highly sophisticated therapies "ups the ante" for the infertile, creating the new burden of "not trying hard enough." [. . .]

In addition, the advent of procreative technologies furthers the medicalization of infertility, constraining options for resolving the crisis of involuntary childlessness (e.g., adoption) and drawing attention away from the medical and social causes of infertility. While expanding possibilities for biological parenting, assisted reproduction also severs connections long thought important between sexuality, procreation, and parenthood. To many, new ways of configuring the family are welcome; still, doubts linger about the extent to which primary biological and genetic relationships can be refashioned without ultimately harming children.

Perhaps most troubling for feminists is the capacity of procreative technologies to "disembody" reproduction. [. . .] Women's previous experience with reproductive technologies suggests that women's own agency is likely to be submerged in the network of multiple experts needed to achieve IVF. Far from accomplishing a liberation from childbearing responsibilities, it can entail "further alienation of our life processes." [. . .] Along with Christian ethicist Lisa Sowie Cahill, I take the view that the human ideal for procreation and parenthood is biological and relational partnership: a couple "committed to one another, as well as to the child-to-be, and who initiate their parental project with a loving sexual act." It is a view that I would defend ultimately on theological grounds, although I believe it is defensible on non-theological grounds. The question posed by reproductive technologies concerns what exceptions to the ideal are justifiable. If the union of sexual intimacy, procreation, and parenthood cannot always be realized—indeed, if sometimes it ought not be—what possibilities for procreation and parenthood are consistent with a commitment to the value of biological and relational partnership?

Also with Cahill, I support the view that reproductive interventions are defensible to the degree that they maintain "the crucial biological relations that undergird the personal and social relations of spousehood, parenthood and childhood." *In vitro* fertilization using gametes from within a marriage is more easily defended from this position, therefore, than IVF using donor gametes; in the former, procreation remains a shared biological endeavor, growing out of a sexual and marital relationship. [. . .]

Reproductive interventions are defensible also insofar as they respect the well-being of offspring as well as the needs and rights of adult parties. [. . .] Reproductive technologies open the opportunity of biological parenting to those for whom it would be impossible, but not without a price; the technologies are both justified and properly constrained by the goal to which they aspire: the bringing forth of new life in loving and nurturing relationship.

[. . .] Although it is reasonable to argue that we do not harm very early embryos by bringing them into existence merely to use them for experimental purposes, to initiate human life in the absence of intentions to care for and sustain it is nonetheless an assault on the character of procreation. It is an extension of the power to remove conception from the body, to manipulate the basic material of reproduction, that moves outside the most compelling justifications for developing and exercising it. As I have argued, reproductive interventions can serve the goods of intimacy, generativity, and commitment to nurture, but interventions carry with them the risk of "further alienation from our life processes" and loss of regard for the embodied and relational character of reproduction. To initiate human embryonic life with the intention of bringing it to fruition is consistent with the best reasons for "paying the price" of intervening in biological reproduction. [. . .] To initiate human embryonic life in the absence of intentions to care for and nurture it is, however, inconsistent with the goals I have argued justify and ought to constrain reproductive interventions.

In excluding as oocyte donors women who are not scheduled to undergo a surgical procedure, the HERP itself recognized a distinction between the intention to initiate a pregnancy and the pursuit of research goals, however important. [. . .]

The goal of bringing about a pregnancy provides a rationale for accepting a degree of risk, for allowing certain kinds of harms to occur, that other goals do not.

Someone might argue that creating embryos for research does not undermine the relational and embodied significance of procreation as long as research embryos are not transferred for implantation. [. . .] Yet initiating human embryonic life with the sole intention of obtaining research material is the appropriation of the power of procreation divorced from the context in which it finds its meaning and focus, whether or not the embryo is brought to personhood. [. . .]

CONCLUSION

In her statement of dissent, panel member Patricia King stated that "fertilization marks a significant point in the process of human development, and the prospect of disconnecting fertilization from the rest of the procreative process in which there is an intent to produce a child is profoundly unsettling." I have tried to suggest here why, indeed, we might find the prospect of severing fertilization from the rest of the procreative process, or, more accurately, from the rest of the parenting project, profoundly unsettling. In the end, King was persuaded that the benefits to be gained through embryo research outweighed the anxieties, although she approved the use of research embryos only where the information needed could not be gained in any

other way. Assessing the risks and benefits somewhat differently than King did, I remain unsettled.

Disagreements over the use of research embryos have centered, on the one hand, on conflicting assessments of the moral status of the preimplantation embryo and, on the other hand, on differing judgments about how to weigh moral anxieties over the treatment of human embryos against the social importance of the research.

I have argued that a narrow focus on moral status abstracts the question of acceptable limits to embryo research from its larger setting. Beyond the question of whether embryos can be harmed is the deeper question of how we justify interventions into the procreative process. Severing fertilization from reproduction, in the full sense, is problematic precisely because it stands outside of the goods and values that medically assisted reproduction most directly and appropriately serves. The risks to be weighed, therefore, involve not only the "interests" of the preimplantation embryo, but also societal interests in women's health and in the integrity of sexuality, reproduction, and parenthood.

I have left an important issue unaddressed. The argument I have offered rests on a particular account of the intrinsic relationship between sexuality, procreation, and parenthood, an account with which many in this society may disagree and one with important theological influences. It is not unfair to ask what weight such arguments should have in public and policy-oriented debates. Should arguments for banning the use of research embryos be accepted that depend on what may constitute a minority position on the goals of medically assisted reproduction?

The limits of this essay make an adequate answer impossible, although it does seem to me that there is an important place in public debate for perspectives that challenge the dominant research ethos, particularly when it concerns issues of such human importance as the limits of research and the nature of reproduction. Here, however, I share Lisa Sowie Cahill's conclusion: The important thing is not how to prevent embryo research or cloning from occurring. Indeed, given the vast commercial potential in reproductive and genetic technologies, I am not optimistic that it will be possible even to contain them well, let alone prevent them from being introduced. What is important is how to open up public discussion to values beyond unexamined scientific progress or self-determination. For now, the important thing is to expand the range of what is taken to be morally important in the debate over the creation of embryos for research or the introduction of human cloning, to resituate the question of what it means to respect human embryos in our ongoing reflection about the meaning of intervention into human reproduction.

Drug Challenge and Drug Washout Studies

59 Drug-Free Research in Schizophrenia

An Overview of the Controversy

PAUL S. APPELBAUM

[...]

WHY THE CURRENT PROMINENCE OF ISSUES RELATED TO DRUG-FREE RESEARCH IN SCHIZOPHRENIA?

In May 1994, the federal Office for Protection from Research Risks [OPRR, now the Office for Human Research Protections, or OHRP—eds.] issued a report on its investigation of complaints against a leading group of schizophrenia researchers at the University of California at Los Angeles (UCLA) Medical School. The subjects on whose behalf complaints were filed had participated in a series of studies using Prolixin decanoate, a long-acting, injectable form of a standard antipsychotic agent.

Subjects in the UCLA studies initially went through a one-year, fixed-dose study in which they received injections every two weeks. On the successful completion of the first study, subjects who were willing to continue in the research were enrolled in a second, more controversial protocol. Each subject was assigned, in a randomized, double-blind fashion, to continue the same dose of Prolixin or to receive a placebo injection. After twelve weeks, the groups crossed-over, with those subjects who had received active medication now getting placebo, and vice versa. Subjects who were still stable after an additional twelve weeks were then assigned to a withdrawal protocol. The medications were stopped and subjects were followed for at least one year, or until a serious exacerbation or psychotic relapse occurred. The goal of the study was to identify predictors of successful functioning without antipsychotic medication.

Two subjects who had been enrolled in the withdrawal protocol ran into trouble. One subject committed suicide

---

Paul S. Appelbaum, "Drug-Free Research in Schizophrenia: An Overview of the Controversy," *IRB: A Review of Human Subjects Research* 18, no. 1 (1996): 1–5.

after completion of the formal one-year drug withdrawal study, while continuing to be followed by the research team in a drug-free state. A second person, a young college student, experienced a severe psychotic relapse that began not long after the medication was discontinued. During this period, he left school, began to hallucinate, and threatened to kill his parents when he became convinced that they were possessed by the devil. He and his parents alleged that, despite repeated appeals to the research team, it took nine months before he was put back on medication. [...]

OPRR's investigation concluded that the design of the research was not unethical, since it comported with current clinical and scientific standards. However, the agency determined that the informed consent obtained from subjects was inadequate because the consent documents failed to describe clearly the differences between being in the research project and receiving ordinary clinical care. Although UCLA's monitoring of subjects' clinical status was deemed to be acceptable, OPRR also found that subjects should have been informed that their clinicians simultaneously were acting as investigators in the study. [...]

WHAT IS SCHIZOPHRENIA AND HOW IS IT TREATED?

Schizophrenia is a major mental disorder characterized by periods of psychosis or detachment from reality. Patients typically experience hallucinations, delusions, disorganized thinking and behavior, and social withdrawal. Psychiatrists only make a diagnosis of schizophrenia after symptoms have been present for at least six months, but most patients will suffer from the effects of the disorder for the rest of their lives. Periods of relative remission [...] are frequently punctuated by acute exacerbations. [...] Persons with schizophrenia experience considerable agony as a result of their disorder; lifetime rates of suicide approximate 10 percent.

Treatment of schizophrenia, once limited to lifetime custodial care, was revolutionized in the mid-1950s by the introduction of the first effective medications for the disorder, the phenothiazine antipsychotics. [...] Administration of the medications can lead to resolution of acute psychotic episodes and a diminished likelihood of recurrence over time. Eighty percent or more of patients with schizophrenia get some benefit from the medication, [but] currently available antipsychotic medications are a mixed blessing. Though they usually are effective in diminishing symptoms, complete remission is uncommon. Even when maintained on medication, most patients will experience periodic breakthroughs of their psychosis. Moreover, the success achieved by the medications is purchased at the price of substantial side-effects. Acutely, many patients experience drug-induced parkinsonism, muscle spasms called dystonias, feelings of inner restlessness associated with a need to move ("akathisia"), and akinetic states in which the motivation to move and even to think is diminished. Less frequently, patients may experience a potentially fatal hypermetabolic state known as "neuroleptic malignant syndrome." [...]

The most profound of the long-term side-effects of the phenothiazine-type medications [...] is tardive dyskinesia. This syndrome is characterized by involuntary muscular movements affecting the face, limbs, and trunk, [and] occurs in 4 to 5 percent of patients on neuroleptic medication each year. [...]

WHY CONDUCT DRUG-FREE RESEARCH IN SCHIZOPHRENIA?

[...] First, it has been known for many years that some schizophrenic patients can have their medication discontinued without experiencing relapse for a substantial period of time. If such patients could be identified in advance, they would be spared the negative effects of the medication, without undue risk of relapse. At this time, though, there are no good predictors for identifying this patient group. [...]

Second, [w]hen these new drugs are tested, subjects' current medications are often stopped for a period of several weeks to allow them to wash out of the body, thus minimizing the risk of adverse drug-drug interactions. [...]

Third, drug-free research may be helpful in elucidating the patho-physiology of schizophrenia. [...]

WHAT ARE THE RISKS OF DRUG-FREE RESEARCH?

The major risk of taking clinically stable research subjects off their antipsychotic medications is that they will suffer a relapse of their disorder. The most recent analysis of studies involving discontinuation of medication in schizophrenia indicates an overall relapse rate of 54.8 percent during an average follow-up period of 9.7 months. In comparison, 16.6 percent of patients maintained on medication are likely to relapse during the same period of time. [...]

Efforts to limit the risk of relapse, for example, by eliminating subjects who may be particularly likely to suffer exacerbation of their conditions, are hampered by the absence of reliable predictors. [...] One factor frequently associated with research protocols, however, appears to magnify the risk of relapse: abrupt discontinuation of medication induces a threefold greater risk of relapse than gradual discontinuation over a period of weeks to months.

The effects of a psychotic episode on patients with schizophrenia are not limited to the profound psychic suffering that often accompanies psychosis. Patients may engage in high-risk behaviors, such as assault and suicide attempts. A relapse may destabilize their psychosocial situations, costing them their jobs, housing, and the support of family and friends. Some evidence suggests intermittent use of medications increases the risk of tardive dyskinesia compared with uninterrupted treatment. [...]

SHOULD WE DO DRUG-FREE STUDIES IN SCHIZOPHRENIA?

Given the risks associated with withdrawal or withholding of medication from patients with schizophrenia, a lively debate is under way about the legitimacy of this form of research. [...] Some advocates for mentally ill persons would ban all studies involving prolonged drug-free periods on the grounds that they threaten subjects with an unacceptable likelihood and level of harm. [...]

Most commentators [...] have not gone so far as to endorse an absolute ban on drug-free research. Not only do they fear that progress on the treatment of schizophrenia will be stymied, but they shy away from the implied stigmatization of persons with mental illness. [...] To suggest that persons with mental illness, alone among other competent adults, should not be permitted to participate in risky research labels them as unable to play an equal role in making decisions about their lives. [...]

Use of Placebo in Medication Trials

[...] Opponents of placebo use argue that medical ethics, as embodied in the Declaration of Helsinki, require that "[i]n any medical study, every patient—including those of a control group, if any—should be assured of the best proven diagnostic and therapeutic method." This statement, it is claimed, "effectively proscribes the use of a placebo as control when a proven therapeutic method exists." [...] A more moderate group of critics is willing to permit subjects to consent to participation in placebo-controlled trials, as long as they are aware of the risks of for-going standard treatment. [. . .] They argue, however, that once potential subjects are well informed about these matters, it is difficult to imagine that many of them would agree to participate in the placebo-controlled study. [. . .]

A variety of methodologic difficulties could underlie the failure to detect real differences between the drugs. [. . .] Alternatively, each medication may have truly failed to have much effect because of peculiarities of the sample. This is a particular problem in schizophrenia research, where study samples seem to be drawn increasingly from treatment-resistant populations. It is, after all, persons who have not benefited from existing treatments who are most likely to seek opportunities to try new medications. Whereas the failure to find a difference between new and current treatments in this population could be interpreted as their being equally effective, in fact the results may be due to the selection of an atypical study sample resistant to the effects of all medications. [. . .]

Mechanisms of Reducing Risk to Subjects

[. . .] The ethics of research demand that attention be given to means of minimizing the risks faced by subjects. [. . .] First, high-risk subjects could be excluded from entry into the study. [. . .] This group might include patients with histories of disastrous consequences from deterioration, or those in marginal social situations. Patients who have done exceptionally well on existing treatment might also be excluded. [. . .]

Who should make these decisions? [. . .] When the potential subject's clinician is also involved in the research, an independent clinical judgment attesting to the appropriateness of including the patient could be required.

[The] research milieux can be designed with enhanced psychosocial treatments available, since these may mitigate the effects of taking patients off medication. They point to the importance of close monitoring for early signs of relapse, since restarting medication will usually, though not always, prevent the development of a full-fledged psychotic episode. Use of the shortest possible medication-free period, and a study design that offers some benefits to all participants, even those receiving placebo, are also suggested. The latter might be accomplished, for example, by offering subjects in the placebo group the opportunity for an open trial of the new medication at the conclusion of the double-blind study. [. . .] Slowly tapering medications,

rather than stopping them abruptly, appears to reduce the risk of subsequent relapse.

Informed Consent Procedures in Drug-Free Research

Much of the criticism of the UCLA studies and similar projects has focused on the procedures they used to get consent from prospective subjects. OPRR's investigation highlighted several inadequacies in the UCLA disclosures. [. . .]

Extra attention from institutional review boards may be warranted to insure that investigators communicate information targeted specifically at [. . .] common problems in investigators' disclosure and subjects' understanding. Persons independent of the research project could be used, for example, to supplement the information potential subjects receive to insure that it is complete and unbiased.

The rationale for allowing patients with schizophrenia to participate in drug-free studies presumes their competence to consent to research. Reassuring data came from a study of a small group of psychiatric patients, most with schizophrenia, showing that their decisions about participation in hypothetical research projects that varied systematically in their risk-benefit ratios were no different from those of a medically ill group. More recent data suggest, however, that hospitalized schizophrenics as a group are at elevated risk of having their capacities to consent impaired, compared with persons with other psychiatric and medical disorders and with matched controls from the general population. [. . .] Indeed, some of the information that should be communicated to subjects in drug-free trials may be particularly difficult for persons with schizophrenia to understand. Denial of the presence or seriousness of their illness, for example, is extremely common in schizophrenics. [. . .]

Given the risks inherent in drug-free studies, and the complexities of the consent process, it may be worth verifying the assumption of subjects' competence by screening potential participants for decision-related capacities. [. . .]

Also of concern is the probability that as subjects in a drug-free condition begin to experience more symptoms, they may lose the decisionmaking capacities they had at the start of the study. [. . .] This suggests the desirability of creating mechanisms (e.g., through a durable power of attorney) whereby substitute decisionmakers can act on patients' behalf, if necessary, when they are unable to do so. [. . .]

60 Psychiatric Symptom–Provoking Studies

An Ethical Appraisal

Franklin G. Miller and Donald L. Rosenstein

[...] In this article we identify and discuss ethical concerns posed by one form of psychiatric research—the "challenge study." In this paradigm investigators administer a psychopharmacologic agent or psychological challenge procedure to patients under controlled conditions to probe psychiatric symptoms and other neurobiological responses. The principal scientific rationale behind this approach is to learn more about the underlying pathophysiological mechanisms responsible for the symptomatic expression of psychiatric illnesses. [...]

In psychiatric research the term "challenge study" encompasses a wide range of pharmacologic and psychologic provocations, such as intravenous amphetamine, inhaled carbon dioxide, and the presentation of a phobic stimulus, and an equally diverse set of outcome measures: e.g., hormonal responses, cerebral blood flow, and behavioral or mood ratings. [...]

Psychiatric symptom–provoking studies offer considerable scientific and clinical promise. For example, challenge experiments with obsessive-compulsive disorder (OCD) patients have contributed to understanding the role of brain serotonin in the pathophysiology of this illness and the mechanism of action of effective drug treatments, such as clomipramine, fluoxetine, and fluvoxamine. [...]

ETHICAL CONCERNS POSED BY PSYCHIATRIC SYMPTOM–PROVOKING STUDIES

The two main ethical concerns with psychiatric symptom–provoking studies are related to informed consent and risk-benefit determinations. [...] Undoubtedly, psychiatric illness—e.g., severe depression and profound thought disorder—can interfere with the understanding, judgment, and volition required to give informed consent. Although the capacity of psychiatric patients to give informed consent to research has not been studied systematically, a recent study of the capacity of psychiatric patients to make treatment decisions found that the majority of the sampled patients

Franklin G. Miller and Donald L. Rosenstein, "Psychiatric Symptom–Provoking Studies: An Ethical Appraisal," *Biological Psychiatry* 42 (1997): 403–9.

with schizophrenia and major depression displayed decision-making capacity. We see no reason to presume that psychiatric patients are incapable of giving informed consent for participation in research. [...]

[P]atients are often invited to participate in these nontherapeutic experiments either before or after receiving treatment. For example, in a number of studies amphetamine and methylphenidate have been administered to schizophrenic patients shortly after psychiatric hospitalization, during a period when they were acutely psychotic and before receiving treatment. We believe that this linkage between treatment and symptom-provoking studies has the potential to interfere with informed consent in two respects: first, the patient-subjects who are seeking treatment may not fully appreciate the nontherapeutic nature of the symptom-provoking experiment; second, the offer of treatment may operate as an undue inducement to patients to agree to participate in symptom-provoking studies. [...]

To be ethically appropriate, symptom-provoking experiments, like all research involving human subjects, must [...] present a favorable or acceptable "risk-benefit ratio." [...]

[...] For most symptom-provoking studies the level of risk is relatively low, since the psychic distress that they produce is typically brief and of mild to moderate intensity: e.g., a panic attack lasting a few minutes, comparable to those often experienced by panic disorder patients; temporary increase in anxiety and obsessive thoughts in OCD patients; short-lived depressive symptoms, etc.; however, some subjects experience more pronounced symptomatic responses. The psychic distress caused by symptom-provoking studies should be assessed against the background of distressing symptoms typical of the psychiatric disorders from which the research subjects suffer. It is the additional, immediately provoked distress resulting from challenge procedures, and any more lasting sequelae, that prompt ethical concern with this type of research.

We present below some examples, derived from published articles of relatively intense reactions to symptom-provoking experiments. [...]

1. A study of metergoline administered to OCD patients:

   The magnitude of the change during the metergoline study period was within the subclinical category as assessed by the National Institute of Mental Health

[NIMH] Global Anxiety Scale (4 to 6) for all but two patients. Over the four-day metergoline period, one patient (patient 5) developed gradually mounting anxiety, which remained unabated for three days after the study was terminated. Another patient (patient 7), who was well-controlled with relatively low doses of clomipramine, reported a similar experience peaking in the evening of day 3 of metergoline administration. She reported being "frantic," "agitated," and very fearful and noted a dramatic increase in compulsive checking. On the evening of day 3, she reported three hours of moving repeatedly in and out of her house during a severe thunderstorm to check on a specific item in her backyard. [...]

2. A study of tryptophan depletion following treatment for depression:

[The patient] began to cry inconsolably and described her emotions as being "out of control." She said that she did not know why she was crying but could not stop. She also described psychic anxiety, difficulty concentrating, loss of energy, loss of self-confidence, and a sense that nothing was worthwhile. She felt as if all the gains she had made over the past few weeks had "evaporated," and her Hamilton Depression Rating Scale [HDRS score—eds.] increased to 34. . . . By the following morning she said that she felt "back to herself," with an HDRS score of 9. She commented that the previous day had been a "nightmare" but that she had learned that the depression was not her "fault." She also noted that although she would not want to repeat the test, it had been worthwhile because of what she had learned about her illness.

3. A study of lactate infusion of Vietnam veterans with post-traumatic stress disorder:

Except for patient 6, all the men became depressed and felt guilty during flashbacks. . . . Patient 7 burst into tears during a lactate flashback as he saw his best friend blown up by a booby-trapped grenade.

4. A study of methylphenidate infusion in patients with borderline personality disorder:

The placebo infusion produced no subjective or objective changes. The methylphenidate response was dramatic; within a few minutes after the infusion Mr. A experienced nausea and motor agitation. Soon thereafter he began thrashing about uncontrollably and appeared to be very angry, displaying facial grimacing, grunting, and shouting. . . . Fifteen minutes after the infusion he shouted, "It's coming at me again—like getting out of

control—it's stronger than I am." He slammed his fists into the bed and table and implored us not to touch him, warning that he might become assaultive. Gradually over the next half-hour Mr. A calmed down and began to talk about his experience. . . . He described the episode as identical to those he had experienced at home. [...]

THE JUSTIFIABILITY OF PSYCHIATRIC SYMPTOM–PROVOKING STUDIES

[...] The potential for psychic distress needs to be evaluated in the context of the benefits that these studies may produce and the process of obtaining informed consent from patient-subjects. [S]pecifically, these studies may produce the following benefits:

1. Help generate and test hypotheses concerning pathophysiology of psychiatric disorders.

2. Identify and discriminate between neurobiologically distinct disorders.

3. Elucidate the mechanism of action of treatments.

4. Aid in predicting treatment response or risk of relapse after discontinuation of treatment.

5. Lead to the development of clinically useful diagnostic tests.

6. Contribute to the design of new treatments.

[...] Participation in these studies may help patients gain a better understanding of the disorders from which they suffer; and recognition of the biological basis of the disorder may help counteract patients' negative self-image. [...]

We hold that symptom-provoking studies are ethically justifiable if three conditions are met: (1) they have genuine scientific merit; (2) the effects of administering challenge agents or procedures are not anticipated to be severe or long-lasting (any discomfort should be relievable by supportive care, reassurance, or brief pharmacologic treatment); and (3) recruitment, screening, contracting, and the process of obtaining informed consent engage subjects who are knowing, voluntary partners in the research enterprise. [...]

RECOMMENDED GUIDELINES FOR DESIGN AND INSTITUTIONAL REVIEW BOARD REVIEW OF SYMPTOM-PROVOKING STUDIES

Scientific Design

[...] Protocols for symptom-provoking studies should either present a reasonable opportunity of making an original contribution to knowledge concerning the etiology, pathophysiology, diagnosis, or treatment of psychiatric disorders, or they should be capable of providing a useful test of hypotheses and findings reported in significant prior research.

Exclusionary Criteria

[...] Since suicide is a risk in various psychiatric disorders, and these studies can elicit or exacerbate distressing symptoms, screening of prospective subjects to assess the risk of suicide is imperative. [...] In addition, evidence of a propensity to violent behavior should be considered as a potential exclusionary criterion. [...]

Selection of Challenge Procedures

[...] For pharmacologic challenge studies, this calls for careful attention to the dose of the challenge agent, its route of administration (e.g., intravenous versus oral), the frequency of administration, and invasiveness of challenge procedures. For a scientifically successful and ethically appropriate experiment, the challenge procedures must be potent enough to elicit transient symptoms, but not so strongly provocative as to cause severe or long-lasting distress. [...] When adequate information is lacking, investigators should err on the side of caution by experimenting with less potent challenge procedures before attempting more strongly provocative interventions.

Subject Monitoring

[...] Reasonable decisions must be made about whether, after receiving challenge agents, subjects should be hospitalized for the likely duration of adverse reactions, or whether it is safe to conduct the experiment with outpatients. In the latter case, careful planning is needed to determine the appropriate frequency and quality of contact to assess the condition of subjects who have received challenge agents. Effective treatments should be available and used as clinically indicated to counteract severe reactions. To the extent practicable, investigators should specify in advance criteria for discontinuing challenge procedures and offering effective symptomatic treatment. [...]

Process of Informed Consent

[...] When psychiatric patients are offered treatment in a research setting, informed consent depends on an understanding of the differences between standard clinical care and research. In initial conversations with potential subjects, investigators should clarify that participation in the challenge study is intended to produce scientific knowledge by eliciting and studying potentially distressing symptoms under experimental conditions and will rarely have direct medical benefits for the subjects. It is vital that research subjects understand the alternatives for treatment and care in clinical practice outside the research program. [...]

[...] Subjects of symptom-provoking studies must be capable of understanding the lack of therapeutic intent and the design to elicit symptoms that may be distressing. [...] Independent assessment of decision-making capacity is recommended if investigators or other members of the research or clinical care teams have any serious doubts about the capability of a patient to give informed consent. [...]

Rationale and Justification for Study

[...] Protocols involving symptom-provoking studies should explicitly discuss the risk-benefit ratio of the proposed research, including a detailed rationale for conducting the study with respect to scientific merit and potential benefits for improving the diagnosis and treatment of psychiatric disorders. [...]

Follow-up with Subjects

To protect human subjects it is important to develop systematic information on the effects of participation in symptom-provoking studies. It is desirable that follow-up studies be conducted to collect data from research subjects on their reasons for participation, their reactions to participation (including assessment of the degree of psychic distress experienced), evidence of any lasting adverse effects, and their willingness to repeat the challenge procedure or participate in other challenge studies. [...]

Section Five

Research with Communities

61   A Model Agreement for Genetic Research in Socially Identifiable Populations

MORRIS W. FOSTER, DEBORAH BERNSTEN, AND THOMAS H. CARTER

[...] There is a long history of the popular or political use of scientific findings about heredity to support racism and other varieties of discrimination. A recent National Research Council (NRC) report on the study of human genetic diversity recognized the possibility that members of socially identifiable populations may be adversely affected if associated with a particular genetic predisposition. [...]

Little consideration has been given, though, to how to address the collective implications that genetic studies may have for the populations that they name. Even the recent NRC recommendations for the study of genetic diversity rely primarily on existing human-subject protections for individuals, rather than suggesting new protections against collective risks to identifiable populations. [...]

[...] Although federally funded U.S. researchers are bound by the doctrine of informed consent for individuals, there is considerable variation in how persons with differing cultural and ethnic identities decide to participate in research studies or make treatment choices. In particular, one should not expect to find everywhere the highly individualistic decision-making process idealized in Euro-American culture and enshrined in Western medical ethics. Indeed, researchers should be aware of the possibility of unintentionally imposing a foreign social structure on members of other cultures. [...] Our approach to negotiating an agreement with a Native American tribe may serve as a model for how genetic researchers can collaborate with diverse, socially identifiable populations and take appropriate account of both biomedical and indigenous ethics.

Morris W. Foster, Deborah Bernsten, and Thomas H. Carter, "A Model Agreement for Genetic Research in Socially Identifiable Populations," *American Journal of Human Genetics* 63 (1998): 696–702.

COMMUNAL DISCOURSE

We used a process of communal discourse to engage the participation of the Apache Tribe of Oklahoma. We began by conducting a health survey through 150 ethnographic interviews (~20 percent of the adult population). The interviews included questions about who was consulted in making health-care decisions. We used the answers to those questions to identify public and private social units that Apaches were accustomed to consult about their well-being. [...]

A related problem was the inclusion of a cross-section of appropriate social units sufficient to represent all segments of the Apache population. Here, we relied on a combination of information from the health-survey interviews and advice from Apache elders. [...] In the Apache community, the major public unit is a five-person Apache Business Committee that is elected by tribal members. It is recognized as having public authority to make formal decisions about matters affecting the well-being of the community as a whole. Everyday private life, however, is ordered by five major extended families, which are the private units within which information about such matters as individual health status is confidential. [...]

We requested that the Apache Business Committee sponsor a series of public meetings, open to all tribal members, in which we explained our research goals. As a result of this initial dialogue, we modified our goals to take account of communal priorities. [...]

The Apache Business Committee [appointed a committee to evaluate the research proposal and to negotiate a subcontract with the University of Oklahoma and] designated this committee as a "tribal institutional review board" [IRB] but that designation may be somewhat misleading. What the Apaches called a "tribal IRB" functioned in a dual role that is not standard in bioethical practice; that is, it both evaluated the research project for its implications for the Apache community and then explained those implications to and negotiated them with researchers. [...] To avoid confusion with more typical IRBs, we will use the term "community review board," or "CRB," to refer to the Apache committee.

The Apache CRB functioned as the public arena for a dialogue in which investigators provided information and answered questions in eight formal meetings over the course of 6 mo. Members of the CRB, in turn, related specific features of the proposed agreement to their extended families. Questions or concerns that arose out of those discourses in private social units were brought up by the CRB when we met. [...]

They asserted a communal interest even for biological specimens that would be individually anonymous, because of the use of the collective name "Apache." Nevertheless, despite potential collective risks, Apaches were strongly motivated to participate in research on diabetes mellitus, which they perceived as a major health problem.

A tentative agreement was reached, and a written draft prepared by the [University of Oklahoma] counsel. The tribal CRB approved it unanimously. However, final approval by the Apache Business Committee was not given for several months, while private discourses continued in the extended families. Only after a consensus in these private social units became apparent did the Apache Business Committee approve the contract. The agreement included funds to compensate the tribe for expenses of maintaining a CRB and helping to recruit volunteers. It does not obligate members to participate in the research. Nor does it supplant standard informed consent by individual participants.

PROVISIONS

Scope of Research

Community members expected the research questions to be specific and to be relevant to communal concerns. [...] If additional questions arise, the researchers must return to the Apache CRB for approval.

Publications

All manuscripts that report project findings will be reviewed by the Apache CRB, which will have 60 days to raise objections to use of the tribal name. In that event, investigators either could revise the manuscript to satisfy Apaches' concerns or could publish the results without naming the Apache tribe. [...]

Intellectual Property

[...] In our agreement, the owner of any intellectual property is the university, the sponsoring institution. [...] The university will deduct 10 percent of royalties for legal and administrative costs. Of the remainder, the university will retain 30 percent, the tribe will receive 30 percent, and investigators will receive 30 percent. The unassigned 10 percent will be retained in a reserve fund for liability or litigation. [...]

Archival Storage and Study

At the conclusion of our project, we will negotiate with the tribal CRB the issue of long-term storage of biological specimens. If we are unable to reach an agreement, those materials will be disposed of in a culturally appropriate manner. [...]

Cultural Concerns

[...] Apaches have restrictions about physical contact that are specific to gender, family, and age. Thus, the tribal CRB decided that blood samples should be drawn by a non-Apache. Apaches also expressed an interest in what is done with biological materials that are not consumed by laboratory analyses. Those materials still are considered part of the body, so investigators and the tribal CRB will review procedures to ensure that the proper respect is accorded. [...]

DISCUSSION

Researchers cannot assume that collective issues can be addressed fully by the informed consent of individuals. [...] We found that Apaches expressed most concern about the culturally specific implications of more general aspects of genetic research. Our findings also indicate that, in some populations, private social units may have a larger role in communal decision making than do public authorities. Thus, the existence of readily identifiable public social units and leaders does not mean that informed communal consensus can be assured simply by seeking approval from a public authority. [...]

Commercialization

The sharing of royalties with a subject population has not been a standard practice. [...] To the extent that genetic research addresses questions that are population specific, the population is the subject. As we have noted, members of socially identifiable populations have demonstrably greater risk for participating in genetic research, as compared with members of the general population. In addition, in an identifiable population, nonparticipants share the same collective risks as do persons who volunteer for research. As a matter of equity, we believe that it is reasonable that such populations should have the opportunity to share in any financial benefits that come from commercial development of a population's unique genetic resources. [...]

Future Studies of Archival Samples

[...] We found [...] that members of the Apache community expressed a desire to see how the research project actually was performed and to hear reports from researchers on its preliminary results before agreeing to archiving samples. As part of our agreement, we will make periodic reports to the Apache community on our findings. Only afterward will they consider entering into a longer-term agreement that might include maintaining a collection for future research. [...] All the collective risks that we outlined for our initial research project also apply to future uses of archival specimens. Thus, in subsequent projects under-

taken with archival material, communal discourse and contractual provisions can provide important human-subjects protections. [...]

Coercion

[...] A communal consensus in support of a research project constitutes a collective willingness to promote the research, not a commitment of individual participation. Apache culture makes a strong distinction between communal and individual action. [...] Our university IRB asked us to strengthen protections for individuals by allowing donors to have their samples withdrawn at any time during the first 60 days after donation. [...]
[Figures omitted—eds.]

62   Groups as Gatekeepers to Genomic Research

Conceptually Confusing, Morally Hazardous, and Practically Useless

Eric T. Juengst

POPULATION GENOMICS
AND COLLECTIVE INTERESTS

[...] It has recently become popular (and politically important) to argue that population genomics puts significant interests of the groups under study at risk, and that those groups should therefore be involved in the decision to conduct any study that would use individual genotyping to generate information about the group as a whole. At one extreme are those who object to any "targeting" of particular groups for study without their consent. [...] At the other extreme are those who recommend preliminary consultation with targeted groups to determine how best to secure culturally appropriate informed consent from individual members. In between the extremes are those who argue that groups, once targeted for genomic study, should be given the opportunity to decline participation on behalf of their members by being asked in advance for permission to contact and recruit individuals from their membership.

These proposals have vast practical and ethical implications. Accepting them would significantly complicate the work of population genomicists. If groups have interests that require protections like those of individual subjects, a layer of research arrangements would be necessary that our individually-oriented biomedical research ethic is ill-prepared to define or delimit. [...]

[...] Does population genomics put important interests of human groups at risk, and could some form of "group consent" succeed in protecting those interests? [...]

THE CASE FOR GROUP RIGHTS
IN GENOMIC RESEARCH

At first glance, the proposal to allow human groups to play a gatekeeping role in population-genomics research seems compelling. [...]

First, advocates argue that people tend to identify themselves through and with the human groups to which they belong, and not as isolated existential atoms. They largely accept their group's values and priorities as their own, and tend to be protective of their group's interests as reflective of their own. [...]

Second, even those who envision human groups as simply free associations of atomistic contractors recognize

Eric T. Juengst, "Groups as Gatekeepers to Genomic Research: Conceptually Confusing, Morally Hazardous, and Practically Useless," *Kennedy Institute of Ethics Journal* 8 (1998): 183–200.

the moral authority of many kinds of groups to make collective decisions about the best interests of their members. After all, the very concept of autonomy, or self-governance, which we now wield in defense of individual freedom, has its roots in efforts to protect the ability of particular human groups to govern themselves. [...]

Finally, there are real interests at stake for human groups in population-genomics research. For some studies, such as those in genetic epidemiology, there are risks analogous to those that individuals and families face in research aimed at identifying genes associated with disease. [...] The resulting stigmatization of members of groups could then be used unfairly to deny them social goods and opportunities, or even to justify coercive and unnecessary medical treatments. As a consequence, the group's own sense of self-worth and solidarity would be undermined. [...]

THE CASE AGAINST GROUPS AS GATEKEEPERS

I am persuaded by the arguments that human groups face significant risks from population-genomics research, and that, ordinarily, autonomous human groups should have the right to decide for themselves whether to take on such risks. Nevertheless, I think that it would be a mistake for scientists and science policymakers to attempt to give groups a gatekeeping role in genomic research. [...] What do we mean by "human groups" in the context of population genomics, anyway? [...]

Demes and Self-Determination

For the last 60 years, population geneticists have defined the groups their science describes as "demes" or groups of individuals more genetically similar to each other than to any other individuals. [...]

[...] With rare geographically isolated exceptions, however, the maps of human groups that would be produced by the field biologist's random sampling approach to genetic diversity would bear little resemblance to a map of the world's self-identified autonomous human groups that are empowered to speak on behalf of their members. The population genomicists have consistently observed that

> the basic conclusion from the study of differences among [self-identified social] groups is that they are small compared with the differences within the groups themselves. The aspiration of "race purity" of classical racism is absurd. A village or small tribe will show almost the same extent of genetic variation among individuals as will the whole world. [...]

Moreover, it is our membership in socially constructed groupings, or "*ethnoi*," not our genetic membership in invisible demic families, that gives us our connections, origin stories, and identifies and also commands our loyalties. [T]he shifting demes of humanity have neither the self-consciousness nor the moral standing to serve as guardians of their members' interests.

Further, given our species' long history of using putative genetic relationships as the basis for nepotism, tribalism, racism, and aggression, aspiring to invest human demes with special moral standing seems wrong-headed in the first place. If we are right in our convictions that our biological roots should be irrelevant to the ways in which humans regard each other, promoting our demes as groups with interests of their own makes no more sense than reviving old eugenic attempts to reify the concepts of "race," "genetic stock," or "germ plasm." [...]

Social Groups as Surrogates for Demes

Of course, advocates of "group approval" for population-genomics studies do not have our silent and invisible demic connections in mind at all in making their proposals; they are thinking of our loud and politically visible social networks. [...]

This focus on self-identified, politically organized *ethnoi* is understandable among proponents of group approval because these *ethnoi* also seem to be the human groups that the scientific community pursuing population genomics are most interested in comparing. [...]

If autonomous social groups are going to be asked to serve as the templates for genomic (demic) studies in this way, then the proponents of group approval seem correct: all the arguments in favor of respecting their autonomy and protecting their interests would appear to apply. But would the practice of obtaining group approval achieve those goals? Such a process may in fact provide the control and protection it promises for many kinds of nongenetic epidemiological and clinical studies of the members of autonomous social groups. However, I do not think that this is true for population-genomics research. [...]

Demic Reductionism and the Denigration of Culture

Ethnoi, like human individuals, have a vital interest in their own perpetuation. Above all, what group members seek for their groups is the survival of their cultural treasures: the languages, customs, beliefs, and values that constitute the identity of the group. Moreover, unlike individual humans, *ethnoi* can aspire to open-ended life spans. [...]

By constructing demes against the boundaries of real social groups and then reinterpreting those boundaries in terms of the demic results, genomic research relocates the group's reality to the genetic level. As anthropologists have long pointed out about previous attempts to biologize social groups in order to undermine racist social policies, "the consequent confusion of biological and cultural characteristics, paradoxically, is the hallmark of racism." Reifying the deme this way makes it easier for the group and its neighbors to stereotype its members, [...] and to set them apart from the rest of humanity [...]. No matter how great the potential of population genomics to show us our interconnections, if it begins by describing our differences it will inevitably produce scientific wedges to hammer into the social cracks that already divide us.

Indeed, historically, the authority of the biological sciences has often been exploited whenever it has appeared to justify social disparities between groups: either by ranking groups hierarchically, using group-specific traits as stigmata, or rationalizing social barriers between groups. Combating this kind of scientific racism has been the goal of heroic social policy efforts over the last century. [...]

Scientific Reconstruction
and Social Self-Identity

Another important interest of groups is to protect their own understanding of who they are. [...] That is why population genomicists are careful to allow groups to identify themselves rather than try to use the labels that others may give them. This approach, however, simply underscores the other predictable harm that the use of social groups as demic surrogates will cause to the interests of those groups: the discovery that, in fact, they are not exactly who they thought they were.

The point of allowing sample donors to "self-report" their ethnicity is to honor their own understandings of their social group membership and the meaning that it provides for their lives. Unfortunately, if we are correct about the mismatch between human demic and social group boundaries, scientists cannot really hope to sustain that form of respect in their relations with their subjects. [...]

The Inherent Limitations of
"Group Approval" to Genomic Research

The irony of asking social groups to serve as proxies for demes by giving permission for their study is that doing so cannot work to protect their interests. The proponents of group approval acknowledge that human social groups are often nested within each other, making it difficult to discern the appropriate levels at which to seek approval and the appropriate "culturally relevant authorities" to approach. They usually recommend extensive preliminary re-

connaissance and local consultation, arguing that "the fairest and most revealing approach would be to solicit the advice of the local populations to identify the level of analysis and the group identifications that would make the most sense to them." Moreover, they insist that

> consent must always be sought from the local community affected. If the researchers are sampling members of a town, village, or a religious unit, they need to explain the project to the members of that community and obtain its permission to seek willing individual participants.

The complexity of human population structure, however, poses more than practical difficulties for the notion of group approval to genetic studies. First of all, no matter how careful researchers are to get permission from the right authorities in a local self-identified social group, as long as that group can be nested within a larger genetic population, its ability to protect itself from the consequences of the research will be compromised by any other subpopulation's decision to participate in that research. [...] Local community consent cannot give people control over findings at that level. [...]

The problem of locating the appropriate "population" to consult is exacerbated by the increasing ability of human groups to scatter across the world and be adopted by other cultures with their own means of approving research. For example, imagine some quite high resolution genetic studies that would only serve to differentiate the Hmong people from their neighbors in Southeast Asia. As long as the Americanized children of recent Hmong immigrants in Minnesota can be successfully recruited, seeking the consent of the Southeast Asia Hmong will not increase the latter's control over their interests in this research. [...]

SUMMARY AND NEXT STEPS

It is hard to resist the demands of autonomous social groups for respect; indeed it would be wrong to do so. To the extent that population genomicists seek to use these self-identified, politically organized groups in their research, even as phenotypic placeholders, they will have to give them the same panoply of rights we give to individual human subjects in biomedical research: free and informed agreements to participate, withdrawal rights, confidentiality protections, control over the disclosure of identifiable research results, and just compensation. Allowing groups to exercise those rights, of course, would kill many population-genomics studies in their cradles. But that is not why it would be a bad idea to involve social groups as gatekeepers for population-genomics research. Such involvement would be a bad idea for three reasons:

(1) It would involve the wrong groups. The human groups that are picked out, described, and compared in the course of population-genomics research are not the named social groups in which we all claim membership. They are the nameless demes which, population genomicists assure us, are the results of mixed lineages that make hash of most of our familial origin stories and social groupings. [...]

(2) It would send the wrong message. Acting as if social groups were the groups under study suggests that they are reducible to the demes we construct around them, setting the stage for new forms of scientific racism and providing new tools for discrimination. [...]

(3) Obtaining group approval would not give groups control over research risks. Our practice of nesting local groups within larger social categories, as well as cross-cultural immigration, means that no one group with the voice to do so can have the moral reach to decide for all those who might participate in such research. [...]

---

63 Protecting Communities in Research

Current Guidelines and Limits of Extrapolation

CHARLES WEIJER, GARY GOLDSAND, AND EZEKIEL J. EMANUEL

[...] To begin the process of determining whether protections for communities are appropriate and what their substance should be, we critically examine well-established guidelines protecting aboriginal communities participating in biomedical research. [...]

EXISTING GUIDELINES FOR PROTECTING COMMUNITIES

So far, most guidelines for the protection of communities in research have been written for research involving aboriginal communities and peoples. [...] These [guidelines] are motivated by three considerations. First, aboriginal communities are often geographically isolated and possess histories, cultures, and traditions distinct from the dominant culture. Second, there is an evolving political consciousness and aspiration to self-determination in aboriginal communities. Third, aboriginal peoples are increasingly concerned that research may adversely affect them and their values. [...]

Historically and conceptually, the guidelines of Australia's National Health and Medical Research Council (NHMRC) are paradigmatic. Distilling from the NHMRC

Charles Weijer, Gary Goldsand, and Ezekiel J. Emanuel, "Protecting Communities in Research: Current Guidelines and Limits of Extrapolation," *Nature Genetics* 23 (1999): 275–80.

guidelines and 16 other documents [...], we identified 23 specific requirements for the protection of communities in research that are organized into five broad themes. The protections are arranged chronologically [...] as follows: consultation in protocol development, consent process and informed consent, involvement in research conduct, access to data and samples, and dissemination and publication of research results. [...]

SUBSTANCE AND CONTENT OF THE GUIDELINES

[...]

Consultation in Protocol Development

Almost all the guidelines require that researchers respect the culture of the community. The fact that each of the four of the specific requirements in this theme [respect for culture; input on protocol; research useful; respect for knowledge and experience] is mentioned in half or more of the guidelines surveyed suggests widespread agreement about the need for consultation early in the research development process. It is this early involvement of the community that lays the groundwork for the partnership between community and researcher.

All but three of the documents require that the community be consulted in the actual development of the study protocol. Consultation on research design is a necessary prerequisite to ensuring that the research itself is useful to the community and respects aboriginal knowledge. [...]

[...] Projects need to take account of the fact that oral tradition is considered an important source of knowledge in many aboriginal communities. The guidelines indicate that researchers ought to collaborate with the community to define how the research problem might be approached and, where relevant, oral tradition and other sources of communal knowledge ought to be used in a respectful manner.

Consent Process and Informed Consent

The guidelines view community consultation and consent as supplementary to but not a replacement of individual consent. [...] Almost all of the documents recognize the need to communicate in a clear and intelligible manner, such as using local languages where necessary. The most comprehensive of the guidelines suggest face-to-face meeting between community and researcher and adequate time for review and consideration of the protocol by the community's leaders. [T]he issue of withdrawal of consent by the community is rarely mentioned. [...]

In some circumstances it may be unclear who speaks for a particular aboriginal community. [...] None of the guidelines discuss how to resolve conflicts between legitimate authoritative bodies.

Involvement in Research Conduct

[...] The community as partner ought to be meaningfully involved in the actual conduct of the research project. [...] First, community members can be trained to help conduct the research, thereby transferring research skills and expertise. Second, individual members of the community may be given employment on the research project, [and] only two documents add that the community should be reimbursed for any costs it incurs through its participation, such as accommodation for researchers, or water, power, or materials used during the conduct of the study. [...]

Access to Data and Samples

[...] The requirement of consent for further uses of data or samples, as a few of the guidelines suggest, promotes trust between the community and the researcher and protects the community from unwanted uses of such materials.

The related requirement of storage of data negotiated refers to the need for researchers and communities to discuss where data or samples will be stored, whether or not any will be destroyed, or who ultimately controls them after the completion of the project. [...]

Dissemination and Publication

[...] Consideration of co-authorship by community members and the circulation of preliminary drafts for comment and criticism allows the community to remain a full partner throughout the research process. In a recent description of research in the aboriginal community of Kahnawake, consensus between community and researcher on data interpretation is sought and, failing this, the competing interpretations will be included in published work. [...]

THE CHALLENGE OF DEVELOPING GUIDELINES FOR NON-ABORIGINAL COMMUNITIES

[...] Further work will require a more nuanced approach and recognize that communities represent a wide variety of human associations, including ethic, cultural, religious, political, artistic, professional, sexual, and disease communities. To define and delineate the substantive, practical protections for the principle of respect for communities, we need to construct a typology of communities matching protection to specific community characteristics. For example, if one is to be able to implement the requirement for community consent or other requirements involving community consent, then the community in question must have a system of legitimate political representation. What constitutes legitimate political representation is itself an issue requiring further analysis. Similarly, to establish health priorities, the community must have a formal organization devoted to its health affairs. [...]

[Tables omitted; subscribers may access them at the *Nature Genetics* Web site: www.nature.com/ng/.—eds.]

64   Protecting Communities in Biomedical Research

CHARLES WEIJER AND EZEKIEL J. EMANUEL

[...]

COMMUNITY CHARACTERISTICS

The term community delineates a wide variety of human associations, from tribes to municipalities to religious adherents. A single set of regulations to fit all types of communities is doomed to failure. What is needed are morally relevant criteria that distinguish communities. Characteristics of particular importance or relevance to communities in biomedical research can be identified and used to delineate seven types of communities.

Communities may be arrayed along a spectrum of cohesiveness, from those that have all the characteristics to those that have only a few. At one end of the spectrum, a cohesive aboriginal community, [and at the other end] a less-cohesive occupational community [...]. [...]

CONNECTING GUIDELINE REQUIREMENTS TO COMMUNITY CHARACTERISTICS

It is possible to identify particular characteristics of communities that are necessary for the implementation of specific protections. In this way, each of the identified community characteristics is linked to one or more of the protections.

For example, if the community is to have input on the protocol, the community must have representatives who can provide this input on behalf of the community. Similarly, if community consent is to be sought before individuals are approached for study participation, the community must have a legitimate political authority that is empowered to speak authoritatively for, and make binding decisions on behalf of, the community; more than mere representation is required. [...]

SYNTHESIZING APPROPRIATE PROTECTIONS

Three general regimes of protection can be delineated, based on the specific protections appropriate to the distinct types of communities: (i) community consent and consul-

Charles Weijer and Ezekiel J. Emanuel, "Protecting Communities in Biomedical Research," *Science* 289 (2000): 1142–44.

tation, (ii) community consultation alone, and (iii) no added protections.

Community consent is only possible if the community has a legitimate political authority, which could be a legislative assembly, mayor, or tribal council that has the authority to make binding decisions on behalf of its members. [...]

Not surprisingly, communities that have legitimate political authorities are among the most cohesive communities and have all or most of the characteristics relevant to the implementation of guidelines requirements. [...] Community consultation encompasses the involvement of community representatives to a limited degree in study planning, informing the community as a whole of the study at its start and as progress is made, consulting with community representatives regarding the disposition of data, and providing them with a draft report on which to comment. Communities that share a religion, a disease, ethnicity, or race may be relatively cohesive and share many, although not all, of the characteristics required for the implementation of guideline requirements. [...]

Occupational and virtual communities are the least cohesive of the communities in the typology. [N]o added protections are required for research involving them.

However, there may be exceptions to these guidelines. Actual communities are diverse and can deviate from the ideal types. For instance, for historical and social reasons, farm workers or coal miners with strong union representation, geographic localization, union-based health insurance, and other social security programs may be more cohesive than typical occupational communities. Their cohesiveness may be so extensive that they have all or most of the characteristics legitimizing the additional protections of community consent and consultation. [...]

POSSIBLE QUESTIONS

How do community protections relate to individual informed consent? [N]o person can be enrolled in research without his or her individual consent. Properly understood, community consent is an additional protection [...]. However, protections for communities are asymmetric: If the community consents to research participation, individuals may still refuse to participate; if the community does not consent, then individuals who are identified because they are members of the community should not be approached for study enrollment. [...]

Is it more appropriate to conceive of a community as a vulnerable group protected by current regulations? [...] Vulnerable groups are socially, economically, and otherwise disadvantaged and, therefore, are more susceptible to exploitation or harm. Regulations protecting such groups include added consent requirements and limits on the nontherapeutic research risk to which they may be exposed. Conversely, the driving issue for protections for communities is not vulnerability, but rather, that communities have interests that are entitled to respect and protection. [...]

Who counts as the community leader? In some communities, a multiplicity of legitimate leaders may make it difficult to discern with whom researchers ought to interact; an aboriginal community may have both a tribal council and an elected mayor. The decision will depend on the values and traditions of particular communities and whose authority encompasses the questions raised. [...]

What if the community wants to suppress adverse or undesirable research findings? This problem is not restricted to research with communities but also exists in relation to research funded by pharmaceutical companies, managed care and other health care institutions, or other research organizations. Experience in research with the aboriginal community provides a useful guide to the negotiation of disparate interests. Researchers and the Kahnawake community have negotiated a mechanism in which consensus between the researcher and the community on data interpretation is sought. If consensus cannot be attained within a reasonable amount of time, the competing interpretations of the study will both be published. [...]

[Two tables omitted; *Science Online* subscribers may access supplemental Web tables at www.sciencemag.org/feature/data/1050363.shl—eds.]

Section Six

International Research

---

65 Unethical Trials of Interventions to Reduce Perinatal Transmission of the Human Immunodeficiency Virus in Developing Countries

PETER LURIE AND SIDNEY M. WOLFE

[In 1994] the [*New England Journal of Medicine*] published the results of AIDS Clinical Trials Group (ACTG) Study 076, the first randomized, controlled trial in which an intervention was proved to reduce the incidence of HIV infection. The antiretroviral drug zidovudine [azidothymidine, or AZT], administered orally to HIV-positive pregnant women in the United States and France, administered intravenously during labor, and subsequently administered to the newborn infants, reduced the incidence of HIV infection by two thirds. The regimen can save the life of one of every seven infants born to HIV-infected women.

Because of these findings, the study was terminated at the first interim analysis and within two months after the results had been announced, the Public Health Service had convened a meeting and concluded that the ACTG 076 regimen should be recommended for all HIV-positive pregnant women without substantial prior exposure to zidovudine and should be considered for other HIV-positive pregnant women on a case-by-case basis. The standard of care for HIV-positive pregnant women thus became the ACTG 076 regimen.

In the United States, three recent studies of clinical practice report that the use of the ACTG 076 regimen is as-

Peter Lurie and Sidney M. Wolfe, "Unethical Trials of Interventions to Reduce Perinatal Transmission of the Human Immunodeficiency Virus in Developing Countries," *New England Journal of Medicine* 337 (1997): 853–56.

sociated with decreases of 50 percent or more in perinatal HIV transmission. But in developing countries, especially in Asia and sub-Saharan Africa, where it is projected that by the year 2000, 6 million pregnant women will be infected with HIV, the potential of the ACTG 076 regimen remains unrealized primarily because of the drug's exorbitant cost in most countries.

Clearly, a regimen that is less expensive than ACTG 076 but as effective is desirable, in both developing and industrialized countries. But there has been uncertainty about what research design to use in the search for a less expensive regimen. In June 1994, the World Health Organization (WHO) convened a group in Geneva to assess the agenda for research on perinatal HIV transmission in the wake of ACTG 076. The group, which included no ethicists, concluded, "Placebo-controlled trials offer the best option for a rapid and scientifically valid assessment of alternative antiretroviral drug regimens to prevent [perinatal] transmission of HIV." This unpublished document has been widely cited as justification for subsequent trials in developing countries. In our view, most of these trials are unethical and will lead to hundreds of preventable HIV infections in infants.

Primarily on the basis of documents obtained from the Centers for Disease Control and Prevention (CDC), we have identified 18 randomized, controlled trials of interventions to prevent perinatal HIV transmission that either began to enroll patients after the ACTG 076 study was completed or have not yet begun to enroll patients. The studies are designed to evaluate a variety of interventions: antiretroviral drugs such as zidovudine (usually in regimens that are less expensive or complex than the ACTG 076 regimen), vitamin A and its derivatives, intrapartum vaginal washing, and HIV immune globulin, a form of immunotherapy. These trials involve a total of more than 17,000 women.

In the two studies being performed in the United States, the patients in all the study groups have unrestricted access to zidovudine or other antiretroviral drugs. In 15 of the 16 trials in developing countries, however, some or all of the patients are not provided with antiretroviral drugs. Nine of the 15 studies being conducted outside the United States are funded by the U.S. government through the CDC or the National Institutes of Health (NIH), 5 are funded by other governments, and 1 is funded by the United Nations AIDS Program. The studies are being conducted in Côte d'Ivoire, Uganda, Tanzania, South Africa, Malawi, Thailand, Ethiopia, Burkina Faso, Zimbabwe, Kenya, and the Dominican Republic. These 15 studies clearly violate recent guidelines designed specifically to address ethical issues pertaining to studies in developing countries. According to these guidelines, "The ethical standards applied should be no less exacting than they would be in the case of research carried out in [the sponsoring] country." [...]

The 16th study is noteworthy both as a model of an ethically conducted study attempting to identify less expensive antiretroviral regimens and as an indication of how strong the placebo-controlled trial orthodoxy is. In 1994, Marc Lallemant [...] applied for NIH funding for an equivalency study in Thailand in which three shorter zidovudine regimens were to be compared with a regimen similar to that used in the ACTG 076 study. An equivalency study is typically conducted when a particular regimen has already been proved effective and one is interested in determining whether a second regimen is about as effective but less toxic or expensive. The NIH study section repeatedly put pressure on Lallemant and the Harvard School of Public Health to conduct a placebo-controlled trial instead [but] eventually relented, and the study is now under way. Since the nine studies of antiretroviral drugs have attracted the most attention, we focus on them in this article.

ASKING THE WRONG RESEARCH QUESTION

There are numerous areas of agreement between those conducting or defending these placebo-controlled studies in developing countries and those opposing such trials. The two sides agree that perinatal HIV transmission is a grave problem meriting concerted international attention; that the ACTG 076 trial was a major breakthrough in perinatal HIV prevention; that there is a role for research on this topic in developing countries; that identifying less expensive, similarly effective interventions would be of enormous benefit, given the limited resources for medical care in most developing countries; and that randomized studies can help identify such interventions.

The sole point of disagreement is the best comparison group to use in assessing the effectiveness of less-expensive interventions once an effective intervention has been identified. The researchers conducting the placebo-controlled trials assert that such trials represent the only appropriate research design, implying that they answer the question "Is the shorter regimen better than nothing?" We take the more optimistic view that, given the findings of ACTG 076 and other clinical information, researchers are quite capable of designing a shorter antiretroviral regimen that is approximately as effective as the ACTG 076 regimen. The proposal for the Harvard study in Thailand states the research question clearly: "Can we reduce the duration of prophylactic [zidovudine] treatment without increasing the risk of perinatal transmission of HIV, that is, without compromising the demonstrated efficacy of the standard ACTG 076 [zidovudine] regimen?" We believe that such equivalency studies of alternative antiretroviral regimens will provide even more useful results than placebo-controlled trials, without the deaths of hundreds of newborns that are inevitable if placebo groups are used. [...]

INADEQUATE ANALYSIS OF DATA
FROM ACTG 076 AND OTHER SOURCES

The NIH, CDC, WHO, and the researchers conducting the studies we consider unethical argue that differences in the duration and route of administration of antiretroviral agents in the shorter regimens, as compared with the ACTG 076 regimen, justify the use of a placebo group. Given that ACTG 076 was a well-conducted, randomized, controlled trial, it is disturbing that the rich data available from the study were not adequately used by the group assembled by WHO in June 1994, which recommended placebo-controlled trials after ACTG 076, or by the investigators of the 15 studies we consider unethical.

In fact, the ACTG 076 investigators conducted a subgroup analysis to identify an appropriate period for prepartum administration of zidovudine. [...] This analysis is somewhat limited by the number of infected infants and its post hoc nature. However, when combined with information such as the fact that in non-breast-feeding populations an estimated 65 percent of cases of perinatal HIV infection are transmitted during delivery and 95 percent of the remaining cases are transmitted within two months of delivery, the analysis suggests that the shorter regimens may be equally effective. This finding should have been explored in later studies by randomly assigning women to longer or shorter treatment regimens.

What about the argument that the use of the oral route for intrapartum administration of zidovudine in the present trials (as opposed to the intravenous route in ACTG 076) justifies the use of a placebo? In its protocols for its two studies in Thailand and Côte d'Ivoire, the CDC acknowledged that previous "pharmacokinetic modeling data suggest that [zidovudine] serum levels obtained with this [oral] dose will be similar to levels obtained with an intravenous infusion."

Thus, on the basis of the ACTG 076 data, knowledge about the timing of perinatal transmission, and pharmacokinetic data, the researchers should have had every reason to believe that well-designed shorter regimens would be more effective than placebo. These findings seriously disturb the equipoise (uncertainty over the likely study result) necessary to justify a placebo-controlled trial on ethical grounds.

DEFINING PLACEBO AS THE STANDARD
OF CARE IN DEVELOPING COUNTRIES

Some officials and researchers have defended the use of placebo-controlled studies in developing countries by arguing that the subjects are treated at least according to the standard of care in these countries, which consists of unproven regimens or no treatment at all. This assertion reveals a fundamental misunderstanding of the concept of the standard of care. In developing countries, the standard of care (in this case, not providing zidovudine to HIV-positive pregnant women) is not based on a consideration of alternative treatments or previous clinical data, but is instead an economically determined policy of governments that cannot afford the prices set by drug companies. We agree with the Council for International Organizations of Medical Sciences that researchers working in developing countries have an ethical responsibility to provide treatment that conforms to the standard of care in the sponsoring country, when possible. An exception would be a standard of care that required an exorbitant expenditure, such as the cost of building a coronary care unit. Since zidovudine is usually made available free of charge by the manufacturer for use in clinical trials, excessive cost is not a factor in this case. Acceptance of a standard of care that does not conform to the standard in the sponsoring country results in a double standard in research. Such a double standard, which permits research designs that are unacceptable in the sponsoring country, creates an incentive to use as research subjects those with the least access to health care.

What are the potential implications of accepting such a double standard? Researchers might inject live malaria parasites into HIV-positive subjects in China in order to study the effect on the progression of HIV infection, even though the study protocol had been rejected in the United States and Mexico. Or researchers might randomly assign malnourished San (bushmen) to receive vitamin-fortified or standard bread. One might also justify trials of HIV vaccines in which the subjects were not provided with condoms or state-of-the-art counseling about safe sex by arguing that they are not customarily provided in the developing countries in question. These are not simply hypothetical worst-case scenarios; the first two studies have already been performed, and the third has been proposed and criticized. [...]

JUSTIFYING PLACEBO-CONTROLLED
TRIALS BY CLAIMING THEY ARE
MORE RAPID

Researchers have also sought to justify placebo-controlled trials by arguing that they require fewer subjects than equivalency studies and can therefore be completed more rapidly. Because equivalency studies are simply concerned with excluding alternative interventions that fall below some preestablished level of efficacy (as opposed to establishing which intervention is superior), it is customary to use one-sided statistical testing in such studies. The numbers of women needed for a placebo-controlled trial and an equivalency study are similar. In a placebo-controlled trial of a short course of zidovudine, with rates of perinatal HIV transmission of 25 percent in the placebo group and 15 percent in the zidovudine group, an alpha level of 0.05 (two-sided), and a beta level of 0.2, 500 subjects would be needed. An equivalency study with a transmission rate of 10 percent in the group receiving the ACTG 076 regimen, a difference in efficacy of 6 percent (above the 10 percent), an alpha level of 0.05 (one-sided), and a beta level of 0.2 would require 620 subjects.

TOWARD A SINGLE INTERNATIONAL STANDARD OF ETHICAL RESEARCH

Researchers assume greater ethical responsibilities when they enroll subjects in clinical studies, a precept acknowledged by [Harold] Varmus recently when he insisted that all subjects in an NIH-sponsored needle-exchange trial be offered hepatitis B vaccine. Residents of impoverished, postcolonial countries, the majority of whom are people of color, must be protected from potential exploitation in research. Otherwise, the abominable state of health care in these countries can be used to justify studies that could never pass ethical muster in the sponsoring country. [...]

---

66   Human Rights and Maternal-Fetal HIV Transmission Prevention Trials in Africa

GEORGE J. ANNAS AND MICHAEL A. GRODIN

[...]

RESEARCH ON IMPOVERISHED POPULATIONS

The central issue involved in doing research with impoverished populations is exploitation. Harold Varmus, speaking for the National Institutes of Health (NIH), and David Satcher, speaking for the Centers for Disease Control and Prevention (CDC), both seem to realize this. They wrote in the *New England Journal of Medicine* last year [1997] that "trials that make use of impoverished populations to test drugs for use solely in developed countries violate our most basic understanding of ethical behavior." However, instead of trying to demonstrate how the study interventions, such as a shorter course of zidovudine (AZT), could actually be delivered to the populations of the countries in the studies, they assert that the studies can be justified because they will provide information that the host country can use to "make a sound judgment about the appropriateness and financial feasibility of providing the intervention." However, what these countries require is not good intentions, but a real plan to deliver the intervention, should it be proven beneficial.

Unless the interventions being tested will actually be made available to the impoverished populations that are being used as research subjects, developed countries are simply exploiting them in order to quickly use the knowledge gained from the clinical trails for the developed countries' own benefit. If the research reveals regimens of equal efficacy at less cost, these regimens will surely be implemented in the developed world. If the research reveals the regimens to be less efficacious, these results will be added to the scientific literature, and the developed world will not conduct those studies. Ethics and basic human rights principles require not a thin promise, but a real plan as to how the intervention will actually be delivered. Actual delivery is also, of course, required to support even the utilitarian justification for the trials, which is to find a simple, inexpensive, and feasible intervention in as short a time frame as possible because so many people are dying of AIDS. No justification is supportable unless the intervention is actually made widely available to the relevant populations. [...]

[T]he mere assertion that the interventions will be feasible for use in the developing countries is simply not good enough, given our experience and knowledge of what happens in Africa now. For example, we already know that effectively treating sexually transmitted diseases such as syphilis, gonorrhea, and chancroid with the simple and effective treatments that are now available can drastically lower the incidence of HIV infection. Yet, these inexpensive and effective treatments are not delivered to poor Africans. For example, a recent study showed that improving the treatment of sexually transmitted diseases in rural Tanza-

George J. Annas and Michael A. Grodin, "Human Rights and Maternal-Fetal HIV Transmission Prevention Trials in Africa," *American Journal of Public Health* 88 (1998): 560–63.

nia could reduce HIV infections by 40 percent. Nonetheless, this relatively inexpensive and effective intervention is not delivered. Vaccines against devastating diseases have also been developed with sub-Saharan African populations as test subjects. Nonetheless, even though vaccines such as the group A meningococcal meningitis vaccine are inexpensive and effective they are not adequately delivered to the relevant sub-Saharan African populations.

CULTURAL RELATIVISM OR UNIVERSAL HUMAN RIGHTS?

In their article in the *New England Journal of Medicine*, Varmus and Satcher sought to bolster their ethical position by quoting the chair of the AIDS Research Committee of the Uganda Cancer Institute, who wrote in a letter to Dr. Varmus:

> These are Ugandan studies conducted by Ugandan investigators on Ugandans. . . . It is not NIH conducting the studies in Uganda, but Ugandans conducting their study on their people for the good of their people.

Two points are especially striking about Varmus's and Satcher's using this justification. First, their justification is simply not accurate. If the NIH and the CDC were not involved in these studies, these agencies would not have to justify them; indeed, the studies would not have been undertaken. These U.S. agencies *are* involved—these trials are not just Ugandans doing research on other Ugandans. Second, and more importantly, the use of this quotation implies support for an outdated and dangerous view of cultural relativism.

Even if it were true that the studies in question were done by Ugandans on Ugandans, this would not mean that the United States or the international community could conclude that they should not be criticized. (This rationale did not inhibit criticism of apartheid in South Africa, genocide in Rwanda, or torture and murder in the Congo.) Human Rights Watch, referring to repression in Central Africa, said in its December 1997 review of the year on the issue of human rights that the slogan "African solutions to African problems" is now used as a "thin cover" for abusing citizens. That observation can be applicable to experimentation on citizens as well.

The other major justification both the NIH and the CDC use for the trials is the consensus reached at the June 1994 meeting of researchers at the WHO. Of the many analogies that have been drawn between the HIV transmission prevention trials and the U.S. Public Health Service's Tuskegee syphilis study, perhaps most striking is their reliance on professional consensus instead of ethical principle to justify research on poor, black populations. [. . .]

Neither researcher consensus nor host country agreement is ethically sufficient justification for choosing a research population. As the National Research Council's Committee on Human Genome Diversity properly put it, in the context of international research on human subjects, "Sensitivity to the specific practices and beliefs of a community cannot be used as a justification for violating universal human rights." Justice and equity questions are also important to the ability of individual research subjects to give informed consent.

INFORMED CONSENT

Research subjects should not be drawn from populations who are especially vulnerable (e.g., the poor, children, or mentally impaired persons) unless the population is the only group in which the research can be conducted and the group itself will derive benefits from the research. Even when these conditions are met, informed consent must also be obtained. In most settings in Africa, voluntary, informed consent will be problematic and difficult, and it may even preclude ethical research. This is because, in the absence of health care, virtually any offer of medical assistance (even in the guise of research) will be accepted as "better than nothing" and research will almost inevitably be confused with treatment, making informed consent difficult.

Interviews with women subjects of the placebo-controlled trial in the Ivory Coast support this conclusion. For example, one subject, Cecile Guede, a 23-year-old HIV-infected mother participating in a U.S.-financed trial, told the *New York Times*, "They gave me a bunch of pills to take, and told me how to take them. Some were for malaria, some were for fevers, and some were supposed to be for the virus. I knew that there were different kinds, but I figured that if one of them didn't work against AIDS, then one of the others would." The *Times* reporter who wrote the front-page story, Howard W. French, said, "For Ms. Guede, the reason to enroll in the study last year was clear: it offered her and her infant free health care and a hope to shield her baby from deadly infection. . . . [T]he prospect of help as she brought her baby into the world made taking part in the experiment all but irresistible."

Persons can make a gift of themselves by volunteering for research. However, it is extremely unlikely that poor African women would knowingly volunteer to participate in research that offered no benefit to their communities (because the intervention would not be made available) and that would only serve to enrich the multinational drug companies and the developed world. Thus, a good ethical working rule is that researchers should presume that valid consent cannot be obtained from impoverished populations in the absence of a realistic plan to deliver the intervention to the population. Informed consent, by itself, can protect many subjects of research in developed countries, but its protective power is much more compromised in impoverished populations who are being offered what looks like medical care that is otherwise unavailable to them.

THE INTERNATIONAL COMMUNITY AND THE AIDS PANDEMIC

If the goal of the clinical trials is to reduce the spread of HIV infection in developing countries, what strategy should public health adopt to achieve this end? It is not obvious that the answer is to conduct clinical trials of short-term zidovudine treatment. [...] A more effective public health intervention to improve the health of women and their children may be to put more efforts into providing clean water

and sanitation. This will help not only to deal with HIV, but also to alleviate many other problems, including diarrheal diseases. [...]

CONCLUSION

Actual delivery of health care requires more than just paying lip service to the principles of the Universal Declaration of Human Rights; it requires a real commitment to human rights and a willingness on the part of the developed countries to take economic, social, and cultural rights as seriously as political and civil rights.

[Table omitted—eds.]

---

67 AZT Trials and Tribulations

ROBERT A. CROUCH AND JOHN D. ARRAS

[...]

CLARIFYING THE ISSUES

It is well established that for a clinical trial to be ethical, a state of genuine uncertainty as to the comparative merits of the treatments under study must exist within the expert clinical community. Given the uncertainty regarding the study treatments—in other words, given that a state of clinical equipoise exists—trials must be conducted with the aim of removing this uncertainty. The aim of the study must be to disturb equipoise and, thus, alter clinical practice. This means, *inter alia,* that conduct of a clinical trial requires that the "compendious effect of a treatment . . . a portmanteau measure including all the elements that contribute to the acceptance of a drug within clinical practice," rather than one discrete measure of a treatment's effect, should be the focus of the research. And, because clinical trials are responsive to and centrally concerned with the realities of clinical practice, it is crucial for the clinical trialists to take the study context into account when designing and conducting such studies. Recognition of these considerations has several consequences for this discussion.

Given the widespread poverty and lack of resources endemic to much of the developing world, to be understood properly the proposed trials must be analyzed within

a framework of extreme fiscal scarcity. Within such a framework, clinical trialists should be concerned with a compendious evaluation of the AZT regimen's effect: reduction of HIV transmission, safety, ease of administration, and, importantly, cost.

In these studies, therefore, the question is not merely whether short course AZT is better than nothing. Rather, the study question is whether the shorter AZT regimen is safe in these populations, and, if so, whether the demonstrated efficacy is large enough, as compared to the placebo group, to make it affordable to the governments in question. For government officials in the developing world to make sound public health policy decisions regarding whether they can provide a treatment to reduce perinatal HIV transmission, trials must demonstrate that AZT is safe for women and their infants and offer convincing evidence as to the treatment difference that exists between short course AZT and placebo.

Unanswered questions about the safety of AZT for populations among whom anemia is prevalent, as is well documented among pregnant women in Africa, and whose immune status is compromised by malnutrition argue against use of the 076 regimen as a control arm in these efficacy studies, as does the real possibility that zidovudine-resistant HIV variants may develop in the mother and be passed on to the fetus.

Further, the use of the 076 regimen (or, indeed, another less intensive AZT regimen) as a comparison, would yield less informative results because there is ample evi-

Robert A. Crouch and John D. Arras, "AZT Trials and Tribulations," *Hastings Center Report* 28, no. 6 (1998): 26–34.

dence to suggest that the mother-to-infant HIV transmission rate is highly variable within the developing world (as well as between developed and developing worlds) and that determinants of this variation are not fully understood and hence cannot easily be predicted. Thus part of the information to be gleaned from a placebo-controlled study is the background rate of perinatal HIV transmission in a particular population which will give researchers a more definite baseline against which to assess AZT efficacy.

This leaves us with the final charge raised by critics of the trials: that it is simply unjust for researchers to operate according to a double standard with regard to the developed and developing worlds. We discern two distinct issues here: are the subjects in placebo-controlled trials morally entitled to more than nothing? And, are these trials unjust because they exploit poor, deprived, developing world subjects largely for the benefit of the more affluent populations of the sponsoring countries?

THE CLAIM OF ENTITLEMENT

The critics of placebo-controlled AZT studies assume, either implicitly or explicitly, that all research subjects were morally entitled to receive the prevailing standard of care in more developed countries. One possible source of such an entitlement would be a theory of health care justice as applied to the host countries in question. Importantly, this approach does not rely on any special research-related features of the situation. Although there are many competing theories of equitable access to health care, the account we present here for illustrative purposes embodies several elements common to a variety of leading theories. According to what we will call "the liberal consensus view," justice is equivalent to the kind and amounts of health care that informed, rational, and prudent individuals would choose for themselves against a background entitlement to a fair share of their society's resources. Realizing that they have a limited but fair amount of resources to spend on health care—and that they have many competing needs both within the health care sphere and in such areas as education, housing, employment, and leisure—individuals would no doubt abandon their usual "spare no cost" attitude toward health care in favor of a much more discriminating, cost-effective approach. Would they opt for a good, solid basic package of health care benefits? Most likely. Would they pay thousands of extra dollars to insure continuing care for years in a persistent vegetative state? Surely not. According to the liberal consensus view, then, health care justice simply is what such real or hypothetical persons would choose against a backdrop of basic equity.

Applying the liberal consensus view to the situation of individuals in developing countries, we must first ask whether their present standard of living would qualify as a fair share of societal resources. If their present shares were deemed to constitute a reasonably just baseline situation, the citizens of most, if not all, developing countries would clearly not choose to purchase, and thus have no right to expensive antiretroviral therapies. Given the extreme shortages of goods, services, infrastructure, and personnel across a wide spectrum of basic needs, individuals and governments would realize that they simply don't have the money to invest in such treatment, and that the meager amount of money that they do control would be better spent on cheaper, more effective interventions that could reach many more people and save many more lives. Instead of the 076 protocol at $800 per person—or even the CDC/Thailand protocol at $50—in a country that currently spends $5 per person per year on health care, they might favor more modest public health measures, such as improved nutrition or water systems. According to this analysis, research subjects randomized to placebos in the recent short course trials were not deprived of anything to which they were already justly entitled.

It is highly debatable, however, whether the current holdings of citizens in most developing countries satisfy the condition of background fairness required by the liberal consensus view. Agreeing with Judith Shklar's perceptive observation that it is always "easier to see misfortune rather than injustice in the afflictions of other people," we are loath to conclude that the current plight of these impoverished peoples is unfortunate but not unjust. Their misery must be due in no small measure to the flagrantly unjust behavior of the former colonial powers, which plundered their natural resources and subjugated their peoples; in many subsequent cases to the rapacious behavior of their home-grown military dictators, who treated their country's natural resources as their own private stock; and more recently to global economic policies that often stifle economic growth under huge debt-servicing policies. In a more just world, the citizens of the developing world would have a more equitable share of their country's resources, and the colonial powers and the generals would have a lot less. Recalculating their social and economic baseline to reflect the demands of compensatory justice, would these people have a just claim to expensive antiretroviral therapy, a claim denied by placebo-driven AIDS trials?

Although we support any and all efforts to narrow the huge economic gap separating developing from more developed countries, we doubt that even taking past injustices into account would yield a moral entitlement to expensive antiretroviral treatments. In the first place, many of these countries are so poor and underdeveloped that even the best efforts at compensatory redistribution would not take them very far. Under the rosiest of estimates, such countries might be able to afford the $50 CDC/Thailand protocol, but certainly not the hugely expensive 076 regimen.

Second, even if compensatory redistribution were required by justice, it will usually be impossible to tell who owes what kind and amount of compensation to whom, and there are currently no authoritative international bodies that could legitimately adjudicate such compensatory claims. As a result, the citizens of these impoverished countries may indeed have a moral right to a better standard of living, but this is almost certainly a claim that will go unredeemed for the foreseeable future. Hence the desirability and feasibility of choosing to pay for expensive antiretroviral therapies must be gauged against the backdrop of their present, admittedly unjust, baseline.

Third, claiming and *per impossibile* securing such a right would surely generate new injustices, as more numerous people with equally pressing needs would be passed over in favor of HIV-infected pregnant women and their children. The families of children and adults dying from diarrhea and lethal parasites in their drinking water could reasonably claim a higher priority on public funds. Their numbers are greater and it would cost far less to mount effective preventive programs in such areas.

Perhaps most importantly, the plausibility of a claimed right to antiretroviral treatment fundamentally depends upon the successful completion of the contested placebo-controlled trials. Even if we assume that the potential subjects' current baseline situation is unjust, any set of more just holdings will perforce be limited, they will have many competing (and expensive) needs, and they will thus be extremely sensitive to the opportunity costs of spending money on expensive AIDS therapies rather than on less expensive and more cost-effective, life-saving interventions. To tell whether they would reasonably choose to spend large sums of money on AIDS therapies, reliable scientific data on their costs, risks, and benefits must first be accumulated so that reasonable and prudent investment comparisons might be made. Thus until we know just how safe and effective the short course of AZT is in these host counties, it makes little sense to say that people there independently have a right to it.

A second approach to justifying an entitlement would focus not on theories of health care justice, but rather on certain role-specific duties of researchers. Whether or not potential subjects have a pre-existing right to antiretroviral therapies, it might be claimed that researchers have a duty to provide it to them based upon their special relationship. One might claim, for example, that participating subjects assume additional burdens by participating in a drug trial and are therefore owed special treatment. Or one could argue that researchers have special fiduciary responsibilities for all those who are placed in their care, responsibilities that include providing all subjects in the control group with the highest standard of care in the world (i.e., with the 076 protocol).

Although both of these arguments contain a large grain of truth, neither succeeds in justifying a claim to the 076 protocol for subjects in the control group. Even if subjects do assume additional burdens by participating in a trial, they also become eligible for important benefits not normally available off study, especially if they end up receiving a safe and efficacious active drug. And even if they end up in the placebo group, they will probably receive better basic medical care than would have been available to them otherwise. Moreover, there are other more realistic ways of compensating them for burdens incurred, especially when this proposed method of compensation would have the undesirable effect of preventing researchers from answering the most meaningful questions that motivated the research in the first place.

This last point is crucial for determining the scope of researchers' fiduciary responsibilities to subjects entrusted to their care. Although researchers undeniably have such role-specific duties, we doubt that they would include entitlements to kinds and amounts of health care services that, first, are unavailable elsewhere in the host country and to which its citizens have no independent right of access, and second, would arguably preclude the timely and successful completion of desperately needed clinical trials. As we argued above, the point of running a clinical trial is to disturb equipoise and thereby potentially change clinical practice. Researchers must therefore show that the proposed short course AZT intervention is both safe and sufficiently effective to warrant large-scale investments on the part of host governments, developed nations, and pharmaceutical companies. In the absence of reliable information on the background vertical HIV transmission rate, information that can only be gained via a placebo group, researchers will be unable to meet this burden of demonstration. Neither the assumption of special burdens nor the enhanced fiduciary responsibilities of researchers for their subjects can ground an entitlement to the best treatment available anywhere.

THE SPECTER OF EXPLOITATION

Even if the research subjects within a host country have no right to expensive treatments available elsewhere in the world, and even if researchers have no moral duty to provide such treatments to controls in trials of less expensive interventions, research undertaken in developing countries may still be deemed unethical if it violates other canons of distributive justice. Specifically, if the results of a clinical trial are not made reasonably available in a timely manner to study participants and other inhabitants of a host country, the researchers might be justly accused of exploiting poor, undereducated subjects for the benefit of more affluent populations of the sponsoring countries.

Two distinct issues bearing on the charge of exploitation need to be distinguished here. First, there is the question of whether the organizers of these studies have an exploitive intent. Are they deploying their studies in developing nations primarily to skirt the stricter research ethics environment in North America and gain access to a vast reservoir of uneducated, undemanding, and compliant research subjects? Is their primary intention to obtain answers in the quickest and cheapest possible fashion and then, as critics charge, export them immediately for use in the sponsoring countries?

In scrutinizing the intentions of the organizers of the contested AZT trials in Thailand, Ivory Coast, and elsewhere, we need to attend both to their words and their deeds. Without exception, the sponsors from the NIH, CDC, and Joint UN Programme on HIV/AIDS [UNAIDS] have stated unequivocally that their primary intention all along has been to respond to local needs for a safe, effective, and affordable treatment regimen in the host country's battle against the catastrophic AIDS epidemic. These same sponsoring agencies have also worked in close collaboration with scientists and public officials in the host countries, an unlikely move for researchers intent upon merely exploiting the local population for their own selfish ends. With regard to the question of intent, we see no reason to second guess the motivations of those responsible for these studies.

The second question, whether these contested trials were exploitive in execution (or in the final analysis), presents greater difficulties. Even if the organizers were well-intentioned, their research may nevertheless violate ethical canons if its positive fruits are not made reasonably available to former research subjects and other inhabitants of the host country. Securing these benefits in the context of developing world deprivation poses daunting challenges to sponsoring agencies. It is hard enough to design a scientifically and ethically sound clinical trial in such settings, but it is harder still to orchestrate such bodies as the United Nations International Children's Emergency Fund [UNICEF], the International Monetary Fund, the World Bank, the involved drug companies, and the national governments of the sponsoring and host countries in a concerted effort to fund the implementation of any positive research findings.

We agree with the Council for International Organizations of Medical Sciences [CIOMS] guidelines and with many observers that in order to be judged ethical and non-exploitive in the final analysis, such research must not only address local problems, but the results must also be made reasonably available to local populations. Assurances of continued provision of reasonable levels of support (financial, infrastructural, technical) from the sponsoring agencies and/or pharmaceutical companies will need to be in place. No doubt due to a long and disappointing history of failure to deploy the results of successful research in the developing world, the CIOMS guidelines state that such mutual understandings must be reached before the study is begun. While the motivation for this requirement is

understandable and commendable, it raises a number of difficult interpretive and normative questions.

First there is the question of the scope of "reasonable availability." Must new pharmaceuticals be made available merely to former research subjects or to the social groups they (loosely) represent, as the Belmont Report seems to require? Or does the scope of this requirement also include the entire town, city, region, or national boundaries in which the study was performed? Although recent commentary appears to favor the notion of a commitment to the country in which a study is done—an interpretation to which we are sympathetic—this gloss raises important questions about the moral relevance of political boundaries. Suppose researchers mount an antiretroviral trial in a northwest province of Tanzania and the results are positive. The nationalist interpretation of this commitment would then dictate an obligation to make the new drug available to people in distant southeast provinces of Tanzania but not to neighbors in nearby Burundi and Rwanda, many of whom might belong to the same regional tribes as the research subjects. Does this result make sense, and will it give sponsoring agencies and pharmaceutical companies a powerful incentive to conduct studies in smaller, less populated developing nations in order to avoid higher costs of implementation elsewhere?

Questions can also be raised about the content of "reasonable availability." Exactly how much access for how many people are we talking about? Suppose a new antiretroviral is deemed effective in a clinical trial in Uganda. Should it be made available to everyone in the country with the requisite medical need [...], or only to a representative sample in certain especially hard-hit geographic regions, or to some intermediate number? Should it be made available immediately after the conclusion of the trial, or merely implemented "with all deliberate speed" or "within the foreseeable future"? And who is to determine the answers to such questions: international bodies, such as the U.N. and CIOMS, or local constituencies?

Additional questions arise about the exactitude and stringency of the required prior assurances. Just how certain must trial sponsors and organizers be that the requisite funding will be forthcoming from drug companies, national governments, and other funding sources? Will it be enough for them to rely upon vague but well intended promissory notes [...] or must there be a written commitment, in advance, binding the various sources to pay for exactly what has been deemed to be "reasonable access" in the circumstances?

Although we are generally in agreement with efforts to wring commitments out of funding agencies before trials are undertaken, we are not sure that this approach must be enshrined and rigidly enforced as a matter of principle. We can easily imagine scenarios in which funders might be initially interested but unwilling to commit themselves on paper in the absence of tangible research results. In such cases, a staged progression from initial contact with funding sources, to estimates of available per capita health care dollars, through collection of safety and efficacy data of a likely-to-be-affordable antiretroviral dose, and on to final negotiations among trial sponsors, researchers, and other funding sources might be a more realistic depiction of what such a process might look like. [. . .] It is an empirical and political question whether such an approach would prove to be more or less effective than the absolutist precommitment strategy in securing desired results. The downside of this approach is that expensive and ultimately successful clinical trials may be run yet fail to gain sufficient financial backing for deployment of their results. The possible downside of the precommitment strategy is that potentially successful clinical trails may not be run at all due to funders' unwillingness to commit vast resources ahead of time in the absence of hard data. To us this looks more like a matter of political strategy than a matter of principle.

Whatever the outcome of this debate, however, we agree that for a trial to be ethical at its inception there must at least be a very strong likelihood that its results will be made available to the population of the host country or region. Researchers know ahead of time what any proposed experimental intervention is likely to cost, at least in the short run, at the completion of the trial. They are thus capable of knowing, in advance, whether any particular intervention is at least in the ballpark of cost-effectiveness for a particular country. If a reasonable economic analysis suggests that the host country in conjunction with outside funding sources hasn't a prayer of widely implementing a suggested drug intervention, we agree that the study should not be done. Absent that kind of broad reassurance, the odds that a trial will merely end up being exploitive of the local population are simply too great.

We fear that this may, in fact, have been the case with regard to the short course AZT trails in Thailand, the Ivory Coast, and elsewhere. At a recent meeting of the Elizabeth Glaser Pediatric AIDS Foundation and Emory/Atlanta Center for AIDS Research devoted to this topic [. . .] not a single person rose up to announce that her or his country had resolved to fund the CDC/Thailand protocol's short course of AZT at $50 per patient. Even the representatives from relatively affluent developing nations such as South Africa and Thailand itself indicated that their countries simply could not afford widespread dissemination of such an expensive intervention. [. . .] Against this background, admittedly with the assistance of hindsight, it appears that the clinical trail conducted in Thailand will prove to be of little if any use to countries in the developing world. If a reliable cost-effectiveness analysis could have determined this beforehand, as we fear it might have done, then the CDC/Thailand study would have arguably been unethical *ab initio.*

THE FUTURE OF INTERNATIONAL RESEARCH

There is clearly an unfinished research agenda in the developing world, with its large, diverse population and enormous public health burden in desperate need of attention and amelioration. Our intention has been to offer a qualified endorsement of the placebo-controlled studies that were planned for the developing world. In so doing, we have articulated the background conditions that we feel must obtain if future international research is to be ethically permissible. First, the collaborative nature of the proposed research, and its need in the underdeveloped country, must be clearly and publicly articulated. Second, a careful distinction must be made between standards of care, on the one hand, and standards of ethical and scientific review, on the other. Thus when we attempt to apply the CIOMS guidelines or the Declaration of Helsinki during the planning phase of international research, we should realize that though the standard of care available in industrialized nations might not be available in underdeveloped nations, ethical and scientific review of the proposed study must be conducted at the highest possible level.

Finally, there should be in place a more nuanced understanding of the requirement that the "best proven" treatment be provided to all research subjects. Treatments should be subject to a compendious evaluation that is multidimensional and responsive to clinical realities and, therefore, more likely to potentially alter clinical practice. Correctly understood, "best proven" should allow for the fact that what is the "best" treatment might itself be in question and the subject of controversy, and must be understood in a locally relevant manner, such that the health care needs of the host country are given their due priority when international collaborative research is conducted within its borders.

Recently proposed research initiatives that aim to decrease vertical HIV transmission in the developing world have clear implications when considered within our analytic framework. For example, participants at a recent workshop convened by the Elizabeth Glaser Pediatric AIDS Foundation and the Emory/Atlanta Center for AIDS Research reached a general consensus about the immediate concerns of developing countries in their quest to reduce vertical HIV transmission and highlighted the following four research priorities: (1) to identify other effective antiretroviral agents that can be feasibly implemented; (2) to define the shortest course (e.g., intrapartum only or newborn only) of antiretroviral that is feasible and effective; (3) to evaluate nonretroviral interventions (e.g., vitamin A supplementation, peripartum birth canal cleansing) that are cheap and effective and that can be implemented for pregnant women without the need for costly HIV counseling and testing; and (4) to evaluate methods of reducing

HIV transmission via breastfeeding. Those conducting research into any of these four areas suitable to randomized inquiry will inevitably be confronted by a fundamental question regarding the appropriate choice of control group. Is a placebo arm justifiable, or should the more affordable but still unfeasible CDC/Thailand AZT regimen be employed instead?

Though the reasoning would be similar with other proposed interventions, consider the case of nutritional supplementation to combat vitamin A deficiency. Epidemiological evidence suggests that vitamin A deficiency in pregnant HIV-infected women is associated with increased vertical HIV transmission. In one study in Malawi, researchers found that women with the lowest serum vitamin A levels had a vertical HIV transmission rate of 32 percent compared to a 7 percent transmission rate among those with the highest serum vitamin A levels. While there are other explanatory variables of importance in this study, and although the way that vitamin A deficiency contributes to increased vertical transmission is not clearly understood, the results of this research have led to at least four clinical trials in sub-Saharan Africa to assess the efficacy of vitamin A or other micronutrient supplementation in reducing the vertical transmission of HIV. Nutritional interventions are appealing in the context of developing world countries because they avoid many of the problems associated with AZT prophylaxis. As [Richard] Semba notes, they are inexpensive, easy to administer, do not require that the HIV status of the mother be known (i.e., can be given as part of routine antenatal care), do not require monitoring, and are safe.

With such attributes, vitamin supplementation could be put forward as an affordable prophylaxis against vertical HIV transmission, provided that randomized evidence exists to support claims of its efficacy. With some developing countries having declared that they will not allow placebo controlled trials to be run in their communities, the alternative is to use some form of active control—such as the CDC/Thailand AZT regimen—in assessing the efficacy of nutritional supplements in reducing vertical HIV transmission. Unfortunately, such a policy merely regenerates the problems initially raised by the debate concerning whether the 076 regimen or a placebo should be used in the control arm. First, the CDC/Thailand results were obtained in a population of non-breastfeeding women, thus making the generalizability of the results to an African breastfeeding population impossible. This point underscores the dubious wisdom of the CDC's initial decision to halt all placebo-controlled studies after the results of the Thailand study were released. Second, a placebo arm would be needed to separate out the effects of the vitamin supplement intervention from any background, secular trends in the vertical transmission rate. Absent a clearly determined baseline rate of vertical transmission, inferences about comparative efficacy are dulled and policy implications accordingly made unclear. More importantly, should the CDC/Thailand AZT regimen prove to be more effective than vitamin supplements, the study would have been conducted for naught since the short-course AZT regimen is unaffordable to most developing nations.

Lest one think that we are practicing "placebolatry," we believe that one could in principle carry out a vitamin supplement study using the CDC/Thailand AZT regimen as a control provided it was within a Thai population comparable to that used in the CDC-sponsored study. Even though Thailand's government can't afford to provide the short-course AZT regimen to its HIV-infected women, one could still glean useful results from such a randomized control trial because the short-course AZT regimen was shown to be safe and effective when run against a placebo arm. The vertical transmission in the vitamin supplement arm, whether less or more than that in the AZT arm, could be in principle interpretable because recent placebo data would exist in a comparable population. The qualifier—in principle—is important here because it will be an empirical matter whether the placebo arm data from the CDC/Thailand study is recent enough, and the populations comparable enough, to overcome concerns about secular trends of vertical transmission in the population which make generalizing study results so tenuous. While the cost-effectiveness of using an expensive AZT control arm would be doubtful, such a study could supply useful results to government officials in the host country.

Like those diligently at work in the public health community, we hope that a truly international effort is mounted to reduce the HIV burden in developing countries and to bring much needed relief to those who have suffered so terribly. To do so will require a collaborative effort to conduct ethically and scientifically sound research that yields results capable of influencing policy decisions within communities of need. Failure to acknowledge both that standards of care between countries can legitimately diverge without compromising the ethical justifiability of a study, and that there is a way to evaluate therapies in a locally relevant and respectful manner, is to be set upon a dangerous path whose terminus would be the aborting of valuable international research. Given the important existing research agenda within the developing world, we believe that this path should not be taken.

Fair Benefits for Research in Developing Countries

PARTICIPANTS IN THE 2001 CONFERENCE ON ETHICAL ASPECTS
OF RESEARCH IN DEVELOPING COUNTRIES

Collaborative, multi-national clinical research, especially between developed and developing countries, has been the subject of controversy. Much of this attention has focused on the standard of care used in randomized trials. Much less discussed, but probably more important in terms of its impact on health, is the claim that in order to avoid exploitation interventions proven safe and effective through research in developing countries should be made "reasonably available" in those countries.

This claim was first emphasized by the Council for International Organizations of Medical Sciences: "As a general rule, the sponsoring agency should agree in advance of the research that any product developed through such research will be made reasonably available to the inhabitants of the host community or country at the completion of successful testing." The reasonable availability requirement has received broad support, with disagreement focusing on two elements. First, how strong or explicit should the commitment to provide the drug or vaccine be at the initiation of the research study? Some suggest that advanced discussions without assurances are sufficient, while others require advance guarantees that include identifiable funding and distribution networks. Second, to whom must the drugs and vaccines be made available? Should the commitment extend only to the participants in the study, the community from which participants have been recruited, the entire country, or the region of the world? While these disagreements have ethical and practical implications, there is a deeper question about whether reasonable availability is necessary, or the best way, to avoid exploitation in developing countries.

What constitutes exploitation? A exploits B when B receives an unfair level of benefits as a result of B's interactions with A. The fairness of the benefits B receives depends on the burdens that B bears as a result of the interaction, and the benefits that A and others receive as a result of B's participation. Fairness is the crucial aspect, not equality of benefits. Although being vulnerable may increase the chances for exploitation, it is neither necessary nor sufficient for exploitation.

ploitation. The potential for clinical research to exploit populations is not a major concern in developed countries since there are processes, albeit haphazard and imperfect, for ensuring that interventions proven effective are introduced into the health care system and benefit the general population. In contrast, target populations in developing countries often lack access to regular health care, political power, and an understanding of research. They may be exposed to the risks of research, while access to the benefits of new, effective drugs and vaccines goes predominantly to people in developed countries and the profits to the bio-pharmaceutical industry. This situation fails to provide fair benefits and thus constitutes the paradigm of exploitation.

By focusing on a particular type of benefit, the reasonable availability requirement fails to avoid exploitation in all cases. First, and most importantly, the ethical concern embedded in exploitation is about the amount or level of benefits received and not the type of benefits. Reasonable availability fails to ensure a fair share of benefits; for instance, it may provide for too little benefit when risks are high or benefits to the sponsors great. Moreover, it applies only to Phase III research that leads to an effective intervention; it is inapplicable to Phase I and II and unsuccessful Phase III studies. Consequently, reasonable availability fails to protect against the potential of exploitation in a great deal of research conducted in developing countries. Furthermore, reasonable availability embodies a narrow concept of benefits. It does not consider other potential benefits of research in developing countries, including training of health care or research personnel, construction of health care facilities and other physical infrastructure, and provision of public health measures and health services beyond those required as part of the research trial. Finally, insisting on reasonable availability precludes the community from deciding which benefits it prefers.

Reasonable availability should not be imposed as an absolute ethical requirement for research in developing countries without affirmation by the countries themselves. Representatives from African developing countries and developed countries proposed a novel alternative to reasonable availability to avoid exploitation in developing countries: Fair Benefits. The Fair Benefits framework would supplement the usual conditions for ethical conduct of research trials, such as independent review by an institutional review board or research ethics committee and individual informed consent. In particular, Fair Benefits relies on

Participants in the 2001 Conference on Ethical Aspects of Research in Developing Countries, "Fair Benefits for Research in Developing Countries," *Science* 298 (2002): 2133–34. A list of the participants may be found at www.sciencemag.org/cgi/data/298/5601/2133/DC1.

three widely accepted ethical conditions and introduces 3 additional principles. First, the research must address a health problem of the developing country population, although, as with HIV/AIDS, it could also be relevant to other populations. Second, the research objectives, not vulnerability of the population, must provide a strong justification for conducting the research in this population. For instance, the population may have a high incidence of the disease being studied or high transmission rates of infection necessary to evaluate a vaccine. Third, the research must pose few risks to the participants, or the benefits to them clearly outweigh the risks.

The Fair Benefits framework requires satisfaction of the following 3 additional fundamental principles to protect developing communities from exploitation:

Fair benefits. In determining a fair level of benefits from research, the population could consider benefits from both the conduct and results of research. Among potential benefits to research participants are additional diagnostic tests, distribution of medications and vaccinations, and emergency evacuation services. Research might also provide collateral health services to members of the population not enrolled in the research, such as determining disease prevalence and drug resistance patterns, or providing interventions such as antibiotics for respiratory infections or the digging of boreholes for clean water. Conducting research usually entails the benefits of employment and enhanced economic activity for the population as well.

Reasonable availability of a safe and effective intervention may provide an important benefit for the population after the completion of some research trials. Alternatively, other post-research benefits might include capacity development, such as enhancing health care or research facilities, providing critical equipment, other physical infrastructure such as roads or vehicles, training of health care and research staff, and training of individuals in research ethics. Furthermore, any single research trial could be an isolated endeavor or form part of a long-term collaboration between the population and the researchers. Long-term collaboration embodies engagement with and a commitment to the population; it can also provide the population with long-term training, employment, investment, and additional research on other health issues. Finally, profits from direct sales of proven interventions or from intellectual property rights can be shared with the developing country. It is not necessary to provide each of these benefits; the ethical imperative is for a fair level of benefits overall—not an equal level.

Collaborative partnership. Collaborative partnership requires that researchers must engage the population in developing, evaluating, and benefiting from the research. Currently, there is no shared, international standard of fair-

ness. In part this is because of conflicting conceptions of international distributive justice. Ultimately, the determination of whether the benefits are fair and worth the risks cannot be entrusted to people outside the population, no matter how well intentioned. They may be ill-informed about the health, social, and economic context and are unlikely to appreciate the importance of the proposed benefits to the host community. The relevant population for collaborative partnership is the community that is involved with the researchers, bears the burdens of the research, and would be the potential victims of exploitation. There is no justification for including an entire region or every citizen of a country in the distribution of benefits and decision-making, unless the whole region or country is involved in the research study. To avoid exploitation, it is the village, tribe, neighborhood, or province whose members are approached for enrollment, whose health care personnel are recruited to staff the research teams, whose physical facilities and social networks are utilized to conduct the study who must receive the benefits from research and determine what constitutes a fair level of benefits. [...]

Transparency. The lack of an international standard for fairness and the disparity in bargaining power between populations and researchers in developing countries and sponsors and researchers from developed countries means that even in the presence of collaborative partnership, the community might agree to an unfair level of benefits. The systematic list in the Fair Benefits framework can be used to catalog benefits provided in diverse research contexts (Table [68.1]). To fulfill the need for an independent as-

Table 68.1

*The Fair Benefits Framework**

Fair Benefits

Benefits to Participants during the Research
    1. Improvements to health and health care
    2. Collateral health services unnecessary for research study

Benefits to Population during the Research
    3. Collateral health services unnecessary for research study
    4. Public health measures
    5. Employment and economic activity

Benefits to Population after the Research
    6. Reasonable availability of effective intervention
    7. Research and medical care capacity development

continued on next page

Table 68.1. Continued

8. Public health measures
9. Long-term research collaboration
10. Sharing of financial rewards from research results

Collaborative Partnership

1. Community involvement at all stages
2. Free, uncoerced decision-making by population bearing the burdens of the research

Transparency

1. Central, publicly accessible repository of benefits agreements
2. Process of community consultations

* It is not necessary to provide each benefit.

sessment, the framework delineates a transparent procedure for determining when the level of benefits is fair.

Transparency can be facilitated by creating a central and publicly accessible repository of all formal and informal agreements on research benefits with an independent body, such as the World Health Organization. This body should develop a program of community consultations that actively informs the communities, researchers, and others in developing countries likely to participate in research about previously negotiated agreements. These consultations would also provide forums in which all interested parties could deliberate on the fairness of the agreements. Over time, such a central repository and the community consultations would generate a collection of critically evaluated benefits agreements that would become a kind of "case law" generating shared standards of fair benefits.

69 Ethical Imperialism?

Ethics in International Collaborative Clinical Research

MARCIA ANGELL

[. . .] Is it proper for Americans to insist that their ethical standards be applied to clinical research performed in other countries? Should ethical standards be substantially the same everywhere, or is it inevitable that they differ from region to region, reflecting local beliefs and custom? And do the answers to these questions depend in any way on the importance of the research to society? Underlying these concerns is the fundamental issue of whether ethical standards are relative, to be weighed against competing claims and modified accordingly, or whether, like scientific standards, they are absolute.

The dominant view in this country is that subjects of clinical research have certain rights that can be abridged only under the most unusual of circumstances. Among these are the right to have their welfare held paramount by the researchers and the right to refuse to participate. Both are protected by institutional and governmental regulations. According to these regulations, the value of research to society does not justify violating the rights of individual

Marcia Angell, "Ethical Imperialism? Ethics in International Collaborative Clinical Research," *New England Journal of Medicine* 319 (1988): 1081–83.

subjects. [. . .] Federal regulations establish the priority of individual subjects implicitly, by defining in detail their right to be informed about a study in which they are asked to participate, to refuse participation, to be informed of findings that may modify their decision as the trial proceeds, and to withdraw without penalty. Thus, in this country ethical standards are not to be relaxed because the study is important.

The federal regulations, as well as institutional guidelines, are explicit in requiring informed consent from all research subjects. Exceptions to this general requirement are extremely limited. Federal regulations, for example, permit exceptions only in unusual situations when the research involves no more than minimal risk. IRBs are to review clinical research studies to see that they conform to ethical standards; their approval is necessary for obtaining federal funding, but it does not generally substitute for informed consent. Obviously, even informed consent cannot justify inherently unethical research—that is, research in which the risks to subjects are known to outweigh by far the benefits to them—and this is made clear in the federal regulations. It is an important constraint, since some patients might consent to nearly anything if asked by a trusted authority.

Contrary to widespread assumption, these restrictions on the use of human subjects in clinical research are not peculiar to this country. They are spelled out explicitly in several international agreements, most notably in the Nuremberg Code [and] the Declaration of Helsinki [...]. Indeed, these international codes are, if anything, more stringent than the U.S. federal regulations. The Nuremberg Code, for example, states that in medical experiments on human beings, "The voluntary consent of the human subject is absolutely essential." No exceptions are mentioned. The Declaration of Helsinki also requires informed consent; if researchers believe an exception is necessary, they must give specific reasons to an independent committee. [...]

It is often argued that, international agreements notwithstanding, insisting on certain ethical standards when doing research in another country is a form of imperialism and therefore inappropriate. Why should we believe that ethical principles that make sense in one culture are necessarily right in another? More specifically, why should researchers be expected to obtain informed consent in a society that places little value on individual autonomy? [...] Any notion of equality among societies, after all, demands that we recognize one another's traditions and not try to impose foreign ones. Many see this position as a step toward countering the long history of exploitation of the Third World by the developed countries. According to this view, if informed consent is not an accepted concept in a society or if a community leader customarily speaks for the members of the community, we should not insist that subjects give informed consent. [...]

The problem with this argument is the implication that ethical standards are matters of custom, like table manners, and that their content is irrelevant as long as they are indigenous. It further presupposes that all members of a community share its dominant values. This ethical relativism gives the same weight to practices that would sharply curtail individual freedom (whether by tradition or by a community leader) as to those that would protect it. Does this make sense? Consider an analogy. Does apartheid offend universal standards of justice, or does it instead simply represent a South African custom that should be seen as morally neutral? If the latter view is accepted, then ethical principles are not much more than a description of the mores of a society. I believe they must have more meaning than that. There must be a core of human rights that we would wish to see honored universally, despite local variations in their superficial aspects. Ethical standards in medicine similarly cannot be relative; they must be judged by their substance. The force of local custom or law cannot justify abuses of certain fundamental rights, and the right of self-determination, on which the doctrine of informed consent is based, is one of them.

Furthermore, if we accept the view that ethical standards in clinical research are relative, we may create a situation in which Western researchers use Third World populations to do studies they could not do at home because they would be tempted to short-circuit the sometimes onerous requirements for protecting human subjects by appealing to this ethical relativism. What would follow, then, would be true imperialism in the sense of exploitation —the very opposite of what the proponents of honoring local traditions would wish.

This is not to say that Western researchers should not make appropriate accommodations to local custom [...]. Local sensitivities should be respected. It may be necessary, for example, to obtain permission from community leaders to enroll members of the community in a clinical study or from a husband to enroll his wife. Such permission should not, however, be a substitute for informed consent from the subjects themselves or be allowed to override a refusal. Similarly, conveying the information necessary to give informed consent may be very difficult and require a good deal of ingenuity, but it must be done. In such ways, the ethical requirements of performing clinical research in Third World societies may be more, rather than less, exacting.

Fundamental principles of human research, however, should not be compromised. Human subjects in any part of the world should be protected by an irreducible set of ethical standards, including the requirements that they not be subjected to unreasonable risks and that they be asked for informed consent to participate. When Western researchers collaborate on studies performed in the Third World, it is particularly important that they adhere to these standards. [...] Just as there can be no compromise in scientific standards based on local traditions, there can be none in ethical standards.

70　Ethics Are Local

Engaging Cross-Cultural Variation in the Ethics for Clinical Research

Nicholas A. Christakis

[...] [T]he basic problem that confronts us is: which ethics should govern transcultural clinical research? By "transcultural" I mean generally the situation that arises when the investigator and the subjects in biomedical research come from different cultural settings. But more particularly, I mean the relatively frequent situation in which the investigator is Western and the subject is non-Western.

I wish to consider four possible practical solutions to the problem of which ethics should govern transcultural biomedical research. Two assume that research ethics are culturally relative and two assume that a unified, universalistic conceptualization of research ethics is possible. All four, I will argue, are to a greater or lesser extent unsatisfactory, largely because of the way that the question itself is configured. This fact militates for a fundamental shift in the way the problem of cross-cultural ethical differences is approached.

NO TRANSCULTURAL BIOMEDICAL RESEARCH

One solution to the problem of which ethics should govern clinical investigation when researchers from one culture use subjects from another is simply to avoid (or prohibit) such research. [...]

There are two fundamental problems with this model. The first one arises from the worldwide ascendancy of Western biomedicine, accepted, as it is, as the official medicine in most countries. Since clinical research itself is generally conducted by physicians who practice Western medicine, the ethics that come to govern such research are largely those of Western biomedicine. This is exacerbated by the fact that physicians in the developing world often identify more with the culture of cosmopolitan medicine than with their own. [...] Much more so than in the West, physicians in the developing world form part of a social

elite, and this fact, coupled with the frequent use of English in training, compounds the cultural distance between doctor and patient, between investigator and subject. The system of medical training in much of the developing world is such as to foster identification with Western norms and expectations regarding such things as specialty choice, language of instruction, patient care, career advancement, and, in all likelihood, research ethics.

Thus, allowing the research ethics of the investigators to prevail in a particular cultural setting will not necessarily solve the problem of appropriate ethics because, arguably, the subject and the investigator will still come from different cultures. The ethics guiding the conduct of clinical research will thus not truly be *local* in the sense that they are not indigenous to the research subjects.

The second problem with this model [...] is that—as an essentially relativistic ethical model—it does not *evaluate* the ethical systems involved. May the members of a given society adhere to a system of clinical research ethics that, by some other standard, is inappropriate?

TRANSCULTURAL RESEARCH SHOULD SATISFY BOTH ETHICAL SYSTEMS

An alternative model is to require transcultural research independently to meet the ethical requirements of the two cultures involved (that is, the culture of the investigator and of the subject). This would entail a commendable respect for the beliefs of the subjects' culture. In addition, it would ordinarily involve adopting a relativistic position towards ethics; no assessment of the ethical systems is made: all are considered to be inherently satisfactory.

The basis for such relativistic thinking about ethics is the contention that nothing is inherently right or wrong, that no moral principles are inherently legitimate. Such thinking supposes that actions are defined as right or wrong by given peoples in specific cultural contexts at specific times and that behavior is culturally relative. As a result, ethical relativity contends that value judgments should be forsworn in assessing foreign systems of belief. Moreover, ethical relativity contends that the impossibility of objectively determining moral action obliges *tolerance* towards other cultures.

Nicholas A. Christakis, "Ethics Are Local: Engaging Cross-Cultural Variation in the Ethics for Clinical Research," *Social Science and Medicine* 35 (1992): 1079–91.

Several practical problems are raised by this position. If research is designed so that it independently meets the ethical expectations of both the subjects and the investigators, then the research, in this model, is perforce ethical and permissible. Yet, it is possible to imagine that research meeting the ethical criteria of both the investigator and the subjects might, under some third standard, be considered unethical. Does this mean that all clinical research projects should meet all possible ethical standards for research, or only the two standards of the involved researchers and subjects? Moreover, this model provides no guidance for resolving conflicting ethical expectations: if neither system is superior and the two conflict, to which one should there be recourse? If the resolution of the conflict is in favor of the subject and is antithetical to the investigator, is the investigator relieved of his ethical duty? Can the research then proceed? If no resolution between conflicting ethics is possible, what is to be done if both societies perceive the research to be essential? Or, if no resolution between conflicting ethics is possible—and the research is therefore impermissible—may the investigators conduct it elsewhere? Finally, to meet the ethical prescription of this model requires a knowledge of local ethical expectations. Who should decide when "all" ethical expectations have been met? A paternalistic feeling on the part of the investigator that the ethical expectations of the subjects have been met would presumably not be enough.

Aside from the foregoing practical problems with this solution, there is a significant theoretical problem as well. The notion of tolerance, to which ethical relativism is linked, is subject to criticism. Ethical relativism is *not* value-free, for a value judgment is contained in its call for tolerance: it asserts that we *ought* to respect other value systems. The problem here is that the evidence regarding cross-cultural variation in basic moral beliefs does not in itself justify tolerance. Though on liberal, humanistic grounds tolerance has some appeal, critics of relativistic thinking, such as Elvin Hatch, have pointed out that tolerance should not be extended beyond its limits. At what point should tolerance stop? Noting that ethical guidelines for judging across cultural boundaries are insufficiently refined, Hatch proposes a "humanistic principle" to address ethical standards cross-culturally. This principle includes two basic assertions: (1) people ought to enjoy a reasonable level of material existence, and (2) human suffering is bad. If these criteria are met, however, other moral principles or other (non-moral) portions of a people's cultural inventory should not be morally evaluated and should be tolerated. Unfortunately, these alone are insufficient guidelines for clinical research. Indeed, if these were the only standards to evaluate the ethics of clinical research, much that is now considered unethical by present standards (at least Western ones) would be deemed ethical.

ETHICS GOVERNING MEDICAL RESEARCH SHOULD BE ABSTRACTED CROSS-CULTURALLY

Thus, a theoretically developed, fundamental, universal principle to guide research could be the humanistic standard. An alternative, empirically based approach would be to examine systems of medical ethics cross-culturally in an effort to identify universal principles. In this manner, an absolutist system of ethics could presumably be developed around the observed common themes. [. . .] The general goal of this model of ethics to govern transcultural biomedical research would be to develop a universal standard through cross-cultural analysis of disparate systems of medical ethics. [. . .]

[I]n this model of ethics to govern transcultural biomedical research, the ethics of Ayurveda and traditional Chinese medicine, along with other systems of medical ethics from throughout the world—such as the Western ones discussed below—would be studied in an effort to develop a universal, cross-cultural standard based on common concerns. A significant problem arises, however, with this familiar cross-cultural approach of looking for universals. Both research and research ethics are singularly Western. Largely because the very notion of clinical research on human subjects is rare, if not absent, in other medical systems, systems of biomedical research ethics *as such* do not exist in any medical system other than Western biomedicine. The systems of medical ethics found in the literate Asian medical traditions, for example, are [. . .] largely professional ethics that include precepts regarding respect for the texts, loyalty to the profession, and commitment to the craft. [. . .] Do the essentially professional ethics of Ayurveda and traditional Chinese medicine permit extension to the case of subjects of research? Can an absolutist conceptualization of biomedical research ethics, based on more general medical ethics, be formulated?

Some aspects of these professional ethics truly *are* relevant to the conduct of human research. The Asian texts generally recognize a special responsibility or duty that physicians have with respect to the sick. The texts recognize that, in addition to a commitment to the discipline of medicine, doctors must be committed to their patients. When the commitment to patients conflicts with the commitment to the texts or to the profession, the resolution is generally, but not always, in favor of the patient. The texts recognize the inherent conflicts sometimes seen in medical practice, between devotion to the profession and desire to help a patient or between a desire for profit and a concern for therapy. Perhaps in response to such conflicts, or perhaps in order to enhance professional status, all the texts articulate that doctors should be "good" or "moral" in some culturally specific way; the texts state that physicians should be held to a higher standard than the rest of society. These concepts could provide a basis for the development of a special code of ethics when the patient happens also to be a research subject; towards such an individual, it could be argued, special commitment must exist. Indeed, the injunction to put oneself in the patient's place would be especially applicable in the case of research.

Beyond this articulation of the special status of physicians because of their special responsibility, the two literate Asian systems of medical ethics tend to articulate a principle of humaneness or beneficence. Akin to the humanistic principle that suffering is bad, this basic principle may also provide a foundation for research ethics. Moreover, the texts recognize the potential for harm inherent in medical practice. [...]

Aside from the two foregoing themes, however, a cross-cultural analysis is unlikely to yield many constant precepts. Indeed, quite a few of the ethical expectations in the literate Asian traditions would be difficult to reconcile with the conduct of modern biomedical research. Comparison of alternative forms of therapy, use of risky invasive procedures, informed consent without deception, use of placebos, tolerance of some risk to the subject for a greater good of society: all these might be differently construed in different ethical traditions. [...]

In sum, this model of ethics to govern transcultural clinical research—that of abstracting a universal system of ethics from cross-cultural analysis—is imperfect on two accounts: (1) the lack of a research tradition in non-Western systems of medicine results in a lack of explicit research ethics, and (2) the concerns raised in systems of professional ethics [...] are not always relevant to the issues raised in the conduct of modern clinical research.

WESTERN RESEARCH ETHICS
SHOULD APPLY UNIVERSALLY

Since non-Western medical systems lack an experimental tradition involving the use of human subjects, should we not therefore use a Western conceptualization of research ethics in conducting transcultural clinical research, a conceptualization which, after all, has been developed to contend with the Western tradition of human experimentation? Such use is supported by the fact that biomedical research is unique to the West and also by the fact that, in some sense, research ethics are *an integral part of research*. [...] This fourth model for transcultural biomedical research ethics generally contends that Western ethics should be the universal standard. [...]

Western codifications of biomedical research ethics, including the CIOMS guidelines, are generally founded, implicitly or explicitly, upon three principles: respect for persons, beneficence, and justice. Application of these principles, however, will be greatly influenced by the cultural setting of the research in a number of critical ways, only some of which are directly addressed in the guidelines.

Respect for persons incorporates a deontologic conception of human beings as ends unto themselves and gives rise to the necessity for informed consent [...]. A very fundamental problem arises, however, in the application of the respect for persons principle because of cross-cultural variation in the definition of personhood. Western societies stress the individualistic nature of a person and put much emphasis on the individual's rights, autonomy, self-determination, and privacy. But this is at variance with the more relational definitions of a person found in many non-Western societies which stress the embeddedness of the individual within society and define a person by means of his relations to others.

From this variation in the definition of a person arise important practical implications. Since the notion of persons as individuals is undermined, the consent of the individual may be viewed as nonessential in certain cultural settings. [...] Thus, in the context of research, it may initially be necessary to secure the consent of a subject's family or social group instead of or in addition to the consent of the subject himself.

Variations in the definition of personhood between societies may also find expression in who precisely is deemed able to give informed consent for others. [...] There will be considerable variation by culture as to who is acknowledged to be a "community leader" and whether such an individual will meet a Western investigator's expectation regarding who can appropriately give consent for another adult. The principle of community leader consent, however, may be the only alternative [...] to individual consent in many cases where beneficial research is essential. But this alternative may not necessarily be disturbing within the society of which the research subject is a member. [...]

In the context of human subjects research, beneficence is the obligation to protect research subjects from harm and to maximize possible benefits and minimize possible harms. The principle of beneficence thus mandates an appropriate risk-benefit ratio. A relational or expansive definition of personhood of the kind described above may result in ethical decisions that, by Western standards, unduly favor the interests of society-at-large at the risk of the individual. Western ethical standards generally accord considerable import to the welfare of the individual in the conduct of research. [...]

The calculus of such balancing will be different in different socio-cultural settings. In some situations, cultural expectations may be that the anticipated benefit to society or to one's community will justifiably outweigh the anticipated risk to the individual. Societal values may be such that the interests of the subject are not perforce precedent over the interests of society. Thus, furthering the interest of society-at-large may not necessarily compromise the rights and interests of the individual research subject [. . .]. Even more fundamentally, a developing world research subject may find it "difficult to see how the interests of the subject conflict with the interests of the society except, of course, if the society is not his own." In this view, the interests of the subject and of the society or the community are necessarily congruent. Problems arise only if the values and expectations of a society of which the individual is *not* a member are imposed. [. . .]

It is thus clear that a simple, straightforward application of Western biomedical research ethics in non-Western settings is problematic. A refined object of this model might therefore be to take a Western standard and modify it in a culturally sensitive way, in recognition of the problems outlined above, rather than apply it as is. But this too is problematic: even if the Western standard is modified to accord with local cultural expectations, the danger of imposing Western perceptions of what is appropriate to consider in ethical decision-making, of stipulating in advance which aspects to emphasize, still remains. Indigenous peoples may have ethical concerns about biomedical research that are difficult for Westerners to appreciate, let alone anticipate or validate. These concerns might not fit easily within the framework of Western codifications, or worse, might escape recognition altogether.

ENGAGING ETHICAL DIFFERENCES

[. . .] The inadequacy of these four models has three causes, all of which have to do with the influence of culture upon the problem itself. This influence is quite profound: culture shapes (1) the content of ethical precepts, (2) the way ethics as a concept is configured (that is, the form of ethical precepts), and (3) the interaction between conflicting ethical expectations (that is, the way ethical conflict is handled). Addressing the first problem (how culture shapes ethical rules) requires careful analysis of indigenous ethical expectations. [. . .]

Addressing the latter two problems (how culture shapes our idea of what ethics is and our idea of how to resolve ethical conflict), however, is more difficult: it requires the development of a special perspective on ethical systems. That is, traditional Western bioethical approaches may well be inadequate to contend not only with the manifest variability in ethical norms across cultures but also with the other two causes of the inadequacies in the models. These models break down in part because they treat ethics in a philosophically orthodox fashion and look for the answer through what *ought* to be done rather than through what is done. Configuring ethics solely as a set of prescriptive and proscriptive rules, and not also as a cultural system of thought that has explicative and creative functions is inadequate. This inadequacy on the one hand is highlighted by the conduct of transcultural clinical research—which, by its nature, brings into direct contact potentially discrepant ethical expectations—and on the other hand must be rectified because of the pressing need for international medical research.

All four models fail to address the culturally defined meaning of ethical systems in that they assume a non-interpretive posture with respect to the concept of ethics. Medical ethics is not the same kind of thing in all cultures. [. . .] Clifford Geertz has observed that a paradox arises when conceptualizing systems of ideas because of the realization that "socio-political thought does not grow out of disembodied reflection but it is always bound up with the existing life situation of the thinker." The solution to this problem, Geertz argues, lies in a more adroit handling of socio-political thought—including ethics, I believe—by conceptualizing it as an ordered system of cultural symbols.

That is, it is not the ethical rules themselves which are so important; it is their *meaning*. The rules, in a sense, may be taken to reflect how a given culture perceives that human beings should be treated by others, how investigator and subject should communicate, or how medical knowledge is to be acquired. Ethics do not just regulate behavior; they construe it. [. . .] In this respect, ethics has something in common with ideology. Though the two are admittedly different, ideological and ethical systems are similar in that both are templates for the organization of social processes. [. . .]

Medical ethics may be different things in different cultures in part because of the activity ethics are viewed as appropriately governing. For example, the distribution of resources that maintain or restore health is configured as necessarily a moral problem within contemporary Western medical ethics. Yet, in other societies, the distribution of such resources might not be configured as a moral issue at all, and the distribution of health-related resources may be seen as requiring no more attention to ethical precepts than the distribution of food.

A culturally sensitive perspective on systems of medical ethics has a further consequence. According to the prevailing view, medical ethics [. . .] consists of rules and principles directed at what ought to be the case. An alternative, contextualist, view of medical ethics, however, focuses on accounting for the phenomena of medical ethics. It seeks to understand the practice of medical ethics by locating its cultural context. A contextualist perspective on morality offers a way out of the thorny methodologic and substantive issues raised by a positivist—and culturally myopic—perspective on morality, issues brought to the fore by the conduct of transcultural clinical research.

A contextualist approach also contributes to a solution to the problem of which ethics should govern transcultural research by broadening the philosophical basis of research ethics. Part of the problem with the foregoing four models—even from a Western point of view—is that the full richness of Western philosophy itself has not been tapped. As Fox and Swazey have argued,

> the paradigm of values and beliefs, and of reflections on them, that has developed and been institutionalized in American bioethics is an impoverished and skewed expression of our society's cultural tradition. In a highly intellectualized but essentially fundamentalistic way, it thins out the fullness of that tradition and bends it away from some of the deepest sources of its meaning and vitality.

Bioethics has, until very recently, based itself almost exclusively on Anglo-American analytic philosophical thought and largely ignored other Western philosophical traditions, such as phenomenology, virtue theory, existentialism, social ethics, and so forth.

Hence, present concepts of medical ethics are too detached from the clinical reality in which ethics come into play. A significant source of ethical meaning is the particular situation in which ethical issues are raised. Clinical research ethics have a concrete existence, expressed in each research setting. Ethical rules such as those pertaining to clinical research, like other socio-political and religious thought, are constructed, fashioned, made. And since both the maker and the situation in which they are applied vary, so will the product. In order to resolve the troubling problems raised by the conduct of transcultural clinical research, an ethnography of the practice of morality in medical contexts in general and in transcultural clinical research in particular will be needed, and social scientists can contribute meaningfully in this respect.

Such a casuistic view of medical ethics has practical implications: it means that understanding the specific, relevant ethical expectations of indigenous peoples will be a prerequisite of transcultural clinical research. It is not the existence of moral standards that varies cross-culturally, it is their form and content. Could we not ask members of a given society a series of ethnographic questions: Is it right for a doctor to try a new or untested therapy on a patient in order to see what happens? How is knowledge acquired in a given medical system? Can doctors do anything other than *treat* a patient? Can doctors misbehave when interacting with patients, and if so, how? How is participation in medical research viewed? How do Western research ethics come to be indigenized? The study of the answers to such questions might provide a strong foundation for evaluating the assumptions underlying what is considered to be ethical care of patients and research subjects in the relatively homogeneous medical system of American culture.

Indeed, the Western system of research ethics is itself a recent creation, largely articulated since World War II. It rests on a medical ethic that was exclusively doctor-patient oriented and which, under pressure of the research endeavor, was expanded to accommodate the investigator-subject relationship. Western medical ethics, that is, were at the outset based on the Hippocratic tradition, and, akin to [certain systems of] Asian medical ethics [. . .], were largely professional in nature. The concept of essential patient rights which in themselves create obligations for professionals is alien to the Hippocratic ethical tradition. This concept found its important expression in the West in the Nuremberg Code. The code abandoned the notion that experimental subjects are protected by professional standards and replaced it with the notion that subjects intrinsically have self-determination and autonomy.

In short, there has been an evolution in medical ethics—in response to the existence of research and to the abuse of research subjects in certain settings—in the West. The indigenous ethics of non-Western cultures, as they apply to professional etiquette or clinical care, are also capable of evolution. [. . .]

But the emergence of non-Western systems of clinical research ethics, such as they might be, must be expected and understood. Indeed, we are at the initial stages of a proliferation of biomedical research in the developing world, a proliferation that includes many collaborative efforts between developed and developing countries. In view of the importance and ubiquity of such research, an understanding of the emergence of research ethics in non-Western countries is of enormous practical significance. As traditional and biomedical practice converges around much of the world, clinical research ethics will be under increased pressure to adapt to local circumstances and local cultures.

Thus, culture shapes both the content and form of ethical systems. It can also be seen to shape how the existence of conflicting ethical expectations is construed and handled. In the United States in particular, we often seem to expect that a solution to ethical problems is indeed possible, if only we were clever or persuasive or patient enough. The expectation, tempered by our culture, is that ethical dilemmas have a solution. However, not all conflicts, especially in such a complex area as research ethics, are resolvable. Resolving ethical dissonance is apt to be especially unlikely when non-casuistic, systematic solutions—those divorced from actual, clinically and culturally specific situations—are applied. The four models considered above are problematic on this account. American bioethics has an inherent bias in that there is an expectation that final and transcendent resolution of ethical disputes is indeed possible. [...]

Ethical systems, however, do not exist in order to eliminate ethical discourse. Instead, they provide a framework for such discourse—a framework for the confrontation of particular situations that pose ethical dilemmas. A discourse between ethical systems requires mutual understanding—not only of the ethical expectations that are being contested and discussed, but also of the very meaning of what ethical systems are and what their function is.

Such a discourse can address which ethics should govern transcultural clinical research. This approach to the problem is similar to the second solution in four critical respects: (1) an ongoing *dialogue* between ethical systems is inherent in it; (2) a *negotiation* between ethical systems about *a particular situation* takes place; (3) proponents of both the dissonant ethical systems *assess and examine* themselves and each other; and (4) a rationale for *tolerance* is thus provided, namely, that ethical conflict is sometimes irresolvable but must nevertheless be handled.

The kind of negotiation between equals that this approach entails would admittedly be difficult to attain in many settings in the developing world where research is conducted—if for no other reason, because of the tremendous difference in education, literacy, wealth, and power between investigators and subjects. The difficulty in achieving such a cross-cultural dialogue, however, does not mean that efforts should be abandoned. Moreover, in such a discourse, the involved parties must accept the existence of alternative ethical systems, and, while not forswearing assessment of the other systems, must still negotiate with them. Such negotiation and mutual understanding also provides the practical advantage of providing a mechanism for dispute resolution. Thus, the hallmarks of such an approach are ethical *pluralism* and humility rather than either ethical relativism or universalism.

[T]he comparative study of research ethics cannot be a matter of reducing concrete differences to abstract commonalties, nor of locating identical phenomena masquerading under different names. Rather, in the thick of ethical differences, the goal should be to *engage* rather than *abolish* ethical conflict. [...]

We must navigate, in short, between the simplicity of ethical universality and the evasion and complexity of ethical relativism, between intellectual hubris and moral paralysis. We should not ask "Is there a single model for research ethics?" but rather "Can there be?" We must face and accept the indeterminacy of ethical variability. That medical ethics cannot be separated from the behavior they are intended to govern in the cultural setting in which they are to govern it means that the search for a single model of transcultural research ethics would be fruitless. Instead of such a search, the varieties of ethical expectations should be turned into commentaries one upon the other, the one illuminating what the other obscures.

---

71 Ethical and Regulatory Challenges in a Randomized Control Trial of Adjuvant Treatment for Breast Cancer in Vietnam

Richard R. Love and Norman C. Fost

[...]

MEDICAL BACKGROUND, THE PROPOSED PROJECT, AND PROPOSED CONSENT PROCEDURES

Standard treatment of breast cancer in the United States (and most Western/developed countries) includes various surgical procedures, usually coupled with adjuvant therapy, in this case surgery. Adjuvant therapy is given in the absence of any obvious evidence of cancer spread, to treat presumed microscopic diseases. [...]

In the treatment of premenopausal women with breast cancer, the place of hormonal therapies is incompletely defined. The physiologic basis is the observation that breast cancer growth is stimulated by estrogen. Thus, removing a major producer of estrogen, such as the ovaries, or providing a drug, such as tamoxifen which opposes the cellular action of estrogen, would possibly be helpful in controlling the growth of breast cancer. While there is evidence that such hormonal treatments have benefit, these observations

Richard R. Love and Norman C. Fost, "Ethical and Regulatory Challenges in a Randomized Control Trial of Adjuvant Treatment for Breast Cancer in Vietnam," *Journal of Investigative Medicine* 45 (1997): 423–31.

come from studies and analyses in which other variables make it difficult to determine confidently their relative contributions to improved outcomes.

While there is considerable scientific support for conducting breast cancer studies of the specific role of hormonal treatments in premenopausal women, it has been difficult to conduct such studies in the United States where the standard adjuvant treatment has been chemotherapy. Whatever the merits of hormonal treatments and the importance of studying them, it is generally acknowledged that mounting a placebo- or a no adjuvant treatment–controlled trial in the United States is not politically feasible at present.

As a result of multiple visits to Vietnam, initially as a representative of the International Union Against Cancer, the first author (R. R. L.) and principal investigator (PI) was familiar with the state-of-the-art of breast cancer care. [...] The lack of resources and systems prevented any well-organized care for these cancer victims. Systematic adjuvant treatments (such as chemotherapy or hormonal treatment with oophorectomy or tamoxifen) were only occasionally used and then in manners unlikely to achieve any benefit to the patient (that is, not with full doses or according to schedules shown to be effective).

The PI conceived of the idea of a clinical trial as a means for technology transfer, education, and immediate improvement of treatment. [...]

The investigator proposed to conduct a randomized, controlled trial of adjuvant surgical oophorectomy and tamoxifen in 350 premenopausal women with operable breast cancer, in collaboration with physicians at 2 major cancer hospitals in the Socialist Republic of Vietnam. [...] A comprehensive protocol was submitted to the institutional review board [IRB], including an extensive discussion of the rationale for conducting the trial in Vietnam. The specific benefits of the proposed trial to the Vietnamese, and also to the international community, was noted.

DIFFERING STANDARDS OF CARE

In developing the proposed research program, the investigator found himself uncertain about the application of American standards of informed consent in the Vietnamese setting. After detailed discussions with Vietnamese physicians and cultural experts [...] it became clear that the American standards would not be acceptable to Vietnamese physicians, political leaders in Vietnam, or the vast majority of Vietnamese patients. [...]

In particular, it is not customary in Vietnam for patients to participate in their own medical decisions in the way that is normative in the United States and other Western cultures. Patients expect and look to their physicians to tell them the appropriate treatment. It is unacceptable for a physician to openly express uncertainty with regard to

what is the best treatment. In practice, given a choice of options, patients virtually always defer to the physician. [...] Thus, while it might be technically possible, though difficult, to inform Vietnamese women about alternative ways of treating breast cancer or options within a research protocol, Vietnamese people do not believe it is the right thing to do, and even if it were done, the informed consent that resulted would not be functionally relevant because patients, in fact, would defer judgment to their doctors. In addition, trying to force this mode of consent on the physicians risked losing their cooperation with the project because of the tone of cultural imperialism that it would convey. In light of these considerations, the PI initially considered waiving some elements of the consent process, namely those that would convey uncertainty by the treating doctor. This would imply not disclosing that the patient's proposed treatment had been determined by a process of randomization.

THE USE OF SURROGATES
IN THE CONSENT PROCESS

The authors anticipated that the IRB would have to consider a proposal for surrogate consent in 2 senses. First, particularly in view of the limited participation of the prospective patients in the consent process, someone had to represent them as a group in deciding to initiate the study. This could be considered especially problematic in view of the intention to use 2 treatment approaches, neither of which would be considered standard treatment in developed countries. We thought it important that the macro decision not be made solely by U.S. agencies, such as the University of Wisconsin IRB. Second, since patients would not be participating actively, by American standards, in the decision to be a research subject, it was unavoidable that the decision would be made by a surrogate. This would typically be the patient's physician. Given the mixture of research and clinical motives, however, we thought it prudent to seek an additional layer of representation for the patients. Toward this end, the PI convened 2 surrogate groups to review the protocol, with particular attention to the proposed consent process.

[...] The process involves identifying a group of laypersons who resemble the prospective research subjects as much as possible. The surrogates are asked to review the proposal, including the consent forms, in an informal, open-ended session, for the purpose of eliciting candid opinions about the study and consent form, as well as to gain impressions as to whether prospective subjects, fully informed, would want to participate, or if not, what the reasons might be. [T]he purpose of the surrogate groups was 2-fold: first, to provide the investigator and the IRB with independent opinions about the project as a whole, including the medical and consent aspects; and second, to provide some protection for individual patients by ensuring that their interests would not be violated by participation in the study. [...]

Surrogate Group 1. Educated, American-Living Vietnamese Immigrants

The PI assembled a group of 4 Vietnamese immigrant women, 2 of their husbands (one Vietnamese, one American), and a visiting Vietnamese Ph.D. sociologist who met for over 2½ hours. The PI indicated that he needed their help to decide the best way to conduct a Special Breast Program for Vietnamese women in Vietnam.

The PI asked them to pretend that they were in Vietnam and developed cancer, or to imagine that their sisters were in this circumstance and sought their advice. [...] The full spectrum of issues normally covered in the consent process was presented: purpose, selection of subjects, procedures, benefits, risks, alternatives, confidentiality. The PI discussed the American way of informing women about the choice of treatment, and group members presented their understanding of the Vietnamese way. They described a paternalistic system in Vietnam, which they believed was best, under which a physician would tell the patient that one or the other treatment was best and recommend it. The PI openly discussed the review process for such programs in the United States and said that he was exploring the possibility that if the group approved, foregoing some elements of individual informed consent might be possible. This discussion led to further very detailed questioning about the treatment choices, benefits, risks, and treatment in the West for such cases, as well as direct questions about the principal investigator's interests and possible benefits for Vietnamese women. [...]

The PI asked each individual for their opinion about the appropriateness of conducting this program in the Vietnamese way, that is without presenting the alternative treatments and randomization details to individual women, and each agreed that they believed this was the best way and said they would approve of a program conducted under these conditions.

Surrogate Group 2. Moral Leaders: Directors of the Vietnamese Women's Union

During a visit by the PI, he arranged to meet with the leaders of the Vietnamese Women's Union, which represents women's interests at all levels of Vietnamese society as a functionally independent entity.

The PI met with the vice president and the chief of the International Relations Department of the Vietnamese Women's Union for 1½ hours. [...] The PI explicitly stated that without their personal approval this program could not be undertaken. These leaders appeared to well understand the ethical and regulatory problems the PI faced and accepted responsibility for passing judgment on the appropriateness of this program.

At the conclusion the vice president consulted with her colleague and then stated her approval of the program to be conducted in the Vietnamese way with the responsible physician telling the patient post randomization that one or the other treatment would be given. [...]

THE REVIEW PROCESS: STANDARDS FOR CONSENT

The second central issue in the review process concerned informed consent. While the international guidelines for research in underdeveloped countries suggest that "every effort will be made to secure the ethical imperative that the consent of the individual subjects be informed[,]" [c]ommentary with these guidelines states:

> For example, when because of communication difficulties investigators cannot make prospective subjects sufficiently aware of the implications of participation to give adequately informed consent, the decision of each prospective subject on whether to consent should be elicited through a reliable intermediary such as a trusted community leader. In some cases other mechanisms, approved by an ethical review committee, may be more suitable.

Other language in the Council for International Organizations of Medical Sciences (CIOMS) guidelines, however, suggests that their authors were considering educational difficulties (such as literacy) most in suggesting acceptable circumstances for alternatives to individual consent and not cultural differences such as the investigator was confronted with in this proposal.

In his initial presentation on proposed consent procedures, the PI argued that surrogate consent could be justified under the CIOMS international guidelines. [...] The PI went on to argue that the standard practice in Western countries of obtaining individual informed consent from each subject was not appropriate and probably not meaningful and feasible in Vietnam, given the widespread resistance to this notion by patients, doctors, and political and community leaders. He requested that the IRB waive the requirement for informed consent, at least with respect to the subject of randomization.

A majority of IRB members rejected this request for partial waiver of consent, based on 3 concerns. First, there was a concern that such an approval could place the institution in jeopardy with the Office for Protections from Research Risks [now the Office for Health Research Protections —eds.] at the National Institutes of Health, the agency with oversight authority for IRBs. Second, IRB members were troubled by the remoteness of their relationship to the treating physicians in Vietnam, implying insufficient knowledge to trust their communications with the patients. One of the strengths attributed to the local control implicit in the IRB system has been its familiarity with the physician-investigators whose integrity is critical to the ethical conduct of experimentation involving human subjects. Third, reviewers felt that only through a written document could they insure that subjects were being informed about critical elements of the research program. While the PI offered assurances that subjects would be informed about critical elements, such as their inability to bear children after oophorectomy, the IRB insisted that presentation of this information in a written document was necessary to assure that such information was transmitted.

The negotiation about disclosure of randomization was more difficult. As stated earlier, the surrogate groups felt strongly that talking about the concept of randomization was wrong for Vietnamese patients. Indeed, the language expressing this concept in the Vietnamese language is especially confusing, even to educated Vietnamese. The surrogate groups felt there would be de facto deferral to physicians over treatment choices, and thus presenting this issue in a written document was functionally meaningless and would serve only to confuse and upset physicians and patients. These arguments were not persuasive to the IRB reviewers, who insisted on the inclusion of this information in a written document. There was a negotiated agreement to use a form that was brief compared to traditional consent forms and that omitted some speculative or minimal risks.

CONSENT MONITORING

The IRB committee also required an independently conducted consent monitoring study. This was accomplished in 13 consecutive subjects queried 3 months after entry into the study (Table [71.1]). The responses showed a high degree of awareness of the critical elements of the study—research, conducted by both Vietnamese and American doctors, and treatment that would prevent future child bearing. As the table shows, subjects were evenly split in answering whether they or the research plan decided treatment and whether they should follow instructions regarding treatment or could refuse proposed treatments.

With respect to the treatment decision (Question 3), the fact that half of the queried women said that they decided (Answer B) in contrast to their physician (Answer C), suggests a greater degree of perceived autonomy than might have been expected. The consent monitors thought there was an alternative explanation, namely, that the third

Table 71.1

Results of Consent Monitoring

---

1. Were you aware that the proposed treatment for breast cancer is part of a research project?
   12, yes
   1, no (but suspected)

2. Who is doing the research?
   0, doctors from the United States
   1, doctors from Vietnam
   12, both of the above (one included Australia)

3. How was it decided which treatment you will receive?
   1, my physician decided which treatment is best for me
   6, I decided which treatment I prefer
   6, the research plan determined my treatment (by random selection)

4. Will this treatment affect your ability to have children?
   0, it will help me to have children if I want them
   13, if my ovaries are removed, I will not be able to have children ever again

5. What happens if you do not want your ovaries to be removed?
   1, I can refuse, but then the doctors will not take care of me any more
   5, I must follow the instructions of the physicians including having my ovaries removed if they tell me to
   7, I can refuse to have my ovaries removed and still receive the other treatments without penalty

6. What do you have to pay for?
   6, my breast surgery
   1, vitamins and other drugs
   0, transportation expenses to the clinic
   6 (no answer given, but noted patient has social insurance)

---

answer (treatment was decided by randomization) involved concepts that were completely foreign and virtually meaningless to many women, so they picked the second answer [presumably] by default. Some sense of perceived autonomy is revealed also in the answers to question 5. Seven subjects said, yes, they could refuse the immediate surgical treatment. However, a great majority of women subsequently enrolling in the study have not shown such willingness. As of November 1996, 186 women have entered the study and been randomized to immediate oophorectomy and tamoxifen; of these, 17 have refused this treatment (9 percent), and of this small group 10 (5 percent of the total) received tamoxifen alone. While this number of refusals possibly suggests more autonomy than the foregoing opinions and discussions predicted, in fact all but 2 of these refusals occurred in one institution where different medical and social/political factors and one physician contributed to this situation. [...]

CONCLUSIONS

[...] The study presented 2 major difficulties for the U.S. IRB. First, both the experimental intervention (oophorectomy and tamoxifen) and the control arm (standard treatment as it existed in Vietnam) were initially considered ethically unacceptable. After extensive discussion, using surrogate groups in the United States and Vietnam, and consultation with experts in the treatment of breast cancer, the IRB accepted the study design, with slight modification, as ethically acceptable. Second, a proposal to use a consent process that was designed to meet the cultural norms and personal values of Vietnamese patients, physicians, and political leaders was considered unacceptable by the IRB. After extensive discussion, again including surrogate groups and Vietnamese political leaders, there was agreement on the appropriate content of the consent process and consent form. In its final form, this included the key elements of informed consent, as required by U.S. standards, though with somewhat less detail than is typical in a U.S. consent form. Consent monitoring suggested that the study participants understood the key elements, namely, that they were part of an American-sponsored research project and that oophorectomy would result in permanent infertility. Some patients appeared to understand that they could refuse to be in the study or to have their ovaries removed. It is unclear whether they understood that their treatment was determined by randomization.

A negotiated agreement acceptable to the investigator and the IRB was reached. It is our impression that the vast majority of patients who have enrolled in this study have not consented in the way that is envisioned by mainstream ethical thought in the United States and as is contemplated by the writers of the U.S. regulations. On the other hand, those Vietnamese patients who wish to make autonomous choices have sufficient information and freedom to do so.

Some might ask what harm would have been done by using the standard American consent form and by insisting on a consent process more in line with American expectations. At the least, the study would have been extraordinarily difficult to conduct, possibly impossible. Failure to respect the cultural norms of the Vietnamese people, including physicians, patients, and political leaders, would have seriously undermined the complex negotiations that are required for any large-scale, randomized clinical trial. The final outcome allowed for respect of both perspectives: traditional Vietnamese physicians and patients have been able to relate in the way they apparently prefer, and more Westernized patients are able to express their autonomous choice. [...]

[Figures omitted—eds.]

Part VIII

The Behavior of Clinical Investigators

Conflicts of Interest

In 1980 the U.S. Congress passed the Bayh-Dole Act, the Patent and Trademark Law Amendments Act, which required closer collaboration of researchers funded by the National Institutes of Health (NIH) with private industry. It was a mandate to commercialize scientific discoveries. The result has been a growing link between researchers and industry, leading to a profusion of reports about researchers' conflicts of interest and the potential adverse consequences for research participants. The Gelsinger case is among the most prominent and tragic examples.[1] In September 1999 Jesse Gelsinger, an 18-year-old male with ornithine transcarbamylase deficiency, a genetic defect that impairs ammonia metabolism, underwent a gene transfer experiment at the University of Pennsylvania's Institute for Human Gene Therapy. Using a special diet and medications, he was in relatively good health with few symptoms. But the day after being injected with an adenovirus carrying the gene for ornithine transcarbamylase, Gelsinger began having serious problems with heart rhythm and mental confusion. Despite intensive care, he died four days after injection of the virus. Among the many ethical issues raised by the case was the fact that the principal investigator and head (until July 2002) of the Institute for Human Gene Therapy, James M. Wilson, had a substantial financial stake in Genovo, the privately held company that had produced the gene-altered adenovirus. Furthermore, Genovo was providing substantial funds to finance research at the Institute for Human Gene Therapy.

The Gelsinger case and other similar cases have prompted substantial reaction. In January 2001 the U.S. Office for Human Research Protections (OHRP) issued interim guidelines on conflicts of interest.[2] Various professional organizations, academic institu-tions, and officials have reexamined their conflict-of-interest policies or issued new statements about conflicts of interest. In December 2001, for example, the Executive Council of the Association of American Medical Colleges (AAMC) approved the first report of its Task Force on Financial Conflicts of Interest in Clinical Research.[3]

The writings excerpted in Part VIII illuminate the current thinking about conflicts of interest in clinical research. The topics examined in these writings include (1) an ethical analysis of conflicts of interest, (2) financial conflicts of interest of investigators in clinical research, and (3) potential remedies.

ETHICAL ANALYSIS OF CONFLICTS OF INTEREST

Our first contributor, Dennis F. Thompson, elucidates the concept of conflict of interest. He argues that a professional has a primary interest as well as myriad secondary interests. A conflict of interest occurs when the secondary interests "unduly influence" the person's "professional judgment concerning a primary interest." In medicine it is classically argued that there are three primary interests: patient health and well-being, clinical research, and education of future health professionals. Secondary interests of researchers include financial gain, promotion, grant renewals for research, publication of research results in prominent journals, desire for fame, interest in avocational pursuits, family obligations, and so on. As Thompson emphasizes, these secondary interests are "usually not illegitimate"; indeed, they are frequently "necessary and desirable." We praise people who are committed to their families; the desire to earn a good income (within limits) is viewed as both necessary and legitimate; and we respect avocational pursuits as the embodiment of a well-rounded person. The problem—the conflict of interest—is not therefore the result of "bad" secondary interests. Instead, a conflict of interest occurs when these secondary interests dominate, unduly influence, distort, or corrupt the integrity of a physician's judgment in relation to patient health, clinical research, or medical education. In other words, problems arise when fortune, fame, or family preference threaten the integrity of the physician's professional judgment.

Conflicts of interest are often distinguished from conflicts of commitment. Conflicts of interest arise between primary and secondary interests, where it is clear that secondary interests are not part of the physician's duties as a physician and should not influence professional judgments. Conflicts of commitment are different because they arise between primary interests; they are conflicts between caring for a patient and educating medical students or between caring for a patient and completing a research study. Although conflicts of commitment can be difficult to deal with, they are not especially problematic from an ethical point of view; conflicts of interest, however, are.

Not all conflicts of interest are of equal concern. As Thompson points out, the severity of a conflict depends on two factors: (1) the probability that judgments will actually be distorted and (2) the potential magnitude of the harm. In evaluating a conflict of interest both factors must be considered. This leads to a sliding scale of conflicts of interest. When the secondary interest is small enough that it is unlikely to corrupt decisionmaking or when the potential harm is transient or of small consequence, concern is lessened. Conversely, if the influence of the secondary interest on professional judgment is likely to be great—say, because the financial incentive is very large—or if the potential harms could be life-threatening or disabling or lead to a significant loss of public confidence, concern is heightened.

Finally, when assessing conflicts of interest it is important to note that appearances matter. First, it is frequently difficult for an external observer to determine when secondary interests have improper influence and when they do not, especially if the observer has no personal relationship with the professional making the judgment. External observers—and sometimes even those directly involved—may not be able to determine when secondary interests are actually influencing a professional's judgment. Second, public confidence in the integrity of professional judgment is important; the public does not want to—and should not have to—examine each and every decision by a professional to determine whether it was distorted by a secondary interest. Instead, people should be able to rely on settled practices that ensure that the professional's judgments are free of illegitimate influences. Because external observers cannot know what influences a person and because the public should not have to investigate each judgment, ensuring that appearances are appropriate is necessary. Suspicion of a conflict is already an ethical problem. Maintaining *appearances*—secondary to dealing with the *reality* of conflicts of interest—is an important mechanism to sustain public confidence.

More generally, as two of our contributors, Joseph B. Martin and Dennis L. Kasper, point out, the public's interest in medical research must be kept in mind when dealing with issues surrounding conflicts of interest. Among other things, as Martin and Kasper argue, the public has a right to know that the research it funds (via taxation) is pursued in a bias-free manner and that the risks they encounter when participating in research will not be heightened by any profit-seeking among study investigators. Ultimately, as Martin and Kasper note, conflicts of interest in clinical research are against the public's interest.

FINANCIAL CONFLICTS OF INTEREST

There is a perception that researcher conflicts of interest are growing and that this is a growing problem in clinical research.[4] Much of the attention has been focused on financial conflicts that arise when clinical researchers have stock ownership or other equity interests, paid consultancies, patent-licensing arrangements, or research grants with pharmaceutical, biotechnology, or medical device manufacturers on whose products they are conducting research. Conflicts arise because these clinical investigators receive—or have the potential to receive—financial rewards that are linked, explicitly or implicitly, to the outcomes of the clinical research. The concern, then, is that this financial reward may compromise the investigators' judgments about their clinical research. As the Gelsinger case shows, this is no mere theoretical worry. Another of the more infamous cases occurred at the Massachusetts Eye and Ear Infirmary and Harvard Medical School in the 1980s.[5] An ophthalmology fellow was conducting a trial on a vitamin A–based ointment for the treatment of "dry eye" syndrome. He owned over half a million shares of the company, Spectra Pharmaceutical Services, that planned to market the ointment if it was proven effective. The fellow's mentor also had stock in the company. Not only were more patients enrolled than the protocol called for, but before making the results public the fellow sold stock when he realized the product was ineffective. This case prompted Harvard Medical School to issue rules on conflicts of interest in March 1990; these were subsequently revised and updated in October 2000.[6]

There were few *harms* in the Harvard case; yet the case does not suffer a shortage of *wrongs*, that is, violations of moral rights. It is arguable that patients were owed the truth about the investigator's financial involvement with the sponsoring company and the way this involvement affected his enrollment practices. While most patients were not harmed, it is true, insofar as they were kept in the dark regarding the financial conflict of interest, these patients were wronged. Although wrongs are often thought to be less weighty than harms, they should nonetheless figure into people's discussion of conflicts of interest and the ills that spring therefrom.

In other cases, however, it is alleged that serious harms resulted from similar conflicts of interest. A case in point occurred at the prestigious Fred Hutchinson Cancer Research Center in Seattle, in which researchers were charged with financial conflicts of interest related to a bone marrow transplantation study.[7] In this study researchers were trying to reduce graft-versus-host disease (GVHD), a serious and sometimes fatal side effect of bone marrow transplantation in which the new bone marrow attacks the patients' cells. In "Protocol 126," a study carried out from 1981 to 1993, T cells were removed from the subjects' bone marrow because they were thought to cause GVHD. Several key researchers at the Fred Hutchinson Center, including the Nobel Prize–winning bone marrow transplantation pioneer Donald Thomas, had stock shares in Genetic Systems, the company that produced three of the eight antibodies used to remove the T cells from the bone marrow. The Fred Hutchinson Center had other financial relationships with Genetic Systems relating to commercial rights to antibodies produced by its researchers. The center's institutional review board (IRB) initially rejected the protocol but later approved it. During the 12 years of the study, 20 out of the 82 patients on Protocol 126 died, allegedly as a direct result of participating in the study, when their T cell–depleted bone marrow failed to engraft and produce blood cells, usually a rare complication of transplantation.[8]

The Harvard, Fred Hutchinson Center, and Gelsinger cases have caused great concern about situations in which clinical researchers have financial interests in the results of their research. But these are not the only types of financial conflicts of interest. There are financial conflicts of interest that arise from paying physicians, who are not necessarily investigators and not linked to the scientific aspects of the research, to enroll patients in research studies.[9] In some cases this compensation is intended to cover costs related to tasks involved in conducting the research that are not otherwise reimbursed—for instance, submitting the protocol for IRB approval, screening potential subjects, providing informed consent, completing clinical research forms documenting outcomes, reporting adverse events, and so on. David Shimm and Roy Spece condemn this practice as "double billing."[10] They argue that, after consideration of the initial setup costs for seeking IRB approval, hiring a data manager, and so on, the marginal cost of each additional enrolled patient is very small; the clinical researcher nonetheless receives the same payment per patient enrolled. This can generate a large profit for physicians (Shimm and Spece estimate that enrolling 100 patients into a research study can net an investigator approximately $475,000) and thus provides a lucrative incentive to enroll larger numbers of patients.[11] They surmise that this payment to cover unreimbursed costs of clinical research "can pose a temptation for the clinical investigator to enter a patient into an experimental study for a condition for which another treatment is known to be effective or even surmised to be superior, thus denying the patient the opportunity to receive the best available treatment."[12]

One of our contributors to Part VIII, Stuart E. Lind, considers the financial incentive of a "finder's fees." In clinical research a finder's fee is usually, but not exclusively, a financial incentive provided to physicians for referring patients to or enrolling them in a clinical research trial. These fees do not cover uncompensated costs of enrolling patients; rather, they are bounties paid per patient enrolled above and beyond the compensation necessary to cover the costs of operating the research studies. Lind argues that these finder's fees in clinical research are equivalent to fee splitting in clinical care. Both practices are wrong, because they allow money to threaten to compromise the determination of what is best for the patients and because "patients may not be able to evaluate [the] recommendation" or referral of their physician.

Conflicts of interest also occur when a company sponsors clinical research and asserts control over the data, especially when the research results run counter to the company's interests. The Olivieri case at the University of Toronto raised this issue.[13] Nancy F. Olivieri, a hematologist conducting research on the use of deferiprone for iron overload in thalassemia, attempted to report that the drug loses potency and can cause liver problems. The company sponsoring the drug trial, Apotex, attempted to prevent publication of the data, claiming breach of contract. Olivieri eventually published the results of this study,[14] but not without employees and paid consultants of Apotex vigorously defending deferiprone in print.[15] Similarly, researchers at the University of California, San Francisco, attempted to publish data showing that a new drug to combat the human immunodeficiency virus / acquired immune deficiency syndrome (HIV/AIDS), HIV-1 Immunogen, was ineffective in preventing HIV progression. The company producing the drug, Immune Response Corporation, refused to release some of the data to the investigators and attempted to prevent publication of the negative finding.[16] The researchers were eventually able to publish their study.[17] Control by companies over research data—and the potential suppression of negative data—may account for publication bias in favor of positive findings.[18]

Another contributor, Baruch A. Brody, takes a broader approach to the issue of conflict of interest. He argues that the harms of financial conflicts of interest may be more insidious than withholding negative data or endangering the health of individual participants. He writes: "[M]any decisions have to be made about both the design and implementation of a clinical trial, and . . . these decisions provide ample opportunity for those with a conflict of interest to make decisions [consciously or unconsciously] that promote their favored treatment." Using studies of thrombolytic agents in the 1980s as an illustration, Brody delineates eight different types of decisions in the design and conduct of clinical research that might be influenced by financial conflicts of interest. These include decisions about

1. which treatments to test in the clinical research trial

2. whether to have a placebo or an active control arm

3. the endpoints of the clinical research trial

4. what inclusion and exclusion criteria to use

5. what information will be provided in the informed consent document and what process will be used

6. the rules for stopping the trial if efficacy is proven or there are adverse events

7. whether the clinical research trial will be stopped due to evidence from other clinical research trials

8. which eligible patients will be enrolled

Brody emphasizes that the design and conduct of every clinical research trial includes "many controversial decisions" that can be influenced by financial conflicts of interest. Because of these multiple decisions, it is very difficult for clinical researchers and physicians—let alone patients and the public—to determine when money has distorted judgments and decisionmaking. It may indeed be the difficulty of perceiving these influences that accounts for the fact that such issues as the ones described above have received less attention than the effects of financial conflicts of interest on the reporting of data.

POSSIBLE REMEDIES

In considering remedies for conflicts of interest it should be noted that some conflicts are not sufficiently problematic to warrant remedy. For instance, when the amount of financial gain is relatively small—at so-called *de minimus* levels—it can be assumed to have little effect on the decisionmaking of clinical researchers, and no remedy is needed. Moreover, as Martin and Kasper note, if the research does not involve human participants (that is, if it is not patient-oriented research) the conflict-of-interest remedies may be somewhat diminished. Because such basic research is carried out at arm's length from human participants, the possibilities of harming humans is far more remote. Nonetheless, as they argue, there should be guidelines in place even for basic research.

For clinical research involving greater financial interests that constitute more serious conflicts of interest, however, there are four types of remedies. First, physicians have long advocated professional self-regulation. Indeed, there have been regular denunciations of conflicts of interest since the turn of the twentieth century, although they have not been formally addressed by professional medical societies until relatively recently.[19] Beyond self-regulation is a formal disclosure of the possible conflict of interest. This is the remedy most commonly adopted by journals that publish clinical research. For instance, the *New England Journal of Medicine* has the following requirement: "Authors of research articles should disclose at the time of submission any financial arrangement they may have with a company whose product figures prominently in the submitted manuscript or with a company making a competing product."[20] Most universities have similar disclosure policies.[21] Some who have written about this topic, such as Shimm and Spece, suggest that "full disclosure requires that patients be told not only the source of funding but also the investigator's potential conflict of interest in receiving industry funding for enrolling patients."[22] However, as Thompson observes, while disclosure gives the affected parties information to evaluate the decisions of the clinical investigators, it may be ineffective and counterproductive. Human research participants may not know how to interpret the disclosure and how to act on the information. Furthermore, this information may only create unnecessary anxiety and distress, undermining the participants' confidence in clinical research.

A third possible remedy is what Thompson calls "mediation." This entails placing the financial incentives in a blind trust or donating the funds to institutions that can then use them for educational purposes or to support research. In both cases, the aim is to prevent the funds from being targeted at individual clinical researchers. Finally, there could be prohibitions on certain financial incentives. These prohibitions would bar clinical researchers from participating in clinical research in which they had any financial interests that were tied to the products being studied. For instance, one cardiac study required that participating clinical researchers "have no equity interest such as stock or stock options in a company sponsor and that there be no remuneration for a consultancy arrangement, expertise, or service during the course of the trial."[23] These prohibitions applied to physicians and to their spouses and financial dependents. Some journals have adopted similar prohibitions for certain kinds of papers submitted. For example, the *New England Journal of Medicine* has promulgated the following guideline regarding review articles and editorials: "Because the essence of reviews and editorials is selection and interpretation of the literature, the *Journal* expects that authors of such articles will not have significant financial interest in a company (or its competitor) that makes a product discussed in the article."[24]

With the growing links between clinical researchers and industry, conflicts of interest are likely to increase and to occur in new situations. Similarly, there will be new attempts to craft rules to regulate them. The articles in Part VIII should provide a framework for thinking about conflicts of interest, when they are unethical, and how they might be regulated.

1. Deborah Nelson and Rick Weiss, "Hasty Decision in the Race to a Cure? Gene Therapy Study Proceeded Despite Safety, Ethics Concerns," *Washington Post,* November 21, 1999, Sec. A, p. 1; and Eliot Marshall, "Gene Therapy's Web of Corporate Connections," *Science* 288 (2000): 954–55.
2. Office for Human Research Protections (U.S. Department of Health and Human Services), "Financial Relationships in Clinical Research: Issues for Institutions, Clinical Investigators, and IRBs to Consider when Dealing with Issues of Financial Interests and Human Subject Protection," available online at: ohrp.osophs .dhhs.gov/nhrpac/mtg12-00/finguid.htm. These are draft guidelines and will likely change in the future.
3. AAMC Task Force on Financial Conflicts of Interest in Clinical Research, "Protecting Subjects, Preserving Trust, Promoting Progress: Policy and Guidelines for the Oversight of Individual Financial Interests in Human Subjects Research," available online at www.aamc .org/members/coitf/firstreport.pdf.
4. Eliot Marshall, "When Commerce and Academe Collide," *Science* 248 (1990): 152–56.
5. William Booth, "Conflict of Interest Eyed at Harvard," *Science* 242 (1988): 1497–99.
6. Faculty of Medicine, Harvard University, Faculty Policies on Integrity in Science, October 2000, available online at www.hms.harvard.edu/integrity.
7. Duff Wilson and David Heath, "Uninformed Consent: What Patients at "The Hutch" Weren't Told about the Experiments in Which They Died," *Seattle Times* 11–15 March 2001, available online at seattletimes.nwsource. com/uninformed_consent; Eliot Marshall, "Fred Hutchinson Center under Fire," *Science* 292 (2001): 25; and Kathryn Senior, "Gene Therapy: A Rocky Start to the New Millennium," *Trends in Molecular Medicine* 6 (2000): 93.

8. Robert M. Nelson, "Protocol 126 and 'The Hutch,'" *IRB: Ethics and Human Research* 23, no. 3 (2001): 14–16.

9. Howard M. Spiro, "Mammon and Medicine: The Rewards of Clinical Trials," *JAMA* 255 (1986): 1174–75.

10. David S. Shimm and Roy G. Spece, Jr., "Industry Reimbursement for Entering Patients into Clinical Trials: Legal and Ethical Issues," *Annals of Internal Medicine* 115 (1991): 148–51.

11. David S. Shimm and Roy G. Spece, Jr., "Conflict of Interest and Informed Consent in Industry-Sponsored Clinical Trials," *Journal of Legal Medicine* 12 (1991): 477–513; citation on p. 484.

12. Shimm and Spece, "Industry Reimbursement for Entering Patients into Clinical Trials," 149.

13. Laura Bonetta, "Inquiry into Clinical Trial Scandal at Canadian Research Hospital," *Nature Medicine* 4 (1998): 1095; and Karen Birmingham, "Controversial HSC Clinical Trials Report Made Public," *Nature Medicine* 5 (1999): 7.

14. Nancy F. Olivieri, Gary M. Brittenham, Christine E. McLaren, et al., "Long-Term Safety and Effectiveness of Iron-Chelation Therapy with Deferiprone for Thalassemia Major," *New England Journal of Medicine* 339 (1998): 417–23.

15. Fernando Tricta and Michael Spino, "Iron Chelation with Oral Deferiprone in Patients with Thalassemia" [correspondence], *New England Journal of Medicine* 339 (1998): 1710; and, under the same heading on the same page of that issue, the letter by Francesco Callea.

16. Catherine D. DeAngelis, "Conflict of Interest and the Public Trust," *JAMA* 284 (2000): 2237–38.

17. James O. Kahn, Deborah Weng Cherng, Kenneth Mayer, Henry Murray, and Stephen Lagakos, for the 806 Investigator Team, "Evaluation of the HIV-1 Immunogen, an Immunologic Modifier, Administered to Patients Infected with HIV Having 300 to 549 × 106/L CD4 Cell Counts," *JAMA* 284 (2000): 2193–202.

18. Richard A. Davidson, "Source of Funding and Outcome of Clinical Trials," *Journal of General Internal Medicine* 1 (1986): 155–58.

19. Marc A. Rodwin, "The Organized American Medical Profession's Response to Financial Conflicts of Interest: 1890–1992," *Milbank Quarterly* 70 (1992): 703–41.

20. *New England Journal of Medicine*, "Instructions for Submission," available online at www.nejm.org/hfa/subinstr.asp#Conflict.

21. Mildred K. Cho, Ryo Shohara, Anna Schissel, and Drummond Rennie, "Policies on Faculty Conflicts of Interest at U.S. Universities," *JAMA* 284 (2000): 2203–8.

22. Shimm and Spece, "Industry Reimbursement for Entering Patients into Clinical Trials," 149.

23. Eric J. Topol, Paul Armstrong, Frans van de Werf, et al., on Behalf of the Global Utilization of Streptokinase and Tissue Plasminogen Activator for Occluded Coronary Arteries (GUSTO) Steering Committee, "Confronting the Issues of Patient Safety and Investigator Conflict of Interest in an International Clinical Trial of Myocardial Reperfusion," *Journal of the American College of Cardiology* 19 (1992): 1123–28.

24. Jeffrey M. Drazen and Gregory D. Curfman, "Financial Associations of Authors," *New England Journal of Medicine* 346 (2002): 1901–2.

72   Understanding Financial Conflicts of Interest

DENNIS F. THOMPSON

[T]he concept of conflict of interest itself has been inadequately analyzed, and consequently its elements, the purposes of regulation, and standards for assessment are still often misunderstood.

ELEMENTS OF CONFLICT OF INTEREST

A conflict of interest is a set of conditions in which professional judgment concerning a primary interest (such as a patient's welfare or the validity of research) tends to be unduly influenced by a secondary interest (such as financial gain). Conflict-of-interest rules, informal and formal, regulate the disclosure and avoidance of these conditions.

The primary interest is determined by the professional duties of a physician, scholar, or teacher. Although what these duties are may sometimes be controversial (and the duties themselves may conflict), there is normally agreement that whatever they are, they should be the primary consideration in any professional decision that a physician, scholar, or teacher makes. In their most general form, the primary interests are the health of patients, the integrity of research, and the education of students.

The secondary interest is usually not illegitimate in itself, and indeed it may even be a necessary and desirable part of professional practice. Only its relative weight in professional decisions is problematic. The aim is not to eliminate or necessarily to reduce financial gain or other secondary interests (such as preference for family and friends or the desire for prestige and power). It is rather to prevent these secondary factors from dominating or appearing to dominate the relevant primary interest in the making of professional decisions.

Conflict-of-interest rules usually focus on financial gain, not because it is more pernicious than other secondary interests but because it is more objective and more fungible. Money is easier to regulate by impartial rules, and it is also generally useful for more purposes. It is therefore a mistake to object to the constraints on financial gain by complaining that there are other kinds of influence [. . .] that can have equally bad or worse effects on professional judgment. Just because we cannot do much about the other

secondary interests, it does not follow that we should do little about financial gain. [. . .]

It is also a mistake to treat conflicts of interest as just another kind of choice between competing values [. . .]. In ethical dilemmas, both of the competing interests have a presumptive claim to priority, and the problem is in deciding which to choose. In the case of financial conflicts of interest, only one of the interests has a claim to priority, and the problem is to ensure that the other interest does not dominate. This asymmetry between interests is a distinctive characteristic of conflicts of interest.

REASONS FOR REGULATING CONFLICTS OF INTEREST

[. . . Among the] basic purposes of conflict-of-interest rules, the first purpose is to maintain the integrity of professional judgment. The rules seek to minimize the influence of secondary interests (such as personal financial gain) that should be irrelevant to the merits of decisions about primary interests (such as the care of a patient or the conduct of research). The rules do not assume that most physicians or researchers let financial gain influence their judgment. They assume only that it is often difficult if not impossible to distinguish cases in which financial gain does have improper influence from those in which it does not. [. . .] Given this general difficulty of discovering real motives, it is safer and therefore ethically more responsible to decide in advance to remove insofar as possible factors that tend to distract us from concentrating on medical and scholarly goals.

Why not simply judge professional decisions by their results? One reason is that many treatment or referral decisions are never reviewed by anyone other than the physicians directly involved. Neither is the market an adequate test of results [. . .]. In the conduct of research, peer review of results offers greater protection. But the objectivity of a particular piece of research is not the only concern [. . .]. The more far-reaching issue, which peer review does not normally address, is the choice of topics and the direction of research—for example, the tendency of industry-sponsored researchers to put more emphasis on commercially useful research than basic research. [. . .]

The second purpose of conflict-of-interest rules [. . .] is to maintain confidence in professional judgment. The aim is to minimize conditions that would cause reasonable

Dennis F. Thompson, "Understanding Financial Conflicts of Interest," *New England Journal of Medicine* 329 (1993): 573–76.

persons (patients, colleagues, and citizens) to believe that professional judgment has been improperly influenced, whether or not it has.

Maintaining confidence in professional judgment is partly a matter of prudence. To the extent that the public and their representatives distrust the profession, they are likely to demand greater regulation of practice and research and are likely to supply fewer resources for both. [...]

STANDARDS FOR ASSESSING CONFLICTS OF INTEREST

[...] The severity of a conflict depends on (1) the likelihood that professional judgment will be influenced, or appear to be influenced, by the secondary interest, and (2) the seriousness of the harm or wrong that is likely to result from such influence or its appearance.

In assessing likelihood, we may reasonably assume that, within a certain range, the greater the value of the secondary interest (e.g., the size of the financial gain), the more probable its influence. Below a certain value, the gain is likely to have no effect; that is why *de minimis* standards (which define that value) are appropriate for some gifts. [...]

[...] Longer and closer associations increase the problem. A continuing relationship as a member of the board or a limited partner of an industrial sponsor, for example, creates a more serious problem than the acceptance of a one-time grant or gift.

The extent of discretion—that is, how much latitude a physician or researcher enjoys in exercising professional judgment—partly determines the range of probabilities. The more routine the treatment or the more closely it follows conventional professional practice, the less room there is for judgment and hence for improper influence. Also, the less independent authority the professional has in a particular case, the less latitude there is for improper influence. [...]

The greater the scope of the consequences, the more serious the conflict. Beyond its effects on the particular patient or research project, a conflict may have effects on the practices of other physicians or on the research projects of colleagues. Questions such as these should be considered: Will this physician's association with a commercial laboratory raise doubts about the objectivity of all the physicians in his or her hospital or health maintenance organization [HMO]? Will the fact that this drug company is sponsoring this research project tend to undermine confidence in the results of the work of other scholars in the institution and their ability to raise funds from other sources? [...]

Finally, the more limited the accountability of the physician or researcher, the more serious the conflict. If the decision of a physician is reviewable by colleagues or au-

thorities (who do not themselves have conflicts of interest), then there is less cause for concern. But the reviewers must be, and must be seen to be, genuinely independent and effective. Even if professionals are accountable for particular decisions, however, they may escape scrutiny for the cumulative effects and broader policy implications of their decisions. [...]

REMEDIES

Historically, the trend has been from less to more extensive control of conflicts of interest [...].

Relying on the good character of individual physicians and scholars to ensure that they avoid conflicts, or deal with them judiciously when they arise, is the least intrusive procedure. It also has the advantage of maintaining conditions of mutual trust between physicians and patients and between scholars and their public. It is, however, more effective in face-to-face relations that continue over time [...]. It is less likely to be adequate in large organizations and in the impersonal encounters or distant relationships that characterize much of the practice of modern medicine and medical research.

Regulation by the profession provides more assurance than individual discretion that conflicts will be avoided. As compared with government regulation, it also has the advantage of involving those who know and care personally about professional practice. Rules are more likely to fit the special circumstances of the clinic and the laboratory when they are written by those who know these circumstances well and who have a personal stake in maintaining the integrity of the profession. The disadvantage of relying exclusively on the profession is that physicians, not only individually but also collectively, confront a conflict between their primary interest in maintaining the integrity of the profession and their secondary interest in promoting the economic welfare of its members. Unlike many other professions, the medical profession did not formally address conflicts of interest in its codes until the 1980s, and even then it in effect left the problem to the discretion of individual physicians. [...]

The growing role of governments in regulating conflicts of interest is in part a response to the failure of physicians and scholars to deal adequately with the problem and in part a result of the greater stake that society has in medical practice and research. [...] The chief advantage of government regulation is that it includes more people in the process of making and enforcing the rules, thereby reducing the problem of conflicts of interest on the part of the profession itself. An important disadvantage is the uniformity and procedural complexity that normally characterize the legal process. [...]

Whether the responsibility for dealing with conflicts of interest falls to individual physicians and researchers, the profession, or governments, disclosure is the remedy most commonly prescribed. [. . .] A scholar is expected to indicate the sources of financial support for the research. Disclosure may be more or less public; the information may be provided to colleagues, hospital or HMO administrators, professional boards, state boards, or the general public. An advantage of disclosure is that it gives those who would be affected, or who are otherwise in a good position to assess the risks, information they need to make their own decisions.

A deficiency of disclosure is that those who receive the information may not know how to interpret it and may not in any case have reasonable alternative courses of action in the circumstances. Disclosure could even exacerbate some of the indirect consequences of conflicts, such as the effects on confidence in the profession or in the research enterprise. By itself, disclosure may merely increase levels of anxiety [. . .]. Disclosing a conflict only reveals a problem, without providing any guidance for resolving it.

[. . .] Other methods (roughly in order of increasing stringency) include mediation (devices such as blind trusts that insulate the physician from the secondary interest), abstention (an analogue to judicial recusal that would have physicians or researchers withdraw from cases in which they have substantial secondary interest), divestiture (which would eliminate the secondary interest), and prohibition (which would have physicians or researchers withdraw permanently from fields in which they have substantial secondary interests). [. . .]

---

73   Finder's Fees for Research Subjects

STUART E. LIND

At a specialty conference, a postdoctoral fellow describing a new study being conducted at a neighboring institution showed a recruiting letter from the investigator, which outlined the study and noted that a $350 finder's fee would be paid to resident physicians who referred patients who subsequently enrolled in the study. [. . .]

FINDER'S FEES

In many settings finder's fees are an accepted and acceptable part of business practice. These incentives, rewards, or payments are basically compensation for services rendered, the unstated implication being that it doesn't matter, in any ethical sense, whether an apartment is located, for example, by a realty office, a newspaper advertisement, or word of mouth. Similarly, there is little wrong when a health club offers its members a discount on their membership fee if they bring new clients into the club. If the business is a medical practice, however, the situation changes. [. . .]

If physicians paid other physicians for bringing them new patients, however, there would be no ambiguity, for the unethical nature of this arrangement can easily be recognized. The practice, known as fee-splitting, has long been banned by major medical organizations. The prohibition against it, which originated at the beginning of the century,

represented an ethical advance, because patients were often sent to poorly trained, if not clearly incompetent, physicians simply because a fee was paid to the referring physician, and not because the consultant could offer good care. It was recognized that patients may not be able to evaluate their doctors' recommendations and may act on trust alone. [. . .]

FINDER'S FEES FOR RESEARCH SUBJECTS

Finder's fees offered to physicians who refer patients to investigators may involve cash or nonmonetary payments and may or may not be contingent on the patient's enrolling in the study. [. . .]

At first glance, finder's fees may seem a good solution to a chronic problem—that of recruiting adequate numbers of patients to participate in clinical studies. [. . .] Closer examination reveals, however, that this practice is flawed because it has the potential to violate the patient's trust in the referring physician, the investigator, or both, and in the process of clinical research. [. . .]

[. . .] Relating the principles of clinical practice to clinical research makes it clear that offering finder's fees for research subjects is very much the same as offering fees for the referral of patients. In fact, the practice may be worse, for it could turn segments of the public—not just individual patients—against clinical research by making them suspicious of the motives of everyone involved. [. . .]

Stuart E. Lind, "Finder's Fees for Research Subjects," *New England Journal of Medicine* 323 (1990): 192–95.

FINDER'S FEES SHOULD NOT
BE A PART OF CLINICAL RESEARCH

That finder's fees may at times be offered and accepted without compromising patient care does not negate the fact that their being offered increases the risk that a physician's judgment will be altered. Although it is not possible to know the exact likelihood that this will occur, it is also not possible to be sure that such instances will be recognized, even by the best intentioned, as is the case in other areas of medicine for which there is no clear standard. Disclosure—i.e., making the patient aware of the finder's fee—is not a good compromise, because of the risk that even knowing of its existence may cause patients to question the validity or worth of the research project. Furthermore, if physician payment is predicated on the assumption that the physician will be responsible for the patient's care, a finder's fee should not be offered or accepted, because the referring physician usually gives up such responsibility temporarily while the patient is being treated by an investigator.

The human studies committee at Massachusetts General Hospital considered the pros and cons of using finder's fees to obtain research subjects. It decided that such fees should not be offered to individual physicians for referring patients. [. . .] For example, an investigator should not take just the house-staff members who referred patients out for pizza, but all house staff who were in a position to do so. Similarly, contributions to libraries, education funds, or other charitable causes should be made without regard to the specific number of patients referred or enrolled. This is only one way of dealing with the question of finder's fees. [. . .]

---

74   Conflicts of Interests and the Validity of Clinical Trials

Baruch A. Brody

[. . .]

CONFLICT OF INTEREST VERSUS FRAUD

The original *Newsday* article that called attention to the stockholding [of some of the clinical investigators] in Genentech [the company that manufactures tPA, tissue plasminogen activator—eds.] discussed the possibility that this type of conflict of interest might lead to fraud in research, that is, to the publication of incorrect data. The report of Congressman Ted Weiss's subcommittee at the end of its hearings, which combined investigations into fraudulent misconduct with investigations into conflicts of interest, was entitled "Are Scientific Misconduct and Conflicts of Interest Hazardous to our Health?" and may also have encouraged the view that conflicts of interest are troubling because they will lead to publication of fraudulent data. But I want to argue that this concern with fraudulent data is not central precisely because the design of contemporary clinical trials makes it difficult to perpetrate frauds.

Instead, the concern should be with how conflicts of interest may lead investigators, perhaps unconsciously, to make inappropriate decisions about the design and conduct of clinical trials. [. . .]

Many standard features of modern clinical trials are designed, at least in part, to protect against fraud. The fact that patients are randomly assigned to the various treatment arms in a clinical trial means that the investigators cannot assign more favorable cases to their favorite treatment. The fact that neither the subjects nor the investigators know which treatment the patient is getting [i.e., that the trial is double-blinded] makes it difficult for the investigators to improve the data on patients getting their favorite treatment. The fact that the clinical data are often gathered and analyzed by an independent group (a central lab and/or data analysis group) prevents investigators from perpetrating fraud in the manipulation of the data. [I]f fraud were our real concern, we would do best to focus on improving these features of modern clinical trials [. . .].

What then are the concerns with conflicts of interest? It seems to me that concerns grow out of the recognition that many decisions have to be made about both the design and implementation of a clinical trial, and that these decisions provide ample opportunity for those with a conflict of interest to make decisions that promote their favored

Baruch A. Brody, "Conflicts of Interests and the Validity of Clinical Trials," in *Conflicts of Interest in Clinical Practice and Research*, ed. Roy G. Spece, David S. Shimm, and Allen E. Buchanan (New York: Oxford University Press, 1996), 407–17.

treatment. This may be a conscious process, in which case we are dealing with personal guilt, or it may be an unconscious process, in which case we are not. In either situation, the social problem of how to minimize these inappropriate decisions remains.

Some of these decisions have to do with the design of the clinical trials. The issues include the following: (1) Which treatments will be tested in the proposed trial, and which ones will not be tested? (2) Will there be a placebo control group as well, or will the treatments be tested against each other or against some active control group? (3) What will be taken as the favorable endpoint (the result of constituting the evidence of efficacy of the treatment), and what will be taken as the adverse endpoint (the result constituting the evidence of the dangerousness of the treatment)? (4) What will be the condition for inclusion or exclusion of subjects from the trial? (5) What provisions will be made for informed consent, and what information will be provided as part of the informed consent? Some of these decisions have to do with the actual conduct of the clinical trial. They include the following: (6) Under what conditions will the trial be stopped or modified because there have been too many adverse endpoints in one or more arm of the trial or because the preliminary data have shown that one of the treatments is clearly the most efficacious treatment? (7) Under what conditions will the trial be stopped or modified because of the newly available results of other trials? (8) Which patients who meet the criteria will actually be enrolled, and which ones will not?

[...] In some cases, the answers to these questions will be straightforward, so the opportunity for biased, flawed decision-making will be modest. In other cases, the answers will be far from obvious, with great potential for conflicts of interest leading, consciously or unconsciously, to flawed decision-making. In either case, however, the actual data are not fraudulent. [...]

ILLUSTRATION OF THE CONFLICT OF INTEREST ISSUE

These are not merely theoretical concerns. In fact, many of these decisions, made in the design and conduct of the clinical trials of the thrombolytic agents, were quite controversial, so the potential for flawed decisions resulting (consciously or unconsciously) from conflicts of interest was real. [...]

[...] In 1980, Marcus DeWood published a study showing that clots (thrombi) in the coronary arteries are usually the immediate cause of myocardial infarctions. This led to a renewal of interest in the treatment of patients undergoing a myocardial infarction with clot-busting (thrombolytic) agents. [...]

The National Institutes of Health (NIH) therefore planned a series of trials (the Thrombolysis in Myocardial Infarction [TIMI] trials) designed to test the efficacy of these drugs. After considerable planning, the strategy adopted was to test streptokinase [SK] against tPA in the TIMI trial, using clot lysis as the endpoint that measured comparative efficacy (as opposed to improved left ventricular ejection fraction or increased survival). The winner was to be tested in a TIMI-2 trial against a placebo to demonstrate absolute efficacy. The TIMI-1 trial was stopped in 1985 because of early impressive results, and tPA was declared the winner. The originally planned TIMI-2 trial of tPA against a placebo was not run [...].

The two major trials of SK against a placebo demonstrated significant efficacy as measured by improved survival. [...]

[...] Questions of type 1 involve deciding which treatments to test and which treatments not to test. [...] The initial decision to take tPA as a serious candidate for study so soon after its synthesis, the decision to run a preliminary TIMI-1 trial and then to run all the rest of the studies involving only the winner of TIMI-1, and the decision to not study anoisylated plasminogen streptokinase-activating complex [APSAC] are all good examples of controversial decisions of type 1. Questions of type 2 involve deciding whether or not to use placebo control groups. Nearly all of the trials provide good examples of such controversial decisions, ranging from TIMI's decision not to run any placebo-controlled trials after the results of the Gruppo Italiano per lo Studio della Sopravvivenza nell'Infarto Miocardio [GISSI] were published in 1986 to those [...] that continued such trials after the publication of the GISSI and the Second International Study of Infarct Survival [ISIS-2] preliminary data. Questions of type 3 involve deciding what to take as favorable and adverse endpoints. In the thrombolytic trials, the choice of the favorable endpoint was quite controversial, with some trials using survival and others surrogates. Of particular significance was the controversial decision of TIMI-1 to use reperfusion (clot lysis) as the favorable endpoint rather than other surrogates such as ejection fraction. Questions of type 4 involve decisions about inclusion and exclusion criteria and are closely related to questions of type 3. Investigators who want large trials, like the European trials [...], must include nearly everyone, but if they are running smaller trials with surrogate endpoints [...], they can employ stricter inclusion and exclusion criteria, and these can be quite controversial. Questions of type 5 involve decisions about informed consent. Nearly all of the trials involved controversial decisions of this type. [...] Questions of type 6 involve decisions about the early stopping of trials in light of their own data. The decision to stop TIMI-1 because of its reperfusion data and the decision not to stop ISIS-2 in spite of its own very impressive survival data are good examples of controversial decisions of this type. Questions of type 7 involve decisions about trial abandonment or modification in light of new data from other trials. The decisions to continue ISIS-2, the APSAC Intervention Mortality Study [AIMS], and the Anglo-Scandinavian Study of Early Thrombolysis [ASSET] even after receiving the GISSI and preliminary ISIS-2 data are good examples of controversial decisions of this type [...].

The thrombolytic trials illustrate how many controversial decisions have to be made in the design and conduct of clinical studies. There is clearly great potential for conflicts of interest to lead, consciously or unconsciously, to flawed decision-making. Therefore, the conflict-of-interest problem is how to develop policies that will minimize that potential.

TWO FLAWED PROPOSALS

Two approaches have emerged. The first is the disclosure approach, as found, for example, in the following policy of the *New England Journal of Medicine*:

> The *Journal* expects authors to disclose any commercial associations that might pose a conflict of interest in connection with the submitted article. All funding sources supporting the work should be routinely acknowledged on the title page, as should all institutional or corporate affiliations of the authors. Other kinds of associations, such as consultancies, stock ownership or other equity interests, or patent-licensing arrangements, should be disclosed to the Editor in a covering letter at the time of submission. Such information will be held in confidence while the paper is under review and will not influence the editorial decision. If the manuscript is accepted, the Editor will discuss with the authors how best to disclose the relevant information.

The second, very different approach was described in an influential article published [... in 1989 by ...] leading investigators in a multicenter trial funded by the NIH. Their approach, the elimination approach, rests on the claim that the best way to deal with the conflicts of interest is to ban the commercial relations that generate the conflicts. The policy is formulated as follows:

> Investigators involved in the post–coronary artery bypass graft [CABG] study will not buy, sell, or hold stock or stock options in any of the companies providing or distributing medication under study . . . for the following periods: from the time the recruitment of

patients for the trial begins until funding for the study in the investigator's unit ends and the results are made public; or . . . until the investigator's active and personal involvement in the study or the involvement of the institution conducting the study (or both) ends. Each investigator will agree not to serve as a paid consultant to the companies during these same periods. . . . Certain other activities are not viewed as constituting conflicts of interest but must be reported annually to the coordinating center: the participation of investigators in educational activities supported by the companies; the participation of investigators in other research projects supported by the companies; occasional scientific consulting to the companies on issues not related to the products in the trial and for which there is not financial payment or other compensation; and financial interests in the companies over which the investigator has no control, such as mutual funds and blind trusts.

This approach has attracted much attention, in part because of its obvious merits. [...] In September 1989, the NIH proposed a policy on this issue that was an expansion of the elimination approach. In addition to banning equity holding and paid consultancies, it required that companies sharing the costs of research with the NIH not be in a position to influence the research plan or get access to information in advance. After much controversy those policies were put on hold, and less draconian Public Health Service regulations [...] were adopted. [...]

[A presupposition of both disclosure and elimination policies] is that the conflict-of-interest problem arises primarily out of the commercial relation between clinical investigators and drug companies whose products they are investigating. [...] But [...] the conflict-of-interest problem extends beyond these commercial relations. [...]

I have argued that the conflict-of-interest problem arises when (1) there are controversial decisions that must be made in the design and conduct of clinical trials, and (2) these decisions may be biased by the investigators' financial interests. It is obvious that condition 1 will be satisfied in many clinical trials whether or not the investigators have commercial relations with any drug companies. But it seems to me that condition 2 may also be satisfied even when these commercial relations are not present, because of problems growing out of grant funding. [...]

To explain why condition 2 may be satisfied even if the investigators have no equity interests, consultancies, or other commercial relations with any drug company, we need to reflect on the grants funding the trial in question.

The clinical centers receive substantial support from the funding source, support that pays the salaries of the staff and investigators, helps cover the administrative expenses of the center, and even offers the possibility of a profit (especially if one considers the marginal, as opposed to the average, cost of running the trial). If that support is cut off, there can be substantial financial losses to the center, as well as career losses to the investigators. This certainly has the potential for influencing decisions involving questions of type 6 or 7—questions of stopping trials. Similarly, investigators may be influenced in their decisions about patient eligibility, decisions involving questions of type 8, since failure to enroll enough patients may lead to a lessening of support or even to elimination of the center from the trial. [...]

AN ALTERNATIVE APPROACH

[...] Conflicts of interest are a matter of concern whenever conditions (1) and (2) are satisfied. Both of these conditions can be satisfied when the investigators have stocks in, or receive consulting fees from, a drug company whose product is being tested, but they can also be satisfied when the trial in question is being funded by a grant either from a drug company or from some public agency. [...]

One discussion that has focused on these broader concerns is the discussion in the policies of the Royal College of Physicians in an important statement on research involving patients. [...]

The main thrust of those policies is to avoid situations in which researchers are induced by financial considerations to pressure patients to participate in clinical trials. That is why the Royal College would totally ban per capita payments to physicians (payments in proportion to the number of subjects recruited). That is also why the Royal College would allow research grants conditional on recruiting a minimum number of patients only if the independent committee reviewing the research protocol determines that it is reasonable to assume that the clinic in question can get that number of volunteers in light of the nature of its patient load and the nature of the research.

All of these are quite reasonable policies, and their adoption would go some way toward minimizing the potential for conflicts of interest in questions of type 8, questions about subject eligibility and subject enrollment. [...] Nevertheless, they are far from complete solutions, since they really focus only on question 8. [...]

At a crucial point in its discussion, when considering payments to institutions as opposed to physicians, [the Royal College] has the following to say:

> Payment for recruitment should not exceed a reasonable estimate of the cost of studying the patient together with any legitimate expenses. There should be no element of profit to the institution or department related to the number of patients recruited.

This is a crucial point. As noted above, grants often cover more than the marginal costs of research so they constitute a source of additional revenue to institutions. This is part of the way in which grants (as well as equity holdings and consultancies) are the source of potential conflicts of interest.

We need better information about income from grants if we really want to minimize the potential for conflicts of interest. In an important recent study, Shimm and Spece estimated that at their institution an investigator can harvest a profit of $75,000–$225,000 from a drug company study involving fifty patients. Their analysis is not entirely convincing, since they derived their estimate by simply subtracting the salary of a data coordinator ($25,000) from the income derived from the drug company (fifty patients at $2,000–$5,000 per patient), not considering other marginal expenses. They themselves point out that the calculation will be different if these other marginal expenses are counted. Moreover, I am not convinced that they are right in their claim (unsupported by data) that there is no similar potential in federally funded research. This skepticism is related to the recent controversies about indirect costs. Nevertheless, Shimm and Spece have done a great service by beginning to identify the true institutional gains from grant income.

[...] The crucial philosophical point is, however, clear. Profits to individuals or institutions from grants can be just as much a source of conflicts of interest as equity holdings or consultancy fees, and the former should be avoided as much as the latter.

One needs to be realistic about how much [...] guidelines [about conflicts of interest arising from grant income] could accomplish. Even if they resulted in grants producing no direct financial profit to institutions or individuals, securing grants and implementing research under them would still be in the professional and/or financial interest of both individual researchers and their institutions. That is both inevitable and probably desirable. [...]

75   In Whose Best Interest?

Breaching the Academic-Industrial Wall

JOSEPH B. MARTIN AND DENNIS L. KASPER

[...] Over the past year, medical research involving human subjects has come under intense scrutiny. The issues of concern include the adequacy of informed consent, the surveillance of research protocols by institutional review boards, the reporting of adverse events, and investigators' conflicts of interest. In this article, we address the last of these issues.

Conflicts of interest arise from investigators' financial relationships with companies whose products they are studying, whether the research is supported publicly or by the company itself. Critics charge that academic researchers are for sale, that their engagement in clinical research can be bartered, and that the outcome of research is biased by academic-industrial liaisons, whether individual or institutional. Allegations have been made that these relationships have affected the quality of research. Government officials have reacted with alarm to the possibility that conflicts of interest may prejudice the outcome of research. [...] The Department of Health and Human Services has proposed fines and penalties to protect patients and to safeguard scientific integrity. [...]

The current Harvard Medical School policy prohibits investigators from having a financial interest, above *de minimis* levels, in a company whose technology and products they are studying, regardless of the funding source. [...]

CONFLICT OF INTEREST
VERSUS THE PUBLIC INTEREST

We have entered a time of unprecedented opportunity for the prevention and treatment of human disease, as was recently highlighted by the sequencing of the human genome. To exploit this opportunity fully, we will need to ensure greater interdependence of those "uneasy bedfellows," academia and industry. The pressures and potential conflicts that will inevitably accompany this more porous interface demand that its operations be clearly evident to the public.

Joseph B. Martin and Dennis L. Kasper, "In Whose Best Interest? Breaching the Academic-Industrial Wall," *New England Journal of Medicine* 343 (2000): 1646–49.

What constitutes the public interest in these matters? First, the public deserves to know that the biomedical research it supports will be a search for truth, uncontaminated by even a perception of bias. Second, the public deserves to see that discoveries with the potential to improve health are translated rapidly into practice by means of clinical trials. Third, the public needs to be confident that participation in the development of new therapies will be safe, with fully informed consent obtained from participants at the outset and access to data about outcome provided to them during follow-up. Fourth, the public has the right to know about any potential adverse effects that might influence patients' decisions about participating in the research. Finally, the public must be assured that neither the decision to ask patients to participate in a clinical trial nor the assessment of the risks patients may incur will be prejudiced by the personal profit motives of an investigator.

A historical perspective on the changing interface between academia and industry reveals a steady erosion of the cultural wall that once separated academic activities from the world of commerce. [...]

[...] The Bayh-Dole Act of 1980 not only encouraged but also mandated the translation of NIH-supported discoveries into practice. [...] The number of clinical trials being conducted has already exploded. CenterWatch, a listing service for clinical trials, estimates that about 60,000 trials were under way in the United States in 1998, as compared with 33,000 in 1990 and 14,000 in 1980.

Among the critical issues raised by the proliferation of clinical trials is the need for research institutions and their faculties to balance two interrelated but competing demands: The recruitment of large numbers of patients to fill the trials and expedite the determination of results and the careful selection of appropriate participants to maximize the probability of obtaining meaningful results. Faculty members are commonly paid for each patient enrolled. These payments are used to balance departmental budgets that have been hit hard by declining revenues from patient care and hospital reimbursements. An awareness of the institutional and personal incentives to generate income from clinical trials, as well as of the time pressure placed on physicians by an increased work load, should inspire increased surveillance of the enrollment of patients in clinical trials.

THE EVOLVING TIES BETWEEN
THE UNIVERSITY AND INDUSTRY

[...] Conflicts of interest become a matter of concern when patients are involved in the research and are thereby exposed to potential harm as well as benefit. Research in which new drugs, biologic agents, or medical devices are tested in patients must be performed in such a way that there is no possibility—or even perception—that the investigators' judgment is clouded by the prospect of financial gain. Medical schools and their faculties are in a difficult position. On one hand, they are the guardians of the public investment in biomedical research; on the other, they are at the forefront of scientific advances that must be translated through industry into benefits to the public.

We believe that, in most cases, the public is the beneficiary of academic-industrial relationships. [...] Academic institutions benefit in other tangible ways, including the receipt of funding for drug-development programs, scientific meetings, graduate education programs, and fellowships for postdoctoral students. Support from industry has given medical schools and teaching hospitals greater flexibility. Another benefit of academic-industrial collaboration is an increased level of understanding between these two "cultures" that, despite (or because of) their differences, can often learn from each other profitably. [...]

[T]here are substantial differences among universities and medical schools in the creation, interpretation, and enforcement of conflict-of-interest rules. Some institutions rely heavily on the monitoring of faculty members' conflicts of interest by committees of colleagues. Others impose virtually no limits on faculty members' income from consulting contracts, speaking engagements, equity in companies, and stock options. The biotechnology boom, with the emergence of start-up companies funded by venture capital, has led both public and private universities to accept equity in the new companies in lieu of royalties on their inventions. [...]

TOWARD A JUST AND PRUDENT BALANCE

What, then, might be a reasonable stance for our institutions and faculty members to take with regard to conflicts of interest? We suggest that the criteria applied to the public sector are equally appropriate in the academic sector. Just as we expect elected officials and governmental appointees to be free from any appearance of bias, so should we expect academic scientists to adhere to the highest standards of intellectual integrity.

First, research that does not require human subjects must be considered separately from patient-oriented research. For basic research, we believe it is permissible, with full disclosure to the institutions, for investigators to receive financial support from companies from which they receive consulting fees. It is considered acceptable by many institutions for researchers to hold equity in sponsoring companies in such situations. Other institutions, such as the Howard Hughes Medical Institute, prohibit investigators from receiving monetary support for their laboratories from any company for which they consult or in which they hold equity. Harvard Medical School's policy, while not limiting consulting fees for research that does not involve human subjects, does limit equity interests to $20,000 and only permits such holdings if the company is publicly traded and the equity is acquired in a manner unrelated to the sponsored research agreement. At the national level, such prohibitions are increasingly unusual, and in general, the breach in the wall is so pervasive that expectations of a return to a stricter code of behavior may be unrealistic. [...]

Nevertheless, a few rules are needed regarding industrial support of basic research. Investigators should have no potential to influence, or be influenced by, the sponsoring corporate entity. They should not hold excessive equity or serve in management roles. [...] Also essential are a guarantee, on the part of the industrial sponsor, of academic freedom within the laboratory; mechanisms to ensure that researchers inform students and fellows working on the research of the industrial link; and disclosure of the relationship in scientific communications, written or oral. Trainees must be permitted to pursue their own research free of the constraints that demands related to industrial support might place on their curiosity or creativity. [...]

Clinical research, in which patients are directly involved and human life and health are at stake, presents an entirely different set of circumstances. We believe there should be minimal financial incentive for an investigator to carry out research linked to potential commercialization of a product. This restriction should apply to all patient-oriented research, broadly defined to encompass not only clinical trials of drugs, biologic agents, and devices, but also any research involving biologic samples or genetic information. We propose that an effective conflict-of-interest policy for academic institutions must have a minimum of three elements: a requirement for regular disclosure to the institution of potential conflicts by faculty members, with appropriate administrative scrutiny of financial interests; monitoring by a standing or specially appointed oversight committee; and a mechanism for granting exceptions to the policy when they are warranted by extraordinary circumstances. [...]

Part IX

Scientific Misconduct

There is no shortage of cases of scientific misconduct in all its many guises. Little of pedagogic use can be served by reciting a long list of instances of scientific misconduct, but a few examples will serve to indicate the different kinds of behavior that fall under this at times fuzzy rubric. Stephen Lock claims that the modern preoccupation with scientific misconduct dates to 1974, when the immunologist William T. Summerlin of the Memorial Sloan-Kettering Cancer Center in New York, was working on skin transplantation in mice with skin cancer.[1] As he was walking through the center's hallways, mice in hand, on his way to a meeting with the center's director, Summerlin used a black felt-tip pen to color the skin grafts of the white mice, "thereby implying a successful experiment."[2] Summerlin's deception was discovered within hours, and although he claimed exhaustion, institutional pressure to publish, and an excessive workload for his lapse in judgment, he was dismissed from the institution.

Not all cases of scientific misconduct are as isolated (and colorful!) as that of Summerlin. One of the most highly publicized cases of scientific misconduct is that of John R. Darsee. In the early 1980s, Darsee was a rising star in medical research, working as a National Institutes of Health (NIH)–sponsored postdoctoral fellow at Harvard Medical School in the Cardiac Research Laboratory of the distinguished cardiologist Eugene Braunwald. Many were skeptical of Darsee's vast output—over 100 articles or abstracts by his early 30s—to such an extent that a few of his colleagues secretly observed him at work in his laboratory one evening and witnessed him forging data. While an internal investigation at Harvard concluded that this was an isolated incident—albeit one not without consequences for Darsee: Braunwald stripped him of his NIH fellowship and withdrew his recommendation that Darsee be given a faculty position at Harvard, but did temporarily let him continue to work in the lab—an NIH committee later found Darsee guilty of multiple instances of data forgery (dating all the way back to Darsee's days as an undergraduate) and barred him from NIH funding for ten years.[3] Many of Darsee's papers were retracted from journals, which brought no small shame to Harvard Medical School and Darsee's famous co-authors. Moreover, Braunwald's hospital, the Harvard-affiliated Brigham and Women's Hospital, was later forced to return over $120,000 to the NIH because of Darsee's actions.

Many more cases of misconduct could be described,[4] but we will conclude this brief survey with a study of U.S. doctoral students and faculty that sought to identify ethical problems in academic research. Judith Swazey and her colleagues conducted a survey of 2,000 doctoral students and 2,000 faculty members at 99 U.S. universities in four disciplines: chemistry, civil engineering, microbiology, and sociology.[5] Respondents were asked about whether they had witnessed, or had direct knowledge of, three different kinds of problematic behavior: (1) scientific misconduct proper (e.g., plagiarism and falsification or fabrication of data), (2) questionable research practices (e.g., keeping poor research records, unearned authorship of papers), and (3) other misconduct (e.g., sexual harassment, other forms of coercive or exploitative behavior, the violation of government research regulations). Their study is thus a measure not of the actual incidence of scientific misconduct, but rather of the exposure to perceived instances of misconduct. Nonetheless, their results were surprising. Between 6 and 33 percent of the respondents had knowledge of at least one instance of plagiarism or data falsification/fabrication, 43 percent of faculty knew of colleagues who had made inappropriate (i.e., personal) use of research funds (among civil engineering faculty this figure was 61 percent), nearly a third of faculty members had direct knowledge of an inappropriate assignment of authorship among their peers (again, among civil engineering faculty this figure was 44 percent), and, finally, a quarter of the respondents had direct knowledge of sexual harassment. While Swazey and colleagues note the differences in responses between faculty and doctoral students and across the four disciplines surveyed, these aggregated results surely give one pause.

What emerges from these three examples—what, in fact, characterizes scientific misconduct—are a host of problematic and related features: dishonesty, deception, and the betrayal of trust, to name just three. Yet defining misconduct has proved very difficult, largely because—bracketing obvious cases like that of Darsee—scientific practice is itself heterogeneous, partly an unscripted "art," and so permeated by error and (some would say)[6] the necessity of error that effecting a clear demarcation between good conduct and misconduct is harder than one would think. One is thus left with the uneasy feeling that although one cannot define misconduct, one simply knows it when one sees it.

Of course, this has not stopped some from trying to define the boundaries of misconduct. And thankfully so. For example, the Commission on Research Integrity, which received its mandate from the U.S. Department of Health and Human Services (DHHS), submitted its report, Integrity and Misconduct in Research, in the winter of 1995.[7] It stands as the most authoritative extant statement on scientific misconduct. The commissioners identify two broad classes of misconduct—viz., (1) research misconduct and (2) other forms of professional misconduct—and define them in the following ways. Regarding research misconduct, the commissioners proffer the following definition:[8]

1. Research Misconduct

Research misconduct is significant misbehavior that improperly appropriates the intellectual property or contributions of others, that intentionally impedes the progress of research, or that risks corrupting the scientific record or compromising the integrity of scientific prac-

tices. Such behaviors are unethical and unacceptable in proposing, conducting, or reporting research, or in reviewing the proposals or research reports of others.

The commissioners then provide the following list of examples:

Misappropriation: An investigator or reviewer shall not intentionally or recklessly

(a) plagiarize, which shall be understood to mean the presentation of the documented words or ideas of another as his or her own, without attribution appropriate for the medium of presentation; or

(b) make use of any information in breach of any duty of confidentiality associated with the review of any manuscript or grant application.

Interference: An investigator or reviewer shall not intentionally and without authorization take or sequester or materially damage any research-related property of another, including without limitation the apparatus, reagents, biological materials, writings, data, hardware, software, or any other substance or device used or produced in the conduct of research.

Misrepresentation: An investigator or reviewer shall not with intent to deceive, or in reckless disregard for the truth,

(a) state or present a material or significant falsehood; or

(b) omit a fact so that what is stated or presented as a whole states or presents a material or significant falsehood.

Regarding the second class of misconduct, the commissioners reason this way:[9]

2. Other Forms of Professional Misconduct

(a) *Obstruction of Investigations of Research Misconduct*

The Federal Government has an important interest in protecting the integrity of investigations into reported incidents of research misconduct. Accordingly, obstruction of investigations of research misconduct related to federal funding constitutes a form of professional misconduct in that it undermines the interests of the public, the scientific community, and the Federal Government.

Obstruction of investigations of research misconduct consists of intentionally withholding or destroying evidence in violation of a duty to disclose or preserve; falsifying evidence; encouraging, soliciting or giving false testimony; and attempting to intimidate or retaliate against witnesses, potential witnesses, or potential leads to witnesses or evidence before, during, or after the commencement of any formal or informal proceeding.

(b) Noncompliance with Research Regulations

Responsible conduct in research includes compliance with applicable federal research regulations. Such regulations include (but are not limited to) those governing the use of biohazardous materials and human and animal subjects in research.

Serious noncompliance with such regulations after notice of their existence undermines the interests of the public, the scientific community, and the Federal Government and constitutes another form of professional misconduct.

The themes of dishonesty and deception are clearly present in the commission's report. Notably absent from the commission's definitions, however, is any reference to "other misconduct," such as sexual harassment, that played a role in the survey study of Swazey and her colleagues. Although sexual harassment is an issue of the first importance, it is unfortunately not unique to the practice of science; put differently, while sexual harassment is clearly *misconduct,* it is not obviously *scientific* misconduct.

Whether misconduct consists of one isolated incident (as in the case of Summerlin) or a pattern of dishonesty over many years (as in the case of Darsee), such behavior is deeply disconcerting, both for those who engage in medical research and for members of the general public. And this is so for three principal reasons. First, medical research is, after all, a scientific enterprise. While there are notable and important differences between the practices and aims of the natural sciences (e.g., biology, physics, and chemistry) and those of the medical sciences, they nonetheless share the defining feature of being engaged in a search for the truth. If this is so, untruthful or dishonest behavior among scientific practitioners seems antithetical to the very enterprise in which they are engaged.

Second, medical research is a humanistic endeavor; that is, while medical researchers aim to discover the truth, they do so not principally for the sake of truth itself, but rather for the well-being of current and future patients. While the natural sciences often proceed without concern for the practical applications of their results, medical researchers should always be concerned with the practical outcomes of their research: "Will this intervention improve patient care?" is a question that should be foremost in the minds of those engaged in such research. But if this is true, any dishonesty in the practice of medical research will, of necessity, slow down the progress of this enterprise and delay any therapeutic improvements for the people who need it most. Moreover, dishonest medical research and what follows in its wake—namely, skepticism about its results—is evidence that the research participants were put in harm's way for naught. This too cuts against the grain of medical research thought of as a humanistic endeavor.

Finally, medical research, like all forms of research, is vitally dependant on trust. Medical researchers must trust that the earlier research results on which they build were themselves gained and reported truthfully. Put differently, given that they were not present in the clinics in which prior medical research was carried out, medical researchers must trust that the results they read in medical journals or hear about at medical conferences are based on truthful and transparent practices. This trust is based on the expectation that the research methods have been clearly explained; that these methods, so explained, were *actually* followed; that all the relevant data have been presented; and that the peer review process—a necessary step for any work to appear in print—was carried out by conscientious and unbiased reviewers; and so on. Moreover, and perhaps most important, patients who enroll in research protocols trust that there are good reasons to carry out the research in which they are participating; that is, they trust that the research question is a clinically important one that is prompted not by wide-eyed curiosity, but rather by the health care needs of present and future patients. Research participants also trust that their medical care is not being unduly compromised by their participation in a research protocol. Finally, an enormous amount of medical research is funded by the general public through taxation. However, only a very small minority of members of the general public have access to the inner workings of the medical research enterprise either as researchers or as research participants. Consequently, the general public has little option but to trust that the medical research that is being performed, and that they themselves fund, is done with honesty and great care. Public outcry in response to research scandals and scientific misconduct is an expression of this violated trust. It is thus no great exaggeration to claim that without trust, medical research would grind to a halt.

The question then becomes, What is to be done? The problem with scientific misconduct is that it has its genesis in the foibles and fragility of our all-too-human nature: the desire for prestige, career advancement, or power and income; the avoidance of painstaking work; and the often hubristic belief that one must surely be right *despite* evidence to the contrary, all of which are on prominent display in cases of misconduct. Yet there are steps that can and must be taken at both the individual and the institutional levels, and the selected readings in this part of the book aim to highlight some of these steps. The readings serve two purposes. First, they serve an educational purpose in that they shed light on problematic practices in medical research, some of which have hitherto been lurking in the shadows, as if beyond ethical scrutiny (e.g., statistical practices). Second, however, they offer proposals regarding how best to deal with, or to prevent, scientific misconduct. Some of the proposals are aimed at the institutional level (e.g., the university or research institute or the editorial board of a journal) but all of the selections, of necessity, also address themselves to individuals. Only if one attends to both levels, the institutional and the individual, will scientific misconduct be rightly understood—what it is, what causes it, and what is to be done about it. As the authors of *Integrity and Misconduct in Research* rightly note, "The Commission's proposed definition of research misconduct and other forms of professional misconduct related to research will reach its full meaning when it is tested with real-world experience,

cases, and commentaries. The Commission is relying on professional societies, research institutions, science ethics scholars, and case law to develop the interpretive context."[10] Just as it is important to locate individual conduct *within* such interpretive contexts when attempting to understand what counts as (and causes) scientific misconduct, so too is it important to locate possible remedies or preventative programs for misconduct within such contexts.

SECTION ONE. ALTERING DATA: FRAUD, FABRICATION, AND FALSIFICATION

Our first section of this part addresses the alteration of data. The first contributor in this section, Patricia K. Woolf, attends to the pressure to publish that is faced by scientists. Her essay is thus, in part, a meditation on the pathogenesis of misconduct. As Woolf rightly notes, the publication of research results is not only a means of communication between scientists, nor simply a form of "repayment" to the public that has funded much of the research and expects scientific progress in return; rather, publication has also become a means of evaluating scientists for the purpose of assessing their merits for professional advancement. The more one publishes, in other words, the more quickly one advances up the professional ladder. Researchers thus have a self-interested motive for fraudulently cutting corners if it will result in more publications; they have a motive, in other words, for engaging in scientific misconduct. While Woolf does not lay all of the blame for misconduct at the feet of the systemic background conditions of institutionalized scientific practice (i.e., the "built-in" pressure to publish), neither is she sanguine about characterizing instances of scientific misconduct as merely being the result of one individual's "flawed personality."

Our next two contributors, John C. Bailar III and James L. Mills, focus their attention on the statistical practices of medical scientists. Generally speaking, medical research is only as valid as the statistical methods that are used to design, analyze, and present the data generated by the research. Central to medical research is the process of inference, that is, drawing more general conclusions based on incomplete or imperfect observations. To draw valid inferences requires that one *honestly* and *transparently* follow well-established statistical practices. According to Bailar, failure to do so is deceptive. Bailar's striking claim is that while wholesale deception in science is universally condemned, "deliberate or careless deception short of lying . . . seems to be universally accepted . . . as part of the culture of science." This, as he explains, is deeply problematic. Thus, for example, the perhaps surprisingly common practice of testing a post hoc hypothesis (a hypothesis that was not disclosed prior to the research and for which there is no statistical basis to test) or the incomplete reporting of methods and results are cases of "deliberate or careless deception." It is such deceptive practices among scientists that damage the inferences that are central to the scientific enterprise. Therefore, Bailar argues, those who are concerned about scientific misconduct should be as concerned about the statistical tests that are used in research as they are about more blatant cases of data fabrication.

Mills also focuses on statistical matters by bringing to light two different ways in which one can "torture" one's data, that is, make the data say what one wants it to say. As Mills summarizes the problem, the "unfortunate result of torturing data is the dissemination of incorrect information to the research community and to patients." The two forms of data torturing that Mills identifies are opportunistic data torturing and Procrustean data torturing. Opportunistic data torturing occurs when researchers "go fishing" through their results for an interesting association; in other words, when a post hoc hypothesis—one that is generated after the results are in—is tested for significance without claiming that it is, in fact, a post hoc rather than an a priori hypothesis. (One may respond: If the data demonstrate an important relationship, why does it matter if the hypothesis was generated after an examination of the data? This is an intuitive question that must be met with an unintuitive response: Unless hypotheses are tested according to statistical procedures laid out in advance of data gathering, test results demonstrating an important relationship have a much higher, and thus unacceptable, probability of being falsely positive than if those hypotheses are tested in ways explicitly planned for at the beginning stages of a research project.)

Procrustean data torturing, on the other hand, occurs when the data are manipulated so that the results appear "much better"—that is, more in harmony with the proposed hypothesis or demonstrating a stronger association—than they actually are. Although Mills admits that data torturing is difficult

to prove, he nonetheless offers guidance on how to identify it and offers helpful suggestions to journal editors that will require more transparent reporting of methods and results, thus forcing data torturing out of existence.

Our final contributor to this section, Douglas L. Weed, invokes the strategies and tools of preventive oncology toward the goal of preventing scientific misconduct. Public health practitioners make a distinction between primary and secondary prevention of disease. For example, a smoking cessation program is a primary prevention intervention for cancer, because it aims to *remove* one of the main causes of cancer, namely, smoking. But primary prevention can also involve the identification of factors that, if present, will reduce the likelihood of occurrence of disease. Thus chemoprevention for those at high risk of cancer or daily low-dose aspirin for those at high risk of heart attack are both primary prevention programs because they aim to *introduce* a protective agent into persons. On the other hand, an early detection program coupled with effective therapy, such as mammography for breast cancer followed by therapy, is an example of secondary prevention because it aims to *detect* the disease as early as possible and thereby *reduce* the negative outcome of the disease (namely, death) through a therapeutic intervention. Weed's innovation here is to use this well-established public health framework for the prevention of scientific misconduct.

On Weed's account, primary prevention of misconduct includes removing both external causes (e.g., institutional pressure to publish) and internal causes (e.g., vanity or financial gain) of misconduct. While he is not very sanguine about the effectiveness of programs to reduce pressure to publish—for example, through an emphasis on the quality rather than the quantity of the publications—he is rather more hopeful about the utility of effective mentoring of junior scientists by senior scientists coupled with a robust ethics curriculum in research institutions. For the secondary prevention of scientific misconduct, Weed proposes a system of auditing or of periodic research review so that cases of misconduct can be detected as quickly as possible. Such auditing or review should then be coupled with institutional investigative procedures and appropriate sanctions. Although he recognizes and assesses the shortcomings of his proposals, Weed argues that only through programs of primary and secondary prevention will scientific misconduct be properly dealt with.

SECTION TWO. RULES OF AUTHORSHIP

Authorship and the criteria that should be used to distribute or "award" it have long been a concern to those involved in research and, in particular, to those who sit on the editorial boards of journals. Given the nature of the research enterprise—one that requires contributions from a great many areas of expertise—medical research papers are almost always written by multiple authors. In certain fields, such as high-energy physics, it is not unheard of to encounter a paper with 200 authors. In such instances, much rides on how high on the list of authors one happens to be placed or if indeed one is counted as an author at all. The contributors to our section on authorship rules, Drummond Rennie, Veronica Yank, and Linda L. Emanuel, offer a helpful proposal intended to ensure that authors of papers are held accountable for being listed as authors.

Although one would think that a determination of who and why one should be counted as an author of a research paper would be straightforward, matters tend to be complicated. For example, in their "Uniform Requirements for Manuscripts Submitted to Biomedical Journals," the International Committee of Medical Journal Editors (the "Vancouver Group") make the following claims concerning authorship:

> Each author should have participated sufficiently in the work to take public responsibility for appropriate portions of the content. One or more authors should take responsibility for the integrity of the work as a whole, from inception to published article.
>
> Authorship credit should be based only on (1) substantial contributions to conception and design, or acquisition of data, or analysis and interpretation of data; (2) drafting the article or revising it critically for important intellectual content; and (3) final approval of the version to be published. Conditions (1), (2), and (3) must all be met. Acquisition of funding, the collection of data, or general supervision of the research group, by themselves, do not justify authorship.[11]

Yet as Rennie and colleagues claim, even this detailed account of the conditions of authorship is insufficient because it underestimates the extent to which highly specialized input into papers has made the original concept of authorship outmoded. Moreover, given that this system of authorship is ambiguous on the question of author contributions, it is prone to abuse.

The proposal proffered by Rennie and colleagues is based on assigning credit and blame to *contributors* (rather than to *authors*) where it is due. Contributors should first give a detailed description of their respective and relative contributions so that contributor order for the publication can be determined. In addition to this, Rennie and colleagues suggest that one of the contributors be designated as guarantor of the integrity of the entire research project; the role of guarantor thus speaks not only to the issue of the contributorship (or authorship) of *one* paper, but more broadly to the integrity of the scientific enterprise. There are a few practical implications of this proposal. First, it will more clearly establish who should be considered a contributor to a research paper and on what grounds. Second, however, given that publication is key to professional advancement, this proposal, if followed, will more accurately reflect the genuine contribution of researchers to their papers, thus enabling others to better gauge the value of someone's work. Rennie and colleagues call on journals, professional societies, universities, and granting agencies to take the lead and implement their proposal.

SECTION THREE. PROBLEMS IN THE PUBLICATION OF RESEARCH METHODS AND FINDINGS

Our final two contributions to this part of the book deal with problems surrounding the selective underreporting (or, more accurately, the nonpublication) of research results and the incomplete reporting of research methods in published reports. Both practices are destructive to the scientific and clinical enterprises because they involve the withholding of information from researchers and, ultimately, from patients. Such withholdings are of concern for a few reasons. First, researchers and practicing physicians alike must have at hand the most complete and up-to-date information so that decisions made in concert with patients and research participants can be maximally informed. Second, one of the ways in which research results gain wide assent in medical circles is through the process of reproducibility. That is, with rare exceptions—one such exception being the ECMO trial discussed in this volume, Part III, Section Two—the efficacy of an intervention is not definitively established by the results of one trial. What is needed for results to take root is, rather, several additional studies that confirm earlier results. Therefore, a necessary condition of good science is the complete and accurate reporting of methods so that others can easily reproduce the study. Without complete and accurate reporting of methods—a dishonest practice regardless of its effects—scientific progress can be curtailed, and so is progress in patient care.

Our first contributor, Iain Chalmers, addresses the issue of publication bias—that is, the nonpublication of "uninteresting" or "disappointing" research results. Publication bias occurs when research studies that *fail* to show a significant difference between the two compared interventions (so-called negative trials) are systematically underrepresented in the medical literature. Put differently but equivalently, publication bias means that "positive trials" are systematically overrepresented in the medical literature.[12] The source of the problem lies both with the researchers who produce these results, who fail to submit them for publication, and with the editorial boards of journals that review the papers for publication, who fail to accept them for publication. Chalmers demonstrates the harms (noted earlier) that flow from publication bias by discussing two cases of perinatal research, one whose publication was delayed for seven years and another that was never published. In response to the phenomenon of publication bias, Chalmers proposes several solutions. First, he argues that both researchers and journal editors must change their behaviors regarding "negative trials." Chalmers does realize, however, that institutional changes must occur as well. He thus proposes a wider compliance with the sub-mission of research proposals to existing prospective registries of clinical research, registries that have the study protocols and up-to-date information about the present stage of the research (e.g., currently under way, completed, report under submission to a journal, report published). Not only will the use of such registries aid the process of transparent communication among researchers; it will also make it easier to track down unpublished research.

Finally, the CONSORT (Consolidated Standards of Reporting Trials) group's statement offers guidance concerning how and what to report when publishing one's research results.[13] The aim of the CONSORT group is to rid the medical literature of incompletely reported research results and to thereby maximize the potential usefulness of the literature for researchers and patients alike. In order to accomplish this aim, the group constructed a checklist of items that one should report when publishing one's research results. This checklist includes a full characterization of the research participants, clearly indicated statistical methods, methods of randomization, and so on. As more individual researchers and more journals adopt the use of this checklist, reporting in medical journals will improve, thus making the medical research literature more complete. For example, the first CONSORT statement was published in 1996 and adopted by several of the world's most prestigious medical journals. In a recent study by the CONSORT group, they found that in the journals that adopted the CONSORT statement as policy, reporting improved significantly two years after the statement was adopted.[14] This is heartening news, and it stands as evidence that through concerted individual and institutional efforts, the medical research literature can be improved, thus ultimately serving the needs of patients.

1. Stephen Lock, "Research Misconduct: A Brief History and a Comparison," *Journal of Internal Medicine* 235 (1994): 123–27.
2. Marcel C. LaFollette, "The Pathology of Research Fraud: The History and Politics of the U.S. Experience," *Journal of Internal Medicine* 235 (1994): 129–35, quote on p. 130.
3. Lock, 124.
4. In particular, that involving the Nobel laureate David Baltimore and his supervisee, Thereza Imanishi-Kari. Daniel J. Kevles, *The Baltimore Case: A Trial of Politics, Science, and Character* (New York: W. W. Norton and Company, 1998).
5. Judith P. Swazey, Melissa S. Anderson, and Karen Seashore Lewis, "Ethical Problems in Academic Research," *American Scientist* 81 (1993): 542–53.
6. James Woodward and David Goodstein, "Conduct, Misconduct and the Structure of Science," *American Scientist* 84 (1996): 479–90.
7. Commission on Research Integrity (chaired by Kenneth J. Ryan), *Integrity and Misconduct in Research: Report of the Commission on Research Integrity* (Washington D.C.: DHHS, 1995). The full text of this report is available at the Web site of the DHHS Office of Research Integrity: ori.dhhs.gov/multimedia/acrobat/commissionreport.pdf.

8. Ibid., 13–14.
9. Ibid., 14.
10. Commission on Research Integrity, 14.
11. International Committee of Medical Journal Editors (ICMJE), "Uniform Requirements for Manuscripts Submitted to Biomedical Journals," *JAMA* 277 (1997): 927–34. The ICMJE keeps an updated, full-text version of this document at their Web site: http://www.icmje.org.
12. Colin B. Begg and Jesse A. Berlin, "Publication Bias and Dissemination of Clinical Research," *Journal of the National Cancer Institute* 81 (1989): 107–15.
13. The complete text of the CONSORT Statement and many important supporting documents are available at the CONSORT Web site: http://www.consort-statement .org.
14. David Moher, Alison Jones, and Leah Lepage for the CONSORT Group, "Use of the CONSORT Statement and Quality of Reports of Randomized Trials," *JAMA* 285 (2001): 1992–95.

Altering Data

Fraud, Fabrication, and Falsification

---

76   Pressure to Publish and Fraud in Science

Patricia K. Woolf

Q. Is there pressure to publish in today's science?
A. Yes, there is.

Q. Is pressure to publish bad for science?
A. Bad or good, we're stuck with it. Since its birth, modern science has had an ethos that called for communications; scientists have felt some pressure to make their results known. Publication is an established way of doing so.

Q. Should there be pressure to publish?
A. Why not? If the public has paid for research, they are entitled to evidence that research has been done.

Q. Are publications the product of research? Doesn't the public pay for new knowledge and ideas?
A. Yes, that's the ideal, but not all experiments work. The public is really paying for a good-faith effort by highly skilled people who collectively have a pretty good chance of coming up with some information that is an advance.

Q. How do we know which scientific results represent advances in scientific knowledge?
A. That's where publication comes in; information known only to the discoverer cannot be evaluated and become knowledge. Some say it isn't even science until it is published. Research reports are evaluated by editors and referees before they are published, and then publication allows other scientists to further evaluate and use the results.

Q. Why is there so much concern about pressure to publish?
A. Many persons in science are worried that their important but complicated system of communication is in jeopardy. Because of undue pressure it may not be working the way it's supposed to.

Q. Why is it complicated?
A. Publication is no longer just a way to communicate information. It has come to be a way of evaluating scientists; in many cases it is the primary factor in professional advancement.

Q. Is that so bad? If articles are refereed, doesn't that ensure a breadth of professional judgment?
A. Some say that the quantity of published papers has become more important for evaluation than the quality of ideas they contain.

Q. Is that true?
A. It's hard to say. The evidence is anecdotal. Promotion and granting committees meet in secret; according to a dean in a major medical school, "Confidentiality fans the flames of paranoia." There are no systematic studies of these deliberations, but some reputable people have criticized the system. We need more systematic information about the relation of publications to professional advancement.

Q. Why are they so critical if the facts are not known?
A. Their experience has led them to be concerned about science. And they are worried that careerism is damaging a very important national resource—our research establishment.

Q. Is there that much pressure to publish?
A. It depends on what sort of pressure you mean.

Q. Is there more than one kind of pressure to publish?
A. There are at least two sorts: the pressure the scientist feels from the tradition of science, and the pressures from institutions.

Patricia K. Woolf, "Pressure to Publish and Fraud in Science," *Annals of Internal Medicine* 104 (1986): 254–56.

Q. Are these pressures the same?

A. How could they be? Institutions and their departments may have different standards for promotion. Requirements are often implicit rather than explicit, and frequently they are misunderstood. Some research fields publish more heavily than others.

Q. Why have so many of the recently disclosed frauds been found in medical schools?

A. No one knows for sure. Their research environments are highly competitive. The heroic nature of their quest directly affects issues of life and death, so there are greater economic and social rewards in medical science. Another possibility is that some fraud occurs in all science, but it is more likely to be detected in a rapidly growing research area like biomedicine.

Q. Is there more pressure on medical scientists than on others?

A. Some say there is. Medical researchers often have clinical responsibilities in addition to teaching, research, writing, and applying for research funds.

Q. Have any studies measured psychological pressures on scientists?

A. I haven't found any in a search of the literature. One study currently underway at a major medical school is trying to find out if persons who are up for promotion really understand the promotion and tenure procedures of the institution.

Q. How can we measure the amount of pressure being put on scientists by institutions?

A. One way is to look at the amount of publishing done by practicing research scientists in our best institutions.

Q. Aren't you just counting papers again?

A. It's not the best way of determining research outcomes, but if becoming a full professor at a good university takes an exorbitant amount of publishing, we probably have a problem on our hands.

Q. How many papers does the average scientist publish?

A. A study by King and colleagues showed that in 1977 the average number of articles published per physical scientist was 0.20/year, up from 0.17/year in 1965. The average number per life scientist in 1977 was 0.40/year, up from 0.30 in 1965. In this period only the social sciences showed a big decline; the average number of papers per social scientist was 0.22/year, down from 0.60 in 1965. But these data include industrial or government scientists who may not be actively publishing. A better definition of scientists is prob-

ably a "publishing scientist." Price and Gursey have determined that among publishing scientists, the average productivity is 1 paper per scientist per year.

Q. What are the rates of publication of scientific faculty in our major universities?

A. They differ among disciplines. In a study of the faculty of nine distinguished universities, rates ranged from 1.8 publications per scientist per year in physics to a high of 2.7 publications per scientist per year in biochemistry. Astronomy, chemistry, and microbiology were the other specialties studied. Publication records of over 1000 faculty members were examined.

Q. What about medical schools?

A. There are many medical schools whose faculty publish very little. In the 1973–1975 period the average rate of publication for privately controlled medical schools was 250 papers per year and for publicly controlled medical schools, 150 papers per year.

Q. What do federal granting agencies expect from their investments in research? Is there unreasonable pressure to produce simply to satisfy these requirements? On the average, how many papers per grant per year are produced?

A. The Office of Program Planning and Evaluation of the NIH has examined the literature output of NIH-supported research. A recent study of faculty in departments of medicine shows that one third of M.D. faculty are not significantly engaged in research at all. The NIH makes between 5,000 and 6,000 competitive grants per year. The average length of the grants is 3.2 years and that amounts to roughly 16,000 to 20,000 grants in force. In the same period and with the predicted lag of 3 years between a grant award and its resultant publication, 16,000 to 20,000 papers per year are produced. These figures are subject to a possible 20 percent to 30 percent increase, because at different periods some journals were not included in the survey. But that amounts to 1 or 1.3 papers per grant year.

Q. If you double that to 2 or even 3 papers a year per grant, would that be too much pressure on a scientist?

A. It doesn't seem like it.

Q. If these institutional expectations are relatively modest, why is fraud associated with pressure to publish?

A. There are two principal reasons. First, several of the most spectacular frauds have taken place in laboratories where the number of papers published every year significantly exceeded the norm. Second, many of the persons involved have mentioned pressure as a factor. The newspapers usually report that view, and pressure has come to be a stock explanation.

Q. Could we look at those two factors separately?

A. That's sensible. "Pressure" has come to be a convenient explanation, for two reasons. The reports of these events have shown how shocked scientists are to discover that one of their colleagues was not playing by the rules. They may explain that fault using a psychological excuse that focuses on the flawed personality of an individual person and not on science in general; it is a less severe condemnatory judgment than, for instance, moral turpitude.

Q. Is that what's called medicalizing the deviance?

A. Yes, it seems to isolate the problem and let the other scientists off the hook. But then questions began to be asked about where the pressure comes from.

Q. Does that bring us round to the publishing practices in laboratories where fraud was discovered?

A. Let's look at just a few. The first of the major recent scandals, that of William Summerlin at the Memorial Sloan-Kettering Cancer Center, was in the research group supervised by Robert A. Good. In the 5 years before 1975, Good had published 342 papers, an average of 68/year (16 as first author, 325 as coauthor with at least 136 coauthors). Several other frauds were associated with medical research groups that have been extremely prolific. In the period 1975 to 1980, which preceded the discovery of fraud in their laboratories, Eugene Braunwald had published 171 papers, an average of 31/year. Ephraim Racker, who is not on a medical faculty, had published an average of 16/year.

Q. How do these pockets of prolific publication compare with similar departments in similar institutions?

A. These scientists have made important contributions, significant far beyond the numbers of their publications. Therefore, comparisons with average productivity have limited value. But, yes, their average levels of publishing are significantly higher.

Q. Should we be worried about such prolific publishing?

A. There is reason for concern on several levels. Simple time-and-motion studies lead to the conclusion that when an author's productivity is extremely high, his participation in each paper has to be low. Or at least there is no clear way of telling which articles the author contributed to significantly. These prolific scientists are clearly operating in ways very different from those in the mainstream of science. One can argue that excellent science has always been out of the mainstream, but when there are significant deleterious effects on younger coworkers in their laboratories and eventual effects on scientific research in the United States as a whole, we have a responsibility to question the wisdom of those research and publishing practices.

---

77 Science, Statistics, and Deception

JOHN C. BAILAR III

In science, lying is condemned, even by some of its few practitioners. Deliberate or careless deception short of lying, however, seems to be universally accepted and sometimes even promoted as a part of the culture of science. I do not suggest that scientists as a group are careless, venal, or otherwise depraved: they may even be above the human average in developing and adhering to detailed, albeit tacit, standards of professional conduct. Those who are clearly violators are drummed out of our ranks, loudly and publicly. But what about less clearcut deception?

My thesis is that our professional norms are incomplete and that several kinds of widely accepted practices should also be widely recognized as potentially deceptive and harmful. Some of these practices also have much value, but at times they are inappropriate and improper and, to the extent that they are deceptive, unethical.

The scientific method is fundamentally concerned with the processes of inference, generally from data that are necessarily inaccurate to some degree, incomplete, drawn from small samples, or not quite appropriate for a specific task. Inference—that is, drawing conclusions or making deductions from imperfect data—provides most of the excitement and intellectual ferment of science. Scientific rewards are probably more closely related to valid inferences established than to such related activities as imaginative hypotheses formulated, elegant experiments designed and conducted, or new methods developed. The rewards for publishing a first-class inference can include income, posi-

John C. Bailar III, "Science, Statistics, and Deception," *Annals of Internal Medicine* 104 (1986): 259–60.

tion and power, professional status, and the respect of colleagues. Such rewards may sometimes count for more than self-respect and the joy of discovery. We must therefore be attentive to scientific norms and activities that may distort the processes of inference.

An example of a deceptive practice is the statistical testing (such as the calculating of *p* values) of *post hoc* hypotheses. It is widely recognized that t-tests, chi-square tests, and other statistical tests provide a basis for probability statements only when the hypothesis is fully developed before the data are examined in any way. If even the briefest glance at a study's results moves the investigator to consider a hypothesis not formulated before the study was started, that glance destroys the probability value of the evidence at hand. Certainly, careful and unstructured review of data for unexpected clues is a critical part of science. Such review can be an immensely fruitful source of ideas for new, before-the-fact hypotheses that can be tested in the correct way with other new or existing data, and sometimes findings may be so striking that independent confirmation by a proper statistical test is superfluous. Statistical "tests" are also used sometimes in nonprobability ways as rough measures of the size of an effect, rather than to test hypotheses. (An example is the column of *p* values that sometimes accompanies a table comparing the pretreatment characteristics of patient groups in a randomized clinical trial.) When either the test itself or the reporting of the test is motivated by the data, a probability statement such as "$p < 0.05$" is deceptive and hence damaging to inference.

Other potential problems are the selective reporting of findings and the reporting of a single study in multiple fragments. These practices can obscure critical aspects of an investigation, so that readers will misjudge the evidential value of the data presented. Such reporting may be deceptive, whether deliberately or accidentally. On the other hand, these practices sometimes have positive value that should be preserved. For example, they can facilitate the tasks of both the investigator and the user when a demand for a monolithic analysis might seriously delay or frustrate the progress of both.

"Negative" conclusions of low statistical power—that is, reporting that no effect was found when there was little chance of detecting the effect—can also distort inference, especially when investigators do not report on statistical power. The concept of power is formally defined in terms of the random variability of results that is inherent in a specific combination of data structure, sample size, statistical models, and analytic method; but I believe that the concept should be substantially broadened to include the likelihood that a particular effect would be detected and reported if it were present to some specified degree. Such an analysis rarely accompanies "negative" findings, and readers may be left with an unjustified sense that an effect not demonstrated is an effect not present. Again, however, there are counterarguments: a report with low power may be better than no report (and no power), or meta-analysis of several low-power reports may come to stronger conclusions than any one of them alone. Reporting negative studies of low power can create ethical problems, but those problems may be largely mitigated if the low power is accurately and clearly reported as well. Too many scientists resist the objective reporting of this kind of weakness in their work, and pressure for "strong" results may be greatest during the formative years of graduate training and career entry. Thus we may be training new scientists in unethical methods.

Despite the occasionally useful roles of these and other practices [. . .], each can seriously distort the processes of inference and should therefore be an object of concern. Where the practices have legitimate applications, they should, of course, be used; but even then they should be fully and explicitly disclosed by the investigator, justified in some detail, and accepted with caution by readers. A combination of restraint in their overall use, limiting their use to clearly appropriate situations, providing full disclosure and justification, and maintaining the readers' skepticism will help to diminish the frequency and severity of ethical problems. Full disclosure here means more than a few words buried in the fine print of a Methods section; it means not just that the author send a message, but that the author also work to ensure that the message is received and correctly interpreted by readers. There are parallels here to the evolving requirements for informed consent by experimental subjects.

Pressures to publish can be great and may account for many [. . .] abuses. I fear that even the constrained use of these potentially damaging practices will leave attractive loopholes for an army of ambitious practitioners of science, each feeling great pressure to publish, who will rush in to explain why his or her situation is different, why full disclosure is inappropriate, and so forth. I am convinced that science, scientists, and society as a whole would benefit from substantially broader concepts, ultimately based on the need to protect the processes of inference, about ethical standards and violations in science.

[Table omitted—eds.]

78   Data Torturing

JAMES L. MILLS

"If you torture your data long enough they will tell you whatever you want to hear" has become a popular observation in our office. In plain English, this means that study data, if manipulated in enough different ways, can be made to prove whatever the investigator wants to prove. Unfortunately, this is generally true. Because every investigator wants to present results in the most exciting way, we all look for the most dramatic, positive findings in our data. When this process goes beyond reasonable interpretation of the facts, it becomes data torturing. The unfortunate result of torturing data is the dissemination of incorrect information to the research community and to patients.

It is impossible to tell how widespread data torturing is. Like other forms of torture, it leaves no incriminating marks when done skillfully. And like other forms of torture, it may be difficult to prove even when there is incriminating evidence. [...]

There are two major types of data torturing. In the first, which I term "opportunistic" data torturing, the perpetrator simply pores over the data until a "significant" association is found between variables and then devises a biologically plausible hypothesis to fit the association. The second, or "Procrustean," type of data torturing is performed by deciding on the hypothesis to be proved and making the data fit the hypothesis—Procrustes, a robber in Greek mythology, made all his victims fit the length of his bed by stretching or cutting off their legs.

OPPORTUNISTIC DATA TORTURING

To understand how opportunistic data torturing works, it is necessary to understand the assumptions that underlie significance testing. In simple terms, significance tests are used to determine whether observed differences between groups, such as medically and surgically treated patients, are greater than one would expect to occur by chance. If survival rates in the two groups differed by 5 percent or 10 percent, for example, how would we know whether the difference was due to chance? For fairly arbitrary reasons, we usually say that a result is not due to chance if the P value is less than 0.05. A P value of 0.05 means that there is a 5 percent chance that we will conclude that the two groups differ when they actually do not (called a type I error). In

James L. Mills, "Data Torturing," *New England Journal of Medicine* 329 (1993): 1196–99.

other words, there is a 95 percent probability that we will correctly conclude that there is no difference when no difference is present. But when many independent tests are performed, that 95 percent probability of a correct conclusion drops drastically. For example, by simple probability calculations it can be shown that for two tests the probability that the "significant" differences found by the investigators will reflect true differences is 90 percent (0.95 × 0.95). For 20 tests, it is only 36 percent (0.95^{20}). Thus, the data torturer can find significant results when none exist simply by making multiple comparisons.

One slightly fictionalized example of opportunistic data torturing is a study of parents' occupational exposures as a risk factor for birth defects in their offspring. Seven major categories of occupational exposure were identified. When no significant relation between these categories and birth defects was found for either the mothers or the fathers (14 comparisons), the categories were split into 64 separate occupations for the mothers and 80 separate occupations for the fathers. Not surprisingly, the authors then found "significant" associations with birth defects. Although the authors mentioned that some positive results could have occurred by chance, the differences were treated as real. The probability that all their "significant" findings were real? Three in 10,000 (0.95^{158}).

It must be a great comfort to practitioners of this technique to know that 1 of every 20 independent comparisons they make will yield a "significant" result (P < 0.05) if—and this is critical—they ignore the need to adjust for multiple comparisons. When this type of data torturing is done well, it may be impossible for readers to tell that the positive association did not spring from an *a priori* hypothesis.

PROCRUSTEAN DATA TORTURING

Procrustean data torturing, or manipulating the data so that they prove the desired hypothesis, requires selective reporting. It can take several forms. First, exposure may be redefined in a way that strengthens the association. One study of adverse effects of oral contraceptives on the outcome of pregnancy defined exposure as presumed use within 600 days before a delivery or miscarriage; the choice of an inappropriately extended period to define exposure produced a positive result by including women not actually exposed during pregnancy. Second, study subjects whose experiences do not support the hypothesis may be dropped. For example, the report on a cancer-therapy trial might include outcomes only for subjects who survive more than three months, on the grounds that earlier deaths were inevitable and unrelated to the experimental therapy. In fact, these deaths could have resulted from toxic effects of the agent being tested. Third, disease outcomes may be lumped together, split, or dropped altogether to produce the desired results. In the cancer trial, for instance, the investigators' original intention might have been to look at differences in survival according to six-month intervals. But if no significant differences were found, the data could be reanalyzed according to longer or shorter time intervals until a significant difference was found. The authors could then report only the significant difference. Finally, normal ranges for laboratory results may be altered (although this must be done with care when common tests are reported). Of course, all these methods of selective reporting require the suppression of contradictory data.

Procrustean data torturing is more difficult to carry out than opportunistic data torturing, but its results are often more believable if one starts with a popular hypothesis. It is also more destructive, because it may produce results that are seen as definitive proof of the hypothesis, whereas opportunistic data torturing is often viewed as only hypothesis generation.

CLUES TO DATA TORTURING

Data torturing can rarely be proved. There are, however, clues that should arouse the reader's suspicion.

In the case of opportunistic data torturing (the search for chance associations), the reader must ask, Is this a chance finding with an *a posteriori* hypothesis concocted to give it credibility, or is this an honest hypothesis-generating study? Tukey points out the need for exploratory studies using "theoretical insights and exploration of past data." Hypothesis-generating studies (sometimes referred to somewhat contemptuously as "fishing expeditions") should be identified as such. To warrant further exploration, findings from such studies should be biologically plausible. If the fishing expedition catches a boot, the fishermen should throw it back, not claim that they were fishing for boots. If a finding has good data from animal studies or related human studies to support it, it is unlikely to have resulted from opportunistic data torturing. If it has neither biologic plausibility nor supporting data, it should be viewed with a jaundiced eye.

Similarly, an honest exploratory study should indicate how many comparisons were made. Although there is disagreement about how (or even whether) to adjust for multiple comparisons, most experts agree that large numbers of comparisons will produce apparently statistically significant findings that are actually due to chance. The data torturer will act as if every positive result confirmed a major hypothesis. The honest investigator will limit the study to focused questions, all of which make biologic sense. The cautious reader should look at the number of "significant" results in the context of how many comparisons were made. In the occupational-exposure study described earlier, nine "significant" findings were reported. Given that 158 comparisons were made, eight of those nine results could easily have occurred by chance.

Identifying Procrustean data torturing (in which the data are made to fit the hypothesis) also requires asking the right questions:

Why were study subjects dropped? One recent study of the health effects of exposure to heat dropped one of the four categories of exposure, changing a nonsignificant effect to a significant effect. One should suspect data torturing whenever subjects are dropped without a clear reason, or when a large proportion of subjects are excluded for any reason.

Does the classification of exposure and disease make sense? Statements such as "We studied those with at least five years of exposure to lead smelters, or those with blood lead levels of 50 μg per deciliter or higher" should raise questions. Why were the data on subjects with shorter exposure or less elevated lead levels not reported? Is it because they did not fit the hypothesis?

Are the cutoff points for laboratory studies reasonable and customary? Some of the bolder data torturers will argue that the clustering of subjects' test values at the upper range of normal is evidence of a pathologic state. Others will take advantage of the lack of a well-established cutoff point to select the point that makes their data produce the most significant results. A study of AIDS could use various CD4 cell counts as cutoff points, then report the one that shows the most impressive effect. The presence of a dose-response relation is evidence that the reported effect is genuine, not the result of arbitrary classification. If a diabetic woman's risk of miscarriage increases 5 percent for each 1 percent increase in her glycosylated hemoglobin level, the association is not likely to be due to data torturing. The key is that the effect is consistent across a wide range of values.

Is the rationale for the subgroup analyses convincing? If a drug works only in women over 60 years of age, the savvy reader should suspect a chance finding. Remember that two sexes, multiple age groups, and different clinical features such as stages of disease make it possible for the investigators to examine the data in many different ways.

Is there a clear biologic mechanism that could account for an effect in one subgroup but not in others, or were multiple comparisons made in order to produce positive results? "The study drug produced significantly increased survival at 18 months" may mean that there were no significant differences in survival at any of the other five periods studied.

In the same vein, it is important to ask whether the data have been censored. As I noted above, looking only at the group that survived at least three months after starting treatment may disguise the fact that the drug under study caused a substantial number of deaths in the first three months. [...]

CAN DATA TORTURES BE STOPPED?

Many, if not all, of these data-torturing techniques have been familiar to experts for years. [...] Unfortunately, little has been done to alert the medical community to these abuses, or to eradicate them.

How can data torturing be prevented? It cannot. However, journals can demand information from authors that will discourage it:

Did the reported findings result from testing a primary hypothesis of the study? If not, was the secondary hypothesis generated before the data were analyzed?

What was the rationale for excluding various subjects from the analysis?

Were the following determined before looking at the data: definition of exposure, definition of an outcome, subgroups to be analyzed, and cutoff points for a positive result?

How many statistical tests were performed, and was the effect of multiple comparisons dealt with appropriately?

Are both P values and confidence intervals reported?

And have the data been reported for all subgroups and at all follow-up points?

Honest answers to these questions will make it much easier for editors, reviewers, and readers to separate honest data analysis from data torturing. Until such steps are taken, we shall remain at the mercy of those who are driven to produce positive findings by fair means or foul.

---

79   Preventing Scientific Misconduct

DOUGLAS L. WEED

[...]

THE NATURE AND EXTENT OF SCIENTIFIC MISCONDUCT

Two definitions of scientific misconduct, one from the National Science Foundation and the other from the DHHS, emerged in the early 1990s. In both, scientific misconduct was defined as fabrications, falsification, plagiarism, or any other serious deviation from accepted scientific practices in proposing, conducting, or reporting research. A debate ensued over the inclusion of the words "other serious deviation." Proponents argued that this broad term permitted scientific communities to define what constituted ethical conduct and appropriate practices specific to their branches of science. Opponents argued that the term was too broad. Although its inclusion appeared to allow sanctions against scientists who undertook innovative, groundbreaking science—which could be construed as a "serious deviation from accepted practice"—no such cases were known. Recently, a federally appointed commission recast the definition in terms of a principle with examples. The commission's report stated that "research misconduct is [a] serious violation of the fundamental principle that scientists be truthful and fair in the conduct of research and the dissemination of research results." It said that unethical conduct includes misappropriation (plagiarism or breaches of confidentiality), interference, misrepresentation (falsification or fabrication), obstruction of investigations of misconduct, and noncompliance with research regulations.

Not everyone agrees with the commission's expansion of the definition of misconduct. Some believe such a broad definition could increase the number of investigations because it includes any type of behavior judged to be untruthful or unfair. On the other hand, some authors have for years insisted that misconduct should be very broadly defined to include behaviors not only beyond falsification, fabrication, and plagiarism, but also beyond the categories included in the expanded definition introduced by the commission. Deceptive scientific practices, such as the misrepresentation of research results, are the most commonly cited behaviors. Failure to explain weaknesses in data, selective reporting of results, failure to publish a study with negative results, and reporting as "negative" a study with low power are a few examples of this less serious form of misconduct. Practices of irresponsible authorship and wasteful (i.e., repetitive) publication have also been designated misconduct.

It is important to distinguish between error and misconduct. Science makes progress because error exists, in measurement and in interpretation of evidence. But these

Douglas L. Weed, "Preventing Scientific Misconduct," *American Journal of Public Health* 88 (1998): 125–29.

are unintentional errors. Misconduct involves intentional misrepresentation or misappropriation. To put the relationship of error to misconduct in perspective, it may be helpful to consider scientists' conduct to range across a continuum. At one end are serious forms of misconduct, followed by deceptive reporting practices and then, toward the middle, what might best be called sloppiness. At the other end of the continuum lies appropriate scientific and professional conduct, including unintentional error.

Estimating the occurrence of scientific misconduct is not made easier by conceptualizing such a continuum. The many published opinions on the topic are polarized between the belief that scientific misconduct is a rare event and the belief that it is rampant [...].

Although quantitative assessments will help answer the question of how much misconduct exists, it is an unfortunate fact that big effects may arise from small numbers. A single well-publicized case of serious misconduct, such as the recent case of fabrication in a large government-sponsored cancer treatment trial, can do considerable damage to institutions, to scientists' reputations, and to the public's already precipitously balanced perception of science. Therefore, scientific misconduct must not be ignored or trivialized, regardless of its prevalence.

A FRAMEWORK FOR PREVENTION

Preventing scientific misconduct is a widely recognized goal. Attainment of this goal may require that we consider misconduct a professional affliction amenable to both primary and secondary prevention efforts. The implications of such an analysis have not been carefully examined.

Primary Prevention of Scientific Misconduct

Primary prevention is typically conceived as identifying and removing causes of events and as identifying factors whose presence (rather than absence) actively reduces the occurrence of those events. Frequently proposed causes of scientific misconduct fall into two categories overlapping those mentioned above, and in some cases overlapping each other. There are causes *external* to the individual scientist, such as publication pressure, competition, the large scale of science (reducing opportunities for effective mentoring), and mentors setting bad examples. There are also *internal* causes, such as personal financial gain, ego or vanity, and psychiatric illness.

Psychiatric illness readily fits the traditional conception of primary prevention. "Remove" it by effective psychiatric treatment and some cases of scientific misconduct, specifically those involving mentally impaired yet employable scientists, could be prevented. How much misconduct is attributable to mental disease is an open and important question. Any answer must consider the possibility that those accused of misconduct may run (perhaps instinctively) to a psychiatrist, claiming illness and thereby avoiding responsibility for what may best be described as a character flaw rather than an uncontrollable personality disorder.

The most frequently posited causes of misconduct are publication pressure and competition. However, it is not clear how reducing—much less eliminating—these factors would reduce scientific misconduct without also reducing some of that which makes science the rigorous and productive enterprise it has become. Perhaps it is a matter of degree. Indeed, to reduce publication pressure, suggested interventions typically involve emphasizing quality over quantity in academic appointments and promotions as well as eliminating honorary authorship. Although these are reasonable proposals, they may have little impact on the publication pressure inherent in science.

Another proposed external cause of scientific misconduct—ineffective mentoring owing to the large scale of science—reflects the idea that having too few senior scientist mentors relative to the number of junior scientists reduces the ability to monitor the (mis)behavior of those mentored. Nor can good examples be set if there are too few mentors. In either case, recommendations to increase opportunities for mentoring by increasing the ratio of senior to junior scientists seem reasonable, assuming resources are available. Nevertheless, providing more mentors and providing good mentors may not be equivalent. Indeed, bad mentoring (a proposed external cause of scientific misconduct) and the proposed internal causes of personal financial gain and vanity [...] together reveal an implicit claim regarding the etiology of scientific misconduct: that many scientists, because of ignorance or by design, are seriously unskilled in ethics, if not morally bankrupt. Indeed, descriptions of some cases make it reasonable to wonder if scientific misconduct is a product of basic flaws in the characters of scientists. To what extent, then, can ethics training shore up what has eroded or was never planted: a coherent and useful professional scientific ethic?

An often-cited approach to teaching ethics within the context of scientific misconduct involves codes of responsible conduct, that is, rules or guidelines for good (appropriate) scientific and professional practice. Yet there are some fundamental problems with teaching ethics as a set of rules, just as it would be seriously deficient to teach science as a set of rules for the laboratory or for the computer. In any professional scientific practice there are thousands of decisions not covered in the rules. [...] Ethics, like science, has its theories and methodologies beyond the rules that help to interpret the rules and to guide practice where the rules are missing. Which of these theories and methods will prove most helpful as a foundation for preventing scientific misconduct is an important question, given the prominent theoretical plurality in contemporary bioethics.

It is beyond the scope of this paper to fully discuss the role of moral theory in ethics education. Nevertheless, one such theory—the theory of virtue ethics or character ethics—may be necessary in any account of the ethics of scientific misconduct and so deserves attention. The virtues are traits of character habitually exhibited and important for attaining the goods internal to a practice. By many accounts, the good internal to the practice of science is the truth; science is a search for the "really real" of the world. Fabrication and falsification, or misappropriation and misrepresentation, are direct affronts to this search, as are deceptive scientific practices. While there are many virtues to consider, those of honesty, self-effacement, and excellence seem best suited to helping scientists stay on their appointed path. Put another way, scientists should develop and habitually exhibit honesty rather than dishonesty, and they should put the interests of the profession and of society (especially those of research subjects) before their personal interests, whether financial gain or fame or both. Scientists should habitually exhibit excellence rather than sloppiness. These virtues provide a moral foundation for preventing not only serious forms of misconduct (e.g., fabrication and falsification) but also the lesser offenses (e.g., misrepresentation of research results) that Bailar and others have argued are part of the continuum of misconduct.

An obvious concern regarding virtue ethics as one pillar of ethics education is how to go about developing character traits within individual scientists. Pellegrino argues that virtue ethics, like all moral theories, can be taught from the literature and from case studies illustrating its dimensions, although the most efficacious approach may be to learn by example—by observing, emulating, and reflecting upon the virtuous behavior of a respected mentor. Clearly, such mentors must not only possess the requisite virtues but also habitually display them in their everyday scientific practice. Judging from recent cases of serious misconduct, remedial ethics education for some senior scientists may be necessary. [. . .] Nevertheless, if the virtues of honesty, self-effacement, and excellence could be instilled in scientists during their training, three of the seven causes of scientific misconduct—mentors' setting bad examples, personal financial gain, and ego or vanity—could potentially be modified.

Problems Emerging within a Framework of Primary Prevention

Three problems deserve scrutiny. First, on what evidentiary and inferential bases have the proposed causes of scientific misconduct been judged? Second, how much scientific misconduct can be attributed to these causes, and how much misconduct remains unexplained? Finally, how can we determine whether suggested preventive interventions, inasmuch as they relate directly to purported causes of scientific misconduct, are effective in reducing the occurrence of misconduct, however broadly defined? These are closely related questions in the public health model. Attribution requires a decision regarding causality. Thus, to attribute cases of misconduct to a particular factor is to assume implicitly that the factor is (or can reasonably be judged to be) causal. In turn, an answer to the intervention question may help answer the question regarding cause. One of the best tests of a causal hypothesis is to remove the cause and observe the effect of the preventive intervention. But to observe preventive effects, surveillance systems must be in place to track the occurrence of misconduct before and after the intervention. In addition, primary preventive interventions in public health are rarely attempted without a reasonable body of evidence supporting the underlying causal hypothesis. The evidence supporting proposed causes of scientific misconduct is extraordinarily weak; it consists solely of expert opinion, an evidentiary category almost always fraught with opposing views. [. . .]

Perhaps it is time to formally study the determinants of scientific misconduct. This task will require behavioral and social science methodologies if scientific misconduct represents, for the most part, deliberate and conscious acts on the part of its perpetrators. Its causes, therefore, are more "historical" than "natural," according to Collingwood's classic categorization of causation. A difficult aspect of such a study will be to tease out the effects of the most commonly cited causes, publication pressure and competition, because they are analogous to universal environmental factors; nearly everyone in science is exposed to them. Furthermore, they are not independent of one another. Nevertheless, it makes sense to undertake surveys of professional groups regarding their knowledge, attitudes, and beliefs about misconduct in science; to obtain better empirical estimates of prevalence and incidence rates of misconduct; and to conduct case-control studies in which cases subjects are those who have committed misconduct. Problems of case ascertainment, recall, and other forms of information bias and confounding should be expected.

Secondary Prevention of Scientific Misconduct

In the classic public health model, secondary prevention involves early detection of disease events coupled with effective treatment. For the secondary prevention of scientific misconduct, early detection involves increasing opportunities of discovering instances of misconduct, and "treatment" refers to procedures for investigating cases as well as the sanctions delivered to those responsible for the misconduct.

Auditing is the most obvious strategy for finding instances of scientific misconduct, although less drastic measures have been suggested: periodic review of scientific records, publications, and workloads. Increasing the ratio of senior to junior scientists, discussed previously, is also a form of secondary prevention, inasmuch as one role for the mentor is to monitor the behavior of junior colleagues. These approaches to early detection require the concomitant acceptance of responsibility on the part of institutions and their leaders and especially on the part of working scientists. This is a responsibility to *do* something about scientific misconduct. Perhaps the most difficult responsibility is to report misconduct perpetrated by colleagues; small wonder so many authors recommend protection for whistle-blowers.

Institutionalization of investigative procedures for handling cases of alleged misconduct is often recommended. On moral and legal grounds, due process is essential to an institutional review process in the same way that informed consent is an essential part of medical research. Fair and public investigative procedures provide a structure for judging the facts of the case so that appropriate penalties—the "treatment"—can be meted out. Kassirer mentioned "how much trouble and disgrace are entailed in misconduct investigations," effects that apply not only to those found guilty but also to those wrongly accused. The regular reports of the Office of Research Integrity detail a common sanction against those convicted of misconduct: ineligibility for federal funding, a serious punishment for any scientists whose livelihood depends upon outside funds. At least one journal has published sanctions to be meted out to authors involved in inappropriate acts; fabrication, for example, brings a penalty of "two years to life" during which time the author may not submit a manuscript to that journal for consideration. [...]

Problems Emerging within a Framework of Secondary Prevention

As in the case of primary prevention, there are some problems in approaching scientific misconduct from the perspective of secondary prevention. If any form of increased surveillance occurs (including formal auditing procedures or the less formal approach of encouraging scientists to take seriously their responsibility to report misconduct), then we can expect an increase in the number of cases of scientific misconduct detected. However, such an increase may represent not a true change in the underlying incidence of events, but rather an apparent change due solely to more intense surveillance. This is a well-known phenomenon in programs designed to detect disease early. For the early detection of scientific misconduct, the inevitable increase in numbers of misconduct cases arising from increased surveillance could be misconstrued by commentators, the press, legislators, and others as indicative of a larger problem than truly exists.

A second problem involves the effects of financial penalties and other sanctions. The extent to which sanctions prevent further incidents of scientific misconduct is an unexplored empirical question. Institutional investigational procedures, monetary and publishing disincentives, and other strategies, such as firing the guilty party, may have a preventive effect by engendering second thoughts about committing misconduct among both would-be repeat offenders and would-be first offenders.

SUMMARY

Disease prevention frameworks sometimes include a category of tertiary prevention, which typically involves rehabilitation and other aspects of long-term care. Tertiary prevention can also be applied to scientific misconduct, inasmuch as those who commit such misconduct may require rehabilitation before they return to scientific practice. A more complete analysis will likely lead, as it did in the case of primary and secondary prevention, to questions with answers based on relatively little empirical information. Indeed, in the foregoing analysis, a host of such questions have emerged. Answers will be difficult to obtain, especially if precise scientific methodologies are to be employed. But then, we are scientists, and solving difficult empirical problems is what we do best. Perhaps the essential question is less methodological than motivational: Are we as scientists willing to study our conduct as scientists? If so, then one day we may discover why we suffer from an important and sometimes disabling professional affliction and what works to prevent it.

I am not suggesting, however, that we should postpone interventions until we fully understand the etiology, including the underlying biological, behavioral, and social mechanisms involved in the range of activities we call scientific misconduct. We need fair investigative procedures. We can accept (perhaps on faith) that the discussion of the role of ethics in the conduct of science and medicine should be expanded. Those of us who act as mentors can and should conduct ourselves virtuously. For the sake of those we train, especially for those whose lives are improved by our scientific results, we must exhibit excellence, self-effacement, and, perhaps above all, an unwavering commitment to the truth.

Section Two

Rules of Authorship

80   When Authorship Fails

A Proposal to Make Contributors Accountable

DRUMMOND RENNIE, VERONICA YANK, AND LINDA L. EMANUEL

THE ETHICAL BASIS OF PUBLICATION LIES IN TRUST AND ACCOUNTABILITY

Published articles are the means whereby new work is communicated between scientists and scholars. However, they also establish priority, reputation, and standing. Publications are necessary for the correct attribution of credit, which we are defining here to mean public recognition of scientific discovery, and they constitute a major coin of the realm by which academics proceed along the toll road of promotion. It is for these reasons that scientists view authorship with so much anxiety and passion.

A foundation of trust underlies the entire publication enterprise. Science requires skepticism on the part of readers, but they should be able to start with the assumption that the investigators' report is an honest representation of what they have observed. Readers are forced to accord authors trust because readers cannot be in the authors' institutions checking their work. This need to trust the authors' honesty is the basis of Lederberg's assertion that "[a]bove all, the act of publication is an inscription under oath, a testimony...."

Trust in science is made possible by accountability. This became clear in the special case of anonymous publication, popular 200 years ago. Anonymous opinion was considered to be more objective, and thus more authoritative, because the writer was thought to be shielded from prejudice. However, as anonymity freed the writer from accountability for the work, its advantages were found to be spurious and the system was abandoned.

In accepting accountability, authors must ensure that the manuscript is a faithful and accurate representation of the work they did, and commit to resolving any questions that arise after publication. The standards they follow are those of telling the truth and nothing but the truth. It is central to our thesis that the collaborators, who are the witnesses of the work, hold each other to these standards of proof. The fulfillment of these duties requires meticulous research, as well as the investigators' faithful representation of the work in manuscripts. The standards must equally apply to attributions in multiauthored manuscripts (the byline and acknowledgments) to make the account of who deserves credit, and takes responsibility, as honest and complete as the report itself.

HISTORICAL CHANGES: FROM ONE AUTHOR TO MANY

The concept of an author developed, like that of a composer, when there was but one accountable for the whole work. Sole, named authorship remained the predominant tradition in science until about 1955. But in science, as elsewhere, there has been a proliferation and specialization of jobs. The total number of scientists has multiplied, as have their total number of publications, and the number of authors per publication. As the proportion of 1- and 2-author publications has fallen, the proportion with 3 and 4 or more has risen. Multiple authorship of articles is now the norm. These changes have had an impact on the circumstances and concept of authorship.

THE PRESENT AUTHORSHIP SYSTEM REEXAMINED

Collaboration Prompts New Questions about Accountability

The extreme example of the trend toward "big science" is that of the large, multicenter clinical trial, a phenomenon

Drummond Rennie, Veronica Yank, and Linda L. Emanuel, "When Authorship Fails: A Proposal to Make Contributors Accountable," *JAMA* 278 (1997): 579–85.

of the 1990s, which may involve hundreds of investigators and institutions. But even in smaller projects, collaborators have different areas of expertise that allow them to make separate contributions to the project and that delineate and limit their accountability for their respective contributions.

The collaborators also have titles that are not tightly linked to their jobs in the project. A scientist with the title of "principal investigator," for example, may do little more than fund the project and provide distant oversight, or may originate the study, design it, and work daily toward its completion. While any system of authorship should recognize credit and accountability based on jobs rather than titles, it seems clear that this is often not the case. Twenty researchers worldwide, more than half being heads of biomedical laboratories, published at least once every 11.3 days throughout the 1980s. It is certainly conceivable that sometimes their contributions were minimal.

It is difficult to give a clear account of who did which part of the research, thereby identifying who is responsible for it, when there is no clear and accepted method of delineating the overlapping, cooperative activities of multiple collaborators. Though the reader must assume that the collaborators have fulfilled their duty to hold each other to standards, ambiguity in the meaning of the byline undermines their practice of this duty. It is for these reasons that we believe that the current system of authorship is inadequate, prone to misunderstanding, and abused.

Authorship Disputes

Authorship disputes now arise frequently, partly because scientists have not addressed the root of the problem: lack of clarity and openness about authorship. Indeed, vagueness in the byline opens the door to unfair attribution. This may explain why disputes about authorship are increasingly common, so wasteful of time, and so poorly resolved. Vagueness results in egregious behavior being left unexamined because roles and expectations are undefined and undisclosed. It is for this reason that, at present, the Office of Research Integrity does not even consider cases of alleged plagiarism if they seem to involve a dispute among coauthors.

Multiple Authorship Diminishes Accountability More than Credit

The coin of publication has 2 sides: credit and accountability. On the credit side, no one has the least idea what the coin is worth, or who should be awarded coins, or how the coins should be lined up for inspection, so everyone takes credit. On the flip side of accountability, the greater the number of coauthors, the less responsibility any will take for the whole. So the expansion in numbers of authors per article has tended to dilute accountability, while scarcely seeming to diminish credit. Promotion systems that place more value on numbers of publications than on actual contributions exacerbate the problem. This tendency may explain why many authors perceive it to be in their self-interest to preserve the status quo. It may also explain, in part, why coauthors of fraudulent scientists so readily defend themselves by denying knowledge of the fabrications.

Misuse of the Current System of Attribution

Given that one of the foundations of the scientific enterprise is trust, it is disconcerting to observe such a disconnect between credit and responsibility, where the author's duty to be accountable is shirked. Some coauthors have been unwilling to take the necessary steps to ensure the integrity of their manuscripts, including their colleagues' work. Others have failed to provide journals with highly relevant facts, though these would change the conclusions of the manuscript. Or they have submitted to journals manuscripts containing data known, after audit, to be fraudulent without telling the editors.

Guest authorship is the practice of inviting those whose contribution has been scientifically trivial to be coauthors, as payment for a service (e.g., referral of a patient) or as tribute (e.g., homage to a department head). The practice of guest authorship is deceptive because the "authors" so named gather credit without being able to account for the work. It is frequent, deceptive, and dangerous to the guests, who are expected to vouch for the work. The cases of Darsee, Slutsky, and Pearce are all examples of fraudulent scientists seeking out coauthors simply to lend legitimacy to their fraudulent publications.

Ghost authorship occurs when those who wrote the article, or contributed in important ways to its production, are not named as coauthors. Known instances are becoming common, as is the practice of paying big names to appear on the byline in place of the ghosts, though they contributed nothing except their prestige.

A variant of the practice is for companies to give grants to academics to write up, and to journals to publish, the results of studies carried out by firms acting for drug manufacturers. None of those who carried out the study appeared as authors so there was no link between authorship and accountability. In another case, the manufacturer who paid for the study blocked the researchers from publishing it, and then published the researchers' results, but with opposite results and with none of the researchers named as authors.

Repeated publication of the same work, with or without minor additions, inflates bibliographies and is common. When similar parts of the same trial are published repeatedly under different authors' names, without cross-referencing, the record is distorted in the name of promotion, and meta-analysis is confounded to the detriment of care.

Disagreement about Who Is Responsible

The scientific community is divided about how to apply current authorship standards where the contributions of collaborators have overlapped. Because Regalado has shown that there has been an increase in articles with very large authorships since 1990, it is unlikely that the debate will diminish.

The chief area of disagreement about responsibility concerns that of a coauthor's responsibility for work done largely by others. Neglect of responsibility was fairly clear in one case when the authors advocating a test did not have the expertise to know that their published figure, prepared by someone else, was factitious. However, other cases have proved more ambiguous. In 1989, 2 researchers at Stanford University were found by a National Institutes of Health (NIH) panel to be guilty of scientific misconduct in relation to several multiauthored articles. Stanford University insisted that all the authors shared responsibility for the whole article. In contrast, the NIH panel felt that the requisite "detailed and in-depth level of knowledge by all collaborators is not feasible in contemporary multidisciplinary research."

The problem was summarized starkly by a recent exchange of letters in *Science* concerning an article on a case of fraud. Wooley wrote, "If you haven't done the work, don't put your name on the paper. If you put your name on the paper, then you are stuck with it," while de Sa and Sagar agreed that "[c]o-authors should bear collective responsibility for their publications, sharing blame as well as credit. It is a contradiction to be a co-author but then plead ignorance (and assume victim status) if there is controversy regarding data in the paper."

In contrast, 4 letters asserted that holding all authors fully responsible for all aspects of a publication would increase the risks of collaboration, especially between different specialties, to suicidal levels; was ridiculous in massive projects; and implied omniscience.

The answer to such controversies seems obvious: those who did the work should explain who did what. It is encouraging to note, therefore, that some researchers on collaborative projects already explain to editors what work each person performed. While this may satisfy the editor, by itself it cannot help those readers or authors who want to see public distinctions in recognition.

Editors have to take the position that since only the investigators know who contributed what, only the investigators can decide on authorship. At the same time, they, as well as indexing services such as those of the National Library of Medicine (NLM), have founded policies on the reasonable assumption that to limit the allowable number of authors for each article will not only save space, but will concentrate the minds of collaborators on deciding who merits authorship.

Huth has argued that only a few persons can truly serve the functions of responsible authors: adding authors beyond the number that can really be responsible for an article's content "debases the currency of authorship." While sympathizing with Huth, we also note that journals vary widely in the number of authors they customarily allow. Moreover, editors are constantly required to make exceptions to their own rules, which weakens the claim that setting a limit on the number of authors can solve the problem of responsibility.

Large, multi-institutional clinical trials highlight the different goals of editors and authors most clearly. On the one hand, the Uniform Requirements of the International Committee of Medical Journal Editors (ICMJE or "the Vancouver Group") have served notice that all members of groups carrying out multicenter trials who wish to be named as authors "should fully meet the requirements" (see below). Kassirer has recently emphasized "that in every paper, each listed author must be able to take public responsibility for its content," a position already taken for the *New England Journal of Medicine* by Relman and by Glass for *JAMA*.

On the other hand, those who carry out large clinical trials (trialists) face an extreme version of the problem of being unable, in the current authorship system, to assign credit fairly and publicly recognize their many colleagues for their work. Trialists in the field believe they work hard but get no respect, because some outsiders characterize them as being ill-trained in the scientific method or lacking a research role beyond that of being technicians or enrollers of patients. Yet the whole depends on their meticulous exertions. Whatever the reason, trialists resent it when editors set up rules that award senior authors alone and exclude them from public acknowledgment. Carbone, noting this indignation, has suggested that limiting authorship severely will have a paradoxical effect: it will reward those who get it wrong by reporting small, nonrandomized trials, and punish those who go to very great trouble to get it right.

RESPONSIBLE AUTHORSHIP: EFFORTS SO FAR AND WHAT IS STILL LACKING

It is clear from this catalog of problems, confusions, and incompatibilities that the scientific community finds the current system of attributing authorship inadequate for describing modern research activities, while scientists also lack consensus on how to apply the system. In response, many efforts have been made to try to resolve these dilemmas.

The Vancouver Definition of Authorship

To focus the attention of scientists on accountability, the Vancouver Group in the mid 1980s codified and began disseminating a definition of authorship that emphasizes the idea of responsibility. In the Uniform Requirements for Manuscripts Submitted to Biomedical Journals of 1993, the definition states:

> Each author should have participated sufficiently in the work to take public responsibility for the content. Authorship credit should be based only on substantial contributions to (a) conception and design, or analysis and interpretation of data; and to (b) drafting the article or revising it critically for important intellectual content; and on (c) final approval of the version to be published. Conditions (a), (b), and (c) must all be met.... Any part of an article critical to its main conclusions must be the responsibility of at least one author. Editors may require authors to justify the assignment of authorship.

Order of Authorship

Recognizing that authorship is "awarded" inconsistently, scientists and editors in all sorts of disciplines have attempted to bring coherence to the order of authors by publishing their view of what is denoted by each position in the list.

Some scientists contend that the names in the byline should be listed in order of seniority, others that an author's place does not matter because credit is equal, or, alternatively, it does indeed matter because the system works like the prizes at a golf tournament: each successive finisher receives half the credit of the one ahead, down to 5 (or 6, or perhaps 8). Research colleagues all seem to "know" that the second author is always the statistician, or the graduate student if the graduate student is not first, or the physician who entered the most patients, but it is never the senior author, who, because of noblesse oblige, usually appears last, unless his or her noblesse has somehow failed to oblige. Burman has produced an especially elaborate outline for placing people on the authorship totem pole.

Similarly, in an American Association for the Advancement of Science survey, only 7 of 39 editors of clinical journals confirmed that they "knew" what the order of authors meant in their articles, because they had written policies on the subject, yet these varied so widely that the first author could be the student, the person who did most of the work, the senior author, or whoever had previously been determined by official protocol. Other editors, taking another approach, have tried to remove any hidden meaning from the order of authors, by insisting that authors be listed alphabetically. They have found for their pains that authors late in the alphabet have avoided their journals.

Everyone is equally sure about their own system; the point is that none of these schemes is actually disclosed, so the readers, to whom this should be addressed, are not let in on the secret: they have not been told which code book to use and how it works. Indeed, Davies et al. have recently shown that only 1 of 16 Canadian departments of pediatrics had "explicit written criteria for evaluating authorship" of scientific articles, and, not surprisingly, the departments demonstrated great variability in their methods of assessing authorship.

The article on order of authorship that makes the best sense is the one by Davis and Gregerman in 1969, and this was written as a joke. These authors suggested allocation of credit on the basis of the fraction of the total work performed. What makes particular sense is that the system is open to the reader and easily understood.

Initiatives to Promote Good Authorship Practices

Other commendable initiatives to promote good authorship practices include efforts, often similar and synergistic, by universities, professional societies, and outstanding researchers, as well as journals.

All journals should keep publishing their criteria for, and policies on, authorship, and they should require authors to sign forms attesting that they take responsibility. Statements and forms give notice (authors cannot later plead ignorance), draw attention, and so educate. Conversely, it may be awkward for an editor to object to a deceptive practice when the journal has never printed the rules of the game. Such criteria may also have prevented the cases of a listed coauthor, after publication, having to dissociate himself from an article he knew nothing about. Journals, in addition, should continue to flush ghost authors into the open by insisting that all who contributed substantially are named, so that they can take credit as well as responsibility. Finally, editors should draw their readers' attention to poor behavior that is discovered only after publication. Embarrassment is a powerful tool. The Rudolf Virchow principle, "In my journal anyone can make a fool of himself," should be used by the editor, for just that: to expose misleading or dishonest practices that have slipped into print.

Although we support these efforts, we believe they do not and cannot resolve existing problems, because specialization of jobs has made the original concept of authorship impractical, and the authorship system's vagueness about contribution makes it prone to abuse. Even when current standards for authorship are strictly applied, they fail to represent accurately who should receive what credit and responsibility for aspects of cooperative projects. It is as obvious to us as it is to Bruce Squires (a long-time member of the Vancouver Group) that the "ICMJE definition is not working," a conclusion backed up by Drenth. With modern research by multiple investigators, the authorship model is outmoded, stretched: it no longer fits.

OUR PROPOSALS

Any new system that will reinforce trust and accuracy in the publication enterprise must convince readers of accountability for articles at 2 levels—for each part, or contribution, and for the whole. The idea that accountability can be divided and overlapping reflects the reality that the many-person, 1-product research article of today is an aggregation of the work of many people, each of whom takes full responsibility for certain parts of the project. But for the system to be able to identify accountability, there must be disclosure to the reader of every participant's contributions to the work and to the manuscript. It is equally necessary that the reader receive assurances as to the quality and integrity of the work as a whole. In the end, the only people who can accept accountability for the entire article are one or more of the coinvestigators.

The Job-Centered Approach: Credit (and Blame) Where It Is Due

Because the current system of authorship is idiosyncratic, ambiguous, and predisposed to misuse, we propose in its place a radical change: a new system that is accurate and discloses accountability. We propose the substitution of the word and concept *contributor* for the word and concept *author*. Like others before us, we are concerned to acknowledge work performed. But the word *author* is too imprecise to delineate the work of those many people named in the bylines of articles today. The word *contributor*, on the other hand, describes someone who provides jointly with others or who writes an article. Contribution is the activity of science that is most relevant to publication because its disclosure can identify who is accountable for what part of the research and allows the reader to assign credit fairly.

Abandoning the concept of author in favor of contributor frees us from the historical and emotional connotations of authorship, and leads us to a concept that is far more in line with the actuality of modern scientific cooperative work. No contributors can shirk responsibility or have credit withheld by avoiding or not having their names and work specified. The critical feature of our model is the idea that contributors describe their actual research activities to the reader. Thus, the plan is a simple one: it discloses what each person has already done.

Describing Contributions

Coworkers should meet, discuss, and decide on their respective contributions to the project, as well as the relative value of the contributions to the whole, and in what order to list them in publications. Joint or overlapping activities should be described as such. We recognize that researchers may find this activity challenging, but it is a duty that should grow easier with practice.

The contributions to be described are more complex, detailed, and accurate than the principal components of authorship activities noted in the Uniform Requirements. The coworkers might start with a general roster of contributions that can be expanded and made more specific. When necessary, these descriptions can be combined in series to clarify further the exact, perhaps multiple, contributions of each person. For example, contributors may agree on descriptions similar to those listed below, which accompanied a manuscript submitted to *JAMA* (the 3 names have been removed):

1. Design of the review, literature search, data extraction, data analysis, production of first draft, revision of subsequent drafts, coordination of communication among all investigators.

2. Literature search, retrieval of articles, creation of data extraction forms, data extraction, data analysis, comments on first draft, creation of first draft of table, comments on subsequent drafts.

3. Generation of the idea for a review on this topic, design of the review, financial support, comments on drafts.

As the practice of using job descriptions to disclose contribution becomes common, it may be helpful to develop predefined job categories that are made clear to the reader. Then phrases can be consistent across many research groups. However, it is important to remember that job categories—such as those seen in film credits ("director," "best boy," "key grip")—are intrinsically more rigid and less useful than phrases that describe the actual duties performed. Before job categories replace job descriptions, therefore, researchers and journals will have to be careful to develop descriptors for contribution that are accurate, flexible, and intelligible.

After agreeing on what jobs each did and how to describe them, the colleagues should determine the relative contribution of each person, perhaps as a percent value, to the project as a whole. Though it may be difficult to assign a numeric value to these estimations and they need not be published, the exercise will be useful in determining the order of contributors (see below).

Guarantors

All contributors are fully responsible for the portions of the work they performed and have some obligation to hold one another to standards of integrity. At the same time, special contributors must be designated and disclosed as guarantors of the whole work. Guarantors are those people who have contributed substantially, but who also have made added efforts to ensure the integrity of the entire project. They organize, oversee, double-check, and must be prepared to be accountable for all parts of the completed manuscript, before and after publication. In this way the role of guarantor is precisely defined and differs from that of "first author" or "corresponding author" or "senior author," there being many examples of these showing themselves unable to vouch for the whole work.

The role of the guarantor is best demonstrated in the contrasting responses of Felig (in 1979) and Collins (in 1996) to charges that their respective junior colleagues had falsified data in articles they coauthored with the senior scientists. A Yale advisory committee found that Felig had exercised "poor judgment" in not aggressively investigating charges that his junior had doctored data. In contrast, it seems that Collins, director of the National Center for Human Genome Research at the NIH [since 1997, the National Human Genome Research Institute (NHGRI)— eds.], responded with dispatch. Accepting responsibility for the aftercare of his work, Collins quickly corrected the published literature by exposing tainted data in 5 articles, thereby preventing other researchers from wasting further efforts in trying to replicate the faulty reports. His last important act as the articles' guarantor thus was publicly and speedily to withdraw his "guarantee" that they were based on honest science.

Such examples illustrate how essential it is, for the integrity of science, that contributors identify those among them who are guarantors and publish the description "guarantor" in the list of contributors (see below).

Order of Contributors

We have been highly skeptical of the order of authorship as a way to convey to the reader the investigators' respective levels of contribution. But we cannot ignore 2 facts: that printing the names requires some sort of listing, and that coworkers will tend to covet positions that lend their names prominence, near the top of the list or in the last place. The colleagues, to address these preferences, and having agreed already on their respective contributions, should list their names systematically—in the byline and in the contributors list—according to the relative importance of their duties: in descending order, starting with the collaborator who made the most substantial contributions.

Disclosure to the Reader: The Contributors List and the Byline

All collaborators must disclose to the reader, and not merely the editor, the contributions and guarantors on which they have agreed. These descriptions should be displayed next to the appropriate names in the *contributors list,* which should appear as a footnote on the first page of the article. Our model thus demands job-driven identification of contribution, determined by the colleagues themselves and displayed by editors.

Each journal editor decides on the exact method used to disclose the contributors list, but should not limit the number of contributors who are named as long as each has added usefully to the work. If the editor notes that no one has accounted for key aspects of the project, he or she can require that the contributors identify the responsible person.

The byline, just below the title of the article, should name only those who contributed most substantially to the work. Journals may set their own rules about how many contributors can be listed in the byline, as they do now. A journal might decide, for example, to name only those participants whose contributions total more than 5% or 10% of the work, or, to use another criterion, all those whose contributions could alter substantive parts of the article. Informed of the journal's policy, the collaborators, again by consensus, identify all those who meet the criteria for being listed in the byline. These contributors should be those then required to sign the contribution (old "authorship") statement, together with the copyright, financial disclosure, and other forms currently used by the journal.

Policies of Indexing Services

Indexing databases such as those of the NLM are second only to journals in their ability to recognize and publicize researchers' names and contributions to science. Like journals, they may establish their own guidelines as to the number of contributors that can be cited. If this seems arbitrary, one should note that the present convention for deciding who gets cited developed in an arbitrary manner. For example, the Vancouver Group initially stated that indexing services should list the first 3 names on articles. But in 1994, endorsing a plan originating with the NLM, it ruled instead that reference lists should name the top 6. More recently, molecular biologists have persuaded the NLM to list the first 24 names, plus that of the last author. In general, journal policies on the number of researchers that are listed in the byline have coincided with the number the NLM indexes will cite. When naming contributors, journals and indexing services should continue to coordinate their respective policies.

In addition, indexing services may consider implementing a mechanism for having each publication record disclose the contributors list of the article, or at least the names and contributions of those people in the byline. Such descriptions, along with an option for searching, by key word, multiple contributors lists, would enable readers to identify colleagues in their specialty or the contributors to whom they should direct specific questions.

Policies at Universities, Agencies, and Societies

Journals and indexing services may lead the way, but academic centers and granting agencies can influence the culture substantially through their hiring, promotions, and grant review committees. These committees should require that the references to each publication on the applicant's curriculum vitae include the description of the applicant's work that appeared on the article's contributors list. Professional societies should also institute consistent policies of disclosure of contribution in their materials: as Hopfield has noted, truth in labeling could be an effective force in science if promoted by leading professional societies.

To change how we recognize credit and responsibility for articles, therefore, a number of influential groups—journals, indexers, academic and funding institutions, and professional societies—must agree to implement this explicit and transparent system for recognizing contribution.

WHY THE PLAN WILL WORK

General Advantages of the Proposal

There are several reasons to think that this system would be an improvement on the current one:

1. It is descriptively precise. Precision encourages a high level of honesty, which has intrinsic merit. It is also likely to bear unanticipated practical advantages, since a foundation that requires exacting levels of honesty is more solid than a foundation that allows for deceptions. Readers will feel able to allocate credit and responsibility accurately.

2. It is fair. Contributors should feel assured that they will be recognized appropriately. It will discourage guest and ghost authorship by forcing putative "authors" to describe their contributions, or else withdraw. Distinctions in the credit given for differential work will remain (for example, for being a guarantor or the first listed contributor), but provided that there is honest attribution, at one blow all the problems of hierarchy, order, and undeclared meaning will vanish.

3. It may discourage fraud. The proposed system is likely to provide additional protection against fraud by specifying responsibilities so that individuals are more effectively and publicly linked to those tasks for which they are accountable. Cross-checking of roles may also inhibit fraud by making it harder for individuals or collaborators to maintain a lie.

Specific Benefits: Why the Proposal Is Useful

1. Academic appointment and promotions committees now will be able to weigh coins that have visible, assessable worth. Institutions frequently, but variably, ask candidates to specify the part they played in their research. The advantage to institutions will be that instead of wondering if an individual has given, in retrospect, a biased view of his or her role, they will be able to look up explicit statements: and the guarantee is that the candidate's colleagues agreed on the identified contributions at the time of the article's publication.

2. Collaborators should obtain better protection from abuse by colleagues. In particular, those who feel increasingly put upon by the current system, junior researchers, may gain because the proposal will make it less easy to defend—to oneself, let alone to others—an inaccurate and inflated statement of contribution.

Skepticisms Addressed

Recognizing that some readers may have doubts about the necessity of this proposal, we have tried to anticipate and answer their concerns here.

1. "This proposal is no different than the present system of authors and acknowledgments." The proposal differs substantively from the present system by eliminating the artificial distinction, mostly of a social nature, between authors and nonauthor contributors—that is, between "authors" and "acknowledgees." The contributions of all (not just those of acknowledgees) are described and disclosed.

2. "Researchers will be reluctant to be on the leading edge of change, especially when the response of promotions committees and funding agencies is still unknown." We acknowledge the possibility of such resistance. At the same time, however, if journals and indexers adopt the plan, this will greatly encourage

researchers to comply. Accompanying changes within academic centers, granting agencies, and professional societies will also promote the transition.

3. "It will not stop 'contributors' from claiming, when problems arise, that they did not understand what another contributor was doing." Authors already deny responsibility. But with responsibility pinned upon them for those contributions they have explicitly identified as their own, contributors will find it harder to make this excuse.

4. "It will not stop those who made minimal contributions from getting their names on articles if they have influence and seniority." Maybe. But we think that in a system that requires people to be explicit, people are less apt to lie by claiming that they performed work done by others.

5. "It is cumbersome." The counterargument to this critique is simply that the time, space, and attention are worth it. The extensive energy already expended on trying to resolve problems in the current system demonstrates that the research community wishes to have the most fair and honest system possible: for what could be a more important precondition for honest reporting of data than honest attribution of credit and responsibility for that data? The space taken up by a footnote in fact would be small. Moreover, giving written accounts of their respective work will be a familiar process for many researchers, who already do so in correspondence with editors.

6. "It will lead to hair-splitting negotiations about the origin of ideas, so often joint, and the amount of work done." This danger should be acknowledged, but with practice researchers should become more used to openly discussing and resolving what their contributions have been. The benefits of a better system will outweigh the effort required for such discussions.

7. "It would have been adopted a long time ago were it a good plan." We are by no means the first to advocate listing the contributions of authors, so the answer to this point is best addressed by looking at the research environment from both an individual and a historical perspective. First, colleagues may continue to perceive themselves to benefit from leaving the question of their contribution ambiguous: if we leave the meaning of the byline obscure, then each of us will be able to claim 95% of the credit, but accept only 5% of the blame, for all our multiauthored articles. As Zuckerman described, when discussing order of authorship and the noblesse oblige of Nobel prize winners, ambiguity makes the evaluation of individual roles impossible, but it also "reduces the stress of collaboration" and so may oil the research wheels. We believe this is a poor excuse to avoid frankness, which may prevent future disputes—and thus future stress—among collaborators. The colleagues of fraudulent scientists must surely wish they had gone through a process of delineating contribution. Second, it is only recently that multiauthor articles have come to dominate biomedical publications; consequently, it has taken some time for scientists to begin to understand that the current system of authorship no longer fits their research reality and cannot meet their needs: with the steady increase in collaborators per article and the ambiguity of the definition of authorship, a new system is needed.

It Has Worked Before: The Example of Large Trials

There is evidence that the proposal of listing contributions is practical, because there are good examples of the contributor, or job-description, approach already in the literature. In fact, it has been adopted before, but only in the case of large trials. For example, an article from the ISIS (International Study of Infarct Survival) Collaborative Group listed roughly 2000 "members," whom we would call contributors, usefully divided by committee (writing, steering, data monitoring, and the like) and by country and hospital, and with the tasks of the overseeing research unit described in detail.

This is an entirely reasonable, job-based approach, treating all participants as contributors, their work being differentiated and displayed: it fits the reality and assigns accountability. We endorse it, with the addition that guarantors be named.

Recent Developments

We presented these ideas at a meeting on June 6, 1996, at the University of Nottingham, sponsored by *The Lancet* and the *British Medical Journal* [*BMJ*]. They formed the main focus of discussion at that meeting, and part of the agenda at the meeting of the Vancouver Group, which followed immediately and which one of us (D. R.) attended. As a result, the Uniform Requirements for authorship have been modified to include the statement: "Editors may ask authors to describe what each contributed; this information may be published." Finally, on July 5, 1997, *The Lancet* adopted a major part of our proposals by requiring publication of the contributions of its various contributors. [. . .]

CODA

The key to realizing this idea of linking credit to responsibility by telling readers what the authors actually contributed was to work through the editors of the clinical journals. This is because in a matter having to do with publication, editors are in the position of being able to enforce standards. Once that happened, scientists would fall into line. First editors had to be convinced that authorship was in trouble, that readers had a right to know who did what, and that it was unrealistic to expect all authors of a manuscript to take responsibility for everything. Given editors' numerous bad experiences, this was not a hard sell. The fact remains, however, that there is an inertia and conservatism in all of us, including editors. Though several major journals had rapidly adopted the system, it required sustained effort by several organizations over five years to spread the concept and convince those who had thought of the existing system as being immutable.

Not only did the International Committee of Medical Journal Editors endorse the plan, but in the U.S., the Council of Science Editors (CSE) did so too. Under the enthusi-astic leadership of Frank Davidoff, editor of the *Annals of Internal Medicine,* the CSE held several workshops and retreats, at which editors, scientists, and university and science administrators discussed the idea. At the last such retreat, held in 2001, as no one had raised any ethical problems, and numerous editors had described their successful institution of the system, it was decided that no further such meetings were necessary as it was highly likely that the system would gradually spread.

It was recognized from the start that journals had to emphatically declare it as being their policy. The prestigious journal *Nature* adopted the plan, but with a fatal flaw: they made it voluntary. All of us want power without responsibility, so it was no surprise to find that few authors accepted the invitation to describe who did what, though numerous authors took it as an invitation to declare that they had had the chief role in the study. Apart from that flaw, the steady adoption of this transparent and ethical system seems to be inevitable.

[Coda contributed by Drummond Rennie, M.D., April 2002—eds.]

Section Three

Problems in the Publication of Research Methods and Findings

---

81   Underreporting Research Is Scientific Misconduct

IAIN CHALMERS

Scientific misconduct is commonly conceptualized as deliberate falsification of data—a sin of commission—but sins of omission may be even more important. [...]

Selective underreporting of research is almost certainly more widespread and more likely to have adverse consequences for patients than the publication of deliberately falsified data. At least there is an accepted mechanism—attempted replication of reported investigations—for

reducing the likelihood of being misled by false inferences based on contrived but fully published reports. No such protective mechanism currently exists with respect to the apparently systematic tendency to underreport certain kinds of valid research findings.

Adequate reporting of clinical trials is required for both scientific and ethical reasons. Failure to publish "disappointing" or "uninteresting" research results, or failure to report results in sufficient detail, may either lead patients to receive ineffective or dangerous forms of care or result in a delay in recognizing that other forms of care are beneficial. Neither of these consequences is in the in-

Iain Chalmers, "Underreporting Research Is Scientific Misconduct," *JAMA* 263 (1990): 1405–8.

terests of patients. In addition, failure to provide adequate, publicly available reports of the results of clinical trials does an injustice to the patients who have participated in them, as well as to others who have collaborated with the investigators and those who have provided funds or other resources.

EXAMPLES OF THE CONSEQUENCES OF UNDERREPORTING CLINICAL TRIALS

[...] Debate has existed for many years about whether routine hospitalization of women with uncomplicated twin pregnancies for bed rest reduces the risk of preterm delivery. The results of two relatively recent surveys of practice in the United Kingdom, for example, suggest that British obstetricians are more or less equally divided on the matter. The issue is not trivial: if a policy of routine hospitalization does indeed decrease the risk of preterm delivery in a group of women at higher than average risk of this outcome, it would obviously be important to know this; on the other hand, if controlled trials could rule out any material advantage of such a policy, then abandoning the policy would avoid disrupting the lives of women who would rather not be admitted to a hospital, as well as allowing redistribution of health service resources.

The first randomized evaluation of hospitalization for bed rest in uncomplicated twin pregnancy was conducted in Harare, Zimbabwe, in 1977. The trial was mounted because pressure on antenatal hospital beds had become so acute that some rationalization of their use had become essential. A preliminary analysis of the trial suggested that, far from reducing the risk of preterm delivery, routine hospitalization was actually associated with an increased rate of this unwanted outcome. The trial fulfilled its immediate purpose—to provide information on which a rational policy decision could be made in Harare—and the policy of routine hospitalization for uncomplicated twin pregnancy was abandoned.

Unfortunately, the investigators did not perceive it as their duty to make the results of their study more generally available for guiding clinical practice and research elsewhere. The results of the trial would have remained unreported had it not been for the fact that, 7 years later, two visitors to Harare "discovered" these unpublished data and helped the investigators to analyze and report their unreported trial. A full account of the trial was subsequently published in *The Lancet*.

The results of this trial, taken together with comparable findings in a similar trial conducted in Finland reported at about the same time, provoked reevaluation of an obstetric policy that has been widely accepted for four decades and led clinical investigators to organize further controlled trials. These responses were postponed unnecessarily by the initial failure to report the results of the Harare trial. At

the very least, this delay led to continued inappropriate deployment of limited resources; at worst, it may have resulted in the continued use of a harmful policy.

The second example from the perinatal field concerns the unresolved question as to whether routine (as opposed to selective) ultrasonography is justified in every pregnancy. Controlled comparisons of routine and selective ultrasonography have shown that routine ultrasonography is associated with a lower incidence of induction of labor in pregnancies deemed to be "postterm," but the published trials have not been large enough to assess whether this effect is associated with any reduction in the frequency of substantive adverse outcomes of pregnancy.

The confusion in this field is compounded by the fact that one large trial of routine ultrasonography, conducted nearly 10 years ago, remains unpublished. If the results of this trial show beneficial effects of routine ultrasonography, this would be important evidence on which to base current policy; if no benefits are demonstrated, this might reflect either technical inadequacies of the ultrasound equipment (or its application) during the era in which the trial was conducted, or the fact that routine ultrasonography has nothing important to offer over selective use of the technology. Either way, a full report of the results of the trial has current relevance.

Assessment of the effects of routine ultrasonography in pregnancy is also bedeviled by inadequate published reports of relevant trials. The only randomized trial to suggest that routine ultrasonography has any beneficial effects on substantive outcomes of pregnancy is that conducted in Ålesund, Norway, by Eik-Nes and colleagues in 1979 and 1980. This potentially important trial has never been fully reported in a scientific journal. The reports that are available are contradictory in a very important respect. The only readily available account of the trial, published as a letter to the editor in *The Lancet*, states that women allocated to routine ultrasonography were compared with controls who "were not examined routinely but could be referred for ultrasound examination on a clinical indication." This description is at odds with an account of the trial presented to and published by the NIH some months earlier. In that report Eik-Nes and Okland state that "[t]he pregnant population was randomized either to have routine ultrasound examination twice in pregnancy or *not to have ultrasound at all* [my emphasis]. . . . The control group with no ultrasound went through routine pregnancy care as had been done before ultrasound was introduced at the hospital. All the problems in connection with the pregnancy were solved without the use of ultrasound."

This inconsistency between the only two reports of this trial is clearly of great importance in any attempt to answer the still inadequately addressed question of whether routine ultrasonography is preferable to selective ultrasonography (as opposed to withholding ultrasonography completely). Again, substantial health service resources are involved, and, furthermore, there is no basis for assuming that routine ultrasonography is innocuous.

DIFFICULTIES IN CORRECTING THE PROBLEM OF UNDERREPORTING AFTER THE EVENT

The two perinatal examples cited above were selected to illustrate how inadequate reporting of clinical research can jeopardize the formulation of well-founded clinical policies. Because of this effect, underreporting operates against the interests of patients, not to mention those who fund health services, including the public. [. . .]

In an attempt to identify unpublished randomized trials, we conducted a survey of over 40,000 obstetricians and pediatricians in the 18 countries in which the vast majority of published perinatal trials had been conducted. However, we were notified of only 18 unpublished trials completed between 1940 and the end 1984, a period during which at least 2300 reports of perinatal trials had been published, a ratio of unpublished to published trials of 1:128. Ratios of unpublished to published trials derived from smaller, more focused surveys of clinical research have been of the order of 1:5. This suggests that we failed to identify substantial numbers of unpublished trials, and we are certainly aware of several unpublished trials that were not reported to us.

Because trials with results that are regarded as "positive" are more likely to be published in the more widely read and cited journals, and because we wished (when possible) to increase the statistical precision of our estimates of the differential effects of alternative forms of care by synthesizing evidence from similar trials in overviews (meta-analyses), we conducted a systematic manual search of about 60 core journals, back to the issues published in 1950. These manual searches yielded about twice the number of trials that could be retrieved through MEDLINE using methodological descriptors.

In addition, we were concerned to reduce the biases that result from selective underreporting of results within studies. This form of underreporting may occur either when the analysis presented has not been based on all the people entered into the trial or when the investigators have selected data for presentation on the basis of the pattern of results observed—for example, because the differences observed were statistically significant. So we contacted investigators, when this was possible, and asked them to provide the missing information.

The results of this work have been published in book form and as a continuously updated electronic publication, the *Oxford Database of Perinatal Trials*. Although we have made considerable efforts to offset the adverse consequences of underreporting of clinical research in our re-

view of evidence about the effects of care during pregnancy and childbirth, we can never know the extent to which implementation of these precautions succeeded in producing unbiased estimates of the effects of care.

HOW MIGHT THE PROBLEM BE REDUCED?

Many people could help to ensure that the likelihood of underreporting clinical trials is reduced.

The main change in behavior is required among clinical investigators, and it is the named principal investigators who have primary responsibility for ensuring that the study is reported in full. Because short-term employment contracts may sometimes compromise the ability of principal investigators to see a project through to completion in the form of a published report, ultimate responsibility for ensuring that a full report is submitted for publication would seem to rest with the heads of the departments with which the principal investigators are, or were, affiliated.

It is surprising that so many research-funding organizations do not make an award of funds to researchers conditional on a full report being prepared and published. Similarly, it is surprising that investigators continue to collaborate in commercially organized research without ensuring that the results of the research will be analyzed and reported by people who have no commercial vested interest in selective underreporting. Matters might improve if the reasonable expectations of all parties were more frequently made explicit in the documents exchanged at the outset of the research. In addition, the parties to these implicit or explicit contracts might make better decisions if they had access to systematically collected information about the track records of specific investigators and commercial research organizations in pursuing their research through to publication.

Research ethics committees, too, have a potentially important role to play. They are only doing half their job if they approve clinical research projects but then fail to assess whether the work was conducted as agreed and then reported appropriately. Ethics committees could help to reduce underreporting of clinical research by exerting pressure on investigators in at least two ways. First, they could identify, in regularly published reports, studies that had received committee endorsement. Second, research ethics committees could help to establish mechanisms for monitoring and recording investigators' compliance with the duty to provide adequate accounts of their research.

Finally, journal editors also have duties in this field. They should ensure that they purge from their practices any tendency to dichotomize reports submitted to them into those that have "positive" and those that have "negative" results. Studies should be accepted or rejected on the basis of whether they have been well conceptualized and competently executed, not on the basis of the direction or magnitude of any differences observed between comparison groups. [...]

In addition, journal editors should acknowledge that shortage of space in printed journals can no longer be invoked as a reason for acquiescing in underreporting of research. Medical scientific publishing must exploit the potential represented by electronic publishing. For example, structured abstracts might be published on paper, and the corresponding full reports published electronically.

THE POTENTIAL ROLE OF PROSPECTIVE REGISTRATION OF TRIALS

Wider adoption of prospective registration of trials at inception could help these various parties to play their respective roles in reducing the prevalence of some of the problems alluded to earlier. Existing registers of controlled trials have been established with a view to improving decision making, not only among investigators and potential participants in collaborative trials, but also by funding organizations, research ethics committees, and journal editors. In line with a tradition going back to the beginning of scientific publishing, such registers could also be used as a basis for assessing who deserves credit for precedence in putting forward a new idea.

As Simes and Dickersin have already demonstrated, however, prospective registration of trials also makes it possible to seek and detect selective underreporting; inferences based on the data available from trials registered prior to their results being known can be compared with inferences based on available data from all trials (registered and unregistered). If the conclusions of these two analyses are in conflict, selective underreporting can be suspected, and inferences based on the results of trials registered at inception (assuming the latter were of acceptable methodological quality) [should be] preferred as being less likely to reflect biased reporting.

The protocols could be made publicly available, in either printed or electronic form, as a part of any prospective registration procedure for controlled trials. This would have at least two important advantages. First, the validity of brief reports of trials could be assessed with greater confidence because some details of the research methods would be publicly available. Second, any suspicion that there may have been selective reporting of certain outcomes and not others could be addressed by consulting the protocol to find out which data items were recorded and which outcomes had been specified in prior hypotheses [...]. [...]

If this activity is to be extended and strengthened to meet the various objectives outlined above, it would seem to be appropriate to look to the national and international bodies that fund clinical research for leadership, organization, and funding, and to the National Library of Medicine to coordinate this activity. But investigators and research ethics committees must obviously play their respective roles. Journal editors can encourage these developments by indicating that registration of controlled trials at inception by investigators will be regarded as evidence of scientific good conduct.

---

82   The CONSORT Statement

Revised Recommendations for Improving the Quality of Reports of Parallel-Group Randomized Trials

DAVID MOHER, KENNETH F. SCHULZ, AND DOUGLAS ALTMAN FOR THE CONSORT GROUP

A report of a randomized controlled trial (RCT) should convey to the reader, in a transparent manner, why the study was undertaken and how it was conducted and an-

David Moher, Kenneth F. Schulz, and Douglas Altman for the CONSORT Group, "The CONSORT Statement: Revised Recommendations for Improving the Quality of Reports of Parallel-Group Randomized Trials," *JAMA* 285 (2001): 1987–91.

alyzed. For example, a lack of adequately reported randomization has been associated with bias in estimating the effectiveness of interventions. To assess the strengths and limitations of an RCT, readers need and deserve to know the quality of its methods. Despite several decades of educational efforts, RCTs still are not being reported adequately. For example, a review of 122 recently published RCTs that evaluated the effectiveness of selective serotonin reuptake inhibitors as [a] first-line management strategy for depression found that only one (0.8 percent) article described randomization adequately. Inadequate reporting makes the interpretation of RCT results difficult if not impossible. Moreover, inadequate reporting borders on unethical practice when biased results receive false credibility.

HISTORY OF CONSORT

In the mid 1990s, two independent initiatives to improve the quality of reports of RCTs led to the publication of the CONSORT (Consolidated Standards of Reporting Trials) statement, which was developed by an international group of clinical trialists, statisticians, epidemiologists, and biomedical editors. CONSORT has been supported by a growing number of medical and health care journals and editorial groups, including the International Committee of Medical Journal Editors (ICMJE, also known as the Vancouver Group), the Council of Science Editors (CSE), and the World Association of Medical Editors (WAME). [...] It can be accessed on the Internet, along with other information about the CONSORT group.

The CONSORT statement comprises a checklist and flow diagram [omitted—eds.] for reporting an RCT. For convenience, the checklist and diagram together are called simply *CONSORT*. They are primarily intended for use in writing, reviewing, or evaluating reports of simple 2-group parallel RCTs.

Preliminary data indicate that the use of CONSORT does indeed help to improve the quality of reports of RCTs. In an evaluation of 71 published RCTs in three journals in 1994, allocation concealment was reported unclearly in 43 (61 percent) of the trials. Four years later, after these three journals required that authors reporting an RCT use CONSORT, the proportion of articles in which allocation concealment was reported unclearly had decreased to 30 of 77 (39 percent; mean difference, −22 percent; [95 percent confidence interval, −38 percent to −6 percent]).

The usefulness of CONSORT is enhanced by continuous monitoring of the biomedical literature; this monitoring allows CONSORT to be modified depending on the merits of maintaining or dropping current items and including new items. [...]

This iterative process makes the CONSORT statement a continually evolving instrument. While participants in the CONSORT group and their degree of involvement vary over time, members meet regularly to review the need to refine CONSORT. At the 1999 meeting, participants decided to revise the original statement. This report reflects changes determined by consensus of the CONSORT group, partly in response to emerging evidence on the importance of various elements of RCTs.

REVISION OF THE CONSORT STATEMENT

Thirteen members of the CONSORT group met in May 1999 with the primary objective of revising the original CONSORT checklist and flow diagram, as needed. The group discussed the merits of including each item in the light of current evidence. As in developing the original CONSORT statement, our intention was to keep only those items deemed fundamental to reporting standards for an RCT. Some items not considered essential may well be highly desirable and should still be included in an RCT report even though they are not included in CONSORT. Such items include approval of an institutional ethical review board, sources of funding for the trial, and a trial registry number (e.g., the International Standard Randomized Controlled Trial Number [ISRCTN]) used to register the RCT at its inception. [...]

The revised CONSORT statement includes a 22-item checklist (Table [82.1]) and a flow diagram [omitted—eds.]. Its primary aim is to help authors improve the quality of reports of simple 2-group parallel RCTs. However, the basic philosophy underlying the development of the statement can be applied to any design. In this regard, additional statements for other designs will be forthcoming from the group. CONSORT can also be used by peer reviewers and editors to identify reports with inadequate description of trials and those with potentially biased results. [...]

COMMENT

Specifically developed to guide authors about how to improve the quality of reporting of simple 2-group parallel RCTs, CONSORT encourages transparency in reporting the methods and results so that reports of RCTs can be interpreted both readily and accurately. However, CONSORT does not address other facets of reporting that also require attention, such as scientific content and readability of RCT reports. Some authors, in their enthusiasm to use CONSORT, have modified the checklist. We recommend against such modifications because they may be based on a different process than the one used by the CONSORT group.

The use of CONSORT seems to reduce (if not eliminate) inadequate reporting of RCTs. Potentially, the use of CONSORT should positively influence the manner in which RCTs are conducted. Granting agencies have noted this potential relationship and, in at least one case, have encouraged grantees to consider in their application how they have dealt with the CONSORT items.

The evidence-based approach used to develop CONSORT has also been used to develop standards for reporting meta-analyses of randomized trials, meta-analyses of observational studies, and diagnostic studies. Health economists also have started to develop reporting standards to

Table 82.1

Checklist of Items to Include When Reporting a Randomized Trial

Section and Topic	Item #	Description	Reported on Page #
Title and Abstract	1	How participants were allocated to interventions (e.g., "random allocation," "randomized," or "randomly assigned").	
Introduction Background	2	Scientific background and explanation of rationale.	
Methods Participants	3	Eligibility criteria for participants and the settings and locations where the data were collected.	
Interventions	4	Precise details of the interventions intended for each group and how and when they were actually administered.	
Objectives	5	Specific objectives and hypotheses.	
Outcomes	6	Clearly defined primary and secondary outcome measures and, when applicable, any methods used to enhance the quality of measurements (e.g., multiple observations, training of assessors).	
Sample size	7	How sample size was determined and, when applicable, explanation of any interim analyses and stopping rules.	
Randomization Sequence generation	8	Method used to generate the random allocation sequence, including details of any restriction (e.g., blocking, stratification).	
Allocation concealment	9	Method used to implement the random allocation sequence (e.g., numbered containers or central telephone), clarifying whether the sequence was concealed until interventions were assigned.	
Implementation	10	Who generated the allocation sequence, who enrolled participants, and who assigned participants to their groups.	
Blinding (masking)	11	Whether or not participants, those administering the interventions, and those assessing the outcomes were blinded to group assignment. If done, how the success of blinding was evaluated.	
Statistical methods	12	Statistical methods used to compare groups for primary outcome(s); methods for additional analyses, such as subgroup analyses and adjusted analyses.	
Results Participant flow	13	Flow of participants through each stage (a diagram is strongly recommended). Specifically, for each group report the numbers of participants randomly assigned,	

Table 82.1. Continued

Section and Topic	Item #	Description	Reported on Page #
		receiving intended treatment, completing the study protocol, and analyzed for the primary outcome. Describe protocol deviations from study as planned, together with reasons.	
Recruitment	14	Dates defining the periods of recruitment and follow-up.	
Baseline data	15	Baseline demographic and clinical characteristics of each group.	
Numbers analyzed	16	Number of participants (denominator) in each group included in each analysis and whether the analysis was by "intention-to-treat." State the results in absolute numbers when feasible (e.g., 10/20, not 50%).	
Outcomes and estimation	17	For each primary and secondary outcome, a summary of results for each group, and the estimated effect size and its precision (e.g., 95% confidence interval).	
Ancillary analyses	18	Address multiplicity by reporting any other analyses performed, including subgroup analyses and adjusted analyses, indicating those prespecified and those exploratory.	
Adverse events	19	All important adverse events or side effects in each intervention group.	
Comment			
Interpretation	20	Interpretation of the results, taking into account study hypotheses, sources of potential bias or imprecision, and the dangers associated with multiplicity of analyses and outcomes.	
Generalizability	21	Generalizability (external validity) of the trial findings.	
Overall evidence	22	General interpretation of the results in the context of current evidence.	

help improve the quality of their reports. The intent of all these initiatives is to improve the quality of reporting of biomedical research and by doing so to bring about more effective health care.

The revised CONSORT statement will replace the original one in the journals and groups that already support it. Journals that do not yet support CONSORT may do so by registering on the CONSORT Web site. To convey to authors the importance of improved quality in the reporting of RCTs, we encourage supporting journals to reference the revised CONSORT statement and the CONSORT Internet address in their "Instructions to Authors." Because the journals publishing the revised CONSORT statement have waived copyright protection, CONSORT is now widely accessible to the biomedical community. [...]

A lack of clarification of the meaning and rationale for each checklist item in the original CONSORT statement has been remedied with the development of the CONSORT explanation and elaboration document, which can also be found on the CONSORT Web site. This document reports the evidence on which the checklist items are based, including the references, which had annotated the checklist items in the previous version. We encourage journals to also include reference to this document in their "Instructions to Authors."

Emphasizing the evolving nature of CONSORT, the CONSORT group invites readers to comment on the up-dated checklist and flow diagram through the CONSORT Web site. [...]

[The omitted flow diagram and the explanation and elaboration document are both available at the CONSORT Web site, http://www.consort-statement.org—eds.]

Part X

Challenges to the Institutional Review Board System

Of late, as Jonathan Moreno observes, institutional review boards (IRBs) have been "under the microscope."[1] In the United States, well-publicized tragedies at prestigious medical centers have made many wonder about the safety of research participation. Moreover, 1998 saw the publication of several U.S. government–sponsored reports that took as their focus the current state of research review by IRBs.[2] For those skeptical of the adequacy of current research review, the results of these reports were not encouraging. In short, IRBs are badly overworked and understaffed. Moreover, the burdens of IRB review across the United States are unevenly distributed. For example, a Bell Associates report funded by the National Institutes of Health (NIH) found that the IRBs that rank in the top 10 percent in terms of their annual protocol review volume—so-called high-volume IRBs—accounted for 37 percent of the national total (284,000 reviews in the study year).[3] In such high-volume IRBs it is often true that insufficient time is devoted to protocol review. Moreover, medical research is proliferating. The increase in multicenter research studies, international research studies, and pharmaceutical company studies in the past 20 years means that the IRB workload stands to increase in the coming years.

Along with a burdensome workload for IRBs comes a huge responsibility. In the United States, as in many other nations, IRBs are charged with two principal tasks: first, they must review a research protocol to ensure that the risks of the study are commensurate with the anticipated benefits, and second, they must ensure that prospective research subjects are adequately informed prior to reaching their decision regarding study participation. It may fairly be said that IRBs are the main protectors of human research participants. Given such important responsibilities, however, the recent worry about the adequacy of IRB review gives one reason for concern, and it is on such concerns that the contributors in Part X focus their attention.

IRBs AND MONITORING

Many IRBs are currently unable to adequately fulfill the multiple duties required of them for the protection of human research participants. Our first contributors to this part, Charles Weijer and colleagues, focus on one such unfulfilled role: that of monitoring ongoing research. In response to critics of monitoring, the authors argue that the monitoring function of IRBs is *not* akin to that of a police force in search of protocol violators, but is rather that of an institution-based educator for the research staff. Thought of in this way, IRB monitoring of ongoing research should not send a message to the research staff that the IRB does not trust them (something that would surely occur if the IRB behaved as a local "fraud squad"). Rather, as the authors argue, IRB monitoring of local research should be part of a systematic research quality assurance program, much as routine medical audit programs are a necessary part of clinical care quality assurance. And although medical auditing and research monitoring by the IRB ultimately serve the interests of patients and research participants, respectively, both forms of quality assurance serve the important preventive goal of educating the institution's staff.

Weijer and colleagues delineate and discuss four different categories of research monitoring: (1) annual review, (2) consent monitoring, (3) monitoring of adherence to protocol, and (4) monitoring of data integrity. Within each category of research monitoring the authors discuss the different characteristics of a study protocol that might trigger specific monitoring activities, along with suggested monitoring interventions for each category. Thus, for example, in addition to the standard reporting of participants accrued, how they fared on protocol, and the incidence of adverse events, study investigators should notify the IRB of any relevant evidence that emerges from concurrent research (carried on outside of the local institution's study) as part of its standard annual report to the IRB. In this way the investigators and IRB members can review all extant evidence and determine if the emerging external evidence warrants premature stopping of the trial.[4]

With regard to the monitoring of consent, Weijer and colleagues argue that if a study poses greater than minimal risk or if the prospective participants are of doubtful competence, the IRB may wish to institute a consent monitoring program, in the first case with a third-party competency assessment, in the second case with a member of the IRB present during consent to particularly risky studies. Elsewhere Myriam Skrutkowska and colleagues describe their experience with a consent-monitoring program for a Phase II breast cancer study that involved treatment with high-dose anthracycline, an investigational cardioprotective drug, two standard chemotherapies, followed by two sequential autologous bone marrow transplantations. While few studies are as intensive and risky as this, the analysis of Skrutkowska and colleagues is highly instructive, especially with respect to the questions that the consent monitors asked of the prospective participants after the participants had discussed the study with the physician, but before they had signed the consent form. For example: "Have you been told that this will certainly cure or halt your disease?" "As you have been told, some people who have undergone this protocol are doing well; others have not done well, and some in fact have died. Do you want to speak to someone who has done well, to someone who has done poorly, or to both?" "Do you understand that this protocol involves more intensive treatment than a person would ordinarily undergo?"[5] Honest discussions, prompted by questions such as these, between IRB members (or a third party designated by the IRB) and prospective research participants serve as an example of the educational role that the IRB can play in a research institution, for researchers and patients alike.

Weijer and colleagues also argue that the IRB has a role to play in monitoring both adherence to the study protocol (even though some local deviations from protocol may well be justified)[6] and the integrity of the research data. Consonant with the view of monitoring as an educational intervention is the authors' argument that the best way to monitor protocol adherence is a form of researcher self-regulation, with input from the IRB or from experts external to the institution. Similarly, the authors argue that study investigators should periodically be asked to sign guarantees of data integrity and to submit these to the IRB for monitoring. Although the monitoring function of IRBs is often given little attention, on July 11, 2002, the U.S. Office for Human Research Protection issued their document titled Guidance on Continuing Review in order to help IRB members interpret the U.S. Department of Health and Human Services' "Common Rule."[7]

CONFLICT OF INTEREST AND NON-INSTITUTIONAL COMMERCIAL REVIEW BOARDS

Trudo Lemmens and Benjamin Freedman, our next contributors, examine the issues that have emerged from the recent proliferation of non-institutional commercial review boards.[8] These authors distinguish between two kinds of non-institutional review boards: (1) freestanding commercial review boards, without institutional affiliation, that review protocols for a fee (what they call non-institutional review boards [NIRBs]) and (2) review boards set up within contract research organizations (CROs) or pharmaceutical companies that review in-house protocols of the company's own product (what they call proprietary IRBs). Through an examination of NIRBs and proprietary IRBs, along with the conflict-of-interest considerations that they prompt, Lemmens and Freedman offer guidance on how best to deal with such conflicts of interest. Moreover, given the increasing corporate presence within the modern research university, the authors draw lessons for academic IRBs from their analyses of NIRBs and proprietary IRBs.

Although NIRBs (in particular) have several advantages over academic IRBs—much faster protocol review, better training of review board members, more consistent review board membership—there are nonetheless problems that clearly beset the very structure of NIRBs and proprietary IRBs. For example, NIRBs are financially dependent on their clients; if one NIRB (perhaps rightly) consistently rejects the protocols it reviews as in violation of extant research regulations, this NIRB may see its client base disappear. Similarly, if a member of a proprietary IRB (perhaps rightly) consistently rejects protocols that she reviews, she may find herself out of a job given that, in rejecting or demanding changes to the protocol, she is thereby erecting barriers to the research endeavors of the company, her employer. Thus, as Lemmens and Freedman argue, there are conflicts of interest inherent in the structure of both the NIRB and the proprietary IRB.

The innovation of the analysis proffered by Lemmens and Freedman is that they draw upon the resources of administrative law—in particular, the way that administrative law deals with bias—in order to suggest how best to deal with such conflicts of interest. Given that IRBs, academic or commercial, have a *public* role to play in the protection of research participants, the authors argue that IRBs bear a family resemblance to public curators and administrative licensing boards. They draw upon the relevant features of such administrative bodies (namely, their independence and impartiality) and argue that these features should be the focus of an inquiry into conflicts of interest. Under American administrative common law, for example, the bases for bias include financial interests, personal involvement in a case, and alleged prejudgment of a case. And the remedies against such forms of bias include disclosure of the conflict, removal of voting rights, and prohibition from participation in a review. The authors discuss these remedies and apply their analyses to the case of non-academic research review boards.

In the end, much like those who are skeptical of reliance on the "virtuous investigator" as a sufficient protection for research participants, Lemmens and Freedman are skeptical of reliance on the virtuous IRB member as a sufficient protection for research participants. Their articulation and defense of specific remedies—including an accreditation program for research review board members[9] and a ban on shopping around for less stringent protocol review (so-called forum shopping)—are important for both academic and commercial review boards given the importance of ensuring public trust in the medical research enterprise.

LOCAL VERSUS CENTRALIZED REVIEW

Out next two contributions address not specific duties of IRBs, but rather the form that IRBs should take given the vast changes that have occurred in the roughly 30 years since IRBs became an institutional commonplace. In particular, both articles address the issue of local versus national (or centralized) review of research protocols. Harold Edgar and David J. Rothman lead off this discussion with a focus on the promises and perils of local research review. As these authors note, local (i.e., in-hospital) review of research protocols by IRBs was eminently reasonable when the U.S. regulatory apparatus regarding research with humans was being constructed in the early 1970s. As they explain, it was in the interest of the institution (and hence of the local researchers) to ensure that sloppy and unethical research not pass through their IRB. Moreover, given the protectionist ethos that reigned at the time in light of research thought to be especially risky and burdensome, local researchers were eager to engage prospective participants in the consent process in order to assuage their skepticism about medical research and to enroll adequate numbers of persons in their research projects. For reasons such as these, Edgar and Rothman claim that "localism" worked well in IRB review given the research context that prevailed at the time.

Yet times have changed, and Edgar and Rothman's article may be read as a critique of the "one-size-fits-all" model of research review. Several factors have contributed to this change in the research context. First, research is widely viewed not as a risky endeavor, but rather as a source of potential benefit. Given this altered research ethos, prospective participants often clamor—rightly or wrongly—for the chance to participate in a research study. Second, medical institutions are no longer the sole domain of medical research; many research studies are now being carried out by pharmaceutical companies or CROs off of university campuses. Finally, there has been a proliferation of multicenter and international research projects; consequently, the principal investigators of a research study are often "strangers" to the medical institution in which the study is being carried out. All of these changes mean that the model of the local IRB reviewing local studies may no longer be appropriate.

Edgar and Rothman highlight three broad areas of reform that are meant to address the problems of research review. First, they suggest the formation of "super committees" at the national level, that is, overarching research-monitoring mechanisms that are staffed by specialists who know most about the clinical science behind the research studies. Second, as Lemmens and Freedman also note, more attention must be focused upon the presence of the corporate element in medical research, especially insofar as conflicts of interest are concerned. Finally, they suggest that IRBs must strengthen their "outside elements," that is, the input and importance of both external scientific consultants and lay IRB members.

Michaele C. Christian and her colleagues close out this debate with a focus on the problems presented by multicenter (or multi-institutional) research protocols.[10] Like Edgar and Rothman, Christian and colleagues are concerned about the problems that attend local IRB approval of research involving multiple institutions. The authors discuss their experience to date with a central IRB (CIRB) and facilitated review process for multicenter research projects recently initiated by the U.S. National Cancer Institute (NCI).[11] (We note here that the United Kingdom initiated a similar program of facilitated review in 1997, the results of which have been imperfect but nonetheless an improvement over the previous situation.)[12]

One of the major problems with multicenter research is the duplication of effort in reviewing the research protocol. Initially a protocol is drafted by the principal investigators for review by a granting agency. Once funding is secured, the protocol is sent to all of the local institutions that wish to participate in the recruitment of research participants, and it must therefore be approved by the local IRB at each of these study sites—in NCI-sponsored studies, as the authors note, 100 sites on average for any given trial. Given that the protocol has already been reviewed and approved by the granting agency, the review that local IRBs must perform—in addition to all of their other review and monitoring duties—is duplicative and wasteful. In light of this, the authors initiated a centralized and facilitated review process in the hope of streamlining the overly burdensome process of scientific and ethical review.

The benefits of the CIRB model are several. First, once a study protocol is approved by an expert NCI panel, local IRBs may engage in facilitated review—that is, in a much faster review of the protocol either by the local IRB's chairperson or by a subcommittee of the IRB. Second, patient access to trials can be accomplished in days rather than months. Third, unburdened of a full protocol review and of the monitoring of adverse events at other institutions, local IRBs can focus their attention on more pressing local monitoring issues. Fourth, as Edgar and Rothman note in their discussion of "'super' committees," the initial protocol is reviewed by an NCI panel that has an expertise in cancer clinical trials that is unmatched by most local IRBs. According to the CIRB model, local IRBs have access to all of the documents associated with the initial review and ongoing monitoring of a study, should they desire them. Moreover, as required by U.S. federal regulations, members of the local IRB may call attention to any relevant features of the local research context that must be dealt with, so local IRBs may decide that a full review rather than a facilitated review is required. The proposal by Christian and colleagues is thus an attempt not to remove local IRBs from the review process—since they are, and will remain, crucial—but rather to free up the time of local IRBs so that they may attend to more important matters.

As all of the contributors to Part X note, the current IRB system is imperfect and in need of repair. Each contributor highlights different weaknesses of the IRB system and points to different solutions for strengthening it. In the end, the safety and well-being of research participants is at stake. And just as there can be no one-size-fits-all IRB, so can there be no one-size-fits-all solution to the current research oversight woes. Considered collectively, however, the contributors to this part point us in the right direction.

1. Jonathan D. Moreno, "IRBs under the Microscope," *Kennedy Institute of Ethics Journal* 8 (1998): 329–37.
2. A list of these reports, along with their Web site addresses, is provided in "Frequently Cited Research Regulations, Guidelines, and Reports," at the beginning of this volume.
3. Available online at ohrp.osophs.dhhs.gov/hsp_report/hsp_final_rpt.pdf.
4. Julian Savulescu, Iain Chalmers, and Jennifer Blunt, "Are Research Ethics Committees Behaving Unethically?" *British Medical Journal* 313 (1996): 1390–93; and Peter Brocklehurst, Diana Elbourne, and Zarko Alfirevic, "Role of External Evidence in Monitoring Clinical Trials: Experience from a Perinatal Trial," *British Medical Journal* 320 (2000): 995–98.
5. Myriam Skrutkowska, Charles Weijer, Stan Shapiro, et al., "Monitoring Informed Consent in an Oncology Study Posing Serious Risk to Subjects," *IRB: A Review*

of Human Subjects Research 20, no. 6 (1998): 1–6, quote is on p. 3.

6. Benjamin Freedman, "Multicenter Trials and Subject Eligibility: Should Local IRBs Play a Role?" *IRB: A Review of Human Subjects Research* 16, nos. 1 and 2 (1994): 1–6.

7. Available online at ohrp.osophs.dhhs.gov/ humansubjects/guidance/contrev2002.htm.

8. Trudo Lemmens and Alison Thompson, "Noninstitutional Commercial Review Boards in North America: A Critical Appraisal and Comparison with IRBs," *IRB: Ethics and Human Research* 23, no. 2 (2001): 1–12.

9. Institute of Medicine, *Preserving Public Trust: Accreditation and Human Research Protection Programs* (Washington, D.C.: National Academy Press, 2001).

10. William J. Burman, Randall R. Reves, David L. Dohn, and Robert T. Schooley, "Breaking the Camel's Back: Multicenter Clinical Trials and Local Institutional Review Boards," *Annals of Internal Medicine* 134 (2001): 152–57; and Robert J. Levine, "Institutional Review Boards: A Crisis in Confidence," *Annals of Internal Medicine* 134 (2001): 161–63.

11. Robert J. Levine and Louis Lasagna, "Demystifying Central Review Boards: Current Options and Future Directions," *IRB: A Review of Human Subjects Research* 22, no. 6 (2000): 1–7.

12. Julia C. Lewis, Susan Tomkins, and Julian R. Sampson, "Ethical Approval for Research Involving Geographically Dispersed Subjects," *Journal of Medical Ethics* 27 (2001): 347–51; Joanna Tully, Nelly Ninis, Robert Booy, and Russell Viner, "The New System of Review by Multicentre Research Ethics Committees: Prospective Study," *British Medical Journal* 320 (2000): 1179–82; and K. G. M. M. Alberti, "Multicentre Research Ethics Committees: Has the Cure Been Worse than the Disease?" *British Medical Journal* 320 (2000): 1157–58.

83   Monitoring Clinical Research

An Obligation Unfulfilled

CHARLES WEIJER, STANLEY H. SHAPIRO, ABRAHAM FUKS,
KATHLEEN CRANLEY GLASS, AND MYRIAM SKRUTKOWSKA

[...]

ARGUMENTS AGAINST AND FOR MONITORING BY RESEARCH ETHICS BOARDS

Robert J. Levine has argued against routine monitoring by research ethics boards [REBs, the Canadian equivalent of institutional review boards (IRBs)—eds.] on several grounds. First, routine monitoring would negatively affect the atmosphere of trust between the REB and the investigator.

Second, Levine believes that monitoring procedures are unduly expensive. He points out that "presumptions of trust are much less costly, whether the costs are expressed in terms of dollars, human resources, or the quality of our social structures." Finally, Levine does not see the use of a program that does not "seem to catch many wrongdoers anyhow," although he does seem to acknowledge the usefulness of review of research in certain cases.

If the purpose of monitoring were to have REBs act as a police force, they would surely be ill-prepared for the task. We believe, however, that the ultimate goal of any institutional commitment to monitoring of research must be the education of its research staff. An effective institutional monitoring program should be coupled with an institution-wide program to educate researchers and other staff about the proper and ethical conduct of research. A monitoring program can help an institution develop an educational program that is responsive to its own needs, to "fill in the gaps." In the unusual case of an investigator with idiosyncratic research practices, a more clearly directed educational program may be appropriate.

In establishing monitoring programs, the perception that they reflect the REB's and institution's lack of trust in researchers is likely to be an important concern. This reaction is understandable, given that, in the past, such programs have been characterized as "police work." Therefore, such programs must be clearly identified as quality-assurance mechanisms. Medical audit is recognized as essential to improving the quality of medical care in an institution; research audit is also an essential step to enhance the quality of research, a goal that researchers certainly endorse. [...]

Education and quality assurance are closely connected with another major goal of research monitoring, namely prevention. [... P]revention of a problem is always desirable; after the problem has occurred, damage control is the only option.

In arguing that the cost of prevention is too great, the critics of monitoring have erred. The fraud involving breast-cancer research has shown how damaging a single case of research fraud can be. Schwarz expresses the problem well:

> If integrity and credibility of the process is called into question, our ability to produce new methods for the diagnosis and treatment of disease will be compromised. The ultimate penalty will be paid in decreased benefits to public health. It's that simple, as well as that serious.

In portraying research audit as solely concerned with the detection of fraud, research monitoring's detractors have failed to recognize the role that monitoring can play in education and quality assurance in an institution.

FOUR CATEGORIES OF RESEARCH MONITORING

Heath has suggested three useful categories of research review by REBs, to which we would like to add a fourth: (1) continuing (annual) review; (2) monitoring of the consent process; (3) monitoring for adherence to protocol; and (4) monitoring of data integrity. We do not intend to review each of these categories in detail, since so much theoretic work is required in several of them. Instead, we will sketch the broad contours of each.

Table [83.1] summarizes our overview of the four categories of monitoring activities that are relevant to REBs. For each category, we list protocol characteristics that may indicate the need for such monitoring. A given protocol may, of course, have characteristics that trigger review ac-

Charles Weijer, Stanley H. Shapiro, Abraham Fuks, Kathleen Cranley Glass, and Myriam Skrutkowska, "Monitoring Clinical Research: An Obligation Unfulfilled," *Canadian Medical Association Journal* 152 (1995): 1973–79.

Table 83.1

Characteristics That Indicate the Need for Monitoring and Avenues of Intervention by Research Ethics Boards (REBs) in Four Categories of Research Monitoring

Category of Monitoring	Characteristics That Indicate the Need for Monitoring	Avenues of Intervention
Annual review	• Expected adverse drug reactions • Other concurrent research on the treatment	• More frequent review by the REB • Recommendation of the formation of a committee to monitor data and safety
Consent monitoring	• Greater than minimal risk to the subjects • Enrollment of members of a vulnerable population (e.g., prisoners or patients with advanced cancer) • Inclusion of incompetent (or potentially incompetent) subjects	• Periodic review of consent documents • Involvement of a third party to assess competence • Involvement of a subject advocate in consent negotiations • Periodic post hoc review of subjects • Periodic assessment, in person, of consent negotiations • Presence of a member of the REB at all consent negotiations
Monitoring of adherence to protocol	• Complex treatment regimen • Safety interventions to prevent serious toxic effects, required by the protocol or the REB	• Review of management plan prepared by researchers • Involvement of a third-party expert • Periodic review of documents (e.g., patient charts or pharmacy records)
Monitoring of data integrity	• Generation of research in which the integrity of data is not monitored by an outside agency	• Requirement that data integrity be guaranteed • Periodic in-house data monitoring • Periodic external monitoring

tivities in several categories. For example, a clinical trial of a novel and potentially toxic drug to treat subarachnoid hemorrhage may prompt an REB to consider continuing (annual) review, consent monitoring and perhaps monitoring of adherence to protocol. In Table [83.1], avenues of intervention are outlined for each category. Because review by an REB must respond to local standards, it is impossible to dictate which interventions a given committee should recommend for a given protocol. However, in considering the protocol for a new therapy for subarachnoid hemorrhage, a hypothetical committee could, for example, ensure that a committee to monitor data and safety exists and that the investigator reports to the REB biannually. Furthermore, the REB may insist that the competence of potential subjects be assessed by a physician who is not involved in the clinical trial. Finally, the REB may ask the investigators to develop and submit for approval an audit program for treatment procedures to ensure that the study protocol is followed scrupulously.

In the following discussion we provide additional detail concerning each of the monitoring categories. Because few committees monitor research adequately and because we had to rely on published reports, many of the circumstances that prompted committees to monitor research are exceptional and dramatic (e.g., the first implantation of an artificial heart). As REBs begin to fulfill [these] requirements [...], however, monitoring will become more commonplace.

Annual Review

Most Canadian REBs (53 percent of those surveyed by the National Council on Bioethics in Human Research [NCBHR]) require that investigators submit a report to the REB each calendar year after the approval of a protocol. A report may also be required (by 36 percent of REBs) at the conclusion of the study. [...T]he investigator should report the number of patients accrued, his or her assessment of the outcome or progress of these subjects and any adverse drug reactions. Furthermore, the investigator must report any new information, generated outside the trial, that may disturb clinical equipoise (i.e., the uncertainty within the community of experts concerning the relative superiority of one of the treatments involved in the trial).

In research studies involving possible serious adverse drug reactions, mortality or serious morbidity, the REB may recommend the establishment of a committee to monitor data and safety (if no such committee exists) or more frequent reports from the researcher. Similarly, more frequent review may be needed because results of other relevant clinical trials in the field are anticipated. If clinical equipoise is disturbed by the publication of results of a closely related research study, the REB may decide to halt a trial.

Consent Monitoring

External audits of research studies have often found that informed consent and its proper documentation are deficient. The U.S. Food and Drug Administration (FDA) documented deficiencies in informed consent in 51 percent of audits conducted from 1977 to 1988. The [U.S. National Cancer Institute (NCI)] found that, at 12 percent of the cooperative-group sites audited, there were deficiencies in the consent obtained from more than 30 percent of trial participants. Audit programs may help to rectify these shortcomings. A recent report from the Cancer and Leukemia Group B (CALGB) trial demonstrated the success of an aggressive audit and education program, which reduced the incidence of inadequacies in consent obtained from 18.5 percent to 3.9 percent of trial participants. [...]

Robertson states succinctly, "Monitoring could be as simple as checking that signed consent forms exist or as complicated as interviewing subjects or observing the investigator recruit subjects." Periodic monitoring of consent documents is a straightforward first step to ensure that the requirements for written informed consent have been fulfilled. Faden, Lewis, and Rimer have shown the feasibility of such a review; they reviewed the following information from the consent documents for 214 research subjects: the protocol number, who solicited consent, where and when consent was obtained, whether the consent form was wit-

nessed, and, if so, by whom. The study required 160 person-hours to complete.

Certain studies—those that involve greater than minimal dedicated research risk (i.e., the risk of interventions done to answer the research question that are not associated with therapy), draw subjects from vulnerable patient populations (e.g., patients with advanced cancer) or include incompetent or potentially incompetent subjects—may require more intensive monitoring by the REB. In the case of studies involving incompetent or potentially incompetent research subjects, the REB may require that a third party assess the patients' competence to consent. Shannon and Ockene describe the deliberations of the REB in their institution concerning the first Thrombolysis in Myocardial Ischemia trial (TIMI-1), for which only patients suffering the first hours of an acute myocardial infarction were eligible. Concerns about voluntary participation and comprehension of consent information led the REB to require that family members be present during the consent negotiation and that they also agree with the subject's decision to enter the trial. The involvement of family members in consent is a creative solution that merits consideration in studies like this one that involve seriously ill patients and immediate treatment. In other studies in which the competence or voluntary participation of subjects [is an issue], the REB may appoint an advocate for the subjects, who must be present during consent negotiations. McGrath and Briscoe describe a research center that employs a full-time patient advocate. In the extreme case of novel research that poses serious risks for vulnerable subjects, the REB may require that a member of the REB supervise, in person, the consent negotiations for all patients enrolled in a trial. In the first implantation of an artificial human heart and in the first case of heart transplantation with a nonhuman heart the REB had a member present during the consent process.

As a means of quality control, REBs may wish to observe consent negotiations in order to monitor prospectively the adequacy of information given to potential research subjects. They may also wish to assess subjects' comprehension of consent information by testing subjects immediately after the informed consent has been given. The results of such testing may lead to efforts to improve comprehension; such efforts may include a 24-hour delay before subjects sign the consent form, audiovisual presentations about the research or a policy requiring subjects to complete a multiple-choice test satisfactorily before enrollment. Testing of subjects' comprehension should be immediate; although testing subjects some time after the informed-consent process may be more practical, difficulties with recollection confound the significance of data obtained in this fashion. Theoretic work is needed to define standards for the recollection of consent information.

Monitoring for Adherence to Protocol

Empiric research shows that it is relatively common for investigators to deviate from REB-approved protocols. A survey of researchers showed that half thought that researchers deviated "at least sometimes" from the original research plan without the approval of the REB. Of 92 researchers, 13 (14 percent) said that they had deviated from their own proposals without approval by making changes to the overall study design, the defined subject samples or the participation required of subjects.

Data from the external audits discussed earlier seem to confirm this finding. During 26 percent of the audits conducted between 1977 and 1988, the FDA discovered major problems with nonadherence to protocol. The NCI uncovered deviations from drug dosages or other protocol regimens in 12 percent of the study sites audited; in 19 percent of the sites monitored, more than 30 percent of the cases had had such deviations. The CALGB audits revealed "major protocol deviations in drug dosing" in 10.8 percent of cases audited.

If protocols involve complex treatment regimens or require critically timed safety interventions to prevent serious toxic effects, REBs may wish to institute monitoring to ensure that approved procedures are being followed. (Pharmaceutical companies, as a rule, aggressively audit adherence to protocols in all studies.) The optimal approach is for REBs to encourage researchers to develop self-monitoring mechanisms, which may involve other experts within or outside the institution. In exceptional cases, procedures may be monitored directly by a member of the REB. Perhaps as a response to procedural violations by Cooley and Liotta in the first mechanical-heart transplantation, the University of Utah IRB appointed a member to ensure that procedures were followed in the subsequent implantation of an artificial heart in Barney Clark.

In conjunction with a monitoring program and as part of a quality-control program, REBs may wish to audit relevant pharmacy and medical records directly to ensure that procedures have been followed.

Monitoring the Integrity of Data

Capturing data of the highest quality is central to the validity of subsequent inference. The pharmaceutical industry has taken great strides, undoubtedly as a result of the FDA approval process, to ensure that all data in clinical trials are independently audited. Pharmaceutical companies typically monitor each site every 6 to 10 weeks during the course of a study. Clinical-trial cooperative groups also have procedures for monitoring data quality and integrity. [...]

Despite the fact that pharmaceutical companies and cooperative groups audit data integrity, REBs have a role to play. To fulfill their obligation to monitor data integrity, REBs most often must simply review the audit procedures proposed by the pharmaceutical company or clinical-trial cooperative group. Therefore, REBs' greatest concern is any research generated in the institution that is not subject to external audit. In these cases, REBs may wish routinely to require investigators to sign guarantees of data integrity, as suggested by DeMets and Meinert. In addition, the institution may wish to establish a program to conduct periodic in-house or external audits of data. To develop such programs, institutions may draw on the substantial body of published articles on data-quality control in clinical trials.

ADMINISTRATION OF REVIEWS AND FINANCIAL ISSUES

An institution that establishes a program to monitor research should consider carefully how the program will be administered and funded. Although a detailed review of administrative models is beyond the scope of this article, [we propose] three possible administrative models. These models are not mutually exclusive, and can be used in combination. As the institution's agent in the review of experimentation involving human beings, an REB must play a central role in such a program. Certain aspects of routine review, such as periodic monitoring of consent documents, periodic observation of consent negotiations, testing subjects for comprehension, periodic document checks for adherence to procedures and data-audit programs for in-house research, may best be handled by an office for research audit (Model C [...]). Such an office, established by the institution in collaboration with the REB, could handle continuing reviews and coordinate institutional education programs to respond to problems discovered through the reviews. However, it must be directly responsible to the REB, which would ultimately deal with any difficulties encountered.

In some cases the REB may wish to monitor research projects directly (Model A). This model may be most appropriate in novel research that presents a serious risk to subjects. In most cases of continuing review, however, good research practice dictates that the investigators develop a monitoring program (Model B). Such a program could involve a system of checks and procedures within the project or third-party supervision of procedures (e.g., third-party assessments of subject competence). Self-monitoring by researchers is the model most consonant with the prime goal of continuing review: education.

Continuing review requires institutions to commit substantial financial resources and personnel to the process. [...] However, pharmaceutical companies and government funding agencies should take into account the additional costs entailed by review when they fund research involving human subjects. Discussions among researchers, institutions and funding agencies are needed to define specific arrangements.

CONCLUSION

The monitoring of continuing research provides institutions with the chance to affirm publicly their commitment to the ethical conduct of experimentation involving humans. When combined with educational programs, monitoring offers the opportunity to prevent problems in the conduct of research. In many cases investigators will develop their own monitoring programs. However, the establishment of institutional programs to review clinical research will play an essential role in regaining the public's trust in research. [...]

[Figure omitted—eds.]

---

84   Ethics Review for Sale?

Conflict of Interest and Commercial Research Review Boards

TRUDO LEMMENS AND BENJAMIN FREEDMAN

[...] In [the] context of increasing need for efficient institutional review board (IRB) review and significant growth in industry funded research, commercial IRBs [have] found their niche. They have become very visible participants at the commercial exhibits of drug or therapeutics conferences, where fast research ethics review has become a marketable item, promoted in the well-designed brochures of contract research organizations (CROs) or commercial IRBs. Commercial research review is gaining importance as research and development of new drugs, particularly phase I studies, increasingly take place in research centers of pharmaceutical companies, in CROs, or through physicians independent from academic research centers. [...]

Commercial IRBs can be divided in two different categories: (1) freestanding commercial committees without institutional affiliation, established for the purpose of reviewing protocols for compliance with ethical and regulatory standards, often referred to as non-institutional review boards (NIRBs) or independent review boards, and (2) research review boards set up by CROs or pharmaceutical companies to review research for products developed or tested by the company itself, which we call proprietary IRBs. Often, the work of proprietary IRBs is an integral part of a wide array of services offered by the CRO. While NIRBs, by definition, review research undertaken elsewhere, proprietary IRBs typically review in-house studies. The division is far from absolute [but for] the sake of clarity, we will discuss proprietary [IRBs] and NIRBs as separate entities.

The purpose of this paper is to discuss one particular aspect of commercial research review that has been mentioned in the literature but has yet to be fully analyzed: the risk that fundamental conflicts of interest undermine the structure of commercial research review. Focusing on commercial IRBs, we point out why conflict-of-interest rules should be better developed and why they should prescribe more clearly what types of relationships are appropriate between IRBs or IRB members and research sponsors. In doing so, we recognize that the issue of the impact of financial interests on the independence of IRBs is not exclusive to commercial IRBs. [...]

COMMERCIAL REVIEW: A THRIVING BUSINESS ESCAPING PUBLIC SCRUTINY

The difference between commercial and academic IRBs lies primarily in the context in which they operate and, to some extent, in the goals of the medical research that these IRBs are reviewing. Traditional IRBs are generally established by non-profit educational and research organizations, such as universities, hospitals, granting agencies, or professional associations. Commercial IRBs, by contrast, review for the most part studies on behalf of for-profit companies, such as CROs. While this distinction is beginning to fade as a result of the significant increase in the proportion of industry sponsored research in academic centers, it remains fair to distinguish private from academic IRBs in light of the former's focus on commercial studies. Even when private IRBs are involved in the review of research undertaken at

Trudo Lemmens and Benjamin Freedman, "Ethics Review for Sale? Conflict of Interest and Commercial Research Review Boards," *Milbank Quarterly* 78 (2000): 547–84.

academic health care centers [. . .] they are primarily involved in the review of commercially sponsored research for these institutions. Moreover, by focusing strictly on commercial IRBs, lessons can be learned about the potential need for restructuring academic IRBs, in the context of increasing academic entrepreneurialism. [. . .]

The keys to the success of NIRBs seem to lie in the increasing demand for review of research protocols from CROs and independent physician-researchers, the speed of the review, the quality and variety of services offered, and the ability to review multisite projects. As Erica Heath, president of one of the largest American NIRBs, puts it: "We certainly cannot market approvals. But we can market in terms of speed, efficiency, expertise, customer relations, and complete information on readable forms." Unlike most academic IRBs, many NIRBs can guarantee a very short review time. The average review time of the NIRBs contacted by the [U.S.] Office of [the] Inspector General was 11 days. One survey found that some NIRBs guarantee review in as little as 5 days. Because of the high volume of protocols they review and the concomitant expertise of their members, many NIRBs are likely capable of giving coherent and clear instructions to improve protocols. Their reviews might be more predictable than that of some academic IRBs with more fluctuating and often less experienced membership. The latter have come under increasing criticism for their members' lack of training, administrative understaffing, and disregard of regulatory requirements. Some NIRBs [. . .] have much stricter educational requirements for their members than many academic IRBs, which often hesitate to impose education on their volunteer members, who are frequently hard to recruit. Finally, many multisite trials can be efficiently reviewed by one NIRB, thus avoiding the lengthy process of going through multiple reviews, which often lead to contradictory instructions.

Proprietary IRBs offer a number of other advantages. They are directly accessible and may be under the authority of the CRO, so that research protocols can be reviewed even faster and upon special request. Setting up a proprietary IRB may be cheaper than paying an outside IRB, particularly if the CRO has a high volume of studies. Finally, a CRO may feel more comfortable in granting access to confidential information to an IRB that has a formal link with the company and adheres to its policies. [. . .]

WHAT CONSTITUTES A CONFLICT OF INTEREST?

While the concept of conflict of interest is clearly in vogue in discussions around health policy and the term is used in many different contexts, it is hard to find a clear definition of it. Conflict of Interest in Academic Health Centers, a 1990 report of the Association of Academic Health Centers

(AHC), mentions the importance of professional norms for determining what conflicts of interest are. It states that a conflict exists "when legal obligations or widely recognized professional norms are likely to be compromised by a person's other interests." James P. Orlowski and Leon Wateska define conflict of interest more narrowly as "a discrepancy between the personal interests and the professional responsibilities of a person in a position of trust." Dennis Thompson defines a conflict of interest as "a set of conditions in which professional judgment concerning a primary interest (such as patient's welfare or the validity of research) tends to be unduly influenced by a secondary interest (such as financial gain)." [. . .]

Secondary interests are not in themselves improper, but they should be subservient to primary interests. Secondary interests are often financial, but they can also be intangible ones, such as gaining professional advancement, prestige, or power. Following [Thompson's] definition, the central questions arise: what are the primary obligations of IRBs, what is the role of IRB members *qua* members, and how seriously can these obligations be affected by other interests? The impact of conflicts of interest can only be understood when the primary obligations of IRBs and IRB members are clarified.

IRBs have a protective public role. "The primary purpose [of IRB review]," according to the Food and Drug Administration (FDA) Rules and Regulations, "is to assure the protection of the rights and welfare of the human subjects." The International Conference on Harmonisation Harmonised Tripartite Guideline—Guideline for Good Clinical Practice [ICH-GCP Guideline, excerpted in Part II of this volume—eds.] refers to "the protection of the rights, safety and well-being of subjects" in its definitions of "independent ethics committee" and "institutional review board." As thus defined, an IRB's primary duty is to protect human subjects of research.

In light of their public policy role, we argue that rules of administrative law ought to inspire us in refining the rules by which IRBs are organized. Rules of administrative law apply to a variety of judicial bodies and governmental agencies and may vary accordingly. It is not easy to determine which of these bodies resembles the IRB most closely. In many respects, the role of IRBs can be situated somewhere between, for example, the roles of public curators and administrative licensing boards. Licensing boards are similar to IRBs in that they often have an important public policy goal, they are given much discretion in the implementation of their policies, and their decisions often have a major impact on the activities they regulate. Moreover, administrative licensing boards are often specialized bodies, dealing with issues that require particular expertise from board members. The same is true for IRBs, which function within highly specialized areas of medical research. On the other hand, the IRB's role is clearly more intimately related to individual people's rights and welfare than, say, a land development, transportation, or liquor licensing board. Because of their protective role and their responsibility with respect to the rights, integrity, and well-being of individual research participants, IRBs have some of the characteristics of public curators. They are first and foremost obliged to look after the welfare and rights of research subjects. In addition, the IRB's mandate also resembles that of human rights commissions, when these are involved in policy rather than litigation. Finally, while specialized knowledge on the part of some IRB members is required, representation by the community and by members of different disciplines is a core requirement for IRB review. Thus, IRBs differ from highly specialized administrative or professional bodies in that there is clearly public involvement and public responsibility directed toward the physical and emotional well-being of individual research participants.

BIAS AND CONFLICT OF INTEREST IN ADMINISTRATIVE LAW

Because of this resemblance to administrative bodies, administrative law on conflict of interest (discussed under the heading "bias") can inspire this debate. The independence and impartiality of judges and administrators are major principles of judicial and administrative review. In common law, an essential principle of natural law is expressed in the adage *nemo judex in causa sua* ("no one ought to be judge in his or her own case"). In American law, conflict of interest falls under the due process clause, enshrined in the 14th Amendment to the Constitution, which guarantees the right to a fair hearing before an *impartial* tribunal.

This is not to say that IRBs ought to be treated entirely as tribunals. The rules on bias and conflict of interest in administrative law are a reflection of the general concern for independence and neutrality as essential ingredients for a good administration, particularly when administrators are given a specific public duty. [...]

As we have pointed out, IRBs are situated on a continuum somewhere in between administrative tribunals and administrative licensing boards. Where they are placed on this continuum [...] is important if we want to apply rules of administrative law with respect to conflicts of interest in research review. While administrative adjudicators are held to the same requirement of impartiality as judges, the interpretation of what constitutes a conflict of interest may differ depending on the type of administrative board involved. Conflict-of-interest rules are context-specific [...]. The closer an entity approaches judicial decision-making, the stricter the rules of conflict of interest are. Clearly, judges presiding in a criminal procedure ought to have the highest level of detachment from financial or personal interest in a case. The same level of detachment is not neces-

sary, possible, or always desirable when we are dealing with highly specialized administrative bodies. [...]

While IRBs are specialized entities, they do have general protective obligations toward the public. IRBs and their members have this protective role in a particular circumstance: research participants are often in a vulnerable position. They may suffer from disease; their financial and social situation may push them to participate in trials; in some cases, they may participate in research to try to obtain access to quality care. This situation warrants careful consideration because of the risk of undue influence or manipulation.

[...] The diligent exercise of responsible review by the boards should compensate partially for the vulnerable position of research subjects. In these circumstances, higher duties of protection are imposed on the party with more power. While IRB members have no direct relation with research subjects, IRBs have special duties as organizations and their members have a professional obligation to fulfill their work in accordance with the mission of the IRB. [...] The fiduciary nature of the doctor-patient relation remains a cornerstone of medicine and should not be abandoned when physicians and patients are involved in research. Likewise, this fiduciary relationship should extend to the institutional bodies that are set up to protect patients and others who participate in medical research.

The need to create trust in IRBs as institutions can also be given a very practical justification. When IRBs function in a transparent way, they inspire public confidence. Public trust in the ethical conduct of trials is essential to the success of medical research, which relies on volunteer participation. Creating public trust in research and research review is therefore essential, not only to respect the subjects of research but also to ensure long-term research participation. [...]

In our view, recent controversies and research analyzing the impact of financial interests on the conduct and outcome of medical research show that financial interests can and do impact the behavior of those involved. These controversies understandably erode public trust. IRBs are supposed to counterbalance the concerns raised by these controversies and scandals by offering a system of independent, qualified, hands-off review. NIRBs and proprietary IRBs are financially dependent on the commercial actors they are supposed to control. It seems odd to hold as reasonable the presumption that financial interests can have a conscious or unconscious impact on these actors while ignoring that there is a serious risk of such impact on those who control them.

We hold that problems of conflict of interest in commercial IRBs are not adequately addressed through simple reliance upon the integrity of IRB members, or the fact that most IRB members are likely to adhere to high ethical standards. [...] Although [...] IRBs perhaps need not submit to the stringent conflict [of interest] rules that courts ought to observe, the significant public interest in protecting trust and maintaining confidence in the system calls for the development of adequate conflict-of-interest rules. [...]

What, then, are the conflicts that should be avoided? The law differentiates among bias as a result of (1) pecuniary interests, (2) personal involvement of the decision maker, and (3) alleged prejudgment of the merits of a particular case. [...]

In the case of a pecuniary conflict, a decision maker will be disqualified if the first two (under common law) or all three (under American law) conditions are fulfilled: (1) The "decision maker must stand to gain or lose personally as a result of his decision." (2) The interest is not remote or does not arise upon a purely speculative series of events. [...] (3) Under American law, the interest must also be substantial. The due process clause requires disqualification of a board member only if the interest is more than "*de minimis.*" In contrast, English and Commonwealth common law prescribe that a minimal interest is sufficient to disqualify a person on the basis of bias. [...]

In contrast to financial interest, personal involvement in a case only leads to disqualification if there is a real likelihood that a hearing will not be fair. A paradigmatic example of this is when there is a close kinship between one of the parties and one of the judges or adjudicators. This type of bias might pose greater risk in academic IRBs, where colleagues have to review protocols of persons with whom they are closely related. Such personal conflicts are less likely to occur in NIRBs.

Prejudgment is an even more flexible concept. Courts recognize that adjudicators, particularly those who serve on specialized boards and have experience in the field, have often formulated opinions on cases or situations similar to the ones they have in front of them. In fact, oftentimes the very motivation for selecting these persons as adjudicators is based on their having expressed opinions on certain issues. In the IRB context, one would hope that special expertise of IRB members would not be in and of itself grounds for disqualification. The opinion of expert members is often invaluable in assessing the validity of a given protocol. These experts will often have expressed authoritative opinions on particular issues in research. [...] One could compare the situation to that of judges: their earlier decisions, and the unavoidable interpretations of the law expressed in them, do not disqualify them from ruling on a similar case in the future.

In conclusion, when reviewers or judges have financial interests, they are disqualified if there is a clear potential for personal loss and if the financial interest is not too remote. Financial interests are identified as creating conflicts, and are more clearly subject to regulation than other types of interest. Scrutiny of financial interests, rather than of personal involvement and prejudgment, seems appropriate for IRB review, in particular when we are dealing with research undertaken entirely within a commercial context. While some cases involving personal involvement and prejudgment may necessitate intervention, they do not require the same stringent regulations because they are often unavoidable and may be counterbalanced by the composition of the IRB. Personal involvement can only be decided on a case-by-case basis, for example, by looking at the specific relationship an IRB member has with a researcher who submits a protocol. We further believe that the public function of IRBs strengthens the need for stringent assessment of the impact of commercial interests on the review process. [...]

THE ROLE OF CONFLICT-OF-INTEREST RULES

[...] Conflict-of-interest rules are particularly important when regulations allow much discretion and rely on the fairness and independence of individual decision makers. This is the case with research regulations. Two major types of rules are available for any type of regulation: procedural rules and substantive rules. Through procedural rules, legislators or regulatory agencies can establish a system of review and licensing. These procedural rules are ordinarily, if not always, accompanied by a set of substantive rules. Substantive rules specify what is allowed and what is forbidden. As applied to research ethics review, substantive rules specify *what* research is acceptable, and procedural rules specify *how* one can decide and *who* can decide that a study is acceptable. Substantive rules describe the qualities the conduct of research itself needs to satisfy; procedural rules describe the qualities required of the decision-making process that validates the research project including the ways in which substantive rules are applied and interpreted.

Research ethics codes and research regulations are characterized by the dominance of procedural rules [and, as such,] IRB members are relied upon to make significant value judgments.

The FDA regulations, for example, contain concrete procedures but only general rules dealing with substantive issues. Issues such as IRB membership, the functioning of the IRB, the keeping of minutes, notification procedures, and so on, are specifically regulated. Yet, not so much direction is provided as to what criteria IRBs should use in rejecting or approving protocols. Research procedure, for example, must be consistent with "sound research design" and should not "unnecessarily" expose subjects to risks. Risks have to be "reasonable in relation to anticipated benefits." Selection of subjects has to be "equitable." [...]

Research regulations, in other words, provide no absolute standards upon which IRBs can rely. Appropriate protocol review requires a fair exercise of intelligence and discretion on the part of IRB members. [...] Procedural rules dealing with the membership and composition of IRBs, including conflict-of-interest rules, are important in research ethics review precisely because there is so much reliance on the fairness of IRB members. Members should be sufficiently detached so that they can be trusted to weigh risks and benefits fairly. There should be no suspicion that objectives other than the protection of research subjects will prevail. Unfortunately, current provisions on conflict of interest, particularly the way they are to be interpreted, are too vague to be helpful. [. . .]

CONFLICT OF INTEREST
IN COMMERCIAL IRBs

The English and Commonwealth decisions holding that an interest as a shareholder or ratepayer is sufficient to create disqualifying bias are very interesting in the context of discussing financial conflicts of IRBs and IRB members. When individual IRB members are paid by a commercial IRB, they have an interest in keeping their contractual relationship with this IRB. NIRBs, in turn, have an interest in obtaining as many contracts as possible from CROs. When NIRBs are financially dependent on their clients, they surely have an interest that is less remote than that of a shareholder or ratepayer. An NIRB's decision to reject protocols submitted by a CRO may affect its client–service provider relationship. This, in turn, could have an impact on the earnings of individual IRB members. American law softens the rule on conflict of interest, by suggesting that an interest must be "substantial." This could imply that one has to look in more detail at the salaries IRB members receive, and what percentage this amount is of their overall income. How do these rules apply to the two forms of commercial IRBs?

In the case of proprietary review, the company that establishes the IRB submits its own research protocols for review. Two situations are causes for concern here. First, individual IRB members may be recruited from among personnel of the company, which means they are employees of the institution submitting protocols for review. Consciously or inadvertently, directly or indirectly, pressure might exist to approve protocols or to be more flexible with respect to required modifications. While this situation also exists within academic IRBs, the pressure can be greater within private companies whose practices are not subjected to the same level of public and academic scrutiny. Respect for superiors is part of the hierarchical corporate culture, and may be less prevalent in a university environment that values academic freedom. There might be fewer, or less reliable, means of protecting employee reviewers from corporate sanctions. In academic environments, where academic excellence and integrity should be core values, profit motives may be less likely to prevail. In a commercial con-

text, profit is of the highest importance and the primary responsibility is to shareholders. By definition, CROs depend financially on the protocols that are submitted for review. Employees know very well that rejection of research protocols leads *de facto* to a loss for the company, since it means that lucrative research cannot be undertaken. They are also aware that when they insist on certain modifications to the protocol, research may be delayed or become more expensive. Moreover, systems of financial incentives within the company might increase the pecuniary consequences of rejecting protocols. [. . .]

Second, even if IRB members are attracted from outside the company, they are appointed by those in charge of the company. The latter have a primary interest in the profit margin of the company. They could easily terminate the appointments of IRB members whose decisions affect the profit margin of the company. Even if the board or president acts in good faith and respects the IRB's independence, the appearance of direct control over the IRB undermines the credibility of proprietary review. It is not unreasonable to expect that members may fear losing the financial advantages linked to membership and thus act accordingly. Certainly, this is also a possibility within a university environment, where deans or hospital and department directors may feel the pressure of corporate investments. But as we have argued, academic scrutiny might be higher and other values prevail, or should prevail, in this setting. [. . .]

[. . .] IRB members who earn little income outside their work as reviewer may have a conflict of interest under the *de minimis* approach, while others who have another substantial source of income would have no conflict, even if they are paid more as members. The relatively small weight of the income they gain from participating in research review could be used to argue that external reviewers are more likely to be independent than, for example, a member of an academic IRB who is reviewing profit-oriented protocols submitted by the chair of her department.

Nevertheless, in the context of the commercial IRB structure, we feel more comfortable with the common law rules, which would see this as a situation in which conflicts of interest are inherent, regardless of the significance of IRB remuneration to a specific member. We have three reasons for holding this to be the case. First, it may not be practical to examine in detail how significant the remuneration is, with respect to the overall income of every individual IRB member. Second, the special role of IRBs within medical research demands that we err on the side of caution and develop policies that enhance public trust. This can only be done if rules on conflict of interest are clear and comprehensive. Third, IRB review requires [. . .] the exercise of much discretion. There is no clear standard to verify whether IRB members did perform their work without undue influence from their financial interests. Because of their particular work, strict detachment is required. [. . .]

REMEDIES AGAINST CONFLICT OF INTEREST

Can these conflicts of interest be avoided? Several procedural remedies have been suggested to solve them. The most common suggestions are disclosure, removal of voting right, and prohibition from participating in the review.

The disclosure remedy is based on the idea that people can make truly informed decisions if they are aware of all factors that could influence their physicians' enthusiasm for the trial. If those who could be harmed by a conflict of interest are informed, the argument goes, they can then freely decide whether to take the risk. While this rings true in some circumstances, it ignores the fact that people are often in situations which make them vulnerable, and dependent upon others to protect them. [...] Furthermore, the mere existence of a protective regime in the area of research, based on control by regulatory agencies and IRB review, indicates that reliance on informed consent is not sufficient. [...] IRBs are themselves supposed to control conflict of interest among researchers. [...] When analyzing the potential conflicts, IRBs might consider that direct disclosure of a researcher's interest in a study is an appropriate remedy. But it seems odd to explain to research subjects that the committee protecting them against conflicts of interest is itself affected by such a conflict.

This is not to say that disclosure of financial conflicts is not a core requirement of conflict-of-interest policies. We support efforts by journals and academic centers to require disclosure of any financial ties with research sponsors. Disclosure of financial interests of IRB members also seems appropriate to enhance public accountability if it is connected to a system of overview and authorization. [...] However, disclosure on its own, particularly the mere disclosure of institutional conflicts of interest to research participants, is insufficient as a remedy.

Would all problems be solved if those who are in an employment relationship with the IRB abstain from participation? We argue that even in that case, there is an inherent conflict of interest in the way commercial IRB review is currently organized. Depending on the payment IRB members receive, they may rely financially on these earnings, and may have a significant interest in keeping their status as a member. More importantly, conflict-of-interest rules are as much about perception of influence as they are about real influence, since they focus on establishing trust. Is there any way, then, to remedy situations of conflict of interest in NIRBs and proprietary IRBs?

First, it seems very difficult to avoid or correct conflicts of interest in proprietary IRBs or NIRBs when employees or full-time paid administrators of the IRB are involved. The perception that secondary interests (financial gain, promotion, employment) may affect the duty of IRB members to protect research subjects is serious. One way to de-

crease conflicts of interest in proprietary review would be to establish a system of accredited reviewers who would have to follow clear substantive guidelines and who would be held accountable for violations of their professional code. The paradigm for such a system is the accredited accountant, who is paid by the company but adheres to professional rules. Presently, neither the procedural rules nor the substantive rules of IRB review are appropriate for such a system of review. [...]

In the absence of a professional code for IRB members, one could argue that when IRB review becomes a core aspect of professional practice, reviewers who participate as members of their profession can be held accountable according to their professional code. When they approve research protocols that contradict standard research and clinical practice, they could be charged with professional misconduct. We are aware of one precedent of an IRB member being held accountable as reviewer by his professional organization. The New Zealand Medical Council found the chairman of an ethics committee, which approved a study in which women with cervical cancer died, guilty of professional misconduct for his role in inadequate review and monitoring of the trial. However, it may not be easy to establish whether those reviewers are participating as members of a profession, and what constitutes a violation of one's professional code in reviewing research, particularly in light of the vagueness of the rules of IRB review. Many members are clearly not bound by professional codes. Bioethicists, for example, who often play an important role in IRB review, have no professional code, and often have no training in research ethics when they start participating in the review of protocols. [...] Consequently, it is naïve to trust blindly in the appropriateness of the membership of IRBs and in their ability to always withstand secondary interests.

NIRBs differ in at least one interesting respect: they are, in theory, independent contractors. If they could be financially independent from large CROs, one would not necessarily fear conflicts of interest. But the only way to guarantee fully that they are not pressured to provide client-friendly review is to implement a system where forum shopping is avoided. [...]

If we want to have a credible system of research review, the possibility of forum shopping for friendly review should clearly be banned, with respect to not only NIRBs but also other IRBs. Forum shopping can be avoided by creating an administrative structure that involves exclusive, mandatory jurisdiction, accreditation, and control. Under such a system, CROs and others involved in medical research would have to pay a licensing fee for submitting protocols. CROs should have no direct financial or other link with the IRB members and should not be able to exercise pressure—directly or indirectly—on decisions made by the IRB.

The disadvantage of separating reviewers from the research sponsor or from the research community where the research takes place is that it becomes even more difficult for the IRB to follow up and monitor research. The National Commission for the Protection of Human Subjects of Biomedical and Behavioral Research recommended in 1978 against a system of regional or national review. It suggested that local review has "the advantage of greater familiarity with the actual conditions surrounding the conduct of research" and allows the IRBs to "work closely with investigators to assure that the rights and welfare of human subjects are protected." Influenced by this policy option, federal agencies involved in human subjects research consider the distance between the NIRBs and the place where research is undertaken as already problematic. [...] However, off-site IRBs seem now to be widely accepted, by the FDA and by many other national regulatory agencies, without proper regulation to safeguard their independence. It is time to review this choice for local review and to think about a more structured review system. [...]

In the absence of stringent rules on forum shopping, conflicts of interest can be reduced somewhat if the contractual relationships between the NIRBs and their clients, or the financing system of the proprietary IRBs, provide for long-term financial stability. For example, if an NIRB has a three-year contract with a CRO to review all its protocols, there is at least some financial guarantee. Similarly, if a proprietary IRB has received a guaranteed budget for several years, the IRB and its members cannot be put under constant pressure. However, this is not a guarantee of full independence. An NIRB can [...] be fully dependent on only a few large contracts. This dependence clearly constitutes a significant conflict of interest. [...]

LESSONS FOR INSTITUTIONAL IRBs

How does this discussion relate to academic IRBs? [S]ome of the conflicts existing in academic review are very particular to the institutional context. Academic IRB members may feel inclined to accept studies of colleagues whom they trust, work with, and share other research interests with. Issues of promotion, future co-authorship, and simple collegiality of the working environment may also create pressure. [...]

More important, although many academic IRBs do function in an environment where profit motives are less immediate, IRBs and IRB members increasingly feel the pressure of corporate sponsorship, particularly in light of the proportional decline of governmental funding. [...]

They may be tempted to accept studies that come with needed research dollars, which will help significantly to improve the research potential of their department or institute. When a lucrative study is rejected, some IRB members may [...] be challenged directly by the "rejected" colleague and may have to face researchers whose employment at the institution depends in part upon their role in obtaining commercial funding.

Academic research centers are increasingly entering into institutional relationships with some major pharmaceutical companies and may become partly dependent on them. This exacerbates pressure within the research centers to actively pursue research proposed by those companies. In other words, the fundamental difference between academic research units and CROs is diminishing and so, too, the difference between academic and proprietary IRBs. Thus, it is essential to introduce institutional policies that address the appropriate independence of IRBs and the need to protect IRB members when developing commercial partnerships. One way would be to reinforce some of the core aspects and values of academic scholarship that are increasingly under stress: academic integrity and independence, the public role of academic researchers, and tenure. [...]

Thus, academic IRBs need stricter conflict-of-interest rules, education, and accreditation of IRB members and greater public accountability as well. The conflicts of interest created by the increasing commercial pressures in academia add to other problems the academic IRB system is encountering.

Overall, George Annas's severe assessment that "IRBs should be radically overhauled" does not seem to be an exaggeration. The loopholes in the system of commercial IRB review are only part of a much larger problem. [Annas's suggestions] seem to support the creation of a more accountable review structure. He proposes to set up a national human research agency that would "set the rules for research involving humans, monitor their enforcement, and punish those who fail to follow them." IRBs would be accountable to this agency, and no longer be supervised only by their own institution. We believe that an intermediary agency or institutional body, exercising a level of authority between that of a national or regional authority and the local IRB, remains a valuable option. Greater local oversight of IRB function, combined with increased surveillance by federal agencies, seems a preferable model. However, this institutional supervision should be set up in a way that enhances the independence of IRBs and their public accountability. [...]

85 The Institutional Review Board and Beyond

Future Challenges to the Ethics of Human Experimentation

Harold Edgar and David J. Rothman

As a political and governance institution, nothing in the regulatory domain resembles the institutional review board (IRB). To invert the classic story about God delegating authority to a committee to perfect His creations and getting a giraffe in return, the IRB *is* the giraffe, so odd is it when compared to other creatures in the jungle.

Despite its many idiosyncrasies, over the past two decades, IRBs have transformed the conduct of research projects involving human subjects. Unquestionably, their very existence has tempered the inevitable propensity of researchers to pursue investigations without dispassionately weighing the risks they are asking others to assume or fully informing their subjects of them. Indeed, IRBs have been so successful as to set an international standard for monitoring clinical research.

Nevertheless, in the American context, the very proliferation of these committees, to the point where they are to be found in every type of institution conducting research, raises critical questions about uniform standards and performance. Is it truly the case that a "one size fits all" approach works well? Are the same general procedures for appointing members and defining their obligations appropriate for reviewing research conducted not only at the Central Intelligence Agency (CIA), the Bureau of Prisons, and the National Institutes of Health (NIH), but also at for-profit hospitals, local community hospitals, and university-affiliated, tertiary-care centers? Does it make sense to give the leadership of an institution, which by its very nature cannot survive without the funds and fame brought in by clinical research, the responsibility for appointing the membership of a monitoring committee? Or, more broadly framed, is the local and institutional basis of IRB organization still appropriate? Are the assumptions that initially underlay that choice still valid? The goal of this essay is to suggest that the answers to these questions may well be no, and to provide some modest, but potentially important, recommendations for change. IRBs can take credit for remarkable accomplishments, but it may be time to revise the framework governing human experimentation.

Harold Edgar and David J. Rothman, "The Institutional Review Board and Beyond: Future Challenges to the Ethics of Human Experimentation," *Milbank Quarterly* 73 (1995): 489–506.

THE IRB STRUCTURE

The IRB system rests on two sets of federal regulations. The first commits various agencies of the U.S. government to securing IRB approval before research is conducted on human subjects, either in house or through the grants they fund for outside projects. Government-supported biomedical research is the paradigm case. Before any federal money can be expended on research involving human subjects, the regulations require that a protocol must be approved by this institutionally based committee, with a membership of no less than five persons, at least one of whom must not be affiliated with the institution. The IRB's central charges are, first, to review whether the benefits of the proposed research outweigh the risks, and second, to make certain that the investigators have explained all the relevant issues so as to secure the subject's informed consent. Although the federal regulations that establish the IRB system apply only to federal activities and federally funded grants, many states require IRB review for all research performed within their jurisdiction, no matter how it is funded. Moreover, the vast majority of academic institutions choose to review all their research protocols through an IRB, rather than reviewing some, but not others, on the basis of who is providing the funding.

Contrary to what many people presume, IRB regulations do not require the review of *all* innovations in medical practice, let alone all instances of physicians following their preferred treatment strategies without ascertaining whether their approach works better than someone else's. The IRB focuses exclusively on activities intended to gain generalizable knowledge, and to the extent that someone, a surgeon for example, forswears an interest in general knowledge and presumes that the best way to treat Parkinson's disease is to burn the brain's pallidum—to take an illustration from the *Wall Street Journal*'s headline story of February 22, 1995—that surgeon need not bring his new technique before an IRB.

Independent of federal funding regulations, the Food and Drug Administration (FDA) requires that protocols involving human subjects and new drugs or medical devices must be approved by IRBs. For example, were a surgeon to use a new commercial medical device in order to accomplish a proposed intervention, FDA procedures would be triggered. Insofar as testing new drugs on human subjects is concerned, FDA regulations are in important respects the same as those imposed by the Department of Health and Human Services (DHHS) on research institutions seeking grants. Yet FDA oversight differs in several important respects. FDA reviewers themselves examine the merits of the protocol and do not leave all decision-making to the IRB. Thus, in ways that overlap or supersede an IRB finding, FDA reviewers may reject research that they consider too risky or may compel investigators to carry out more animal studies before beginning clinical trials. At the same time, the FDA may impose strict regulations on the manufacture of drugs and biologics *before* they are tested, again going well beyond the IRB's usual safety concerns.

The FDA procedures do provide a degree of national oversight for clinical research. In addition, some funding agencies may conduct their own reviews of a protocol's research ethics; NIH study groups, for example, have been known to do this on occasion, rejecting a proposal on ethical grounds that a local IRB has already approved. But many human experiments do not come under either FDA or NIH study group purview, leaving decisions about the ethics of research solely in the hands of the IRB.

Thus, the power to approve or disapprove research on ethical grounds is granted to a local institutional committee, composed of members of the same institution (with the one necessary exception) that is seeking the funding. Moreover, by all reports, the members who dominate the IRB discussions are these insiders, not the outsiders (who are everywhere a distinct minority). So, in effect, the key decision-makers on the IRB are colleagues who must live with any disappointed applicants whose protocols they have rejected. Furthermore, most IRB committee members are themselves researchers and the standards they set for others will come back to bite them too.

To be sure, the IRB is uniquely well protected from formal institutional domination. Unlike most committees, which are structured to exercise power delegated by a parent and are ultimately responsible to that parent, an IRB decision to disapprove research may not legally be overturned by the institution. For example, if it believes it has grounds to do so, an IRB can effectively terminate a researcher's career at a particular institution by rejecting his protocols or by insisting on such close supervision that it becomes impossible for him to carry out investigations. [...]

Nevertheless, the IRB's autonomy and isolation are largely theoretical, in that no federal controls or regulations exist on how the institution decides who gets appointed to the committee, how long those persons stay, or on what grounds a member may be dismissed or not reappointed. Indeed, powerful people within an institution have myriad largely untraceable ways for punishing an obstructionist IRB member: from withholding or delaying promotion to blocking his or her access to other grants—a fact that no IRB member can fail to recognize. Similarly, there are no formal controls on the selection of the outside and unaffiliated members, whose professional qualifications thus may not always be clear. While many of these outsiders may understand and appreciate the scientific or ethical dimensions of research, there is no way to ensure that they are anything other than a friend of a trustee, looking for an opportunity to participate in an institutional activity.

Finally, not only the formal structure but also the actual workings of the IRB leave room for dissatisfaction. Despite the amount of time that IRBs devote to examining the language of the consent form, they are not required to investigate whether the consent language they hammer out either is actually used on the floor or serves to educate the patient about the nature of the research he or she has consented to. It is rare for an IRB to leave the confines of its committee room and examine what actually occurs in the consent process.

In effect, then, the regulations governing the IRB are, to say the least, a permeable shield, with no strong framework to ensure that subjects' interests take precedence over institutional ones. The judgments that will be made on this basis need not be so flagrant as to eventually provoke a scandal. Balancing research risks against benefits is complicated, and a committee that consistently makes the calculus in favor of the research will hardly ever be identified. On occasion, a glaring miscalculation will command headlines; the decision of the UCLA IRB to allow investigators to withdraw medication from schizophrenic patients in the course of a trial may be one such instance. But the overriding point is not how typical the UCLA actions are, but how the IRB system provides so few bulwarks against this tilt in decision making. To put the case bluntly, if one were to look at the IRB exclusively in terms of formal structure and organizing principles, it would seem to be a paper tiger. An individual serving on the body and an institution organizing it may fulfill the highest ethical standards; any one participant may claim, with full justice, that his or her IRB is exemplary in its functioning. Nevertheless, there are very few provisions in the regulations that protect against bodies that might be sloppy, venal, or subservient to the institution. Put another way, the quality of an IRB's work depends to an inordinate degree on the conscience and commitment of its volunteer members. The fact that the NIH has created an Office for Protection from Research Risks [OPRR, now the Office for Human Research Protections, or OHRP—eds.] in no way mitigates this point. OPRR is empowered to review the membership roster on local IRBs, but because the formal requirements are so minimal, such review is of limited effect. Nor does OPRR have the funds or personnel to conduct regular and ongoing examination of how individual IRBs normally function. [...]

THE LOCAL CHARACTER OF THE IRBs

Although the scandals in human experimentation drove the decision to regulate research, they hardly explain why the results placed such heavy reliance on local, institution-based procedures. One major reason was that the research community was ahead of the curve of public demand, regulating itself before others did so. Local, institutional review was the least intrusive means of allaying public fears. Ask anyone in the pharmaceutical industry whether they fear more their review by an IRB or their fate with an investigational new drug (IND) at the FDA, and you will learn that the IRB is vastly more flexible than the FDA. An IRB is far more apt to communicate quickly what troubles it and how those troubles may be overcome. The public interest, it should be noted, often gains significantly from this flexibility, but it comes, as we shall see, with a price.

The preference for localism drew as well on a whole set of assumptions about the research enterprise and those who conduct it. First, when the IRB mechanisms were put into place over the 1970s, everyone, at least at the NIH, assumed that funds were readily available to do research. The inevitable result of IRB review was to delay things, but the costs of delay could be absorbed in a generous overhead allotment; moreover, the researcher who had to move more slowly on project A could always find support for project B. In other words, by making review local, the penalties of regulation were minimized.

Second, regulators presumed that IRBs would almost always operate within a university teaching hospital where a shared commitment to the ideals of good science would far outweigh any tendency for persons to trade favors or elevate concerns for the financial viability of the institution above their loyalty to the integrity of science or the well-being of subjects. [...] Thus, once science incorporated ethical principles in human experimentation into its own system, scientists would effectively enforce them, offsetting any dangers in localism. Moreover, the forces motivating researchers were promotions, prizes, and grants, all of which depended upon the respect of peers. No one would, therefore, risk imperiling the prestige of his or her institution by letting sloppy or unethical research slide by. Thus, it seemed as though the local character of IRB review secured all the advantages that came with being close to or part of the action, without running the risk of having regulators captured by the regulated.

Third, the designers of the IRB system expected that the subjects themselves were likely to be suspicious about human experimentation, adopting a cautious, self-protective stand against involvement. Participation was perceived as both burdensome and risky; experiments were dangerous, and subjects were fully alert to the implications of being a guinea pig. Discussion of research ethics spoke of the need to distribute fairly the *burden* of participation, not re-

lying on and exploiting the poor. All the while, the attention devoted to the specific wording of consent forms was a way to guarantee that subjects would be able to act so as to promote their own self-interest. Well-informed subjects would never put themselves at undue risk. Where subjects were for one or another reason not capable of giving consent (owing to the debilitating effects of illness, mental disability, youth, or confinement to a prison), it seemed right to bar them from being used as subjects. The one exception was in the event that they had a special stake in the research mission; research on retardation, for example, might well require that persons with retardation be the subjects—even then, additional protections had to be employed. Research carried such danger that, although the policy was rarely made explicit, women, particularly women of child-bearing age, also seemed to require special protection. [...]

THE LIMITS OF LOCALISM

Each one of these three premises has now been substantially undercut, with the end result that the localism of the IRB appears to generate more problems than it solves. The confidence that IRB delay or disapproval carried no penalties because a surfeit of research opportunities was available has weakened—really disappeared. Money for research has become very scarce, and researchers have no confidence that there will always be another grant if this one is delayed.

Even more important, many potential subjects no longer regard participation in experiments as a dangerous activity. The line between experiment and therapy has blurred, and human subjects do not necessarily greet departures from accepted procedures, even exceptionally risky ones, with suspicion. Accordingly, the IRB presumption that a well-crafted consent form was a meaningful protection has weakened: subjects may well be simply too eager to obtain what they see as the most advanced and potentially therapeutic intervention. [...]

So too, the proportion of research that is industry funded, rather than government supported, has increased dramatically, which carries several critical implications for IRB reviews. Researchers may have entrepreneurial interests in products being tested at their home universities. Indeed, the academic institutions face major issues of conflict of interest because medical entrepreneurialism has become a goal of the university itself. [...]

Indeed, some institutions now function economically as packages of patients with rare diseases. The concentration of patients at the institution makes feasible corporate-sponsored research protocols that could not otherwise be done; the institution profits handsomely by providing experimental options to those sponsors, in effect matching sponsors and volunteers who would not otherwise efficiently find one another. [...]

In fact, for these reasons, and others as well, the academic center, which served as a paradigm for the IRB, is likely in the future to lose what was once a near monopoly over research. Its role is being usurped from at least two sides. On the one hand, huge multistate and international trials have been, and will be, organized, bringing thousands of patients into a single trial, run by a coordinating group. With research becoming more national, ethics review on the local level makes still less sense. Second, the managed care plan provides a perfect site for many trials. To the extent that health maintenance organizations and other providers develop information bases linking different physicians' treatment patterns to patient outcomes, they are the natural place to conduct research on how much of a difference, if any at all, an intervention brings. Indeed, if we are prepared to insist as part of the managed care revolution that cost-containment measures be researched rather than imposed (which we may not be), then an in-house IRB model is hardly equipped to serve as guardian of patient interests.

One final point about the locus of research activity has recently assumed exceptional importance. The original 1960s assumption that the university was the site of most human experimentation minimized the importance of the fact that a number of government agencies, including the Department of Energy (DOE) and the CIA, were already heavily invested in such activities. Although there were discussions and hearings on whether so local and internal a system made sense in this context, and these agencies in time did agree to come under the regulations and establish their own IRBs, not until the 1994 exposé of cold war radiation research did the disadvantages of this arrangement become the center of public attention and policy analysis. Is it truly meaningful for the DOE or the CIA to run its own IRB? In light of what we now know about their activities, the local basis for the regulation of their human experimentation seems less satisfactory.

TAKING THE "I" OUT OF THE IRB

If the old paradigms no longer hold, what revisions should be made in public policy? Where do we go from here?

The IRB system has worked reasonably well, and to dismantle it would be a mistake. Nonetheless, IRBs were a "one size fits all" solution. Obviously, no single reform or institutional structure will be able to provide adequate oversight of all biomedical innovations. Accordingly, public policy innovations should move forward simultaneously on a number of fronts. We mention three.

IRB procedures are completely inadequate to protect the public interest from the ends of research, or to assure sufficient lead time to permit political focus on the limits, if any, that should accompany the development of new technologies. Mechanisms must be found to assure that proposed research that crosses frontiers achieves public visibility and provides opportunity for political choice before it is implemented. In contemplating how to accomplish this end, one is drawn inevitably to the establishment of a "super" committee or committees, charged at the minimum with a monitoring function, at the maximum with the right to veto research deemed unacceptable.

How can this be done? Throughout the world, various countries have established national ethics committees to serve as ongoing advisors on difficult ethical issues associated with research, and medical practice more generally. [. . .] But, in the past, initiatives have floundered on the question of who gets to appoint whom to do what [. . .].

Three principal and interrelated issues must be addressed in the design of an overarching monitoring mechanism:

First, whether to constitute one committee, endowing it with visibility and prestige because of its singularity, or several committees, distributing responsibility among members selected for their particular expertise. The NIH's recombinant DNA advisory group is the prototype of the special committee. And it has worked. Researchers complain about its delays, but it has had a profound impact on securing public consensus that gene research is an appropriate end, and one that can be safely pursued. [. . .]

Second, to determine how expansive a committee's jurisdiction should be: whether it will be limited to reviewing funded grant proposals and issuing advisory opinions, leaving the ultimate decisions to local IRBs and researchers, or whether its approval will be required before research is undertaken.

Third, to decide who should appoint such a committee, and what kind of staff it should have, questions that obviously become more or less sensitive depending on what powers the committee is granted.

Our own preference is to seek multiple committees of specialists, appointed by DHHS-NIH officials, whose responsibilities would extend to their particular fields of research—neurobiology, genetic therapy, reproduction—without regard to the sources of the research funding, governmental or private.

[W]e would not grant the committee formal power to halt research. Adding another layer to the review of human investigation would incur too much expense and delay. Instead, we prefer to have such committees stay abreast of research methods and issues, making public the significant questions and providing general guidance to local IRBs about particular protocols. Yes, investigators who can persuade their own IRBs of the propriety of their work will be able to take the first research steps in advance of such review [. . .]. But two considerations seem to us to reduce the potential risks. For one, frontier research is usually incremental, in the sense that the relevant professional community knows who is involved with research near the boundary and what the likely pace of advance will be. The presence of professional leaders on a committee with high visibility will encourage people in the field who have doubts about their own or their colleagues' agendas to ask whether and to what extent the issues that concern them have already been analyzed and considered. For another, expert committees will have ready access to the media and to policy makers, for biomedical research is (and will continue to be) in the public spotlight. Accordingly, expert committees will have time to foster debate about the research and ultimately provide the opportunity for an informed political decision on its desirability. In short, controversies about the stopping points in particular lines of research—whether they involve cloning, genetic enhancement, or other novel procedures—will have to be decided ultimately in the political arena, and administrative mechanisms cannot avoid that fact.

The second broad area of reform involves improving the present IRB system to take account of the newly entrepreneurial character of biomedical science that we have described.

Many of the concerns we raised are the appropriate object for formal legal rules. For example, conflict-of-interest guidelines can, and should, specify the limits on researchers and institutions that are simultaneously financially invested in the development of products and the testing of those products. We would, for example, preclude investigators from recruiting patients and conducting clinical evaluations where the product being tested is one in which they hold a commercial stake. So too, patients should be told of any financial commitments that would motivate the investigator to select this treatment for the patient rather than the others on hand.

The third direction that reform must take is to strengthen the "outside" elements of the IRBs, while leaving review based in the institution itself. Localism has the advantage of accomplishing review not only more quickly but also with the knowledge, informal as it is, of the character of the investigators. Most important, it greatly facilitates learning that something is going wrong: nurses, residents, physicians do not have to cross institutional lines to inform someone of their concern that a protocol is not being followed.

IRBs processing a substantial number of protocols should, however, include experts drawn from scientific groups outside the institution. Moreover, there must be more focus on the appointment and renewal process. We should also seek to quasi-professionalize the role of outside members, linking them in groups that could come together to study common issues, so that there might be greater uniformity given to concepts like minimum risk. [...] The proposition that outside members can represent a relevant "community" has always seemed suspect to us; and we would prefer to see on each IRB a member who felt loyalty to a newly constituted community of research ethics advisors.

These stipulations about strengthening the outside role in IRB review take on special importance when the research is being conducted by the government itself. To make certain that such bodies as the DOE and the CIA remain well within the bounds of ethical research, it is vital that outsiders play an even more important role in their reviews than elsewhere. To accomplish this change would not be easy, not only because these bodies are very insular, but because outsiders also might well require security clearances and have to assume burdens of confidentiality that would hamper their effectiveness in bringing abuses to light. But were a commitment to extrainstitutional review made, strategies for at once protecting the national interest and the subjects' well-being could be designed.

Finally, and most certainly, we should have far more effective oversight mechanisms. It would be entirely feasible, for example, for an NIH office to sample (in the technical sense) protocols from research settings (not only universities, but also companies and government agencies), and to include in this effort interviews with the subjects of the research (reviewing the process by which they gave consent, what they understood the experiment to be, and how the research itself was conducted). The very existence of such a procedure might help improve IRB performance.

In sum, it is time to take the superintendence of human research to a different, and more national, level. Whether this change can be accomplished within the current political climate is debatable. The necessity for such a shift is not.

86   A Central Institutional Review Board
for Multi-institutional Trials

MICHAELE C. CHRISTIAN, JACQUELYN L. GOLDBERG,
JACK KILLEN, JEFFREY S. ABRAMS, MARY S. MCCABE,
JOAN K. MAUER, AND ROBERT E. WITTES

These are difficult times for the nation's system of protection for human subjects in research. On the basis of a series of reports, the Office of the Inspector General of the Department of Health and Human Services concluded that institutional review boards (IRBs) are now forced to "review too much, too quickly, with too little expertise," and with inadequate resources. One consequence is that there is minimal, often perfunctory, review of ongoing research. In addition, IRB members have become disillusioned as a result of both public criticism concerning the perceived failures of the boards and the increasing amount of time required to perform duplicative tasks that add little to the safety of patients.

We believe that the effectiveness of IRBs has been undermined by many factors that are, in part, the consequence of a system that has failed to adapt to major changes that have occurred in the research environment since the IRB system was established in the 1970s. These changes include a shift from predominantly federally funded studies performed at single academic centers to large multicenter trials of complex treatments involving both federal and private sponsors. The Bell Report for the National Institutes of Health described the staggering annual workload facing 491 IRBs, including an estimated 284,000 reviews: 105,000 initial reviews, 116,000 annual reviews, and 63,000 amendments. It also noted that the annual full-board meeting time ranged from 9 to 50 hours and that the average time devoted to discussion of the initial review of a protocol was 21 minutes for low-volume IRBs and 3 minutes for high-volume IRBs. [...] We describe a possible solution to some of these problems—namely, a novel model, now in the pilot phase, for the review of multicenter phase 3 trials that involves the use of a central IRB (CIRB) and a facilitated review process. The model was developed by the National Cancer Institute (NCI), in collaboration with the Office for Human Research Protections [OHRP], as part of a larger initiative to improve the NCI's clinical-trials program.

Michaele C. Christian, Jacquelyn L. Goldberg, Jack Killen, Jeffrey S. Abrams, Mary S. McCabe, Joan K. Mauer, and Robert E. Wittes, "A Central Institutional Review Board for Multi-institutional Trials," *New England Journal of Medicine* 346 (2002): 1405–8.

ORIGINS OF THE CENTRAL REVIEW BOARD

The CIRB project arose as a means of increasing patients' access to and enrollment in NCI-supported clinical trials. NCI is the largest sponsor of clinical trials of treatment for cancer in the United States, but only 2 percent of patients with newly diagnosed cancer (30,000) participated in NCI-sponsored cancer-treatment trials in 2001. Patients are more likely to participate in a trial if their physicians are investigators, but physician-investigators argue that the burdens associated with securing approval from the local IRB for these studies limit their interest in participation, particularly if only a small number of patients will be enrolled at a particular site. These burdens include long and complex application and review processes and the substantial time required to obtain approval, estimated to be 5 to 14 hours. The recent imposition of fees for review by some IRBs creates yet another obstacle.

The burdens that IRB review places on investigators are neither unique to the NCI program nor necessarily persuasive that change is needed. Nonetheless, in the context of large multicenter trials, they call attention to serious problems of duplication of effort and inefficiency associated with numerous local reviews of the same trial—problems that have also been noted by others. For example, the NCI has a total of more than 10,000 registered investigators at almost 3,000 individual sites. Each year, there are approximately 160 ongoing phase 3 trials, of which 30 are new trials. Conservatively estimated, the average number of clinical sites participating in each trial is about 100 (range, 4 to 809), although many trials have several hundred sites; thus, at a minimum, 16,000 IRB reviews of NCI phase 3 trials are conducted each year (3,000 initial reviews and 13,000 annual reviews of ongoing trials). In addition, IRBs perform an estimated 20,000 reviews of protocol amendments and thousands of reviews of adverse events each year. These numbers will only increase as the NCI implements additional initiatives designed to expand patients' access to clinical trials. At a time of growing concern about the adequacy of an overburdened system for the protection of research subjects, the benefit of these obviously duplicative and seemingly wasteful efforts must be weighed against the cost, especially the distraction of local IRBs from the essential task of effectively monitoring local research. The CIRB project has been structured to address many of these concerns.

THE CENTRAL REVIEW BOARD AND FACILITATED REVIEW

The CIRB pilot project provides an expert IRB review of NCI-sponsored trials at the national level before protocols are distributed to local investigators. Local IRBs can then approve the protocols rapidly, using a facilitated review process based on the CIRB review. A number of regulatory agencies, including the Food and Drug Administration (FDA) and the OHRP, have agreed that this approach is in compliance with relevant federal regulations. Furthermore, the OHRP has made the important determination that a facilitated review may be conducted by the chairperson of the local IRB or by an IRB subcommittee after the CIRB materials have been reviewed. Thus, the protocol can be approved quickly and efficiently. Locally, facilitated review could make it possible for many more physicians and their patients to participate in trials by making them accessible within days rather than months. If this approach were instituted throughout the national IRB system, it would reduce vast amounts of duplication of effort and allow IRBs to address truly local matters, such as oversight of local studies.

The CIRB is composed of 16 members with expertise in cancer from across the country. None are NCI employees, most attend the monthly CIRB meetings in person (some participate by teleconference), and each receives a $200 honorarium for attending meetings. Drawn from both academic and community organizations, the members include physicians, nurses, and pharmacologists with expertise in the treatment of cancer; ethicists; and patient advocates. The composition of the board satisfies federal regulatory requirements and the recommendations of the National Bioethics Advisory Commission, which specify that at least 25 percent of the membership should represent the perspective of research participants, be engaged primarily in nonscientific activities, or both. The work of the CIRB is coordinated by an experienced NCI administrator and five full-time staff members. The pilot program initially involved 22 local institutions and is currently expanding to include 100. The division of responsibilities between the CIRB and each local IRB is spelled out in a formal agreement between the two entities and also in detailed standard operating procedures (available at http://www.ncicirb.org).

The CIRB has reviewed all NCI-sponsored phase 3 treatment trials involving adults with cancer that have been initiated since January 2001. The board's review functions are essentially identical to those of a local IRB. It performs an initial review of each new protocol; discusses any issues with the sponsor, coordinating cooperative group (an NCI-funded multicenter organization that develops protocols and conducts research), and study chair for the protocol; and makes a final decision whether to approve the protocol. The CIRB also reviews annual study reports, reports of serious adverse events, protocol amendments, reports by data and safety monitoring boards, and other documents. All review materials, including the application for approval of the study, protocol reviews, relevant correspondence, and minutes of meetings, are made available to the local IRBs participating in the pilot program.

The OHRP requires that IRB reviews of federally sponsored research involving human subjects, such as NCI trials, reflect an understanding of the local context in which the research occurs. This requirement must be met even if one IRB reviews protocols on behalf of another IRB. To comply with the local-context requirement, the CIRB uses a local-decision-maker approach, in which the local IRB decides, on a protocol-by-protocol basis, whether there are relevant issues involving the local context that must be addressed and whether a facilitated or full local review is warranted. A decision to perform a facilitated review makes the CIRB the review board of record responsible for annual reviews and for reviews of adverse events and protocol amendments. As appropriate, the local IRB may specify local restrictions, stipulations, or substitutions in protocols and informed-consent documents that have been approved by the CIRB. However, deletions or substantive changes that affect the meaning of CIRB-approved protocols or consent documents are not allowed. Changes in consent documents are monitored as part of periodic audits of NCI-sponsored trials.

The local institution and IRB are required to ensure that the research is performed safely and appropriately. They must assess the suitability of the local research environment for the proposed research; make sure that the investigators and other research staff receive training in the protection of human subjects and meet the institution's standards for the conduct of research; monitor the conduct of the study; review serious adverse events occurring at the local institution; and provide a mechanism for handling complaints by local subjects or others. The CIRB must be notified of steps taken to address problems in these areas.

In theory, the CIRB model should also substantially improve the review of adverse events in multicenter trials. In the current scheme, a local IRB must review reports of serious adverse events that occur at all participating sites; the sheer volume of these reports and the administrative burden may distract the IRB from the serious adverse events that actually require its attention. In the CIRB model, the central board evaluates all individual adverse events in the context of the entire clinical trial and on the basis of supplemental toxicity information provided by the

NCI. Such a comprehensive review is seldom possible at the local level.

EARLY EXPERIENCE WITH
THE CENTRAL REVIEW BOARD

In its first year, the CIRB reviewed 20 protocols; 17 were approved with modifications, 2 required substantive revisions before they were approved, and 1 is still being reviewed. For reasons unrelated to the CIRB program, most of these studies have not been initiated at the 22 local institutions participating in the pilot program. Because access to protocols has been based on membership in specific cooperative groups, local investigators have not sought approval from their local IRBs for many of the 19 approved protocols that were not developed by their cooperative group. As of March 2002, local IRBs had performed facilitated reviews 15 times (at six institutions) and had elected to conduct full reviews 25 times. With the planned expansion of the CIRB program to include 100 local sites over the next several months and the availability of all new trials to any cooperative-group investigator by June 2002, more useful data on the rate of utilization and on satisfaction with facilitated review should be available in 12 to 18 months. A formal evaluation of the process by the participating IRBs will be performed at that time.

The members of the CIRB are satisfied with the board's operation in its first year. The CIRB reviews only two or three new protocols each month. This workload allows for in-depth discussion of each protocol, annual reviews of ongoing trials and adverse events, and educational sessions during regularly scheduled meetings. The diverse perspectives and expertise of the board's members have resulted in a rich discussion of issues that is unmatched by many local IRBs. For each study it reviews, the CIRB has ready access to the study chair and to experts at the NCI who can answer questions during the review process. This level of access is rarely available to local IRBs, which must usually rely on information provided by local investigators who may have had little to do with developing the study and may therefore have a less thorough understanding of the rationale for the study, its design, or other issues that IRBs often address.

The logistic difficulties and complexity of communicating rapidly and effectively with all parties involved in large multi-institutional trials pose substantial challenges. The pilot experience has resulted in the implementation of a detailed communications plan to help ensure that the CIRB communicates as required with local IRBs, data and safety monitoring boards, local investigators, cooperative groups, the NCI as the sponsor of the trials, and others. A controlled-access Web site (http://www.ncicirb.org) has been developed to provide reliable electronic access to the many documents that the CIRB generates.

FUTURE CHALLENGES

A major challenge facing this new system is to define and adjudicate overlapping responsibilities. All proposed NCI protocols undergo several layers of scientific and ethical review by committees within the cooperative group and the NCI, as well as by the FDA (if an investigational agent is involved). These reviews address the scientific hypothesis, the study design, ethical issues, and the informed-consent document. In addition, all NCI-sponsored phase 3 trials are monitored by independent data and safety monitoring boards. These boards and the IRBs explicitly share responsibility for ensuring the safety and well-being of enrolled subjects, though the data and safety monitoring boards have a more comprehensive view of accumulating data, since they have exclusive access to unblinded data on efficacy, as well as data on adverse events and safety. The data and safety monitoring boards have a key role in ensuring the safety of subjects and assessing the relative risks and benefits of participation throughout the clinical trial. Lack of clarity about the appropriate division of responsibility between IRBs and data and safety monitoring boards is an important issue that has not been fully resolved. In any case, the hope is that better communication between the data and safety monitoring board for a particular study and the CIRB will address the problem of overlapping responsibilities, further improve the protection of subjects, and ensure that informed-consent processes and protocols are modified appropriately to reflect relevant new knowledge.

The scientific expertise of many of the CIRB members raises the question of the boundary between a review of the scientific aspects of a study and a review of the ethical aspects. Some believe that the CIRB should address only safety and ethical issues, because all NCI-sponsored trials of cancer treatment pose reasonable scientific questions and have reasonable designs or they would not have survived the extensive scientific review to which they have already been subjected. Others argue that scientific merit and trial design are directly related to the risk-benefit assessment and are appropriate areas for review by either a local IRB or a CIRB. Although the CIRB should avoid imposing its views when dealing with issues about which reasonable people may disagree, the disease-specific scientific expertise of the board members increases the likelihood of controversies in the gray zone between safety and science. During its first 16 months of operation, the CIRB has already confronted these issues (as well as conflict over its role in ongoing reviews versus that of a data and safety monitoring board). Because the CIRB is the final committee through which all NCI-sponsored phase 3 trials must pass before they are activated, it has unprecedented power and authority. It will be crucial to pay careful attention to these issues. The selection of CIRB members with extensive IRB experience may help diminish conflicts in this realm.

The success of the CIRB pilot program ultimately depends on the extent to which local IRBs use the facilitated review process; at present, their willingness to do so is uncertain. If large numbers of local IRBs decide to perform full rather than facilitated reviews, the CIRB will simply be another layer of review in an already multilayered process. In the increasingly complex regulatory environment of clinical research, local IRBs, or the institutional officials responsible for them, may be reluctant to relinquish responsibility to an independent body. Institutional concern about legal liability and indemnification may work against full participation in the new program, even though it is clear that fundamental changes in the system for the protection of research subjects are necessary.

As Steinbrook points out, a high-quality IRB review, although necessary, is unlikely to guarantee the full protection of research subjects. This responsibility is truly shared, depending on the efforts of tens of thousands of persons throughout the country. The extent to which the many parties involved acknowledge this shared responsibility and work collaboratively may ultimately determine whether the complex review system actually improves the protection of research subjects. Local IRBs will remain a key component of the system, however, and it is clear that we need a more effective approach than the current one, which places too large a burden on local IRBs. We believe that the facilitated-review model for large national trials is a promising approach that preserves local autonomy and responsibility with regard to local matters, reduces the workload of local IRBs, and eliminates duplication of effort. An expert central review of planned and ongoing research frees local IRBs to oversee the performance of studies at the local level, thus capitalizing on the strengths of both the central and the local systems and improving the overall protection of research subjects.

Appendixes

Informed Consent Forms

According to the principle of respect for persons, individuals should have the opportunity to freely decide whether research participation is compatible with their interests or goals and to provide their informed consent for research (see Part V of this volume). Informed consent is a process that includes the presentation of information to prospective participants who have the capacity to consent, assessment of their understanding of the information, and their making of a voluntary decision about enrolling or remaining in a study. In clinical research this process typically includes the presentation and signing of a written consent form, a document that summarizes both the details of the study and the rights of the prospective participant. According to the U.S. federal regulations found in the Common Rule (45 CFR §46.116, included in Part II), a consent form should include at least the following elements: (1) a statement that the study involves research, (2) an explanation of the purposes of the research and the nature of the procedures, (3) any reasonably foreseeable risks or discomforts, (4) any benefits to be expected; (5) alternative procedures or courses of treatment, (6) the extent of confidentiality protections, (7) an explanation as to whether any compensation for injury is available, (8) whom to contact with questions about the research or participants' rights, and (9) a statement that participation in research is voluntary.

Although consent forms are believed to be a vital part of the process of informed consent, there are many questions about the role and effectiveness of the written consent form in enabling the participant to provide his or her informed consent. First of all, many consent forms are extremely long and include complex, often unfamiliar, scientific concepts. The crux of the difficulty here is how to include all the information that might reasonably bear on a person's decision

whether to participate in research without overwhelming the reader with information. A second and related problem is the level of the language and technical jargon used in many consent forms. It has been recommended that important documents, including consent forms, be written at or below an eighth-grade reading level in order to accommodate the diverse reading skills and competencies of most research participants. Empirical evidence shows, however, that consent forms are often written in language and a style more appropriate for college graduates.[1] There are alternative strategies for making documents easier to read (e.g., the use of active voice, short sentences, large fonts, headings, and white borders, as well as diagrams, charts, and other graphics), but they are only sporadically found in consent forms. Third, there is widespread concern about a "therapeutic misconception" in research. Some claim that written consent forms contribute to this misconception by glossing over the purpose or nature of research, making investigational agents sound like proven treatments, or by exaggerating the possible benefits of the research. (See the discussion of this in Part V.) Fourth, there has been increased attention to legal aspects of clinical research and institutional risk management. In an effort to avoid liability, consent forms have increasingly included legalistic language about participants' rights, confidentiality, and compensation for injury, among other things. Despite the problems found in many consent forms, these forms are reviewed and approved by institutional review boards (IRBs) before they are presented to prospective participants,[2] and it has been claimed that IRBs spend a disproportionate amount of time reviewing and revising specific words or phrases in consent forms.

In this appendix we have included eight anonymized actual written consent forms and one suggested

445

template for use in forms for Phase I studies. Two of those included are consent forms for Phase I oncology studies, and the template is a suggestion for a more straightforward description of the purpose and design, risks and benefits of a Phase I study. (We also encourage readers to peruse the online informed consent template produced by the National Cancer Institute, the Office for Human Research Protections, and the Food and Drug Administration.)[3] The others include a consent form for the use of nitric oxide inhalation therapy for myocardial ischemia, a form used for a crossover and withdrawal study of psychiatric medication, one for a study involving genetic testing for hemochromatosis, another for the research use of tissue obtained during biopsy or surgery, a form for the review of one's medical records, and a script for oral consent for an interview study. Each of these consent forms was written for a specific research project, approved by an IRB, and used in the process of obtaining consent from research participants. Although the forms included in this appendix differ with regard to subject matter, each can be used as an exercise in assessing the readability, comprehensibility, tone, and message of typical consent forms. We encourage the readers of this volume to carefully examine these sample forms and evaluate their respective strengths and weaknesses.

Investigators developing a consent form are challenged to write a clear and comprehensive summary of a considerable amount of complex scientific information, and to do so using lay terminology and an accessible style. Members of an IRB or other review body who have access to the research protocol should evaluate the degree to which the study and its risks and benefits are accurately described in the consent form. Prospective participants do not usually have access to the research protocol, and therefore must rely solely on the consent form to provide all the information they will need to make their decisions about participation. In reality, the information in the consent form typically is and should be supplemented by discussion with the principal investigator or other members of the research team. We invite the readers of this volume to identify what is done well and what could be done better in the consent forms we have included and then try their hand at modifying them or writing different consent forms of their own.

1. Kim A. Priestley, Claire Campbell, Christopher B. Valentine, David M. Denison, and Nigel P. Buller, "Are Patient Consent Forms for Research Protocols Easy to Read?" *British Medical Journal* 305 (1992): 1263–64; and Stuart A. Grossman, Steven Piantadosi, and Charles Covahey, "Are Informed Consent Forms That Describe Clinical Oncology Research Protocols Readable by Most Patients and Their Families?" *Journal of Clinical Oncology* 12 (1994): 2211–15.
2. Dale E. Hammerschmidt and Moira A. Keane, "Institutional Review Board (IRB) Review Lacks Impact on the Readability of Consent Forms for Research," *American Journal of the Medical Sciences* 304 (1992): 348–51.
3. Available online at www.cancer.gov/templates/ page_print.aspx?viewid=5fca4dc5-b6a7-4272-be96-b489f23022e5#english.

Appendix A

Phase I Treatment of Adults with Recurrent Supratentorial High-Grade Glioma with Gliadel Wafers Plus Temodar®

CONSENT FOR RESEARCH FOR ADULTS

Phase I Treatment of Adults with Recurrent Supratentorial High-Grade Glioma with Gliadel Wafers Plus Temodar®

IRB #: _____

You are being asked to take part in a research study entitled "Phase I Treatment of Adults with Recurrent Supratentorial High-Grade Glioma with Gliadel Wafers Plus Temodar®." Your physicians at [the medical institution] study the nature of disease and try to develop better methods of diagnosis and treatment. This is called clinical research. In order for you to decide whether you should agree to be part of this study, you should understand enough about its risks and benefits to make an informed decision. This process is known as informed consent.

This consent form contains detailed information about the clinical study that the person doing the research will discuss with you. Once you understand the study, you will be asked to sign this form if you agree to take part in the study. You will be given a copy of the signed form to keep as a record.

By signing this document you give your consent to the medical procedures to be performed and to take part in the research study. Please read this consent form carefully. Do not hesitate to ask questions about any of the information in it.

This study has been designed to evaluate the drug Temodar® in combination with Gliadel wafers (containing BCNU chemotherapy). The purpose of this study is to define the maximum dose of Temodar® that can be safely administered in combination with Gliadel wafers (approved by the U.S. Food and Drug Administration [FDA]). Response to treatment and side effects will be evaluated.

You are being asked to consent to participate because you have a recurrent high-grade glioma brain tumor (glioblastoma multiforme, anaplastic astrocytoma, or gliosarcoma).

Your physician has told you that standard therapies are no longer controlling your tumor. For this reason, your physician is asking you to participate in this investigational study with Gliadel wafers plus Temodar®. This study will attempt to make clear what dose of Temodar® is likely to be the best dose to use in future studies when the drug is used with Gliadel wafers. Therefore, you may get a dose that is later shown to be too low, and therefore not helpful. Or you may get a dose that is too high, and therefore very toxic. Or the treatment that you are considering may be helpful to control your disease temporarily. However, the treatment is investigational, and therefore it is not possible to predict the likelihood of benefit to you at this time.

Treatment with Gliadel wafers (containing BCNU chemotherapy) is based upon the implantation (placement) of the wafers in the cavity created during surgery. You will have as many Gliadel wafers as possible (maximum of 8) placed at the time of surgery.

Treatment with Temodar® is based upon a 28-day cycle that will begin two weeks after the implantation of the Gliadel wafers. You will receive the drug on days 1 through 5 of the 28-day cycle. The treatment will be repeated every 28 days. Temodar® is an oral capsule; the actual number of capsules you receive will vary depending upon your weight and any side effects that you may experience throughout

Patient initials: _____

CONSENT FOR RESEARCH FOR ADULTS

Phase I Treatment of Adults with Recurrent Supratentorial High-Grade Glioma with Gliadel Wafers Plus Temodar®

IRB #: _____

the study. It is recommended that you not eat for a minimum of one hour prior to each dose and for two hours after each dose.

The actual duration of therapy will depend upon your response to the treatment and the development of side effects. No more than 12 cycles (12 months) of therapy will be given.

Various routine tests are required in this study. These include urinalysis, laboratory blood tests, and a physical and neurological examination. These are considered routine evaluations and would most likely have been ordered by your physician to evaluate your health status whether or not you were considered for participation in this study. Other tests that will be done as a part of this study are MRI brain scans, chest x-rays, and ECGs (heart tracings). Pretreatment evaluations particular to this study include, if applicable, a pregnancy test within 24 hours prior to starting study drug therapy. In addition, a breast exam will be done on males and females. (Rats given Temodar® in toxicity studies have developed cancerous tumors of the breast. The significance of this finding for humans is not known presently.)

Approximately every month, you will be seen in the clinic for a physical and neurological examination and blood laboratory tests. An MRI scan of your brain will be done after every cycle. Blood laboratory tests (about 1 teaspoon each) will be required on days 1 and 21 of every 28-day cycle. Additional tests may be done at the discretion of your physician as part of your regular care throughout the study.

Your participation in this study may or may not result in any direct benefit to you. The treatment you receive may decrease the size of your tumor and extend your life. However, it is not possible to predict or guarantee a favorable response to this treatment.

You have been told that should the disease become worse, should side effects become very severe, should new scientific developments occur that indicate that the treatment is not in your best interest, or should the doctor feel that this treatment is no longer proper, the Temodar® treatment would be stopped and a different type of treatment would be discussed. The Gliadel wafers will not be removed once they are placed at the time of surgery.

Both the disease and the treatment are associated with potentially life-threatening complications and side effects. Those side effects are uncomfortable, and some are potentially dangerous or even life-threatening, but will usually clear up once the treatments have ended. There is also the risk of very uncommon or previously unknown side effects occurring. The most common side effects of the treatment to be used in this study are listed below:

Gliadel wafers: seizures, brain edema (swelling), healing abnormalities, wound infection, and body pain.

Temodar® can cause decreases in blood counts. This can lead to: decreased white cells, which may make you more vulnerable to infection; a lower number of red cells, which may result in anemia and give you symptoms of shortness of breath, weakness, and fatigue; a lower number of platelets, which may result in easy bruising or bleeding for a longer time. The medication's effect on the blood counts is usually temporary, and some of the decreases in cell counts can be helped with transfusions of blood or blood products until your blood counts recover.

Patient initials: _____

CONSENT FOR RESEARCH FOR ADULTS
Phase I Treatment of Adults with Recurrent Supratentorial High-Grade Glioma with
Gliadel Wafers Plus Temodar®
IRB #: _____

Nausea and vomiting occur occasionally and can be severe in some people. Medications may be given either to prevent these symptoms or to treat them. If nausea and/or vomiting occur, you will be given medications to treat them. Other side effects include headache, rash, kidney problems, elevated liver function tests (which may cause your skin to be yellow), hair loss, diarrhea, constipation, high blood sugar (which may make you dizzy), and loss of appetite. Additional rare side effects include itching and burning, decreased energy, and sleepiness.

The collecting of blood samples throughout this study may cause mild discomfort or pain from the needle puncture and possible bruising or mild bleeding. The risk of infection is slight and will be further reduced by keeping the puncture site clean and dry.

Side effects not yet known to researchers may occur. Every effort will be made to minimize side effects and ease your discomfort. Your doctor will examine you regularly and order tests necessary to monitor side effects and determine response.

Treatment with chemotherapy may involve unforeseeable risks to an unborn child, and it is not known whether taking these drugs now can have effects on any future children that you may have. If you are a woman and are pregnant or breast feeding, you cannot take part in this study. You will be given a blood pregnancy test before you begin the study to make sure that you are not pregnant. If there is a chance you could become pregnant during this study, you should not participate in the study, or you must use a highly effective means of birth control while you are taking part. For women of childbearing potential, medically acceptable contraceptives include (1) surgical sterilization, (2) approved hormonal contraceptives (such as birth control pills, Depo-Provera, or Depolupron), (3) barrier methods (such as a condom or diaphragm) used with a spermicide, or (4) an intrauterine device (IUD). If you become or are found to be pregnant while you are taking part in this study, you must notify us immediately so that management of the pregnancy and the possibility of stopping treatment can be discussed.

If you are a man, you should also use a means of birth control while you are taking part in this study, because we do not know what effect the study drug may have on your sperm and what effect this would have upon the development of an unborn child.

Alternatives to this therapy that could be considered include the use of drugs or other therapies that have been previously tried in the treatment of this disease, including starting radiation therapy now, or investigational drugs. An additional alternative is to take no further therapy, which would almost certainly result in the continued progression of the disease. The physician can provide detailed information about the disease and the benefits of the various treatments available. You have been told that you should feel free to discuss the disease and outlook for the future with the physician.

During this research project, new information regarding the risks and benefits of the study may become known to the investigator. If this occurs, they will tell you about this new information. New information may show that you should no longer participate in the research. If this occurs, the person supervising the research will stop your participation in it. In either case, you will be offered all available care that suits your needs and medical conditions.

Patient initials: _____

Your privacy and research records will be kept confidential. However, authorized research investigators and agents of the FDA have the right to inspect the records involving you. Health care providers involved with your care will have access to research-related information contained in your medical records. Privacy and confidentiality of the records will be protected to the extent provided by law. The results of this research may be published. Published reports will not include your name or any other information that would identify you.

By signing this form, you consent to this review and also to the release of medical records, imaging studies, and laboratory and pathology specimens, as necessary, for evaluation of your disease and therapy.

Participation in this study is voluntary.

No compensation for participation will be given. You are free to withdraw your consent for participation in this treatment program at any time without prejudice to subsequent care. Refusal to participate will involve no penalty. If you do not take part in or withdraw from the study, you will continue to receive care.

Temodar® is commercially available. You or your third-party insurance carrier will be responsible for the costs of hospitalization, the Gliadel wafers, clinic visits, x-rays, laboratory or other tests. How much you will have to pay depends on whether or not you have insurance and what costs your insurance will cover. Insurance coverage cannot be guaranteed for all tests and treatments related to this study. However, you may discuss this issue with the [medical institution admission staff (telephone number)] and/or your insurance company before you agree to participate. Treatment to help control side effects may also result in added costs.

Immediate, necessary care is available if an individual is injured because of participation in a research project. However, there is no provision for free medical care or for monetary compensation provided by [the medical institution]. Further information concerning this and also your rights as a subject in a research study can be obtained from [the hospital risk management staff (telephone number)]. Further information on this study can be obtained by contacting [the study physician] in [the clinical department at (telephone number)].

"I have read all of the above, had the opportunity to ask questions, and willingly give my consent for participation in this study. Upon signing this form, I will receive a copy."

_____   _____

Patient Signature   **Date**

_____   _____

Person Obtaining Consent   **Date**

Appendix B

A Phase I Study of Intra-arterial Onyx-015 for Squamous Cell Cancer of the Head and Neck

RESEARCH CONSENT FORM

[Name of Medical Institution]   [Patient ID Number]

Protocol Title: A Phase I Study of Intra-arterial Onyx-015 for Squamous Cell Cancer of the Head and Neck

Principal/Overall Investigator: [Name]

Site-Responsible Investigator(s)/Institution: [Name(s)/Institution]

Co-investigator(s)/Study Staff: [Name(s)]

Description of Subject Population: Adult

For Patients Receiving Onyx 015 Plus PF

INTRODUCTION

This is a clinical trial (a type of research study). Clinical trials include only patients who choose to participate. Please take your time to make your decision, and discuss it with your friends and family.

You are being asked to take part in this study because you have squamous cell cancer of the head and neck that has grown or come back after the use of standard drugs and therapies used to treat your disease (such as chemotherapy, surgery, or radiation).

Subject Population: Adult patients with Squamous Cell Carcinoma of the Head and Neck Receiving Onyx-15 Plus PF

IRB Protocol Number: _____   Sponsor Protocol Number: _____

Consent Form Approval Date: _____   Amendment Number Approved: _____

IRB Expiration Date: _____   Amendment Approval Date: _____

With this treatment you will be receiving a genetically modified virus, related to the common cold virus, called Onyx-015. Onyx-015 has been designed to enter your tumor cells and cause the cells to die. Onyx-015 should only work in cells that have mutated (your cancer cells) because it does not have the right structure to work in healthy cells. Onyx-015 has undergone testing for humans in both head and neck cancer and ovarian cancer.

WHY IS THIS STUDY BEING DONE?

The purpose of this study is to find the highest dose of Onyx-015 that can be given into an artery feeding your head and neck tumor without causing severe side effects, then to test the safety and usefulness of PF (cisplatin and 5-fluorouracil, types of chemotherapy) when given with Onyx-015, and to see what effects (good and bad) these treatments have on you and your head and neck cancer when combined.

This research is being done to learn more about the use of Onyx-015 in the treatment of your type of cancer.

HOW MANY PEOPLE WILL TAKE PART IN THE STUDY?

About 24–35 people will take part in this study.

WHAT IS INVOLVED IN THE STUDY?

[Figure [B.1] is a flow chart that depicts the course of the study.—eds.]

Medical tests: If you take part in this study, you will have the following tests and procedures:
Medical tests that are part of regular cancer care and may be done even if you do not join the study:

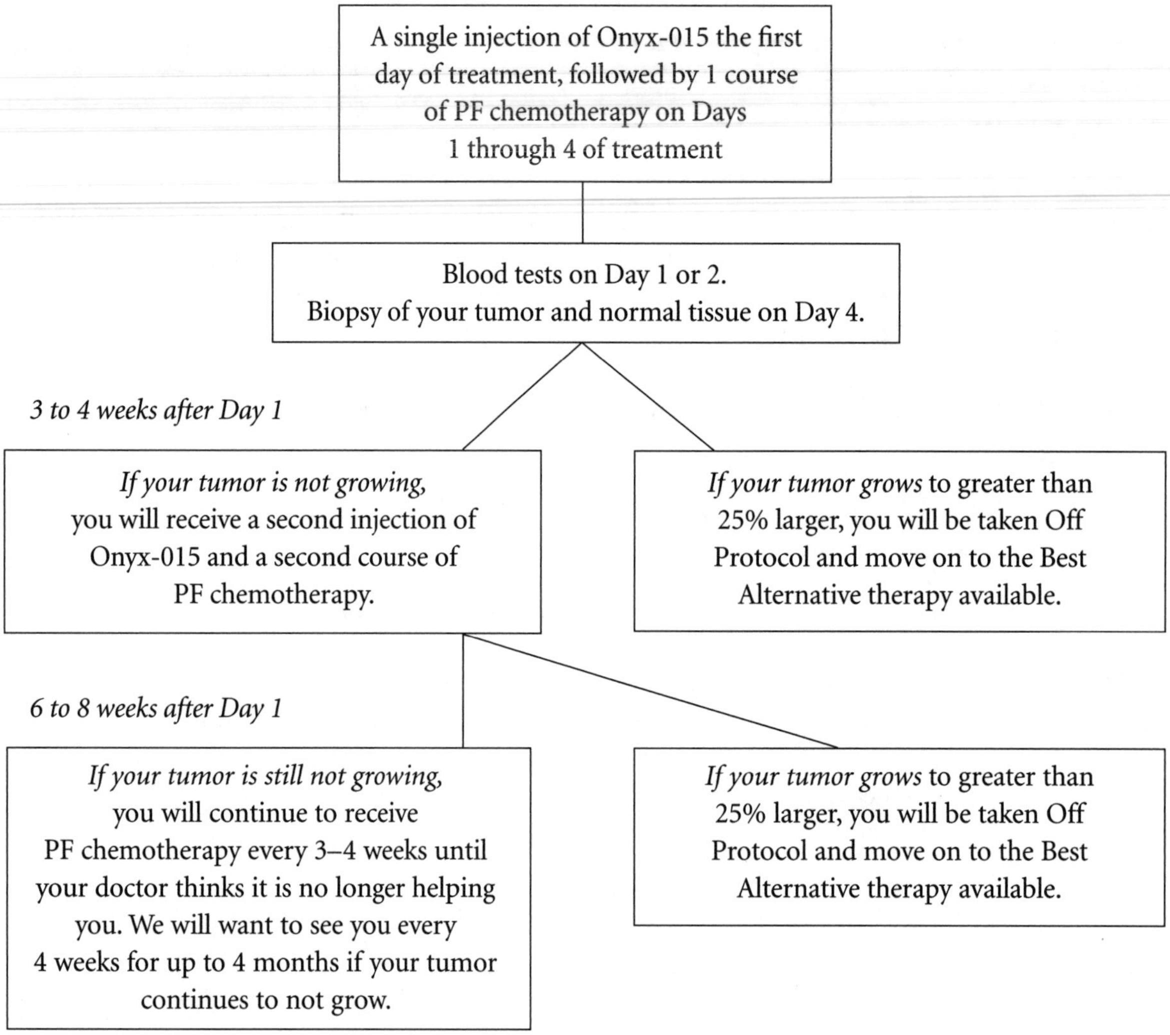

A single injection of Onyx-015 the first day of treatment, followed by 1 course of PF chemotherapy on Days 1 through 4 of treatment

Blood tests on Day 1 or 2.
Biopsy of your tumor and normal tissue on Day 4.

3 to 4 weeks after Day 1

If your tumor is not growing, you will receive a second injection of Onyx-015 and a second course of PF chemotherapy.

If your tumor grows to greater than 25% larger, you will be taken Off Protocol and move on to the Best Alternative therapy available.

6 to 8 weeks after Day 1

If your tumor is still not growing, you will continue to receive PF chemotherapy every 3–4 weeks until your doctor thinks it is no longer helping you. We will want to see you every 4 weeks for up to 4 months if your tumor continues to not grow.

If your tumor grows to greater than 25% larger, you will be taken Off Protocol and move on to the Best Alternative therapy available.

Figure B.1

- Complete physical exam
- Chest x-ray
- CT or MRI scan (uses sophisticated computers and magnetic fields or radio waves to take pictures of your body)
- Blood tests

Many of the tests which are part of regular cancer care are done more frequently because you are on this study.

Standard procedures being done because you are in this study:
- Porta-cath (a device placed under the skin of your chest, giving access to a major vein in your chest and into which a needle can be inserted to deliver chemotherapy)
- Photographs of tumor
- Biopsy of the tumor and normal tissue before and 4 days after treatment
- Arterial catheterization (a needle is placed in an artery in the groin which allows the radiologist to view the blood supply to the tumor using an injected contrast dye called angiography. Local anesthesia will be used, and the procedure will take up to four hours. Your x-ray exposure during this procedure is estimated as about one-half (50%) of the maximum annual exposure that a person who works with radiation is allowed to receive).

Procedures (treatment):
If you are eligible and agree to take part in this study, you will receive an investigational drug called Onyx-015 and two standard chemotherapy drugs: cisplatin and 5-fluorouracil (5-FU). Onyx-015 is a genetically modified virus, similar to what spreads the common cold, that attacks cancer cells and causes them to die.

Onyx-015 will be injected in a small volume of fluid into the arteries in your head and neck near the location of your tumor using arterial catheterization, a process which takes up to four hours. A biopsy will be taken of both your tumor and normal tissues before and after your injection and later looked at to see how well the virus is getting into your tumor and your normal cells. A blood sample will also be taken before and after treatment and stored so that we can later look at how the virus affects you.

The cisplatin is given one to two days after the injection. The 5-FU will be given over four days through a portable pump starting the same day as the cisplatin.

You will be monitored both by clinic visits and by blood tests for 3 to 4 weeks. If your tumor is getting smaller then you will receive a second injection of Onyx-015, another dose of cisplatin and 5-FU, and monitored for another 3 to 4 weeks. If your tumor is still responding after two cycles, you will continue to be treated with cisplatin and 5-FU only.

HOW LONG WILL I BE IN THE STUDY?

We think you will be in the study for a total of between 5 and 6 months minimum, or for as long as your tumor continues to respond (gets smaller). This involves between 4 to 8 weeks of treatment with Onyx-015, continued treatment with chemotherapy alone, followed by once-a-month visits to the outpatient clinic for four months.

The investigator and/or your doctor may decide to take you off this study if:

- You are unable to tolerate treatment

- The treatment does not work on your cancer

- You are unable to meet the requirements of the study (for example, you do not return for follow-up visits)

- Your doctor no longer believes further treatment would be beneficial

You can stop participating at any time. Your decision to withdraw from the study will not affect in any way your medical care and/or benefits. If you decide to stop participating in the study, we encourage you to discuss your decision with your doctor.

WHAT ARE THE RISKS OF THE STUDY?

While on the study, you are at risk for the side effects described below. You should discuss these with the researcher and/or your doctor. There may also be other side affects that we cannot predict. You may receive other drugs to make side effects less serious and uncomfortable. Many side effects go away shortly after the drugs are stopped, but in some cases side effects can be serious or long-lasting or permanent.

Reproductive risks
Because the drugs in this study can affect an unborn baby, you should *not* become pregnant or father a baby while on this study. You should also not nurse your baby while on this study. If you have any questions about the reproductive issues or about preventing pregnancy, please discuss them with the investigator or your doctor.

Risks and side effects related to the Onyx-015 we are studying include:

Very likely:
- Flulike symptoms (fever, chills, fatigue, muscle aches, weakness)

- Pain in the tumor area

Less likely:
- Infection at the tumor site (if the tumor dies rapidly, tissue could break off that would raise the risk of infection)

- Breathing problems (you may have breathing problems if the tumor is located in your mouth and pieces break off, lodging in your airways. You may also have breathing problems if there is an inflammation or swelling around your tumor near your breathing passage, which makes the passage smaller).

- Infection of "normal" (noncancer) cells from Onyx-015 that could cause coughing, fever, shortness of breath, upset stomach, diarrhea, nausea, and vomiting (slight chance)

- Irregular heartbeat (observed in only one previous patient)

- Death (very rare; in a separate study, one patient died after an injection into an artery in the liver of a similar virus at a higher dosage than you will receive in this study)

Risks and side effects related to the standard chemotherapy Cisplatin and 5-Fluorouracil include:

Very likely:
- Nausea

- Vomiting

- Mucositis (mouth sores)

Less likely:

- Kidney damage (rare and potentially permanent)
- Nerve damage (most commonly in arms or legs, or high-frequency hearing loss, potentially permanent)
- Hair loss (rare and temporary)
- Diarrhea
- Skin rashes
- Phlebitis (irritation of the veins)
- Infection at the tumor site (if the tumor dies rapidly, tissue could break off which would raise the risk of infection)
- Breathing problems (if the tumor is located in your mouth and pieces break off, the tissue could lodge in your airways)
- Irregular heartbeat (observed in only one previous patient)
- Chest pain
- Blindness (rare and permanent)
- Death (very rare)

Risks and side effects related to the standard angiography (arterial catheterization) procedure include:

Very likely:
- Pain in the tumor area
- Discomfort from needles for blood draw and tumor injections

Less likely:

- Stroke (rare and permanent)
- Blindness (rare and permanent)
- Nerve injury (rare and permanent)
- Reaction to the injected contrast dye (very rare)
- Death (very rare)

Risks and side effects related to the standard biopsy procedure include:

Very likely:

- Pain in the tumor area
- Discomfort from needles for blood draw and tumor biopsies

For more information about risks and side effects, ask the investigator.

ARE THERE BENEFITS TO TAKING PART IN THE STUDY?

If you agree to take part in this study, there may or may not be direct medical benefit to you. This study may even be harmful. We hope the information learned from this study will benefit other patients with your type of cancer in the future.

WHAT OTHER OPTIONS ARE THERE?

Instead of being in this study, you have these options:

- Other chemotherapy drugs and drug combinations
- Chemotherapy with radiation
- Other studies of new anticancer therapies
- No therapy at this time with supportive care to help you feel more comfortable

Please discuss these and other options with your doctor.

WHAT ABOUT CONFIDENTIALITY?

Please refer to the last two pages of this form for information about confidentiality issues.

WHAT ARE THE COSTS?

Taking part in this study may lead to added costs to you or your insurance company. Please ask the investigator and/or your doctor about any expected added costs or insurance problems.

You will not be charged for Onyx-015, biopsies, arteriography, and special blood tests done for the research part of this study. You or your insurance company will, however, be charged for any other portion of your care that is considered standard care.

In the case of injury or illness from this study, emergency medical treatment is available but will be provided at the usual charge. No funds have been set aside to compensate you in the event of injury.

You or your insurance company will be charged for continuing medical care and/or hospitalization.

You will receive no payment for taking part in this study.

WHAT ARE MY RIGHTS AS A PARTICIPANT?

Taking part in this study is voluntary. You may choose not to take part or may leave the study at any time. Leaving the study will not result in any penalty or loss of benefits to which you are entitled.

We will tell you about new information that may affect your health, welfare, or willingness to stay in this study.

WHOM DO I CALL IF I HAVE QUESTIONS OR PROBLEMS?

For questions about the study or a research-related injury, contact [the principal study investigator] at [telephone number and page number], or contact your research nurse at [telephone number]. Patients at the [hospital] can contact Dr. [name] at [telephone number].

For questions about your rights as a research participant, contact the [medical institution's] institutional review board (which is a group of people who review research studies to protect your rights) at [telephone number].

WHERE CAN I GET MORE INFORMATION?

[Study sponsor information omitted—eds.]
You will get a copy of this form. You may also request a copy of the research study.
The following paragraphs contain standard information that generally applies to persons involved in a research study and are required on all consent forms.

CONFIDENTIALITY

Medical information produced by this study will become part of your hospital medical record unless specifically stated otherwise in this consent form. Information that does not become part of your medical record will be stored in the investigator's file and identified by a code number only. The code key connecting your name to specific information about you will be kept in a separate, secure location. Your medical record is available to health care professionals at [the medical institutions involved in the study], and may be reviewed by appropriate [study hospital] staff members in the course of carrying out their duties; however, they are required to maintain confidentiality in accordance with applicable laws and the policies of the [study hospitals]. Information contained in your records may not be given to anyone unaffiliated with the [study hospitals] in a form that could identify you without your written consent, except as described in this consent form or as required by law.

It is possible that your medical and research record, including sensitive information and/or identifying information, may be inspected and/or copied by the study sponsor (and/or its agent), the Food and Drug Administration (FDA), federal or state government agencies, or hospital accrediting agencies, in the course of carrying out their duties. If your record is inspected or copied by the study sponsor (and/or its agents), or by any of these agencies, the [study hospitals] will use reasonable efforts to protect your privacy and the confidentiality of your medical information.

The results of this study may be published in a medical book or journal used for teaching purposes. However, your name or other identifiers will not be used in any publication or teaching materials without your specific permission. In addition, if photographs, audiotapes, or videotapes were taken during the study that could identify you, then you must give special written permission for their use. In that case, you will be given the opportunity to view or listen, as applicable, to the photographs, audiotapes, or videotapes before you give your permission for their use if you so request.

REQUEST FOR MORE INFORMATION

You may ask more questions about the study at any time. The investigator(s) will provide their telephone number(s) so that they are available to answer your questions or concerns about the study. You will be informed of any significant new findings discovered during the course of this study that might influence your continued participation.

If, during the study or later, you wish to discuss your rights as a research subject, your participation in the study and/or concerns about the study, a research-related injury with someone not directly involved in the study, or if you feel under any pressure to enroll in this study or to continue to participate in this study, you are asked to contact a representative of the [institutional review board at one of the study hospitals at the following telephone numbers: _____]. A copy of this consent form will be given to you to keep.

REFUSAL OR WITHDRAWAL OF PARTICIPATION

Participation in this study is voluntary. You do not have to participate in this study. Your present or future care will not be affected should you choose not to participate. If you decide to participate, you can change your mind and drop out of the study at any time without affecting your present or future care in the [study hospitals]. In addition, the doctor in charge of this study may decide to end your participation in this study at any time after he/she has explained the reasons for doing so and has helped arrange for your continued care by your own doctor, if needed.

INJURY STATEMENT

If you are injured during the course of the study and as a direct result of this study, you should contact the investigator at the number provided. You will be offered the necessary care to treat that injury. This care does not imply any fault or wrong-doing on the part of the [study hospitals] or the doctor(s) involved. Where applicable, the [study hospitals] reserve the right to bill third-party payers for services you receive for the injury. The [study hospitals] will not provide you with any additional compensation for such injuries.

SIGNATURE

I confirm that the purpose of the research, the study procedures, and the possible risks and discomforts as well as potential benefits that I may experience have been explained to me. Alternatives to my participation in the study also have been discussed. All my questions have been answered. I have read this consent form. My signature below indicates my willingness to participate in this study.

_____   _____
Subject/Patient   **Date**

_____   _____
Witness/Advocate/Minor/Legal Guardian (if required)   **Date**

_____   _____
Additional Signature (if required)   **Date**

_____

(Identify relationship to subject)

I have explained the purpose of the research, the study procedures, identifying those that are investigational, the possible risks and discomforts as well as potential benefits, and have answered any questions regarding the study to the best of my ability.

_____   _____
Study Representative   **Date**

Appendix C

Cohort-Varying Information Insert for Form for Consent to Participate in a Phase I Study

[Here we quote an article in which Benjamin Freedman suggested a template to be used for a more straightforward description of the purpose and design, risks and benefits of a Phase I study.—eds.]

COHORT-VARYING INFORMATION INSERT FOR CONSENT FORM TO PARTICIPATE IN PHASE I STUDY

Insert in section on Purpose and Design of Study

In testing new drugs and combinations of drugs for cancer treatment, the first study is designed to establish the highest dose that may safely be given. This is such a study. Underlying this trial is our understanding that, most commonly, drugs to treat cancer are most effective when given at the highest safe dose. The highest safe dose is the dose just smaller than that which produces unacceptable reactions.

A group of subjects is enrolled and given a very small dose. Their progress is followed, and if those patients do not develop unacceptable reactions to that dose, a new group of patients is enrolled at a higher dose. This process continues until a dose is reached that commonly produces an unacceptable reaction. [*For cohort at highest dose substitute for last sentence:* This process continues until a dose is reached that produces an unacceptable reaction in two subjects of the three enrolled at that level. If this unacceptable toxicity is repeated in one person from a further group of three subjects, [at]] At that point the study is complete: It has shown us what the maximum tolerated dose of the drug or combination is.

In this trial, up to nine groups of subjects will be enrolled, at gradually increasing doses of [(drug) A] [(drug) A and (drug) B]. The earliest group of subjects (Group 1) will be [was] given the lowest dose, at a level that should not produce unacceptable toxicity but may also not be sufficiently potent against the cancer. The later the group into which a subject is enrolled, the higher the dose given. It is often, but not always, true that the higher the dose, the more powerful are the effects against cancer, but also the more likely to produce unacceptable side effects.

If I agree to participate in this trial, I will be in the [Nth] group of 9 planned groups.

Insert in section on Risks and Benefits

The likelihood and severity of side effects depends in part on the dose given, although even then these are not completely predictable. Some side effects may occur in patients given a low dose of drug (that is, patients enrolled in an early group), but are more likely to occur and to be more serious when [the drug is] given in higher doses. These side effects are [*insert toxicities that continuously vary at the dosages given cohorts*]. Other side effects are unlikely to appear at low dosages, but may appear at higher ones. These side effects are [*insert toxicities with an expected threshold for appearance*]. These side effects are more likely to occur in subjects of groups [N] through nine. Again, though, we cannot predict well an individual person's reaction to a dose, so it is quite possible that [a] subject in a late group may experience less harmful drug effects than a subject in an earlier group. [. . .]

Adapted from Benjamin Freedman, "Cohort-Specific Consent: An Honest Approach to Phase I Clinical Cancer Studies," *IRB: A Review of Human Subjects Research* 12, no. 1 (1990): 5–7.

Appendix D

Nitric Oxide Inhalation Therapy for Myocardial Ischemia in Patients with Coronary Artery Disease

STUDY NUMBER: _____

STUDY TITLE: Nitric Oxide Inhalation Therapy for Myocardial Ischemia in Patients with Coronary Artery Disease

INTRODUCTION

We invite you to take part in a research study.

First, we want you to know that

Taking part in [this] research is entirely voluntary.

You may choose not to take part, or you may withdraw from the study at any time. In either case, you will not lose any benefits to which you are otherwise entitled. However, to receive care at [the institution] you must be taking part in a study or be under evaluation for study participation.

You may receive no benefit from taking part. The research may give us knowledge that may help people in the future.

Second, some people have personal, religious or ethical beliefs that may limit the kinds of medical or research treatments they would want to receive (such as blood transfusions). If you have such beliefs, please discuss them with your doctors or research team before you agree to the study.

Now we will describe this research study. Before you decide to take part, please take as much time as you need to ask any questions and discuss this study with anyone at [the medical institution] or with family, friends, or your personal physician or other health professional.

Purpose of Study

You have been diagnosed as having coronary artery disease, which is caused by atherosclerosis (build-up of cholesterol and scar tissue within the walls of arteries) and has affected segments of the large arteries of your heart. If atherosclerosis narrows the opening of the artery in a particular segment, blood flow may be limited, particularly during exercise or other stress. This can result in not enough oxygen in blood delivered to the heart muscle dependent upon that artery. As a result, you may experience shortness of breath and chest pain (angina pectoris) during your daily activities. You have previously received treatment for coronary artery disease with medications and with an attempt at revascularization, either by angioplasty or by surgery. Because you continue to be limited by chest pain so that even routine activities are difficult to accomplish, we invite you to volunteer for participation in a research study that is designed to determine whether inhalation of a gas (nitric oxide) mixed with room air may improve blood flow to your heart. Up to 25 patients with coronary artery disease will participate in this study.

The duration of this study is one month, with one week of inhalation of room air mixed with nitric oxide using a portable delivery device, and one week of room air alone from an identical-appearing delivery device, with two weeks separating the two treatment periods. You will not know, nor will we, the identity of the air mixture (that is, whether or not nitric oxide is present) in the delivery devices.

PATIENT IDENTIFICATION: _____

However, the [specified person] will know at all times which air mixture you are breathing, and will also assign to you, by chance, the delivery device for your first treatment. However, you will receive the delivery device containing nitric oxide during one of the two treatment periods. Although we hope that you will complete both treatment periods of the study so that we can learn whether nitric oxide inhalation therapy can help patients like you, you are free to withdraw from the study at any time.

We will inform you of any significant findings discovered in the course of this study that might influence your decision to continue participation.

Description of Study

You have already undergone a heart scan that was performed during the previous year because of chest pain symptoms, and more recently a treadmill exercise test. Based on those results and lab work, you have been found eligible to participate in this study. We want to provide you with all the information you need, and answer all the questions you might have, before you sign this consent form and enroll in this study. During both of the one-week treatment periods, you will be hospitalized [in the study hospital] and you will continue your current medications throughout the entire study. You will be placed on a heart monitor so that we can follow your heart rate and rhythm throughout both treatment periods. We will measure your pulse, blood pressure, and breathing rate at least 3 times daily. We will also measure the oxygen in your blood by means of a clip device that fits over your finger. On the first day, you will exercise on a treadmill, just as was done to determine eligibility for the study, and ask you to tell us when you experience moderately uncomfortable chest pain (5 out of 10 in severity, with 10 being the worst chest pain you have experienced), at which point you will stop exercise. After that test, you begin the inhalation treatment with a small tank that you can carry with you and delivers a burst of air (with or without nitric oxide) through nasal prongs every time you inspire. If you have a cold and your nose is congested, we will postpone the treatment period until you can comfortably breathe through your nose. You will wear this device day and night, and remove it only to shower or bathe. You are free to walk around the nursing unit as you wish. If you commonly breathe through your mouth at night, as is often the case in persons who snore, the nasal prong delivery device cannot deliver air (with or without the nitric oxide) into your nose. This will cause a beeping sound on the monitor attached to the gas delivery system. If this happens with you at night, we will use instead of the nasal prongs a face mask attached with an elastic strap around your head. In this way, you will inhale the gas regardless of how you breathe.

At 2 hours and 24 hours after beginning inhalation therapy, we will draw a blood sample to make sure that there is no harm from breathing nitric oxide (this risk will be described later in the consent form).

On the morning of the second day, you will exercise once again on the treadmill, stopping when you experience moderately uncomfortable chest pain (5 out of 10 in severity). You will wear a face mask for gas delivery during this test.

On the morning of the 5th day additional electrodes will connect you to a monitor device that you carry with you as you walk around and records your heart rate and rhythm for 24 hours. You may be as active as you wish, including excursions off the nursing unit, but you must remain within the [medical institution].

On the morning of the 6th day, you will have a special echocardiogram with imaging of your heart during an infusion of dobutamine, a medicine that increases heart rate and contraction and serves to stress the heart. This manner of stress testing is commonly used in hospitals around the country. Imaging your heart during stress can tell us whether the walls of the heart are receiving sufficient blood supply. The cardiologist performing this study will stop the dobutamine infusion either when you have reached a target heart rate (based on your age) or when you experience moderately uncomfortable chest pain (5 out of 10 in severity), just as was the case for the treadmill exercise tests. Your heart rate and rhythm will be continuously monitored during this study. You will wear a face mask for gas delivery during this test. That afternoon, you will undergo a magnetic resonance imaging (MRI) study of the blood flow in your heart and the contraction of your heart while receiving the same dosage of dobutamine as was used earlier in the day. At peak stress, an imaging agent called gadolinium will be injected into your vein in order to allow measurement of blood flow distribution within the heart. You will wear a face mask for gas delivery during this test.

On the morning of the 7th day, you will undergo another treadmill exercise test, stopping when you experience chest pain that is 5 out of 10 in severity, as before. You will wear a face mask for gas delivery during this test. Later that morning you will undergo a cardiac catheterization during which a long tube (catheter) will be placed into a vein of your neck, your arm, or your groin, depending on your preference and the physician's recommendation, after the skin has been numbed with xylocaine. This tube will be positioned within the right atrium of your heart and into a tubelike structure called the coronary sinus, where venous blood exits the heart muscle. A small catheter will be placed in an artery of your upper forearm after the skin has been numbed with xylocaine. Blood samples will be drawn through the tube in the heart and through the small tube in the artery at the beginning of the study and during infusion of dobutamine to stress your heart, using the same dose as was used in the previous day's stress studies. These blood samples will allow us to measure nitric oxide transported in your blood as well as measure levels of several substances that are important in atherosclerosis and that we believe might be reduced by nitric oxide. You will wear a face mask for gas delivery during this test.

After completing this week's worth of testing, you will go home for two weeks and then return to [the medical institution] for a week of identical testing with the alternate inhalation device to the one that you were assigned during the first week of the study. The total amount of blood required for this study is 300 cc (10 oz. or 20 tablespoons), which is two-thirds of the volume of blood donated by individuals to the Red Cross and to hospitals.

Explanation of the Procedures and Tests

1. *Nitric oxide administration.* Nitric oxide is a colorless, odorless gas which has been studied by us and other groups to determine whether this gas can dilate (enlarge) blood vessels of the lungs as well as the rest of the body. This gas is actually produced by the lining cells (endothelium) of healthy arteries, and keeps arteries dilated. However, production of this gas and the potency of this gas within arteries is markedly reduced in patients with atherosclerosis and coronary artery disease. Nitric oxide inhalation is approved by the U.S. Food and Drug Administration (FDA) for use in newborn infants with severe respiratory problems. Nitric oxide is also used on occasion to treat adults with severe respiratory problems in intensive care units, often for several weeks, without known complications from the gas itself. We have previously conducted studies in volunteer subjects with nitric oxide inhaled at 80 parts per million (80 molecules of nitric oxide per million molecules of air gases) without harm. The delivery system that you will be using delivers between 20 and 40 parts per million of nitric oxide mixed with

room air. During those periods of time when you wear a face mask for gas delivery, the delivery of nitric oxide is set at 40 parts per million.

2. *Treadmill exercise testing.* The treadmill testing we will use for this study will be very familiar to you, as it was important in determining your eligibility for the study. Your heart rhythm will be continuously monitored, as will your oxygen saturation using a finger clip device, and blood pressures will be measured approximately every 3 minutes. A nurse and a doctor will be in attendance throughout the study. In national statistics, the risk of a heart attack or death is approximately one in 10,000 exercise tests. The nurse and doctor are trained in the use of resuscitation equipment, which is kept next to the treadmill.

3. *Ambulatory monitoring.* Monitoring of your heart rate and rhythm will be done for 24 hours by having you wear a portable device with wires attached to sticky patches placed on your chest. Other than possible irritation of the skin, there is no risk to this test.

4. *Echocardiogram.* This test involves holding a small probe against the chest wall and allows the physician specialist to obtain pictures of the heart in order to assess the function of the various chambers of your heart. It uses sound waves to distinguish the various structures of the heart and does not involve any radiation. A small tube will be placed in the back of your hand or arm in order to give fluids into your vein, and to infuse dobutamine. This may cause a small bruise, and may cause you to feel briefly lightheaded and nauseated (faint). Echo measurements will be made before and during an infusion of dobutamine, which is a medicine commonly used in echocardiography laboratories around the country in order to stress the heart by increasing the heart rate and contractions. Imaging of the heart during this stress can help us determine whether sufficient blood flow is getting to heart muscle. The dobutamine will be infused until you experience moderately uncomfortable chest pain (5 out of 10 in severity) or until you achieve a standardized heart rate, based on your age. Some patients (less than 5 out of 100) experience headache, nausea, or anxiety during dobutamine testing. In national statistics, the risk of heart attack or serious heart rhythm problems requiring administration of medicines or an electroshock to the heart is approximately 3 out of 1,000 tests.

5. *Magnetic resonance imaging (MRI).* This test will provide pictures of the heart and measurement of blood flow in the heart during the administration of gadolinium. MRI does not use radiation, but instead uses the effects of magnets and radiowaves in order to provide pictures of the heart. On the day of the scan you will be taken to [the research institute] where the MRI instrument is located. After you arrive in the MRI area, you should use the bathroom before being placed in the machine, as the test can take about an hour. You will be asked to lie on a stretcher, which is inserted into a long, donut-shaped scanner that some people may find confining. The test is also quite noisy, but you can communicate through a microphone with the people performing the test. Your heart rate and blood pressure will be monitored during the study. If for any reason you feel that you cannot complete the MRI study, the scanning can be stopped and you can be removed immediately from the scanner. During the MRI examination you will receive an injection by vein of gadolinium. Gadolinium is approved by the FDA for the purposes of brightening areas of the heart, which we expect with increased blood flow to various areas of the heart. Experience with many thousands of patients here and elsewhere has shown that gadolinium is safe and without side effects in most patients. When side effects do occur (less than 5 out of 100 patients), they are usually mild and last for a short period of time. These include a feeling of coldness in the arm during the injection, headache, and nausea. More severe reactions (shortness of breath, wheezing, or lowering of blood pressure) have occurred in a small number of patients (fewer than 1 out of 100) and can be treated

very easily. Some patients (less than 5 out of 100) describe a sensation of twitching in their legs that is caused by the stimulation of nerves of the extremities. In most cases this is not painful, but should it become painful to you, we can stop the study. At this time, there are no known health risks of MRI itself. However, there are certain medical conditions that can interfere with your MRI study and some can be hazardous. Therefore, in the interest of your safety, please tell us whether or not you have any of the following items in your body:

Artificial heart valve	Yes _____	No _____
Cardiac pacemaker	Yes _____	No _____
Automatic implantable defibrillator (AICD)	Yes _____	No _____
Neural pacemaker	Yes _____	No _____
Aneurysmal clips on arteries on the brain	Yes _____	No _____
Shrapnel	Yes _____	No _____
Foreign bodies in the eye (e.g. metal shavings)	Yes _____	No _____
Surgical clips	Yes _____	No _____

You may have had placement of a stent within one or more arteries of your heart. MRI is safe in patients with stents, although we require that at least 6 months elapse from the time that the stents were placed.

6. *Cardiac catheterization.* This test involves inserting small tubes into the artery of the arm and a long tube into the venous side of the heart by way of an arm or neck vein after numbing the skin with xylocaine, so that blood samples can be obtained before and during the infusion of dobutamine. There is a small (1 in 500) chance of injury to the right side of the heart, which could result in leakage of blood out of the heart and into the sac (pericardium) in which the heart is located. If this happens and if your blood pressure falls because the heart is compressed by blood in the sac, a needle will be inserted under the rib cage to draw the blood out. There is a less than 1 out of 100 chance of puncturing the lung, requiring placement of a chest tube to remove the excess air. Placement of the tube into the heart requires about two minutes of x-ray exposure. The radiation exposure from the two cardiac catheterizations required during the study is for research purposes only, totalling 1.26 rem to the skin, 0.146 rem to the heart, and 0.125 rem to the left lung. This radiation exposure is less than the 13-week (3 rem) radiation dose to each tissue of the body usually permitted to adult research subjects at [the research institute], and less than the 5 rem limit allowed per year for research purposes. Please tell us if you have participated in other research studies, here or elsewhere, so that we may make sure that your total radiation exposure from all studies is not too much. The [safety staff of the research institute], a group of experts on radiation safety matters, has reviewed the use of radiation in this study and has approved the use as necessary to obtain the research information desired. Potential long-term risks from the radiation doses used in this study are uncertain, but these doses to date have not been associated with any definite adverse effects. Thus, the risk to you at this time is estimated to be slight.

Risks

The risks associated with treadmill exercising testing, echo testing with dobutamine stress, MRI scanning with dobutamine stress, and cardiac catheterization with dobutamine stress have been discussed previously in this consent form. Thus, in this section we will discuss the risk associated with the treatment that is the focus of our study, nitric oxide inhalation.

PATIENT IDENTIFICATION: _____

To the best of our knowledge, nitric oxide has not been administered as a gas to patients with coronary artery disease or other forms of cardiovascular disease. However, nitric oxide has been used in normal volunteers and in patients for several years and without harm. At 20-40 parts per million, the dose that you will be given for a week, inhaled nitric oxide rarely (less than 1 in 1,000) causes adverse effects. Some of the possible adverse effects include bronchospasm (rapid contraction and relaxation of the muscles around your breathing tubes) and pulmonary edema (fluid in the lungs). We will minimize the likelihood of such adverse effects by properly caring for the equipment used to deliver the nitric oxide. At high doses, inhaled nitric oxide can react with oxygen in your red blood cells, forming methemoglobin. High levels of methemoglobin can be dangerous because of the inability of this molecule to transport oxygen in blood. Methemoglobin formation is not expected to be a problem at the dose of nitric oxide you will receive for one week. During our previous studies with normal volunteers and patients with sickle cell anemia, methemoglobin was no greater than 1% of all hemoglobin when nitric oxide was administered at 80 parts per million for approximately 3 hours. In published studies of patients with pulmonary disease receiving nitric oxide for several weeks, no elevation in methemoglobin greater than 2% has been reported. We will measure your methemoglobin at 2 hours and at 24 hours during the treatment phases of the study to ensure that the levels are maintained at a safe range less than 2% of total hemoglobin. If methemoglobin levels exceed 2% of the total hemoglobin, we will stop your participation in the study. Also, we will monitor the oxygen saturation of your blood throughout the week by means of a device that fits on your finger. If we see any harmful effect of nitric oxide on your blood pressure, heart rhythm, breathing, or oxygen saturation of your blood, we will stop your participation in the study. There is also a possibility that nitric oxide gas combined with nitroglycerin (a drug that releases nitric oxide into blood vessels) may have additive effects, which could lower blood pressure and cause you to feel lightheaded or have chest pain. For this reason, we will monitor your blood pressure and heart rate frequently after beginning the gas therapy. Further, we will give you a standard dose of nitroglycerin to take under the tongue while you are using the gas therapy in order to be sure that your blood pressure does not fall to such a level that you feel lightheaded or feel chest pain. If you should feel these symptoms with a fall in blood pressure, we will stop your participation in the study. During those periods of time when you must wear a face mask, you may experience some irritation (redness and itching) where the face mask comes in contact with skin. The effects of nitric oxide inhalation on blood glucose levels are not known, and may cause fluctuations of blood sugar levels in patients with diabetes mellitus. If you are diabetic, we will obtain blood sugar levels each morning and afternoon, and make adjustments in your diabetes medication if necessary. This may require the occasional administration of insulin by injection while you are undergoing testing, even if you are only taking pills for blood sugar control.

Benefits

Based on what we know about nitric oxide in studies performed in animals and in humans, we believe that nitric oxide may benefit your heart disease by improving blood flow to the heart muscle during stress. However, it is possible that nitric oxide either does not help the heart or that the number and location of atherosclerotic blockages in the arteries in your heart are too severe for nitric oxide to be of benefit. Based on our experience to date and that of other physicians and scientists who have studied nitric oxide, we do not believe that nitric oxide will harm you. However, we will watch you very closely on our inpatient ward while you use the inhalation device to maximize the safety in this study. Your safe participation is also ensured by maintaining the medications that you were taking prior to enrollment. As an alternative to participating in this study, you may be able to undergo additional angioplasty or surgical revascularization procedures. Also, there are other experimental procedures being performed at other medical centers, including injection or infusion into the heart of substances [that] may grow new blood vessels, and laser treatment of heart muscle to create new blood vessels. It may not be possible to supply you with nitric oxide gas for continued inhalation therapy after you complete the study, as use of this approach to treatment of patients like you has not been approved by the FDA, the government agency responsible for approval and supervision of drug therapies. However, should this study prove the benefit and safety of nitric oxide inhalation therapy for patients with coronary artery disease, this therapy may possibly be available in the future.

Confidentiality

The Federal Privacy Act protects the confidentiality of your medical records. However, you should know that the Act allows release of some information from your medical record without your permission, for example, if it is required by the Food and Drug Administration (FDA), members of Congress, law enforcement officials, [the study sponsor] or their representative, or other authorized people.

Monetary Compensation

You will receive payment for the inconvenience and time spent on our inpatient ward during the study. Compensation includes $200 for each of the one-week treatment periods in the [medical institution]. Furthermore, you will receive an additional $100 for completing the study. Thus, a total of $500 of compensation will be given to you upon completion of the study.

Patient Representative

If you have further questions or concerns regarding your participation in this research study, you may contact the patient representative.

[A consent form for non-study-related intervention was omitted—eds.]

OTHER PERTINENT INFORMATION

1. *Confidentiality.* When results of [a medical] study are reported in medical journals or at scientific meetings, the people who take part are not named and identified. In most cases, the [research staff] will not release any information about your research involvement without your written permission. However, if you sign a release of information form, for example, for an insurance company, the [research staff] will give the insurance company information from your medical record. This information might affect (either favorably or unfavorably) the willingness of the insurance company to sell you insurance.

2. *Policy Regarding Research-Related Injuries.* The [medical institution] will provide short-term medical care for any injury resulting from your participation in research here. In general, no long-term medical care or financial compensation for research-related injuries will be provided by the [medical institution]. However, you have the right to pursue legal remedy if you believe that your injury justifies such action.

PATIENT IDENTIFICATION: _____

3. *Payments.* The amount of payment to research volunteers is guided by the [medical institution guidelines]. In general, patients are not paid for taking part in research studies at the [medical institution].

4. *Problems or Questions.* If you have any problems or questions about this study, or about your rights as a research participant, or about any research-related injury, contact the Principal Investigator, [name (telephone number)].

Other researchers you may call are [_____].

You may also call the [medical institution's] patient representative at [telephone number].

5. *Consent Document.* Please keep a copy of this document in case you want to read it again.

Complete Appropriate Items Below:

A. Adult Patient's Consent	B. Parent's Permission for Minor Patient
I have read the explanation about this study and have been given the opportunity to discuss it and to ask questions. I hereby consent to take part in this study.	I have read the explanation about this study and have been given the opportunity to discuss it and to ask questions. I hereby give permission for my child to take part in this study.
_____ _____	_____ _____
Signature of Adult Patient/Legal Representative Date	Signature of Parent(s)/Guardian Date

C. Child's Verbal Assent (If Applicable)
The information in the above consent was described to my child, and my child agrees to participate in the study.

_____ _____
Signature of Parent(s)/Guardian Date

This consent document has been approved for use from _____ to _____
[applicable dates]

_____ _____   _____ _____
Signature of Investigator Date   Signature of Witness Date

Appendix E

Double-Blind Drug Crossover and Withdrawal Project

[Date] Informed Consent Document

Double-Blind Crossover and Withdrawal Protocol

[Name and Address of Medical Institution]

Informed Consent Agreement for Patients (Version 1)

Double-Blind Drug Crossover and Withdrawal Project

I hereby agree and consent to participate as a research subject in a project entitled "Double-Blind Drug Crossover and Withdrawal," which is part of the ["Name of research project"]. I understand that the purpose of this study is to take people like me off medication in a way that will give the most information about the medication and its effects on me, on others and on the way the brain works. I understand that the reason for my inclusion in this study is that I had a previous psychotic episode and have now been stably recovered for several months.

I understand that in the first 24 weeks (approximately 5½ months) of this study, I will continue to have an injection given to me every 2 weeks. I understand that during some of this time, the injection will contain an inactive substance (placebo) and that at other times will contain the same dose of medication that I have been receiving for the last 6 months. I understand that neither I nor my doctor will be told whether I am on my usual medication or on the placebo. I understand that following the first part of the study, all medications will be stopped and that I will continue to receive regular care at the [medical institution clinic]. During the entire study, psychotherapy will continue as before.

During the study, I understand that, in order to understand the relationship between the amount of medication in my blood and its effect on me, I will have a blood test every 2 weeks; 25 cc (or less than one ounce) of blood will be drawn each time.

I agree to continue to take part in the following procedures both in the beginning of the study and at regular intervals throughout the study. I understand that these procedures are the same that I have been doing in the [medical institution clinic] during the past year:

1. I will complete several questionnaires which will ask about my attitudes and behavior.

2. I will participate in role-played interpersonal scenes with another person. I consent to have audiotapes made of my performance during role-playing, on the understanding that the tapes will be used for research purposes only and will not be played to anyone other than immediate staff on this project and that my identity will not be disclosed. I will be allowed to listen to these audiotapes if desired. I understand that the tapes will be destroyed when their use in this research project is completed.

Date of Expiration: _____

Principal Investigator: _____

Consent for Patient (Version 1) Revised: _____

3. I will have measurements taken from my hands of my skin response while listening to tones over loudspeakers. These measurements will be taken from recording disks placed on the surface of two of my fingers.

4. I will look at a projection screen and identify numbers and letters as they appear on the screen.

5. I will have measurements taken of the movements of my eyes as I rest comfortably. The eye movements will be measured using recording disks on both my temples and on my forehead.

6. I understand that I will receive $15.00 after I have completed all of the tests every 6 weeks for the first 24 weeks. I will receive $15.00 after I complete all of the tests each of two times in the subsequent year and a half. The total amount of compensation is $105.00.

All interviews and various test measures will be administered by various members of the staff of the [medical institution clinic].

I understand that during blood drawing I may experience pain from the needle prick, a small amount of bleeding, infection, or black-and-blue marks at the site of the needle mark which will disappear in about 10 days.

I understand that because of the withdrawal of active medication, I may become worse during this study and that either a relapse of my initial symptoms or new symptoms may occur. I understand that I will not be charged for the active medication or the placebo that I am provided during this study. If I do show a significant return of symptoms, I understand that the clinic staff will use active medication again to improve my condition. If I would require hospitalization during this study, although this is not likely, I understand that the clinic staff would help to arrange an appropriate hospitalization, but the research project would not pay for the hospitalization.

I understand that I may benefit from this study by being taken off medication in a careful way while under close medical supervision. The potential benefits to science in this study are that it will increase my doctor's knowledge of the relationship between the medication, its effect on people such as myself, and on the way the brain functions in certain forms of mental illness.

I understand that my condition may improve, worsen or remain unchanged from participation in this study.

Any questions I have about any aspects of this study or my participation in it will be answered at any time by a member of the [medical institution clinic] staff or [the research investigators] who may both be reached at [address], [phone number]. If the study design or use of its information is to be changed, I will be so informed and my consent reobtained. I understand that I have the right to participate or to withdraw from this research at any time without prejudice.

I understand that all information gained from me will remain confidential, and my identity will not be released without my specific consent or except as specifically required by law.

Date of Expiration: _____

Principal Investigator: _____

Consent for Patient (Version 1) Revised: _____

[Date] Informed Consent Document
Double-Blind Crossover and Withdrawal Protocol

I understand that circumstances may arise which might cause the investigator to terminate my participation before the completion of this study.

I understand that if I am injured as a direct result of research procedures not done primarily for my own benefit, I will receive medical treatment at no cost. The [university] does not provide any other form of compensation for injury.

I understand that if I have any further questions, comments, or concerns about the study or the informed consent process, I may write or call the office of [research program contact person, address, telephone number].

In signing this consent form, I acknowledge receipt of a copy of this form, as well as a copy of the "Subject's Bill of Rights."

Date: _____   Signature: _____

Date: _____   Signature: _____

Date of Expiration: _____

Principal Investigator: _____

Consent for Patient (Version 1) Revised: _____

Appendix F

Information and Consent Letter for Hemochromatosis Study

Information and Consent Letter for [Study Sponsor] Hemochromatosis Study

(Date)

Dear [name of patient],

As I mentioned in my brief note at the front of your [health clinic] questionnaire, I would like your help in a medical research project that may help you directly and is likely to advance medical knowledge. I think you'll find the whole project interesting, regardless of whether you decide to participate or not.

You probably know that iron deficiency commonly causes anemia. But you probably do not know that the opposite condition, *too much* iron, can also cause anemia. Iron overload also causes some cases of diabetes, arthritis, impotence, infertility, congestive heart failure, cirrhosis, chronic fatigue, and menstrual irregularity. Iron deficiency is more common, but iron overload is more important.

The most common cause of iron overload is a genetic disorder called hemochromatosis. Hemochromatosis is far more widespread than better-known hereditary diseases like sickle cell disease, cystic fibrosis, or muscular dystrophy. Only in the past several years have doctors discovered that hemochromatosis occurs in one out of every 250 Americans.

Hemochromatosis and related diseases of iron overload are important to identify for two reasons:

- Early diagnosis and treatment can totally *prevent* organ damage from iron overload.

- Early diagnosis can help identify affected family members before they become ill.

In the past few years we have tested over [numbers] members in [name of city] for iron overload. Because of the significant number of people we have found with this disorder, measuring blood levels has recently become a standard test carried out on everyone going through the [health clinic] office.

In late 1996, a blood test was developed for the actual gene causing most cases of iron overload. As with any new test, we are not yet sure what limitations it has. We need to compare its accuracy with already existing tests for iron overload. Then we need to determine which of the tests is the best to use when screening large numbers of patients for iron overload. We would appreciate your help in answering this question by agreeing to let a few drops of your blood be tested simultaneously with all of these tests, including the new DNA test that can recognize the gene itself. We already have good biochemical tests for this genetic disease. Now we need to see if a genetic test for this genetic disease offers any advantage over what already exists.

You might be wondering why I am explaining this in so much detail. There are no risks in the usual sense of the word. There are no medicines to take and no experimental treatments to undergo. Genetic testing involves using just a few drops of your blood that probably would be left over anyway. However, DNA testing is new and concerns some people so I want to be sure you understand why we are asking you to volunteer to help.

What if we learned that you had hemochromatosis before it made you sick? Most people would probably be pleased to have the preventive benefit of early treatment. But not everyone would. Some people do not want advance warning of trouble, particularly of a hereditary disorder. Others might feel that their insurance or their job might be threatened by advance news of a problem that has not yet occurred. Still others might not want to share the news of their problem with anyone in their family, lest relatives be upset with them for bringing news of illness.

Here is what would happen if the screening tests indicated that you had hemochromatosis or some iron overload–related disease. First of all, we would want to reconfirm the test results. Then we would want to determine the actual amount of iron overload you have, because it is iron overload that actually causes the damage. The best way we have of doing this is by weekly removal of that amount of blood that a person would donate at a blood bank. If this demonstrates iron overload, then treatment has already begun. We would continue this for as many weeks as it would take to reduce the amount of iron in your body to normal. This is important because early treatment of hemochromatosis can prevent all signs of disease from developing. We would carefully check to see whether any disorders related to iron overload already were present.

Now, might this affect your future life insurance or job prospects? Yes. Possibly it might, just as being found to have diabetes or heart disease might. However, is it a better alternative to have a problem that is *not* recognized? We will be happy to provide letters to any insurance company indicating that there is no effect of treated hemochromatosis on health or longevity. You certainly will not lose your [health plan] coverage because of it. We will all be better off to have you diagnosed and treated rather than undiagnosed with the risk of becoming ill.

How might knowledge of a hereditary disorder like hemochromatosis affect your family? Our experience is that most, but not all, families are happy to have early warning of a problem while it is still treatable. If you turn out to have iron overload, we urge you to share the information with your family so that they can be tested. However, that is *your* decision. It is up to you to decide whether you will notify your family members. Medical information about you is confidential and will not be shared with anyone unless you ask us to. We will protect your privacy to the limits of the law.

Some people worry that genetic testing will invade their privacy and that it might be used to test for traits like homosexuality, criminal tendencies, and so forth. Not only is such testing not possible, but the only genetic testing we perform on your blood will be for hemochromatosis and diseases associated with iron overload. Moreover, although the DNA analysis of your blood will be performed at the [medical institution], you will have your privacy ensured because we will use only a code number, not your name, to identify your blood specimen. In other words, no identifiable medical information about you will leave the [medical institution]. Last, we will never use your blood to develop a process that will be sold or that will be patented. Some people worry about such things. They will not happen in this study.

I hope we have made all of this clear and that you will agree to help us to learn the most efficient way to use the currently available tests for iron overload. If you participate and are found to have iron overload or conditions related to iron overload, we will go to great lengths to be sure that you understand the implications for your family and offspring.

If you have reservations about any of this, it would simply be best not to participate. After all, this is a voluntary study. Whether you decide to participate or not to participate in the genetic study of iron overload disease, your decision will in no way affect your medical care or your insurance with your [health plan]. I hope you can help. Your participation in the study may help to set an improved pattern of health care everywhere.

If you understand what I have described and want to help, please sign the consent form below. Then give this paper to the person drawing your blood at your upcoming visit to the [health clinic]. Do not take any vitamin or mineral supplements for 24 hours before you come in.

Sincerely yours,
[Name of physician]

CONSENT

I acknowledge:

1. No patient-identifiable information obtained as a result of participation in this study will be released without patient consent, except possibly to the [Study Sponsor] or their designee, the Food and Drug Administration, and/or other federal or state agencies that review medical records during the course of their audit responsibilities.

2. My consent to participate in this study may be withdrawn at any time without affecting future medical care.

3. My questions regarding this study have been answered. If I have any additional questions about this study, I may contact [name of study contact person; telephone number]

   If I have any additional questions about my rights as a research subject, or in the event of a study-related injury, I may contact [name of contact person; telephone number].

4. In the event complications arise as a result of participation in this study, the physicians and/or employees of the [medical institutions] will render necessary medical care and treatment in accordance with the patient's contract with [his or her health plan]. However, no financial remuneration is available.

I have read the entire consent, consisting of [_____] pages, and voluntarily consent to participate in the research study of the [Study Sponsor] Hemochromatosis Study conducted by the physicians and/or employees of the [medical institutions].

Date: _____   Patient: _____

Date: _____   Witness: _____

Appendix G

**National Action Plan on Breast Cancer (NAPBC) Consent Form
for Use of Tissue for Research**

National Action Plan on Breast Cancer (NAPBC)
Consent Form for Use of Tissue for Research
[Name of tissue repository, address, phone number]

ABOUT USING TISSUE FOR RESEARCH

You are going to have a biopsy (or surgery) to see if you have cancer. Your doctor will remove some body tissue to do some tests. The results of these tests will be given to you by your doctor and will be used to plan your care.

We would like to keep some of the tissue that is left over for future research. If you agree, this tissue will be kept and may be used in research to learn more about cancer and other diseases. Please read the question-and-answer sheet called "How Is Tissue Used for Research?" to learn more about tissue research. [Not included in this volume, but available online at www.4woman.gov/napbc/catalog.wci/napbc/q&a.htm—eds.]

Your tissue may be helpful for research whether you do or do not have cancer. The research that may be done with your tissue probably will not help you. It might help people who have cancer and other diseases in the future.

Reports about research done with your tissue will not be given to you or your doctor. These reports will not be put in your health record. The research will not have an effect on your care.

THINGS TO THINK ABOUT

The choice to let us keep the leftover tissue for future research is up to you. *No matter what you decide to do, it will not affect your care.*

If you decide now that your tissue can be kept for research, you can change your mind at any time. Just contact us and let us know that you do not want us to use your tissue. Then the tissue will no longer be used for research.

In the future, people who do research may need to know more about your health. When the [study staff] gives them reports about your health, it will *not* give them your name, address, or phone number.

Sometimes tissue is used for genetic research (about diseases that are passed on in families). Even if your tissue is used for this kind of research, the results will not be put in your health records.

Your tissue will be used only for research and will not be sold. The research done with your tissue may help to develop new products in the future.

BENEFITS

The benefits of research using tissue include learning more about what causes cancer and other diseases, how to prevent them, how to treat them, and how to cure them.

RISKS

There are very few risks to you. The greatest risk is the release of information from your health records. The [study staff] will protect your records so that your name, address, and phone number will be kept private. The chance that this information will be given to someone else is very small.

MAKING YOUR CHOICE

Please read each sentence below and think about your choice. After reading each sentence, check "Yes" or "No." *No matter what you decide to do, it will not affect your care.* If you have any questions, please talk to your doctor or nurse, or call our research review board at [IRB's phone number].

1. *My tissue may be kept for use in research to learn about, prevent, treat, or cure cancer.*

   ❑ Yes

   ❑ No

2. *My tissue may be kept for research about other health problems (for example, causes of diabetes, Alzheimer's disease, and heart disease).*

   ❑ Yes

   ❑ No

3. *Someone from [name of institution] may contact me in the future to ask me to take part in more research.*

   ❑ Yes

   ❑ No

Please sign your name here after you check your answers.

Your Signature: _____ Date: _____

Signature of Doctor/Nurse: _____ Date: _____

Witness: _____ Date: _____

[Date last revised]
[Available online at www.4woman.gov/napbc/catalog.wci/napbc/consent.htm]

Appendix H

Patient Written Consent Form for Review of Medical Records

Patient Written Consent Form for Review of Medical Records (will be included in mailing with [Study Sponsor] Patient Survey)

CONSENT TO ACT AS A SUBJECT IN A RESEARCH STUDY

Thank you for completing the [Study Sponsor] Patient Survey. You are now asked to participate in phase two of [the study project], a study conducted by researchers at [names of participating universities/research centers]. May we remind you that you were selected as a possible participant in this study because you were diagnosed with breast cancer or colorectal cancer in [year].

PURPOSE OF THE STUDY

The purpose of this study is to learn about the treatment that patients with breast and colorectal cancer are receiving. The goal of this study is to develop a national system that can help doctors to improve cancer care in the United States.

PROCEDURES

Signing this consent form will allow a member of the [Study Sponsor] research team to obtain a copy of your medical records from each of the doctors' offices where you received care for your cancer. This information will be combined with information from the survey you completed.

POTENTIAL RISKS AND BENEFITS

Participation in this study would pose no health risks to you and in no way affect the health care that you receive or the status of your health insurance. The only potential risk to you would result from a breach of confidentiality, which we will make every effort to prevent, as we describe in the "Confidentiality" section of this letter.

No direct benefits will come to you as a result of your participation in this study. The information you provide may help health care providers understand the ways in which we can improve the medical care received by patients with cancer.

PAYMENT FOR PARTICIPATION

As a token of our appreciation for your consideration, we are including $10.00 with this mailing. This in no way obligates you to participate in the study.

CONFIDENTIALITY

The research team will protect the confidentiality of information obtained during the research if it may identify you. We will not disclose this information to anyone outside of the research team, except with your permission or as required by the law. To protect your confidentiality, all patients will be assigned a confidential study number. All data will be kept in locked file cabinets and on password-protected computers that can only be accessed by the research project staff. Your doctors are not members of the research staff and will not have access to your confidential information. All reports or publications of the results of the study will be reported by grouping the data in such a way that it is not possible to identify individual patients.

RIGHTS OF RESEARCH SUBJECTS

Your participation in the [research project] is entirely voluntary and will have no effect on your relationship with your doctors or your ability to obtain medical care. You may withdraw your consent and discontinue further participation in this study at any time. You are not waiving any legal claims, rights, or remedies because of your participation in this research study. Your decision whether or not to participate will not affect your relationship with your physicians. Your decision not to participate or to withdraw from this research is also confidential. The investigator may withdraw you from this research if circumstances arise that warrant doing so (for example, if after enrolling in the study you found out that you do not have the type of cancer we are studying).

IDENTIFICATION OF INVESTIGATORS

If you have any questions or concerns about the research, please feel free to contact any of the following people: [names of research staff, telephone numbers].

SIGNATURE OF RESEARCH SUBJECT OR LEGAL REPRESENTATIVES

My signature indicates that I have read and understand the information provided above, and that I willingly agree to participate in this research study. I have received a copy of this form and a copy of the "Subject's Bill of Rights."

_____

Name of Subject or Legal Representative

_____   _____

Signature of Subject or Legal Representative   Date:

If you are not the subject but are signing on their behalf because they cannot sign, please specify your relationship to the subject:

_____

Relationship of Legal Representative (Signatory) to Subject

**A Descriptive Study of the Views and Experiences
of Persons Involved in a Measles Vaccine Study**

A DESCRIPTIVE STUDY OF THE VIEWS AND EXPERIENCES
OF PERSONS INVOLVED IN THE MEASLES VACCINE STUDY

Written version of consent form—to be read orally

The following information will be read to mother or guardian of child in [study area] by the interviewer.

Because you joined the measles vaccine study, we invite you to participate in a research interview that is separate from the measles vaccine research study.

WHY ARE WE DOING THIS STUDY?

We are interested in finding out what people who joined the measles vaccine study think about the study. We hope that this information will help to conduct better research studies in the future.

WHAT IS THE STUDY ABOUT?

We plan to invite about three hundred mothers who joined the measles vaccine study to answer our research questions. If you agree, we will ask your thoughts about the measles vaccine study. The interview will last about 15 minutes.

WHAT ARE THE RISKS AND BENEFITS OF ANSWERING THE QUESTIONS?

Although very unlikely, it is possible that answering some of the questions may cause you to feel upset or worried. You will receive no direct benefits from answering our questions. However, you may find that by answering these questions you understand the measles vaccine study better.

CONFIDENTIALITY

We will not put your name on the paper that has your answers, and we will not let other people see how you answered the questions. No one at the [health clinic] will see your personal answers. We will be able to have a look at your enrollment questionnaire at the clinic to find information about your baby's age and previous history.

VOLUNTARY PARTICIPATION

Answering our research questions is your choice. If you decide not to answer the questions, it will not affect your baby's care or your joining the measles vaccine study in any way. Also, you can stop answering the questions at any time and can skip any questions that you do not want to answer.

COMPENSATION

We will provide a small article of clothing, such as a t-shirt or socks, for your baby for answering the questions.

DO YOU HAVE ANY QUESTIONS?

Index

Page numbers in *italics* refer to entries within tables.

discussions of, xiii, 27, 28, 141, 179, 234, 247
equivalent protections and, 40
exemptions from, 39–40
minors in, 53–55, 243–47
pregnant women, fetuses, and neonates in, 48–51
prisoners in, 51–53
research with existing data in, 40
scope of, 39
text of, 39–55
communities
alternative ethical systems of, 335
consultation with, 66–67, 202, 279, 280, 281, 282, *287*, 288, *294*, 335, 336, 339, 340, 341, 342, 355, 356, 357, 360, 361
impoverished, 67–68, 190. *See also* international research
informed consent and, 279, 280, 282, 335, 336, 337, 339, 340, 341, 352, 360
involvement in research of, 66–67, 337, 340, 341, 347
levels of consultation with, 280
as research gatekeepers, 279–80, 337–40, 342
research permission from, 146, 339, 342, 357
risks to, 66–67, 279–80, 288, 335, 336, 337, 338, 340, 342, 343
types of, 280, 343
as vulnerable populations, 280, 343
See also vulnerable populations
community review boards (CRBs), 193, 335, 336
Conference on Ethical Aspects of Research in Developing Countries, 281–82
confidentiality
and biological samples, 305, 307
in CIOMS Guidelines, 60, 61, 62
in Declaration of Helsinki, 31
and genetic information, xiv, 62, 78, 273, *286*, *287*, *288*, 288, 289, *293*, *294*, *295*, 295, 296, 297, *299*, 309, 311
in ICH-GCP guideline, 81, 85
informed consent and, 198, 200, 233, 339
in informed consent documents, 449, 457, 466, 469, 473, 476–77, 478
in medical records, 12, 77, 296
in physician-patient relationship, 77–78
and scientific misconduct, 386, 399
conflicts of interest, 326, 428
administrative law and, 376, 421, 430, 431, 432, 433
assessment of, xiv, 59, 298, 376, 379, 380, 381, 382, 400, 420, 438
definitions of, 430

disclosure of, 31, 58, 59, 62, 148, 149, 190, 201, 273, *288*, *295*, *299*, 370, 371, 373, 377, 378, 380, 382, 408, 434
forum shopping and, 434, 435
primary versus secondary interests and, 159, 369–70, 375, 389, 401, 430, 434
prohibition of investigator participation due to, 373, 377, 380, 434
public interest and, 203, 370, 376, 382, 383, 431, 432, 435
remedies for, 58, 372, 380, 413, 434
rules for minimizing, 371, 372, 373, 375, 376, 381, 383, 431, 432, 433, 434, 435, 440
trial design and, 58, 148, 372, 378–79
conscientious investigator
importance of, 10, 20, 191, 192, 203, 236, 237, 421
and scientific misconduct, 372–73, 376, 387, 408
See also Beecher, Henry K.
conscription. *See* participants, conscription of
consent. *See* assent; informed consent
consequentialism, 124, 323. *See also* utilitarianism
Consolidated Standards of Reporting Trials (CONSORT), 391, 414–18
CONSORT. *See* Consolidated Standards of Reporting Trials
contract research organizations (CROs), 87, 183, 184, 421
and conflicts of interest, 420, 429, 433, 434, 435
Council for International Organizations of Medical Sciences (CIOMS), 137
Council for International Organizations of Medical Sciences (CIOMS) Guidelines
discussions of, 27
international research and, 345
mentally impaired persons in, 75–76
minors in, 74–75
text of, 56–80
women in, 76–77
Council of Science Editors (CSE), 415
CRBs. *See* community review boards
CRFs. *See* case report forms
critically ill persons
altruism and, 119, 214, 215
autonomy and, 165, 202, 210, 214, 235, 331
informed consent and, 115, 124, 190, 202, 207, 210, 213–16, 220, 235, 331, *426*
remuneration and, 179, 185
as vulnerable populations, 73–74,

75–76, 124, 145, 146–49, 152, 160, 165, 199, 438
See also Phase I trials; vulnerable populations
CROs. *See* Contract Research Organizations
cross-cultural research, 282, 358, 364, 365. *See also* communities; international research
Crouch, Robert A., 153, 171, 281, 348
CSE. *See* Council of Science Editors
cultural relativism, 282, 347, 356–57, 358–59, 363, 367

Danish Council of Ethics, 289
Darsee, John R., 385, 386, 387, 404
data
access to, 59, 62, 113, 114, 341, 343, 350
integrity of, 87–88, 396, 397–99, 407, 425, *426*, 428. *See also* scientific misconduct
monitoring of, 45, 57, 88, 92, 118, 120, 371, 372, 401, 407, 415, 419, 420, 425, 426, *426*, 428
data and safety monitoring board (DSMB), 245, 426, *426*, 427
purpose of, 66, 71
deception, 29, 63–64, 134, 162, 190, 195, 199, 201, 203, 212, 266, 360, 386, 389, 395, 400, 404
cases of, 15, 23
debriefing after, 63–64, 134, 201
ethical review committee approval of, 63–64
Declaration of Geneva, 30, 201
Declaration of Helsinki, 40, 56, 66, 69, 72, 73, 80, 84, 99, 105, 124, 145, 148, 173, 209
discussions of, 26, 28, 127, 352
purpose of, 30
revisions of, 26
text of, 30–32
deontology. *See* Kantian ethics
Department of Defense, 260, 261
Department of Energy (DOE), 439, 440
Department of Health and Human Services (DHHS), 27, 39, 40, 106, 111, 145, 147, 167, 177, 191, 210, 233, 243, 249, 382, 399, 420, 439
Commission on Research Integrity of, 386, 388
Special Standing Panel (SSP) for research with persons with mental impairments of, 225, 230–31
Department of Health, Education, and Welfare (DHEW), 20, 26, 33, 244. *See also* Department of Health and Human Services

developing nations. *See* international research

DHEW. *See* Department of Health, Education, and Welfare

DHHS. *See* Department of Health and Human Services

disclosure, 15, 36, 46
    of conflicts of interest, 31, 58, 59, 62, 148, 149, 190, 201, 273, *288, 295, 299,* 370, 371, 373, 377, 378, 380, 382, 408, 434

discrimination, 170, 242, 307
    racism, 23, 153, 169, 209, 279, 335, 338, 339, 340
    sexism, 153, 168, 175
    See also Tuskegee Syphilis Study

DOE. *See* Department of Energy

Donagan, Alan, 5

Dresser, Rebecca, 153, 166, 171, 192, 194

drug studies. *See* Food and Drug Administration, drug trials of

DSMB. *See* data and safety monitoring board

ECMO trial. *See* extracorporeal membrane oxygenation trial

EG cells. *See* embryonic germ cells

Eisenberg, Leon, 4

Ellenberg, Susan S., 100, 137, 140

Elliott, Carl, 154, 226, 237

Emanuel, Ezekiel J., 100, 140, 340, 342

Emanuel, Linda L., 390, 403

embryonic germ (EG) cells, 277, 319, 320, 321, 322, 323

embryonic stem (ES) cells, 276, 277, 319, 320, 322, 323, 324

embryos
    abortion and, 167, 213, 276, 320, 321, 322, 323, 324
    creation of, 276, 277, 278, 316, 317, 318, 319, 324, 325, 326, 327, 328
    federal funding and, 313, 315, 317, 319, 324, 326
    from in vitro fertilization (IVF), 277, 278, 314, 315, 316, 320, 323, 324, 325, 327
    human beings and, 277, 317, 323, 325
    informed consent for use of, 278, 313, 319, 322, 323, 325
    moral status of, 276, 277, 278, 314, 315, 317, 323, 324, 325, 326, 327, 328
    and National Institutes of Health (NIH) Human Embryo Research Panel, 277, 313, 317, 324, 328
    research on, 276, 277, 278, 313, 315, 316, 317, 318, 319, 320, 325, 326, 327, 328
    restrictions on use of, 314, 315, 324
    risks to, 46, 76, 85
    somatic cell nuclear transfer (SCNT) and, 278, 319, 320, 326

symbolic significance of, 321, 325, 326
    See also personhood

emergency/rescue situations, 25, 57, 64–65, 111, 157, 165, 199, 210, 245, 355, 450

employees
    commercial IRBs and, 433
    as vulnerable populations, 73, 271, 262

Environmental Protection Agency (EPA), 183

EPA. *See* Environmental Protection Agency

equipoise. *See* clinical equipoise

ES cells. *See* embryonic stem cells

ethical pluralism and international research, 282, 347, 356–57, 358–59, 363, 367

Ethical Principles and Guidelines for the Protection of Human Subjects of Research. *See* Belmont Report

Ethical Principles for Medical Research Involving Human Subjects. *See* Declaration of Helsinki

ethical relativism and international research, 282, 347, 356–57, 358–59, 363, 367

ethical review committees, 15, 31
    conflicts of interest and, 58
    duties to vulnerable populations of, 60
    emergency compassionate care and, 57, 64–65
    lay members and, 58
    membership in, 57–58
    national versus local review and, 57
    records of, 57
    responsibilities of, 57, 59, 64, 66–67, 73
    role of, 56
    sanctions by, 58–59
    See also institutional review boards

"Ethics and Clinical Research," xiii, 3–4

ethics education, 400–401, 425, 427, 428, 429, 430, 435

euthanasia, 148

experimentation, self-, xiii, 1, 16, 152, 159, 165, 259. *See also* Jonas, Hans; Nuremberg Code; yellow fever

"Experimentation in Man," 9–10

exploitation
    of incompetent subjects, 65, 236, 438
    informed consent and, 209
    of minorities, 35. *See also* Tuskegee Syphilis Study
    of patients, 180
    placebo-controlled trials and, 70, 281
    of pregnant women, 320
    of prisoners, 35, 265, 266
    reasonable availability and, 70, 281
    subject recruitment and, 151, 153, 165, 179, 181–82, 184, 185
    of undereducated persons, 35

See also international research, exploitation and

extracorporeal membrane oxygenation (ECMO) trial, 98, 121–26

Faden, Ruth R., 2, 7

fairness. *See* justice

family members. *See* genetic information, family members and

Fauci, Anthony, 113, 114

FDA. *See* Food and Drug Administration

Feinberg, Joel, 325

fetal tissue. *See* fetuses

fetuses, 27, 46, 48–51, 76–77, 85, 153, 167, 200, 277, 291, 292, *293,* 314, 315, 320, 321, 322, 325, 326

financial concerns, 89, 135, 189, 194, 221, 369, 370, 371, 380, 433, 434
    double billing, 371
    finder's fees, 190, 371, 372, 377–78, 381, 382
    funding, 236, 242, 278, 313, 381, 385, 394, 404, 436
    Phase I trials and, 129, 147, 148, 149
    placebo-controlled trials and, 135, 136, 139, 372, 379
    remuneration, 181, 182, 184, 185, 199
    for research participants, 310, 336–37, 348–49
    study size and, 129, 139, 170, 173
    See also conflicts of interest; remuneration; undue influence

Food and Drug Administration (FDA)
    access to research results of, 449, 457, 473
    drug approval of, 95, 101, 148, 209, 223, 242, 438, 443, 447
    drug trials of, 194, 223, 236, 438
    classification of, 96, 104–5
    informed consent and, 191, 201, 210, 260, 261, 445
    IRB review and, 302, 427, 428, 436, 442
    Phase I studies and, 147, 223
    placebo-controlled trials and, 99–100, 128, 129, 130, 131, 139
    regulations of, 41, 145, 147, 167, 171, 432, 437
    responsibilities of, 27

Food Quality Protection Act, 183

45 Code of Federal Regulations 46 (45 CFR 46). *See* Common Rule

Fred Hutchinson Cancer Research Center, 371

Freedman, Benjamin, 96–99, 107, 117, 123, 130, 153, 172, 173, 175, 191, 192, 201, 203, 226, 247, 297, 322, 420, 421, 422, 429, 459. *See also* clinical equipoise

Fried, Charles, 117, 120, 124, 217

Fuks, Abraham, 96, 107, 153, 175, 226, 247, 425

Jenner, Edward, 1
Jewish Chronic Disease Hospital case, xiii, 3, 11–12, 14–15, 19, 26, 197
Johnson Controls, 167
Jonas, Hans, 151, 152, 153, 155, 165, 186, 202, 225
journal editors, obligations of, 389, 390, 391, 393, 399, 405, 411, 413, 414
Juengst, Eric T., 279–80, 337
justice, 152, 161, 163, 164, 165, 180, 182, 206, 261, 263, 360
    in Belmont Report. *See* Belmont Report, justice in
    compensation and, 175
    equitable distribution of benefits and, 57, 73, 152
    and international research, 80, 281, 347, 349, 350, 361
    as motivation for research participation, 161
    participant (subject) selection and, 35, 38, 45, 57, 72, 151, 169, 170, 172, 185, 242, 259, 262, *287, 299,* 313. *See also* access to research
    recruiting impoverished persons and, 179

Kantian ethics, 97, 114, 124, 155, 197, 198, 201, 211, 360
    as applied to embryo research, 317, 324
Kass, Leon, 113
Kassirer, Jerome, 402, 405
Katz, Jay, 3, 8, 11, 103, 146, 193, 195, 198, 210, 220
King, Patricia A., 317, 328
knowledge, generalizable, 33, 41, 66, 103, 111, 153, 173, 185, 211, 220, 243, 245, *287, 294, 417, 436*
Kopelman, Loretta M., 249, 251, 308
Krimsky, Sheldon, 326
Krugman, Saul, 4. *See also* Willowbrook hepatitis study

Lasagna, Louis, 4, 5
Lazear, Jesse, 1
Lebacqz, Karen, 285
Lederer, Susan E., 2, 7
legal issues
    Common Rule and, 28
    confidentiality and, 77, 109, 296, 312
    conflicts of interest and, 376, 440
    informed consent and, 189, 191, 197–98, 200, 201, 203, 402, 445
    legally authorized representatives, 75, 84–86, 231–33, 257, 437, 477
    regulations and, 388, 421, 430
    vulnerable populations and, 177–78, 238, 251, 259, 302, 315, 322
Leikin, Sanford, 227, 252

Lemmens, Trudo, 154, 285, 291, 297, 420, 421, 422, 429
Levine, Carol, 2, 167, 168
Levine, Robert J., 95, 103, 110, 177, 189, 190, 191, 197, 198, 212, 245, 247–48, 425
liberation theory, 180
Lidz, Charles W., 216, 274, 289
Lind, James, 1
Lind, Stuart E., 371
Lipsett, Mortimer B., 101, 144
Lurie, Peter, 280, 281, 343

Macon County, Alabama. *See* Tuskegee Syphilis Study
malaria experiments, 1, 7, 184
Mandel, Emanuel E., 3, 15
Martin, Joseph B., 370, 372, 382
Massachusetts Eye and Ear Infirmary, 370–71
Massachusetts General Hospital, xiii, 378
McCabe, Mary S., 441
McDermott, Walsh, 4, 5
McNeill, Paul, 154, 185
medical records
    confidentiality and, 12, 77, 296
    informed consent for use of, 61, 85, 90, 308
    use of, 61, 79, 85, 312, 428
Meilaender, Gilbert, 326
Memorial Sloan-Kettering Cancer Center, 385, 395
mentally impaired persons
    Belmont Report and, 27, 36, 199
    CIOMS Guidelines and, 60, 75–76
    Declaration of Helsinki and, 26
    informed consent and, 25, 36, 60, 75–76, 145, 190, 199, 200, 347, *426,* 438
    in National Bioethics Advisory Commission report, 226, 229–33, 234–37
    risks to, 237–40
    unethical trials with, 4, 17, 19
    as vulnerable populations, 225, 270, *287, 294,* 438
    See also psychiatric research
Merz, Jon F., 276, 311
Michels, Robert, 226, 234
military personnel, 3, 8, 16, 73, 164, 199
Mill, John Stuart, 114
Miller, Franklin G., 100, 140, 279, 332
minimal risk, 35, 53, 60, 65, 187, 192, 208, 225, 226, 231, 232, 269, 270, 271, 274, 275, 314, 356, 366, *426,* 427, 440
    biological samples and, 61, 276, 309
    deception and, 201
    definition of, 41, 226, 235, 246, 247, 248–49, 273, 304

minor increment over, 54, 67, 110, 199, 226–27, 255–56, 243, 246, 247, 249, 250–51, 258
    research with minors and, 54, 106, 149, 226, 243, 245, 246, 247–52, 256, 257
minority group members, 20, 35, 73, 209, 211
    representation in research, 38, 152–53, 166–71, 172, 179
minors
    assent of, 74, 226, 252–58, *294*
    Belmont Report and, 35
    CIOMS Guidelines and, 58, 60, 73
    Common Rule and, 27, 53–55, 106, 226
    consent and, 67, 74–75, 190, 205, 226, 227, 250, 257, 258, *287,* 427
    Declaration of Helsinki and, 26
    dissent of, 74, 252, 255, 257, 258
    drug studies for, 105, 149, 166, 179
    ECMO trials for, 126
    emancipated, 74–75, 227, 257–58
    exclusion from research of, xiii, 25, 28
    minimal risk and. *See* minimal risk, research with minors and
    short stature trials and, 240–48
    unethical research with, 19, 20
    as vulnerable populations, 145, 165, 225, 226–27, 270, *293,* 347
misconduct. *See* scientific misconduct
monitoring
    of adherence to protocol, 91–92, 258, 298, 401, *426,* 428, 429
    of data. *See* data, monitoring of
    of mentally impaired participants, 331, 334, *426,* 427
    See also data and safety monitoring board
Montefiore Hospital, 7
Moreno, Jonathan D., 2, 7, 227, 258, 419
multi-center research, 58, 88, 93, 176, 182, 380, 403, 405, 419, 421, 422, 430, 439, 441–44. *See also* international research

NAPBC. *See* National Action Plan on Breast Cancer
National Action Plan on Breast Cancer (NAPBC)
    informed consent document of, 474–75
    and stored biological samples, 275
National Bioethics Advisory Commission (NBAC), 442
    Ethical Issues in Human Stem Cell Research of, 277, 278, 319–24
    report on mentally impaired persons of, 225, 226, 229–33, 234–37
National Cancer Institute (NCI), 147, 296, 427, 428, 445

nonpublication, 390, 391, 399, 412, 413, 414

plagiarism, 385, 386, 399

prevention of, 391, 400, 401, 402, 409, 413

remedies for, 388, 391, 396, 399, 413

statistical practices and, 129, 388, 389, 391, 396, 397–99, 401, 408

withholding research materials/methods, 386, 390, 391, 399

See also conscientious investigator

scientific value of research, 23, 56, 57, 69, 80, 97, 109, 142, 172, 189, 265, 278, *287*, 292, *299*, 311, 333–34

SCNT. *See* somatic cell nuclear transfer

self-experimentation, xiii, 1, 16, 152, 159, 165, 259. *See also* Jonas, Hans; Nuremberg Code; yellow fever

self-sacrifice/supererogation, 158, 159, 161, 164, 165, 166

Shapiro, Stanley H., 285, 291, 297, 425

Shimkin, Michael B., 9

Snow, John, 1

somatic cell nuclear transfer (SCNT) and embryos, 278, 319, 320, 326

Southam, Chester M., 3, 12–14, 190–91, 192

special research populations. *See* participants, classes of. *See also* vulnerable populations

Spectra Pharmaceutical Services, 371

sponsors
  auditing by, 92–93
  monitoring by, 91–92
  multi-center research and, 93
  records of, 88, 89, 90, 93
  responsibilities of, 68, 79–80, 87–93, 195, 233
  suspension/termination of a trial by, 88, 93

statistical practices, 117, 120, 126, 129, 141, 159, 173, *286*, *299*, 346, *416*
  ethics and, 388, 391, 397–99
  post hoc hypotheses and, 175, 389, 396, 398
  subgroup analysis, 174

Steinbock, Bonnie, 326

stem cells, 276, 277, 319, 320, 322, 323, 324

students, 58, 187, 190, 199, 202, 207, 225, 227–28, 258, 259, 261, 262, 266–67, 270–72

"studies in nature," 21. *See also* Tuskegee Syphilis Study; Willowbrook hepatitis study

Subject Interview Study of the Advisory Committee on Human Radiation Experiments, 193, 213–16

subjects. *See* participants

Tauer, Carol A., 226, 240

Taylor, Telford, 2

Temple, Robert, 100, 137, 140

theoretical equipoise. *See* clinical equipoise, versus theoretical equipoise

therapeutic misconception, 180, 193, 194, 195, 210–11, 217, 218, 220
  clinical trial brand names and, 194, 221–23
  See also informed consent

Thompson, Dennis F., 369–70, 373, 375, 379–80, 430

Thrombolysis in Myocardial Infarction (TIMI) trials, NIH, 372, 427

TIMI trials. *See* Thrombolysis in Myocardial Infarction trials

Truog, Robert D., 98, 121, 192, 207

trust, 10, 58, 160, 215, 216, 220, 221, 230, 235, 370, 375, 376, 377, 378, 382, 383, 386, 387–88, 403, 404, 421, 431, 432, 433, 435

Tuskegee Syphilis Study, xiv, 26, 35, 169, 189, 197, 209, 262, 281, 347
  apology for, 4–5
  DHEW and, 4, 20, 22–23
  exploitation and, 22, 234
  history of, 4, 21–22
  informed consent and, 22
  Oslo study of untreated syphilis and, 4, 21
  racism and, 4, 22

UCLA. *See* University of California, Los Angeles

Uganda Cancer Institute AIDS Research Committee, 347

undue influence, 31, 34, 36, 44, 62, 64, 65, 81, 146, 151, 206, 223, 288, 289, 431
  in psychiatric research, 332
  remuneration as, 65, 81, 154, 179, 181, 182, 184, 187, 199, 206, 207, 264, 269

Uniform Requirements for Manuscripts Submitted to Biomedical Journals of the International Committee of Medical Journal Editors, 390, 405–6, 407, 410, 411

United States v. *Karl Brandt et al. See* Nuremberg Code

Universal Declaration of Human Rights, 348

universalism, 282, 358, 359, 360, 363

University of California, Los Angeles, schizophrenia study, 234, 278–79, 329, 437

University of Pennsylvania Institute for Human Gene Therapy, 369

utilitarianism, 5, 114, 116, 145, 155, 160,

164, 189, 197, 246, 318, 323, 346, 360, 361 *See also* consequentialism

vaccine research, 59, 69, 73, 80, 254, 263, 279, 346, 347, 354, 355
  for cowpox/smallpox, 1
  for HIV/AIDS, 63, 72, 77, 345, 355

Vancouver Group, 390, 405–6, 407, 410, 411

Varmus, Harold, 346, 347

VCU. *See* Virginia Commonwealth University

Vietnam, breast cancer study in, 282, 283. *See also* international research

Virchow, Rudolf, 406

Virginia Commonwealth University (VCU), 274, 302, 304

virtuous investigator. *See* conscientious investigator

voluntariness, 25, 26, 158, 159, 179, 181, 187, 197, 200, 225, 227–28, 255, 260, 262, 266, 269, 319, 357, 456, 460, 473, 477, 478
  effect of family pressure on, 227, 273, 274, *287*
  informed consent and, 36–37, 85, 189, 190, 191, 199, 202, 253, 258, 427

volunteers, 8, 16, 20, 31, 152, 155, 159, 161, 164, 165, 166–84, 187, 193, 202, 206, 259, 260, 261, 264, 266, 269, 335, 347, 431, 437, 471–72
  healthy, 16, 26, 31, 66, 95, 101, 105, 110, 142, 179, 180, 181, 183, 184, 185, 186, 244, 245, 261, *286*, *293*, 465

vulnerable populations
  appropriate participation of, 26, 48–55, 67, 73, 227, 266, 272
  "descending order of permissibility" of using, 38, 149, 152, 159–60. *See also* Jonas, Hans
  competence of, 9, 64, 65, 67, 190, 198, 199–200, 203, 206, 226, 230, 232, 233, 234, 235, 237, 239, 240, 248, 253, 254, 255, 257, 258, 331, 334, *426*, 438, 445
  duty to exclude, 153, 177, 178
  exclusion of, xiii, 72, 152, 177, 178, 262, 358, 438
  impoverished, 35, 72, 136, 165, 179, 181–86, 199, 202, 206, 207, 211, 227, 263, 264, 266, 346, 347, 348, 349, 350, 352, 438
  minimal risk and, 67
  overprotection of, 228
  overrepresentation in research of, 35, 38, 72, 179, 182, 183, 259
  portrayals of, 259
  protection of, 28, 30, 31, 34, 36, 38, 45, 65, 72–73, 81, 85–86, 124, 136,